ORGAN TRANSPLANTATION 1990

DEVELOPMENTS IN SURGERY

VOLUME 11

The titles published in this series are listed at the end of this volume.

ORGAN TRANSPLANTATION 1990

edited by

G. M. ABOUNA

M. S. A. KUMAR (*Associate Editor*)

and

A. G. WHITE (*Associate Editor*)

Department of Organ Transplantation
Kuwait University
Kuwait City, Kuwait

and

The Division of Transplantation
Department of Surgery
Hahnemann University
Philadelphia, PA. U.S.A.

SPRINGER–SCIENCE+BUSINESS, MEDIA, B.V.

Library of Congress Cataloging-in-Publication Data

Organ transplantation 1990 / edited by G.M. Abouna, M.S.A. Kumar, A.G. White.
p. cm. -- (Developments in surgery ; v. 11)
Includes index.
ISBN 978-94-010-5497-3 ISBN 978-94-011-3386-9 (eBook)
DOI 10.1007/978-94-011-3386-9
1. Transplantation of organs, tissues, etc. I. Abouna, George J. M. II. Kumar, M. S. A. III. White, Arthur G. IV. Series: Developments in surgery ; 11.
[DNLM: 1. Organ Transplantation. W1 DE998S v. 11 / WO 660 O684]
RD120.7.O715 1991
617.9'5--dc20
DNLM/DLC
for Library of Congress 91-7057

ISBN 978-94-010-5497-3

Printed on acid free paper

This Book is Dedicated
to the Staff of Hamed Al-Essa Transplant Center,
the Department of Organ Transplantation,
Kuwait University, Kuwait; and
to the people of Kuwait who suffered the injustices
and the destruction of the Gulf War of 1990–1991

Contents

Foreword by Anthony P. Monaco xv
Preface by George M. Abouna xvii
List of contributors xix

Part One: *Historical Reflections*

1. Reflections on the development of organ transplantation
H.M. Lee 1

Part Two: *Immunology of Organ Transplantation*

2. Cellular and molecular mechanisms of allograft rejection
Pekka Häyry 5
3. What does the alloreactive T cell see?
J.R. Batchelor, G. Lombardi and R.I. Lechler 11
4. HLA matching and organ transplantation
David W. Gjertson and Paul I. Terasaki 17
5. An effective strategy for transplantation of highly sensitized patients
F.H.J. Claas, L.P. de Waal, J. Beelen, P. Reekers, P. van den Berg-Loonen, E. de Gast, J. D'Amaro, G.G. Persijn, F. Zantvoort and J.J. Van Rood 29
6. Rapid lymphocyte crossmatching for renal transplantation
A.G. White, K.T. Raju, M.S.A. Kumar, E.M. Philips and G.M. Abouna 39

Part Three: *Organ Allograft Rejection*

7. Fifteen-year experience with fine needle aspiration biopsies at the University of Helsinki
Pekka Häyry, Eeva von Willebrand and Irmeli Lautenschlager 43

8. Study of antibody specificity in highly sensitized patients using human monoclonal antibody technology
Ibrahim A. Al-Muzairai, Barbra K. Weber and David A. Power 51

9. Idiotypic-Antiidiotypic antibody interaction and renal transplant survival
I.A. Al-Muzairai, A.A. MacLeod, M. MacMillan, K.N. Stewart and G.R.D. Catto 59

Part Four: *Immunosuppression*

10. Transplantation and blood transfusion in 1990
Robert J. Corry 65

11. Quadruple-drug immunosuppressive induction treatments for immunological high-risk patients in cadaveric renal transplantation using poly- and monoclonal antibodies
H. Schneeberger, S. Schleibner, L. Friedl, M. Schilling, W.D. Illner, D. Abendroth and W. Land 71

12. Sequential combination immunotherapy for cadaveric renal transplantation: OKT3 versus rabbit ATG induction
M.P. Posner, H.F. Henriques, A.L. King, Y. Berlatzky, C. Klosterman, B.A.D. Cook and H.M. Lee 83

13. Multi-organ transplant experience with OKT3 and strategies for use at the University of Cincinnati Medical Center
Timothy J. Schroeder, M. Roy First and Israel Penn 91

14. Cyclosporine withdrawal in renal transplant recipients maintained on azathioprine, prednisone and cyclosporine
M. Kalawi, N.A. Al-Sabawi, M. Samhan, D. Panjwani, M.S.A. Kumar, E.M. Philips and G.M. Abouna 101

15. Early experience with FK 506 in liver transplantation
Robert D. Gordon, Satoru Todo, John J. Fung, Andreas C. Tzakis, Noriko Murase, Ashok Jain, Mario Alessiani and Thomas E. Starzl 109

16. Deoxyspergualin. A novel immunosuppressant: experimental and clinical studies
H. Amemiya, S. Suzuki, K. Ota, K. Takahashi, T. Sonoda, M. Ishibashi, R. Omoto, I. Koyama, K. Dohi, Y. Fukuda and K. Fukao 123

17. Preliminary results with FK 506 in pancreas grafting in a non-human primate model
G. Kootstra, B.G. Ericzon, R. Wijnen, T. Tiebosch, K. Kubota and C.-G. Groth 129

18. The effect of DST on graft outcome — the Turkish experience
S. Sert, H. Gulay, M. Koç and M. Haberal 135

19. Induction of specific unresponsiveness (tolerance) to experimental and clinical allografts using polyclonal antilymphocyte serum and donor-specific bone marrow
Anthony P. Monaco 141
20. Comparison of cyclosporine assays using radioimmunoassay, fluorescent polarization immunoassay and high-performance liquid chromatography
A.G. White, D. Panjwani, M. Angelo Khattar, A.S. El-Deen, M.S.A. Kumar, E.M. Philips and G.M. Abouna 159

Part Five: *Renal Transplantation*

21. Long-term outcome in renal transplantation
H. Brynger 163
22. Ten-year experience with 500 renal transplants
G.M. Abouna, M.S.A. Kumar, A.G. White, M. Samhan, O.S.G. Silva, I.H. Al-Abdullah, M. Kalawi, S. Al-Dadah, N. Al-Sabawi, P. John and E. M. Philips 167
23. Long-term results in recipients of cadaveric renal allografts under cyclosporine therapy
S. Schleibner, H. Schneeberger and W. Land 189
24. Transplantation of single and double kidneys from pediatric donors
David E.R. Sutherland, Rainer W.G. Gruessner, Arthur J. Matas, Goncal Lloveras, David S. Fryd, David L. Dunn, William D. Payne and John S. Najarian 201
25. ABO-incompatible living related donor transplantation
M. Haberal, H. Gulay, S. Sert, G. Arslan, M. Koç and N. Bilgin 203
26. The use of single pediatric cadaver kidneys for transplantation into adult recipients
G.M. Abouna, P. John, M.S.A. Kumar, A.G. White, O.S.G. Silva, E. Shuwaikh, M. Samhan, E.M. Philips and S. Al-Dadah 211
27. Living unrelated donor renal transplantation
S. Sert, H. Gulay, M. Koç and M. Haberal 217
28. Renal transplantation in Tunisia — a three-year experience
H. Ben Ayed, A. El-Matri, T. Ben Abdallah, C. Kechrid, H. Ben Maiz, A. Kheder, F. Ben Moussa, S. Smerlie, M. Ayed, M. El-Ouakdi, K. Ayed and R. Bardi 221
29. Renal transplantation in children
M. Samhan, P. John, M.S.A. Kumar, A.G. White, O.S.G. Silva, E. Shuwaikh, E.M. Philips, S. Al-Dadah and G.M. Abouna 225

30. Kidney donors — long-term follow up
P. John, M.S.A. Kumar, H. Abdul Karim, M. Samhan, N. Al-Sabawi, S. Al-Dadah, T. Eche, O.S.G. Silva, E. Shuwaikh, A. Kobryn, E.M. Philips and G.M. Abouna 233
31. Current techniques for permanent vascular access surgery — experience with 930 procedures
S. Al-Dadah, M. Kalawi, M. Samhan, P. John, M.S.A. Kumar and G.M. Abouna 237
32. Results of 319 consecutive renal transplants from living related and living unrelated donors in Iran
A.J. Ghods, I. Fazel, B. Nikbin, K. Rahbar, E. Abdi, H.N. Ghashti and F. Prooshani 247

Part Six: *Liver Transplantation*

33. Liver transplantation: current status
Robert D. Gordon 253
34. An overview of liver transplantation therapy for children
R. Patrick Wood, Byers W. Shaw Jr, Robert J. Stratta, Alan N. Langnas and Todd J. Pillen 263
35. Current anesthetic management in clinical liver transplantation
Yoogoo Kang 279
36. Risk factors in adult liver transplant recipients
R. Patrick Wood, Byers W. Shaw Jr, Robert J. Stratta, Alan N. Langnas and Todd J. Pillen 289
37. The concept of reduced-size liver transplantation, including split-liver and living related liver transplantation
X.M. Rogiers, J.C. Emond, P.F. Whitington, T.G. Heffron, K.L. King, M.D. Yang and C.E. Broelsch 295
38. Immunological factors contributing to outcome in liver transplantation
Robert D. Gordon 301
39. Transplantation for hepatobiliary malignancies
R. Patrick Wood, Byers W. Shaw Jr, Robert J. Stratta, Alan N. Langnas and Todd J. Pillen 307
40. The diagnosis and management of massive blood loss during liver transplantation
Yoogoo Kang 313
41. Early clinical experience with cluster resection and transplantation for right upper quadrant abdominal malignancy
Robert D. Gordon, Satoru Todo, Andreas G. Tzakis and Thomas E. Starzl 323

Part Seven: *Heart/Heart-Lung Transplants*

42. Lung transplantation: current techniques and outcomes
R. Morton Bolman III 329
43. Heart-lung transplantation at the University of Minnesota
R. Morton Bolman III 337
44. Specificity and sensitivity of the cytoimmunological monitoring (CIM): differentiation between cardiac rejection, viral, bacterial, or fungal infection
C. Hammer, D. Klanke, P. Dirschedl, B. M. Kemkes, B. Reichart, M. Gokel and F. Krombach 345

Part Eight: *Pancreas Transplantation*

45. International Pancreas Transplantation Registry report
David E.R. Sutherland, Kristin Gillingham and Kay C. Moudry-Munns 353
46. Techniques and experience of pancreatic transplantation with bladder drainage
Robert J. Corry and John L. Smith 359
47. Pancreas transplantation in non-uremic diabetic recipients
David E.R. Sutherland, David L. Dunn, Kay C. Moudry-Munns, Kristin Gillingham and John S. Najarian 365
48. Early observation with pancreas transplantation using the bladder drainage procedure
W.D. Illner, D. Abendroth, H. Schneeberger, S. Schleibner, M. Stangl, J. Theodorakis, R. Landgraf and W. Land 371
49. Results of pancreas transplantation with irradiated spleen and segment of duodenum
G. Kootstra, J.P. Van Hooff, H. Peltenburg, C.J. van der Linden, R. Wijnen, P. van den Berg-Loonen, J.A.M. de Jong, T. Verschueren and G. Heidendal 377
50. Experience with pancreas transplants from living related donors
David E.R. Sutherland, Frederick C. Goetz, David M. Kendall, R. Paul Robertson, Kristin Gillingham, Kay C. Moudry-Munns and John S. Najarian 383

Part Nine: *Islet Cell Transplantation*

51. Islet transplantation — the World Transplant Registry
R.G. Bretzel, B.J. Hering and K.F. Federlin 389

52. Prevention of rejection of islet allografts and xenografts without continuous immunosuppression of the recipients
Paul E. Lacy and David W. Scharp 397
53. Effect of islet transplantation on diabetic secondary complications
R.G. Bretzel 405
54. Does pretreatment of islets of Langerhans with deoxyguanosine improve allograft survival without immunosuppression?
I.H. Al-Abdullah, M.S.A. Kumar, M.S. Al-Adnani and G.M. Abouna 409

Part Ten: *Bone Marrow Transplantation*

55. Current status of allogeneic bone marrow transplantation
Rainer Storb 415
56. New approach to bone marrow transplantation in thalassemia
G. Giardini, G. Lucarelli, M. Galimberti, P. Polchi, E. Angelucci, D. Garonciani, S.M.T. Durazzi, F. Agostinelli, M. Donati, C. Giorgi and M. Filocamo 425
57. Autologous bone marrow transplantation as treatment for bad-risk first remission acute lymphoblastic leukaemia
R.L. Powles, C.L. Smith and S. Milan 429
58. Conditioning regimens in bone marrow transplantation
R. Storb, F. Appelbaum, C. Badger, I. Bernstein, C.D. Buckner, F.B. Petersen, P. Martin, J. Hansen, C. Anasetti, B. Sandmaier, J. Bianco, F. Schuening and E.D. Thomas 437
59. The antileukaemic action of melphalan and total body irradiation in bone marrow transplantation
R.L. Powles, C.L. Smith, C. Tiley, M. Findley and M. O'Brien 443
60. Antifungal prophylaxis with fluconazole in bone marrow transplantation
R.L. Powles, C.L. Smith and S. Milliken 447

Part Eleven: *Xeno-Transplantation*

61. Mass islet isolation from the pancreas of higher mammals: a potential source for islet transplantation in diabetic patients
R.G. Bretzel, B.J. Hering and K.F. Federlin 453
62. The relationship of eicosanoids and complement components to hyperacute xenogeneic rejection and its modification by the PAF-antagonist WEB 2086BS

David M. Saumweber, Rolf Bergmann, Claus Hammer and Walter Brendel 459

63. Antibody-induced rejection of established pig proislet xenografts in $CD4^+$ T cell depleted diabetic mice
J. Dennis Wilson, Charmaine J. Simeonovic and Rhodri Ceredig 469

Part Twelve: *Complications in Organ Transplantation*

64. Occurrence of malignancies in immunosuppressed organ transplant recipients
Israel Penn 475

65. Transmission of cancer with donor organs
Israel Penn 485

66. Long-term experience with surgical repair for transplant renal artery stenosis
M.P. Posner, A.L. King, K.B. Brown and H.M. Lee 491

67. Lymphoproliferative disorders after liver transplantation (OLT): a recent experience
T.G. Heffron, J.C. Emond, J.R. Thistlethwaite, X.M. Rogiers, M.D. Yang, K.L. King and C.E. Broelsch 497

68. Experience with Kaposi's sarcoma in recipients of renal transplants in Tunisia
T. Ben Abdallah, A. El-Matri, C. Kechrid, R. Bardi, F. Ben Hamida, F. El-Younsi, H. Ben Maiz, F. Ben Ayed, Y. Gorgi and H. Ben Ayed 501

69. Urological complications in 510 consecutive renal transplants
H. Abdul Karim, M.S.A. Kumar, M. Samhan, P. John, I.M. Hassan, S. Abdul Basit, E.M. Philips and G.M. Abouna 505

Part Thirteen: *Organ Procurement and Preservation*

70. Preservation of the kidney and other organs into the nineties
G. Kootstra, R. Wijnen and J.G. Maessen 511

71. Clinical experience with liver preservation
Robert D. Gordon and Satoru Todo 519

72. Management of the organ donor
Yoogoo Kang 525

73. The role of the National Kidney Foundation in cadaveric transplantation in Saudi Arabia
S. Aswad, S. Taha, M. Babiker and A. Qayum 531

Part Fourteen: *Ethical, Legal and Religious Aspects*

74. The position of the Transplantation Society on commercialization in organ transplantation
J.R. Batchelor 537
75. Ethics and transplantation: an analysis of 'rewarded gifting'
John B. Dossetor 539
76. Moral, ethical and medical values sacrificed by commercialization in human organs
G.M. Abouna 545
77. Commerce and trade in human organs
B.N. Colabawalla 555
78. Some ethical concerns in organ transplantation
C.J. Vas 559
79. Islamic view on organ transplantation
Mohammed Ali Albar 573

Index of subjects 579

Foreword

This volume is based on a very successful meeting on organ transplantation that was held in Kuwait in 1990 under the auspices of the Middle East Society for Organ Transplantation. An international group of organ transplant experts attended this conference and their contributions and deliberations have been recently updated to produce this definitive and authoritative summary of current clinical practice in organ transplantation.

The initial chapters appropriately focus on the immunology of organ transplantation with special emphasis on the initial events in the induction of alloreactivity, the mechanisms of rejection, and the potential for tolerance induction. A strong emphasis is placed on the diagnosis of rejection by cellular analysis. The section on immunosuppression deals with several new areas of clinical therapy. The section on renal transplantation is unique in several respects, the long-term results from various countries, including the Middle East, are summarized, the use of living unrelated donors and of ABO incompatible donors — all strategies to maximize organ availability — are presented. The latest clinical practice of liver, lung, and heart-lung transplantation are summarized. An excellent update of whole organ pancreas and islet transplantation is presented including advances in technique and improvements in complications of diabetes post-transplantation are cautiously identified. Newer aspects of bone marrow transplantation are considered in detail, especially in regard to new conditioning regimens for allotransplantation, and the use of autologous marrow transplantation in certain forms of leukemia. The section on organ transplant complications appropriately focuses on two of the most important complications of clinical transplantation, i.e. spontaneous malignancy, especially lymphoproliferative disease, and cytomegalic virus infection.

One of the most outstanding aspects of this volume is the in depth analysis of ethical, legal, and religious aspects of clinical organ transplantation and donation. The major 'world' problems in organ donation and procurement are discussed in detail, particularly the concerns of the entire transplantation community on commercialization in organ transplantation, and the values lost when such negative commerce occurs. It is fitting and appropriate after a conference held in the Middle East, that the Islamic view of organ transplantation is presented in rich detail. Readers of all cultures and faiths will see the similarities of this view with their own. Indeed, this volume not only identifies the rapid and successful development of all forms of clinical organ transplantation in many countries but also emphasizes that organ transplantation is an international effort and that the organ transplant community is an international one, united in common concern for the application of organ transplantation for the well-being of all patients. Professor Abouna and his colleagues have succeeded in bringing together many of the advances and controversial issues of organ transplantation in a comprehensive and well written book that deserves to be read widely throughout the world.

Boston, July 1991 ANTHONY P. MONACO

Preface

During the past decade, Organ Transplantation has rapidly evolved into a very successful therapy for irreversible vital organ failure. The factors responsible for this revolutionary progress are many and include major advances in immunobiology of graft rejection, surgical techniques, patient management, immunosuppressive therapy, preservation technology, and public attitude towards organ donation. As a consequence of this success, the indications for transplantation of organs have become more liberalized with many older patients being transplanted and many high risk grafts being successfully used. The volume of transplants as well as the number of transplant centers has been rising every year in all parts of the world including many developing countries. This book is a comprehensive review of many of these advances and of the current concepts and clinical practices in organ transplantation in the 1990s, by a distinguished team of contributors and recognized experts from all over the world who had initially participated in a very successful International Congress held in Kuwait in the Spring of 1990. It was after that Congress that the idea of compiling this work emerged. The material presented in this book by all the authors, has been expanded and updated in late 1990 and early 1991.

The book covers 79 chapters in 14 major sections dealing with a large variety of general and specific issues in organ transplantation including historical developments; immunobiology and histocompatibility; organ allograft rejection, immunosuppression including the recent clinical use of FK 506 and deoxyspergualin, sequential drug therapy and the indication for safe cyclosporine withdrawal; the induction of experimental and clinical tolerance; organ procurement and preservation including the use of non-heart beating cadavers for renal transplantation; donor management; transplant complications and the future prospect of using xenografts for human transplantation.

The book also contains comprehensive chapters on specific organs including kidney, liver, pancreas, islet cells, multi-visceral organs, heart, lung and bone marrow. The section on renal transplantation deals especially with the use of genetically unrelated living donors, of ABO incompatible donors and of double and single pediatric cadaver kidneys in adult recipients. The part dealing with liver transplantation besides reviewing the current clinical results, describes the latest techniques of split-liver transplantation and of liver-segment transplantation from living related donors. The current excellent results obtained with whole pancreas transplantation from major world centers are reviewed together with the updated results of the two international registries, whole pancreas and islet transplant registries. The section on bone marrow transplantation reviews the latest method of conditioning, of immunosuppression and of management of complications in allogeneic transplantation for leukemia, thalasemia and other non-malignant disorders and also in autologous marrow transplantation. The recent successful techniques of lung transplantation are reviewed.

A unique feature of this book, besides addressing the medical advances and future trends in transplantation, are detailed chapters dealing with the religious, moral and ethical issues as they prevail today among different cultures of the world, including the Middle East, the Far East and the Indian subcontinent which, undoubtedly, will have profound effect on the development of transplantation in those areas of the world.

We hope that the book will be an important source of information on current knowledge and practice in the field of organ transplantation for the practising clinician, the transplant research scientist and the medical and surgical fellows in training. The book may also be a valuable reference for other medical and paramedical personnel involved in transplantation, including nurses, coordinators, ethicists, hospital and health care administrators and planners in different parts of the world.

The realization of this work was made possible through the excellent co-operation and hard work by all the authors who spared no effort in expanding and updating their contributions, often at short notice. I am grateful to the staff of the Department of Organ Transplantation of Kuwait University for their support and dedication in the early stages of the preparation of this book, particularly Dorothy Temudo, E. M. Philips and Reema Antos and also to the secretarial staff at Hahnemann University, Division of Transplantation, for their help in the final stages of this work. Finally, I am grateful to my associate editors for their support, to my wife, Cathy Abouna, for the painful task of transcribing, indexing and compiling the many manuscripts of this work and to our publisher, Kluwer Academic, for their advice and patience and for their commitment to excellence in the production of this book.

Philadelphia, July 1991 GEORGE M. ABOUNA

List of contributors

ABDI, E., M.D.
Hashmi Nejad Kidney Center
University of Medical Sciences of Iran
Tehran, Iran

ABDUL, Basit, S., M.D.
Anesthetist
Hamed Al-Essa Organ Transplant Center
Kuwait City, Kuwait

ABDUL, Karim, H., M.D.
Fellow
Hamed Al-Essa Organ Transplant Center
Kuwait City, Kuwait

ABDUL-QAYM, M.D.
Medical Co-ordinator
National Kidney Foundation
Riyadh, Saudi Arabia

ABENDROTH, D., M.D.
Assistant Professor
Division of Transplantation
Klinikum Grosshadern
Munich, Germany

ABOUNA, G.M., M.D.,
F.R.C.S., (C), F.A.C.S.
Prof. of Surgery
Director
Division of Transplantation
Hahnemann University
Philadelphia, Pennsylvania U.S.A.
former Professor and Chairman,
Department of Organ Transplantation
Kuwait University and Hamed Al-Essa
Organ Transplant Center
Kuwait City, Kuwait

AGOSTINELLI, F., Ph.D.
Lecturer
Division of Hematology
University of Pesaro
Pesaro, Italy

AL-ABDULLAH, I.H., Ph.D.
Assistant Professor
Division of Organ Transplantation
Hahnemann University, Philadelphia
Pennsylvania, U.S.A.

AL-ADNANI, M.S., M.D. F.R.C. Path
Professor of Pathology
Kuwait University
Kuwait City, Kuwait

AL-DADAH, S., M.D.
Fellow
Hamed Al-Essa Organ Transplant Center
Kuwait City, Kuwait

AL-MUZAIRAI, I.A., M.D.
Research Fellow
Department of Medicine
University of Aberdeen, Forrest Hill
Aberdeen, Scotland, U.K.

AL-SABAWI, N.A., M.D.
Nephrologist
Department of Organ Transplantation
Hamed Al-Essa Organ Transplant Center
Kuwait City, Kuwait

ALBAR, Mohammed Ali, M.D.
Consultant in Islamic Medicine
King Fahd Medical Research Center
King Abdul Aziz University
Jeddah, Saudi Arabia

ALESSIANI, Mario, M.D.
Research Fellow
Department of Surgery
University of Pittsburgh
Pittsburgh, Pennsylvania, U.S.A.

AMEMIYA, H., M.D.
Director
Department of Surgical
Research National Cardiovascular Center
Suita-Shi, Osaka, Japan

ANASETTI, C., M.D.
Assistant Member
The Fred Hutchinson Cancer Research Center
Seattle, Washington, U.S.A.

ANGELO, Khattar M., Ph.D.
Assistant Professor
Department of Pharmacology
Kuwait University
Kuwait City, Kuwait

ANGELUCCI, E., M.D.
Assistant Professor
Division of Hematology
University of Pesaro
Pesaro, Italy

APPELBAUM, F., M.D.
Professor of Medicine
University of Washington &
The Fred Hutchinson Cancer Research Center
Seattle, Washington, U.S.A.

ARSLAN, G., M.S.
Assistant Professor of Anesthesiology
University of Hacettepe &
The Turkish Transplant Foundation
Ankara, Turkey

ASWAD, Saleh, M.D.
Director
National Kidney Foundation
Riyadh, Saudi Arabia

AYED, K., M.D.
Professor of Pathology & Immunology
Tunis University Faculty of Medicine
Tunis, Tunisia

AYED, M., M.D.
Professor of Urology
Charles Nicolle University Hospital
Tunis, Tunisia

BABIKER, Moawia, M.D.
Medical Coordinator
National Kidney Foundation
Riyadh, Saudi Arabia

BADGER, C., M.D.
Instructor in Medicine
University of Washington &
The Fred Hutchinson Cancer Center
Seattle, Washington, U.S.A.

BARDI, R., M.D.
Department of Pathology & Immunology,
University of Tunis
Tunis, Tunisia

BATCHELOR, J.R., Ph.D.
Professor and
Head Department of Immunology
Royal Post-Graduate Medical School
Hammersmith Hospital
London, England, U.K.

BEELEN, J., Ph.D.
Transplant Immunologist
Tissue Typing Laboratory
University of Groningen
Groningen, The Netherlands

BEN Abdallah, T., M.D.
Prof. of Medicine
Department of Nephrology
Charles Nicolle University Hospital
Tunis, Tunisia

BEN Ayed, H., M.D.
Professor of Medicine,
Charles Nicolle University Hospital
Tunis, Tunisia

BEN Hamida, F., M.D.
Professor of Medicine
Department of Nephrology
Charles Nicolle University Hospital
Tunis, Tunisia

BEN Maiz, H., M.D.
Professor of Medicine
Charles Nicolle University Hospital
Tunis, Tunisia

BEN Moussa, F., M.D.
Assistant Professor
Ag. Department of Medicine
Charles Nicolle University Hospital
Tunis, Tunisia

BERGMANN, Rolf, M.D.
Institute of Medical Research
University of Munich
Munich, Germany

BERLATZKY, Y., M.D.
Research Fellow
Division of Transplantation
Medical College of Virginia
Richmond, Virginia, U.S.A.

BERNSTEIN, I., M.D.
Professor of Pediatrics
University of Washington &
The Fred Hutchinson Cancer Research Center
Seattle, Washington, U.S.A.

BIANCO, J., M.D.
Senior Fellow in Oncology
The Fred Hutchinson Cancer Research Center
Seattle, Washington, U.S.A.

BILGIN, N., M.D.
Professor of Surgery,
Hacettepe University &
Turkish Transplant Foundation
Ankara, Turkey

BOLMAN, R. Morton III, M.D.
Professor of Cardiothoracic Surgery
Department of Surgery
University of Minnesota
Minneapolis, Minnesota, U.S.A.

BRENDEL, Walter, M.D.
Professor
Institute of Surgical Research
University of Munich
Munich, Germany

BRETZEL, R.G., M.D., Ph.D.
Professor of Medicine
3rd Medical Clinic and Polyclinic
University of Giessen
Giessen, Germany

BROELSCH, C.E., M.D.
Professor of Surgery
Department of Surgery
University of Chicago
Chicago, Illinois, U.S.A.
Professor & Head
Department of Surgery
University of Hamburg, Germany

BROWN, K.B.
Assistant Professor
Department of Surgery
Medical College of Virginia
Richmond, Virginia, U.S.A.

BRYNGER, H., M.D.
Professor of Surgery
University of Goteborg
Goteborg, Sweden

BUCKNER, C.D., M.D.
Professor of Medicine
University of Washington &
The Fred Hutchinson Cancer Research Center
Seattle, Washington, U.S.A.

CATTO, G.R.D., D.Sc., F.R.C.P.
Professor of Medicine
University of Aberdeen
Aberdeen, Scotland, U.K.

CEREDIG, R.
Institute de Chimie Biologique
Faculté de Médicine
Strasbourg Cedex, France

CLASS, F.H.J., M.D.
Professor of Immunology
Department of Immunology
University Hospital
Leiden, The Netherlands

COLABAWALLA, B.N., M.D.
Consultant Urological Surgeon
Bombay, Maharashtra, India

COOK, B.A.D., Ph.D.
Professor of Immunology & Microbiology
Medical College of Virginia
Richmond, Virginia, U.S.A.

CORRY, ROBERT J., M.D.
Professor and Head
Department of Surgery
University of Iowa
Iowa City, Iowa, U.S.A.

D'AMARO, J., Ph.D.
Professor of Immunology
Department of Immunology
University Hospital
Leiden, The Netherlands

DE GAST, E., Ph.D.,
Professor of Immunology
Tissue Typing Laboratory
University Hospital
Utrecht, The Netherlands

DE JONG, J.A.M., M.D.
Head of Radiotherapy
Department Institute of Radiotherapy
De Weven Hospital
Heerlen, The Netherlands

De WAAL, L.P., Ph.D.
Blood Transfusion Service Red Cross
Amsterdam, The Netherlands

DIRSCHEDL, P., M.D.
Research Associate
Institute for Medical Research
University of Munich
Munich, Germany

DOHI, K., M.D.
Professor of Medicine
Second Department of Surgery
Hiroshima University
School of Medicine
Hiroshima, Japan

DONATI, M., Ph.D.
Division of Hematology
University of Pesaro
Pesaro, Italy

DOSSETOR, John B., M.D. F.R.C.P. (C)
Professor of Medicine
Department of Bioethics
University of Alberta
Alberta, Canada

DUNN, David L., M.D.
Assoc. Professor
Department of Surgery Medical School
University of Minnesota
Minneapolis, Minnesota, U.S.A.

DURAZZI, S.M.T., M.D.
Assistant Professor
Division of Hematology
University of Pesaro
Pesaro, Italy

ECHE, T., M.D.
Assistant Professor
Faculty of Medicine
Kuwait University
Kuwait City, Kuwait

EL-DEEN, A.S., M.D.
Assistant Professor
Pharmacology Department
Kuwait University
Kuwait City, Kuwait

EL-MATRI, A., M.D.
Professor of Medicine
Charles Nicolle University Hospital
Tunis, Tunisia

EL-QUAKDI, M., M.D.
Professor, Service d'urologie
Charles Nicolle University Hospital
Tunis, Tunisia

EL-YOUNSI, F., M.D.
Assistant Professor
Department of Nephrology
Charles Nicolle University Hospital
Tunis, Tunisia

EMOND, J.C., M.D.
Associate Professor
Department of Surgery
Liver Transplant Service
University of Chcago
Chicago, Illinois, U.S.A.

ERICZON, B.G., M.D.
Department of Transplant Surgery
Huddinge Hospital
Stockholm, Sweden

FAZEL, I., M.D.
Minister of Health
Tehran, Iran

FEDERLIN, K.F., M.D. Ph.D.
Professor
3rd Medical Clinic & Polyclinic
University of Giessen
Giessen, Germany

FINDLEY, M., M.D.
Leukemia Unit
Royal Marsden Hospital
Sutton, Surrey, U.K.

FILOCAMO, M., M.D.
Division of Hematology
University of Pesaro
Pesaro, Italy

FIRST, M. Roy, M.D.
Professor of Medicine
University of Cincinnati Medical Center
Cincinnati, Ohio, U.S.A.

FRIEDL, L., M.D.
Division of Transplantation Surgery
Klinikum Grosshadern
Munich, Germany

FRYD, DAVID S., M.D.
Associate Professor
Department of Surgery
University of Minnesota
Minneapolis, Minnesota, U.S.A.

FUKAO, K., M.D.
Associate Professor
Department of Surgery
Institute of Clinical Medicine
University of Tsukuba
Ibaragi, Japan

FUKUDA, Y., M.D.
Associate Professor
Department of Surgery
Hiroshima University School of Medicine
Hiroshima, Japan

FUNG, John J., M.D.
Assistant Professor of Surgery
University of Pittsburgh
Pittsburgh, Pennsylvania, U.S.A.

GALIMBERTI, M., M.D.
Division of Hematology
University of Pesaro
Pesaro, Italy

GARONCIANI, D., M.D.
Assistant Professor
Division of Hematology
University of Pesaro
Pesaro, Italy

GHASHTI, H.N.
Hashmi Nejad Kidney Center
University of Medical Sciences of Iran
Tehran, Iran

GHODS, A.J., M.D.
Transplant Immunologist
Hashmi Nejad Kidney Center
University of Medical Sciences of Iran
Tehran, Iran

GIARDINI, G., M.D.
Associate Professor
Department of Hematology
University of Pesaro
Pesaro, Italy

GILLINGHAM, Kristin, M.D.
Associate Professor
Department of Surgery
University of Minnesota
Minneapolis, Minnesota, U.S.A.

GIORGI, C., Ph.D
Division of Hematology
University of Pesaro
Pesaro, Italy

GJERTSON, David W., Ph.D.
Assistant Professor of Surgery
University of California, U.S.A.

GOETZ, Frederick C.
Professor
Department of Medicine
University of Minnesota, U.S.A.

GOKEL, M., M.D.
Professor of Pathology
University of Munich
Munich, Germany

GORDON, Robert D., M.D.
Associate Professor
Department of Surgery
University of Pittsburgh, Falk Clinic
Pittsburgh, Pennsylvania, U.S.A.

GORGI, Y., M.D.
Professor of Pathology
Department of Pathology & Immunology
Tunis University Medical School
Tunis, Tunisia

GROTH, C.G., M.D.
Professor of Surgery
Karolinska Institute, Huddinge Hospital
Stockholm, Sweden

GRUESSNER, Rainer, W.G., M.D.
Research Assistant
Department of Surgery
Medical School, University of Minnesota
Minneapolis, Minnesota, U.S.A.

GULAY, H., M.D.
Assistant Professor of Surgery
Hacettepe University &
Turkish Transplant Foundation
Ankara, Turkey

HABERAL, M., M.D., F.A.C.S.
Professor of Surgery & Director
Hacettepe University &
Turkish Transplant Foundation
Ankara, Turkey

HAMMER, Claus, M.D.
Professor
Institute for Surgical Research
University of Munich
Munich, Germany

HANSEN, J., M.D.
Professor of Medicine
University of Washington &
Associate Director
The Fred Hutchinson Cancer Research Center
Seattle, Washington, U.S.A.

HASSAN, I.M., M.D.
Fellow
Department of Nuclear Medicine
Hamed Al-Essa Organ Transplant Center
Kuwait City, Kuwait

HÄYRY, Pekka, M.D.
Professor of Transplantation
University of Helsinki
Transplantation Laboratory
Helsinki, Finland

HEFFRON, T.G.
Assistant Professor
Department of Surgery
University of Chicago
Chicago, Illinois, U.S.A.

HEIDENDAL, G., M.D.
Internist
Department of Nuclear Medicine
University Hospital
Maastricht, The Netherlands

HENRIQUES, H.F., M.D.
George Washington University
Division of Transplantation
Washington, D.C., U.S.A.

HERING, B.J., M.D.
Professor of Medicine
3rd Medical Clinic and Polyclinic
University of Griessen
Griessen, Germany

ILLNER, W.D., M.D.
Division of Transplantation Surgery
Klinikum Grosshadern
Munich, Germany

ISHIBASHI, M., M.D.
Lecturer
Department of Urology
Osaka University
Osaka, Japan

JAIN, Ashok, M.D.
Research Fellow
Department of Surgery
University of Pittsburgh
Pittsburgh, Pennsylvania, U.S.A.

JOHN P., M.D.
Fellow in Transplant Surgery
Hamed Al-Essa Organ
Transplantation Center
Kuwait City, Kuwait

KALAWI, M., M.D.
Fellow
Department of Organ Transplantation
Hamed Al-Essa Organ Transplantation Center
Kuwait City, Kuwait

KANG, Yoogoo, M.D.
Associate Professor
Department of Surgery
University of Pittsburgh
Pittsburgh, Pennsylvania, U.S.A.

KECHRID, C., M.D.
Professor of Medicine
Department of Nephrology
Charles Nicolle University Hospital
Tunis, Tunisia

KEMKES, B.M., M.D.
Professor of Cardiovascular Surgery
University of Munich
Munich, Germany

KENDALL, David M., M.D.
Assistant Professor
Department of Surgery
University of Minnesota
Minneapolis, Minnesota, U.S.A.

KHEDER, A., M.D.
Assistant Professor
Service de Médicine et de Nephrologie
Charles Nicolle University Hospital
Tunis, Tunisia

KING, A.L., M.D.
Assistant Professor of Medicine
Medical College of Virginia
Richmond, Virginia, U.S.A.

KING, K.L., M.D.
Associate Professor of Medicine
Medical College of Virginia
Richmond, Virginia, U.S.A.

KLANKE, D., M.D.
Institute of Surgical Research
University of Munich
Munich, Germany

KOBRYN, A., M.D.
Assistant Professor
Kuwait University &
Hamed Al-Essa Organ Transplant Center
Kuwait City, Kuwait

KOÇ, M., M.D.
Assistant Professor of Surgery
University of Hacettepe
Ankara, Turkey

KLOSTERMAN, C., M.D.
Transplant Coordinator
Medical College of Virginia
Richmond, Virginia, U.S.A.

KOOTSTRA, G., M.D., Ph.D
Professor of Surgery and
Director of Transplantation
University Hospital
Maastricht, The Netherlands

KOYAMA, I., M.D.
Professor of Surgery
Department of Surgery
Saitamu University Medical School
Saitamu, Japan

KROMBACH, F., M.D.
Institute for Surgical Research
University of Munich
Munich, Germany

KUBOTA, K., M.D.
Fellow in Transplant Surgery
Department of Transplant Surgery
Karolinska Institute
Huddinge Hospital
Stockholm, Sweden

KUMAR, M.S.A., M.D., F.R.C.S.E.
Assistant Professor
Department of Surgery
Hahnemann University
Philadelphia
Pennsylvania, U.S.A.
Former Associate Professor
Department of Organ Transplantation
Kuwait University
Kuwait City, Kuwait

LACY, Paul E., M.D.
Professor of Medicine
University of Washington
St. Louis, Missouri, U.S.A.

LAND, Walter, M.D.
Professor and Head
Division of Transplantation Surgery
Klinikum Grosshadern
Munich, Germany

LANDGRAF, R., M.D.
Professor of Diabetology
University of Munich
Munich, Germany

LANGNAS, Alan N., M.D.
Assistant Professor
Department of Surgery
University of Nebraska
Ohama, Nebraska, U.S.A.

LAUTENSCHLAGER, Irmeli
Transplant Immunologist
Transplantation Laboratory
University of Helsinki
Helsinki, Finland

LECHLER, R.I., Ph.D.
Reader in the Department of Immunology
Royal Postgraduate Medical School
Hammersmith Hospital
London, England, U.K.

LEE, H.M., M.D.
Professor of Surgery and Chairman
Division of Transplantation
and Vascular Surgery
Medical College of Virginia
Richmond, Virginia, U.S.A.

LLOVERAS, Goncal, M.D.
Assistant Professor
Department of Surgery
University of Minnesota
Minneapolis, Minnesota, U.S.A.

LOMBARDIM, G., Ph.D.
Department of Immunology
Royal Postgraduate Medical School
Hammersmith Hospital
London, England, U.K.

LUCARELLI, G., M.D.
Professor of Hematology
University of Pesaro
Pesaro, Italy

MACLEOD, A.A., M.D., M.R.C.P.
Senior Lecturer
Department of Medicine
University of Aberdeen
Aberdeen, Scotland, U.K.

MACMILLAN, M., M.D., M.R.C.P.
Physician
Renal Unit
Stobhill General Hospital
Glasgow, Scotland, U.K.

MAESSEN, J.G.
Resident
Department of Surgery
University Hospital
Maastricht, The Netherlands

MARTIN, P., M.D.
Associate Professor of Medicine
University of Washington, and
The Fred Hutchinson Cencer Research Center
Seattle, Washington, U.S.A.

MATAS, Arthur J., M.D.
Associate Professor
Department of Surgery
University of Minnesota
Minneapolis, Minnesota, U.S.A.

MILAN, S.
Statistician
Computer Department
Royal Marsden Hospital
Sutton, Surrey, England, U.K.

MILLIKEN, S.
Bone Marrow Transplant Coordinator
Leukemia Unit
Royal Marsden Hospital
Sutton, Surrey, England, U.K.

MONACO, Anthony P., M.D.
Professor of Surgery
Harvard University and
Director Cancer Research Institute
Deaconess Hospital
Boston, Massachusetts, U.S.A.

MOUNDRY-MUNNS, Kay C., B.S.N., R.N.S., C.C.R.N.
Coordinator
International Pancreas
Transplant Registrar
Minneapolis, Minnesota, U.S.A.

MURASE, Noriko, M.D.
Assistant Professor of Surgery
University of Pittsburgh
Fifth Avenue
Pittsburgh, Pennsylvania, U.S.A.

NAJARIAN, John S., M.D.
Professor and Chairman
Department of Surgery,
Medical School
University of Minnesota
Minneapolis, Minnesota, U.S.A.

NIKBIN, B.
Hashmi Nejad Kidney Center
University of Medical Science of Iran
Tehran, Iran

O'BRIEN, M., M.D.
Leukemia Unit
Royal Marsden Hospital
Sutton, Surrey, England, U.K.

OMOTO, R., M.D.
Department of Surgery
Saitama Medical School
Saitama, Japan

OTA, K., M.D.
Professor of Surgery
Director of Kidney Center
Tokyo Women's Medical College
Tokyo, Japan

PANJWANI, D., M.D.
Clinical Tutor
Department of Organ Transplantation
Kuwait University
Kuwait City, Kuwait

PAYNE, William D., M.D.
Associate Professor
Department of Surgery Medical School
University of Minnesota
Minneapolis, Minnesota, U.S.A.

PELTENBURG, H., M.D.
Assistant Internist
Department of Medicine
University Hospital
Maastricht, The Netherlands

PENN, Israel, M.D.
Professor of Surgery
University of Cincinnati
Medical Center
Cincinnati, Ohio, U.S.A.

PERSIJN, G.G., M.D.
Euro Transplant Foundation and
University Hospital
Leiden, The Netherlands

PETERSEN, F.B., M.D.
The Fred Hutchinson Cancer Research Center
Seattle, Washington, U.S.A.

PHILIPS, E.M., M.D.
Research Assistant
Department of Organ Transplantation
Kuwait University
Kuwait City, Kuwait

PILLEN, Todd J., M.D.
University of Chicago,
Chicago, Illinois, U.S.A.

POLCHI, P., M.D.
Assistant Professor
Division of Hematology
University of Pasaro
Pasaro, Italy

POSNER, M.P., M.D.
Associate Professor of Surgery
Medical College of Virginia
Richmond, Virginia, U.S.A.

POWER, David A., M.D.
Senior Lecturer
Department of Medicine
University of Aberdeen
Aberdeen, Scotland, U.K.

POWLES, R.L., M.D.
Consultant Physician
Leukemia Unit
Royal Marsden Hospital
Sutton, Surrey, England, U.K.

PROOSHANI, F., M.D.
Hashmi Nejad Kidney Center
University of Medical Sciences of Iran
Tehran, Iran

QAYUM, Abdul, M.D.
Central Coordinator
Kidney Foundation
Riyadh, Saudi Arabia

RAHBAR, K., M.D.
Hashmi Nejad Kidney Center
University of Medical Sciences of Iran
Tehran, Iran

RAJU, K.T., B.S.C.
Research Assistant
Hamed Al-Essa Organ Transplant Center
Kuwait City, Kuwait

REEKERS, P., Ph.D.
Tissue Typing Lab
Nijmegen, The Netherlands

REICHART, B., M.D.
Professor of Cariovascular Surgery
University of Munich
Munich, Germany

ROBERTSON, R. Paul, M.D.
Professor, Department of Medicine
University of Minnesota
Minneapolis, Minnesota, U.S.A.

ROGIERS, X.M., M.D.
Associate Professor
University of Brussels
Brussels, Belgium
Department of Surgery
University of Chicago
Chicago, Illinois, U.S.A.

SAMHAN, M., M.D., F.R.C.S.E.
Clinical Instructor
Department of Organ Transplantation
Kuwait University &
Hamed Al-Essa Transplant Center
Kuwait City, Kuwait

SANDMAIER, B., M.D.
Clinical Research Association
The Fred Hutchinson Cancer Research Center
Seattle, Washington, U.S.A.

SAUMWEBER, David M., M.D.
Institute for Surgical Research
University of Munich
Munich, Germany

SCHARP, David W., M.D.
Associate Professor
Department of Surgery
University of Washington
St. Louis, Missouri, U.S.A.

SCHILLING, M., M.D.
Division of Transplantation Surgery
Klinikum Grosshadern
Munich, Germany

SCHLEIBNER, S., M.D.
Division of Transplantation Surgery
Klinikum Grosshadern
Munich, Germany

SCHNEEBERGER, H., M.D.
Division of Transplantation Surgery
Klinikum Grosshadern
Munich, Germany

SCHROEDER, Timothy J., M.D.
Assistant Professor of Pathology &
Laboratory Medicine
University of Cincinnati
Medical Center
Cincinnati, Ohio, U.S.A.

SCHUENING, F., M.D.
Clinical Research Associate
The Fred Hutchinson Cancer Research Center
Seattle, Washington, U.S.A.

SERT, S., M.D.
Assistant Professor of Surgery
Hacettepe University &
Turkish Transplant Foundation
Ankara, Turkey

SHAW, Beyers W. Jr., M.D.
Professor, Chief of Transplantation Service
Department of Surgery
University of Nebraska
Omaha, Nebraska, U.S.A.

SHUWAIKH, E., M.D.
Anaesthesiologist
Hamed Al-Essa Organ Transplant Center
Kuwait City, Kuwait

SILVA, O.S.G., M.D.
Consultant Anaesthesiologist and
Clinical Instructor
Department of Organ Transplantation
Kuwait University &
Hamed Al-Essa Organ Transplant Center
Kuwait City, Kuwait

SIMEONOVIC, Charmaine J.
Division of Clinical Science
The John Curtin School of Medical Research
Australian National University
Canberra, Australia

SMERLIE, S., M.D.
Charles Nicolle University Hospital
Tunis, Tunisia

SMITH, C.L.
Bone Marrow Transplant Co-ordinator
Leukemia Unit
Royal Marsden Hospital
Sutton, Surrey, England, U.K.

SMITH, John L., M.D.
Assistant Professor
Department of Surgery
University of Iowa
Iowa City, Iowa, U.S.A.

SONODA, T., M.D.
Professor
Osaka University
Department of Organ Transplantation
Biomedical Research Center
Osaka, Japan

STANGL, M., M.D.
Department of Surgery
University of Munich
Munich, Germany

STARZL, Thomas E., M.D., Ph.D.
Professor of Surgery
University of Pittsburgh
Falk Clinic
Pittsburgh, Pennsylvania, U.S.A.

STEWART, K.N., F.I.L.M.S.
Research Fellow
University of Aberdeen
Aberdeen, Scotland, U.K.

STORB, Rainer, M.D.
Professor of Medicine
University of Washington
Head of Transplantation Biology,
The Fred Hutchinson Cancer Research Center
Seattle, Washington, U.S.A.

STRATTA, Robert, J., M.D.
Assistant Professor
Department of Surgery
University of Nebraska
Ohaha, Nebraska, U.S.A.

SUTHERLAND, David E.R., M.D.
Professor
Department of Surgery
Medical School
University of Minnesota
Minneapolis, Minnesota, U.S.A.

SUZUKI, S., M.D.
Department of Surgery Research
National Cardiovascular Center
Osaka, Japan

TAHA, Saleh, M.D.
Medical Co-ordinator
National Kidney Foundation
Riayadt, Saudi Arabia

TAKAHASHI, K., M.D.
Associate Professor
Department of Urology
Tokyo Women's Medical College
Tokyo, Japan

TERASAKI, I., Ph.D.
Professor of Surgery
University of California
Los Angeles, California U.S.A.

THEODORAKIS, J., M.D.
Department of Urology
Klinikum Grosshadern,
University of Munich
Munich, Germany

THISTLETHWAITE, J.R.
Associate Professor of Surgery
Department of Surgery
University of Chicago
Chicago, Illinois, U.S.A.

THOMAS, E.D., M.D.
Professor of Medicine
University of Washington
and former Associate Director
The Fred Hutchinson Cancer Research Center
Seattle, Washington, U.S.A.

TIEBOSCH, T., M.D.
Assistant Pathologist
Department of Pathology
University Hospital
Maastrich, The Netherlands

TILEY, C., M.D.
Leukemia Unit
Royal Marsden Hospital
Sutton, Surrey, England, U.K.

TODO, Satoru, M.D.
Associate Professor of Surgery
University of Pittsburgh
Falk Clinic
Pittsburgh, Pennsylvania, U.S.A.

TZAKIS, Andreas C., M.D.
Associate Professor of Surgery
University of Pittsburgh
Falk Clinic
Pittsburgh, Pennsylvania, U.S.A.

VAN HOOFF, J.P., M.D.
Associate Nephrologist
Department of Internal Medicine
University Hospital
Maastricht, The Netherlands

VAN DER LINDEN, C.J., M.D.
Associate Surgeon
Department of Surgery
University Hospital
Maastricht, The Netherlands

VAN DEN BERG-LOONEN, P., Ph.D.
Transplant Immunologist
Tissue Typing Laboratory
University of Maastricht
Maastricht, The Netherlands

VAN ROOD, J.J., M.D., Ph.D.
Professor of Immunology
University Hospital
Leiden, The Netherlands

VAS, C.J.
Consultant Neurologist
Dr. B. Nanavthi Hospital
Bombay, India
Chairman
International Commission for Health Professionals
Geneva, Switzerland

VERSCHUEREN, T., M.D.
Radiologist
Department of Radiology
Institute of Radiotherapy
De Weven Hospital
Heerlen, The Netherlands

VON WILLEBRAND, Eeva, Ph.D.
Assistant Professor
Transplantation Laboratory
University of Helsinki
Helsinki, Finland

WEBER, Barbra, K., M.D.
Research Fellow
Department of Medicine
University of Aberdeen
Aberdeen, Scotland, U.K.

WHITE, A.G., Ph.D.
Associate Professor
Department of Organ Transplantation
Kuwait University and
Hamad Al-Essa Transplant Center
Kuwait City, Kuwait

HITINGTON, P.F.
Associate Professor of Pediatrics
Department of Surgery
University of Chicago
Chicago, Illinois, U.S.A.

IJNEN, R., M.D.
Department of Surgery
University Hospital
Maastricht, The Netherlands

WILSON, J. Dennis, M.D.
Department of Endocrinology
Woden Valley Hospital
Woden, Australia

WOOD, R., Patrick, M.D.
Associate Professor
Department of Surgery
University of Nebraska
Omaha, Nebraska, U.S.A.

YANG, M.D., M.D.
Assistant Professor of Surgery
Department of Surgery
University of Chicago
Chicago, Illinois, U.S.A.

ZANTVOORT, F., M.D.
Eurotransplant Foundation and
University Hospital
Leiden, The Netherlands

1. Reflections on the development of organ transplantation

H.M. LEE

Obviously, it will not be possible to go through all aspects of the development of organ transplantation in this brief space. The following review will, therefore, be a personal reflection of some of the highlights of this medical miracle of the twentieth century.

Modern medicine generally accords Dr Ullman, the Hungarian surgeon in Vienna, with some priority of performing the first kidney transplant in the animal model in 1902. The same year, Alexis Carrell, a young French surgeon in Lyon published an article on suturing techniques of blood vessel anastomosis. He emigrated to Canada and then to America, working on kidney transplantation in animal models and applying this suture anastomosis technique. He received the Nobel Prize in 1912 for his contribution in establishing the possibility of transplanting an organ by blood vessel anastomosis.

The immunological nature of tissue and organ transplantation had been suggested by some workers early in this century. It took the late Sir Peter Medawar to establish the immunological background for transplantation with his work in the skin graft study in 1943 and the study of acquired immunological tolerance in 1953. He also received the Nobel Prize for these contributions.

The modern era of human renal transplantation recorded a case of a cadaver kidney transplant performed by Dr Voronoy of Russia in 1933, the results of which were published in an obscure medical journal in 1936. A series of kidney transplants performed in Boston from 1950 to 1953 were reported in detail in 1955 by Hume, Merrill, Miller and Thorn. This opened up the new beginning of clinical investigation in this field.

The basic understanding of immunology and clinical feasibility of organ transplantation began to move together. In 1954, the first identical twin kindney transplants were performed in Boston and in Paris. In 1958 and 1959, with the use of total body irradiation as an immunosuppressant, non-identical twin transplants were also performed in Boston and Paris. The first long-term survival of a patient for 22 months with this method was reported by Professor Hamberger.

The difficulties with total body irradiation as an immunosuppressive modality were enormous. More practical immunosuppressive methods were therefore needed.

In 1958–59, Schwartz and Damshek reported studies showing the inhibition of antibody production and 'drug induced immunological tolerance' using the antimetabolite 6-mercaptopurine. This possibility of manipulating the immune response with a 'drug' for kidney transplants was explored by two surgical groups independently.

In 1960, Professor Calne, working in London and Boston, and Dr Zukowski in Richmond, reported prolongation of kidney transplants in the dog with the use of 6-mercaptopurine. In 1963, Dr Hitching of Burroughs-Wellcome developed a derivative of 6-mercaptopurine with less toxicity, later to be known as azathioprine (Imuran). Dr Hitching and his colleague, Dr Elion, received the Nobel Prize in 1988 for their contribution, including the development of this drug.

Thus began a new era of chemotherapy as an immunosuppressive modality in organ transplantation and, in 1964, Hume reported 20 kidney transplants in 15 patients. In 1964, the First International Histocompatibility Workshop also was being held, organized by Dr Amos of Duke University, which highlighted the earlier works by Professors Gower, Daussett, Walford and Back.

In 1965, Starzl reported his experience of kidney transplants including the effect of leucocyte antigen matching. The same year, Reemtsma reported the first 'long term' survival of a xenograft in the human recipient (chimpanzee kidney). Collaboration of basic laboratory research and clinical surgery rapidly emerged producing new clinical scientists who became known as 'surgical biologists' or 'immunologist-surgeons'. In 1967 the term 'immunological adaptation of organ grafts' was suggested by Professor Woodruff — a more practical goal than 'immunological tolerance'. In the same year, Starzl reported successful liver transplants in children and Christiaan Barnard performed the first cardiac transplant in humans. These surgical advances gave a sense of urgency to immunobiological research. Thus the 'brain death' concept began to be discussed in relation to organ donation and, in 1971, Steinmuller and his colleagues reported the role of 'passenger leukocytes' as an initial antigenic stimulus and Monaco reported the use of bone marrow in producing 'tolerance'. In 1972, organ preservation received a big boost with Belzer's report of the continuous pulsatile perfusion machine.

By now, kidney transplantation was becoming a clinical reality. That year, The First International Clinical Transplantation Symposium, organized by Hume, was held in Richmond, gathering basic scientists and clinicians worldwide. In 1973, the salutary effect of transfusion in graft survival was reported by Opelz and Terasaki, ushering in the 'transfusion era'. Later, this was extended into the donor specific transfusion protocol by Salvatierra, reporting excellent results in the living related donor transplantation in 1980.

In the field of immunosuppression, many agents have come to practical use such as antithymocyte globulin, total lymphoid irradiation and monoclonal antibody. The real change came with Borel's report of cyclosporine in 1976.

After encouraging results in the animal model by Green and White, Professor Calne reported preliminary results in human kidney transplants in 1978. Thus began another epoch of organ transplantation with a momentous improvement in survival results leading to enormous expansion of the indications for transplantation of many organs including heart, liver and pancreas and a heightened expectation of society.

2. Cellular and molecular mechanisms of allograft rejection

PEKKA HÄYRY

Excluding hyperacute rejection, two main patterns of rejection have been identified: (a) acute rejection and (b) chronic rejection, designated for 'cellular' and 'humoral' mechanisms of the immune response, respectively. Obviously, however, both arms of the immune response contribute in both major rejection patterns. Thus 'rejection' is not one and the same, but a given clinical situation may result from various pathophysiological mechanisms.

Cellular and molecular cascades of the in situ inflammatory response

The major events occurring inside the allograft upon induction of rejection have been summarized on several occasions (1). An allograft (like all other organs in the body) is continuously flushed by white cells (Figure 1). If immunosuppression is inadequate, the donor-directed recipient lymphocytes recognize the alien transplantation antigens, presented by the so-called antigen-presenting cells (APC), and immunization occurs. At least the vascular endothelial cells and the so-called 'dendritic' macrophages can function as APC. In addition also shedded antigens cause sensitization in the host lymphoid system.

At least two types of lymphocytes (CD4 and CD8) collaborate in the induction process. Triggered 'blast' cells express a variety of receptors, including the receptor for interleukin-2 (IL-2), and produce a variety of factors, lymphokines, including IL-2, IL-3 (M-CSF), IL-4 (BSF-1), IL-5 (TRF), IL-6, and gamma-interferon. The lymphokines drive antigen-responding T cells to 'autocrine' proliferation and to the production of specific effector cells, B cells to produce antibodies, and activate non-specific effector mechanisms, including donor non-directed lymphoid cells, the large granular lymphocytes (LGL) or 'NK effector cells', mononuclear phagocytes and platelets.

The steps summarized below should not be considered as a switch-on — switch-off system, but rather as a cascade where all components are generated in an escalating manner (Figure 1).

One of the first events in a rejecting allograft is an increase in leukocyte influx and outflux and proliferation of inflammatory cells in situ. Concomitantly,

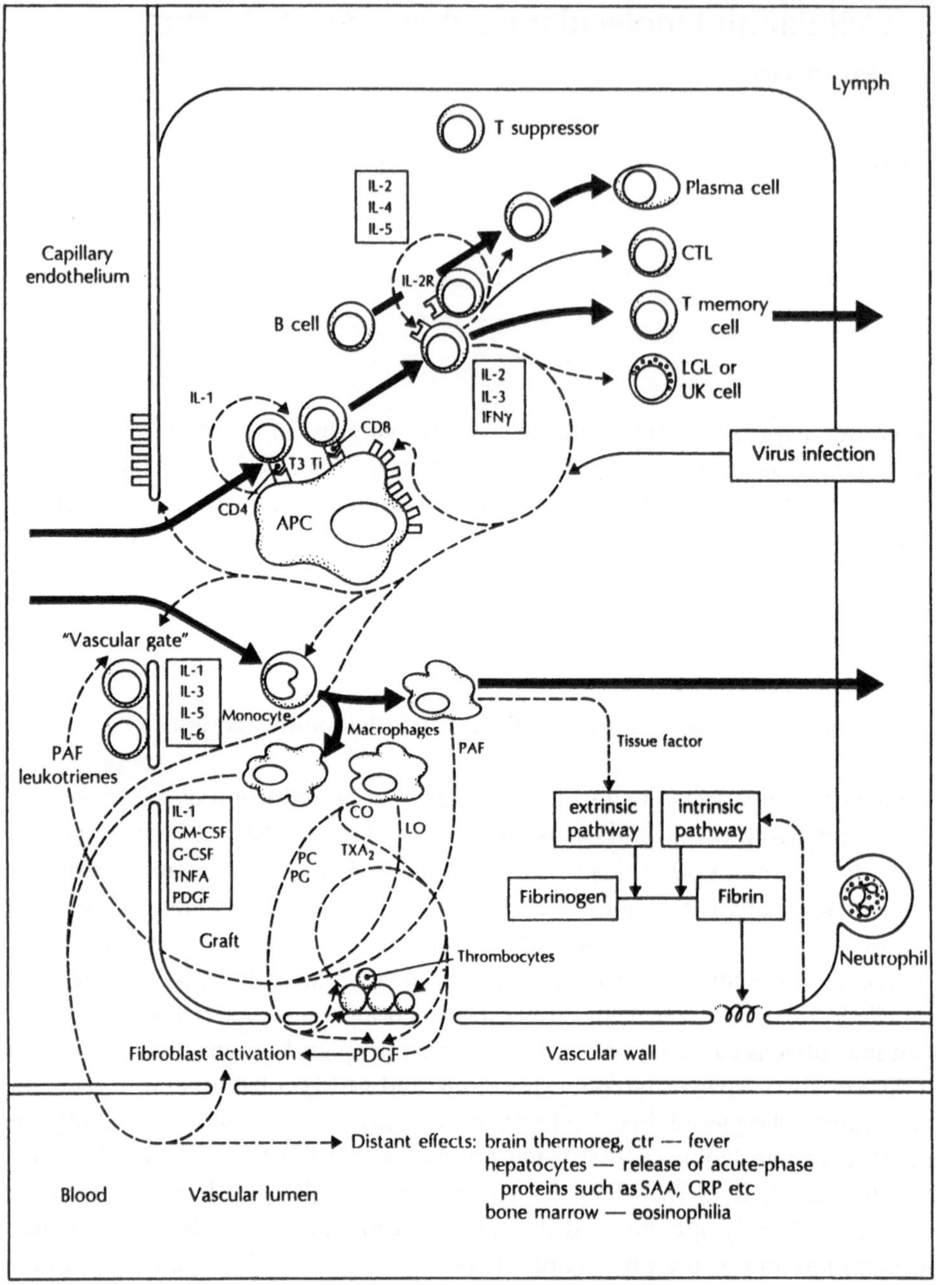

Fig. 1. Major cellular and molecular pathways in allograft rejection. The antigen-presenting cells (APC) have transplantation antigens on their surface and provide a 'second signal', interleukin (IL)-1 alpha and beta to resting T cells possessing receptors (T3, Ti) to this antigen. Both dendritic cells and endothelial cells can function as APC. Obviously, at least two types of T cells, CD4+ and CD8+, collaborate in the induction of transplantation immunity. As a result of antigen presentation, the antigen-reactive T cells display the IL-2 receptor (IL-2R) and secrete a variety of lymphokines including IL-2, −3, −4, −5 and interferon (IFN)-gamma. The net effect of these lymphokines is to induce T and B cell proliferation, including the generation of antibody-secreting

the graft (re-)expresses the transplantation antigens, particularly the class II, in an exaggerated manner especially in the microvascular endothelium. These major components of (acute) rejection generate a 'vicious cycle' inside the allograft: increased antigen expression increases graft immunogenicity, increased immunogenicity increases the immune response, and increased immune response increases the vascular permeability and inflammation.

The lymphokines deriving from the 'primary encounter' with the graft, activate the endothelial cells. The effect of gamma-IFN on class II antigen expression by the endothelial cells seems to be a direct one, regulated via protein kinase C. The effect is counteracted by prostaglandins generated by the endothelial cells. Instead, the effect of gamma-IFN on vascular permeability seems to operate via the 5-lipoxygenase pathway of eicosanoids, whereby 5-lipoxygenase products seem to open the 'vascular gate' and act as chemotactic molecules. Similar effects have been recorded also with the platelet activation factor (PAF), resulting in leukocyte influx and edema. In a renal allograft, the site of entry of white cells is the intertubular capillary venous endothelium which during acute rejection acquires the morphological and functional features of the 'high endothelium' of the lymph nodes.

The lymphokines (secreted in situ?) seem to be responsible also for the major systemic manifestations of acute rejection: IL-5 (eosinophil differentiation factor) might be responsible for blood eosinophilia seen in context of acute rejection, and IL-1 and IL-6 for the generation of fever (via their effect on the brain thermoregulatory center), and of the release of acute phase proteins (such as CRP and SAA). GM-CSF and/or IL-3 (M-CSF) may be responsible for the

---

plasma cells, cytotoxic lymphocytes (CTL) and memory lymphocytes, as well as to activate the natural killer (NK) cells. Several of these lymphokines, most notably IL-1, IL-2 and particularly IFN-gamma, also affect the APC, upregulating major histocompatibility complex (MHC) antigens on these cells and causing them to secrete more of the 'second signal'. This generates a vicious cycle, which is the driving force that keeps rejection going. Induction of MHC antigens on the APC is also a likely mechanism whereby cytomegalovirus and other virus infections can induce graft rejection. More 'peripheral' consequences of the lymphokine response are blood eosinophilia, probably caused by IL-5, and activation of the mononuclear phagocytes. An important consequence of mononuclear phagocyte activation is the induction of eicosanoid synthesis. The various eicosanoid cascades, including the cyclo-oxygenase (CO) and lipoxygenase (LO) cascades, are generated by IL. The activation of mononuclear phagocytes leads to the secretion of more lymphokines, or 'monokines', including IL-l alpha and beta, tumour necrosis factor (TNF), platelet-derived growth factor (PDGF), granulocyte colony-stimulating factor (G-CSF) and granulocyte/macrophage colony-stimulating factor (GM-CSF). In acute rejection, prostacyclin (PC), prostaglandin (PG)-E2, PG-D2 and PG2-F alpha seem to operate as 'good' prostacyclins, down-regulating the class II expression. The 'bad' prostacyclins, particularly thromboxane A2 (TxA_2) and lipoxygenase products, LTA4-F4, are 'pro-inflammatory' prostacyclins inducing vascular permeability and platelet deposition in the graft. Some of the clinical manifestations of rejection, particularly fever and the activation of acute-phase proteins, are caused by IL-1 alpha and beta. These lymphokines, together with the 'bad' prostacyclins, particularly TxA_2 and platelet-activating factor (PAF), also collaborate in the generation of graft atherosclerosis and fibrosis, the basic manifestations of chronic rejection. (LGL=large granular lymphocytes.)

activation of the pluripotent stem cells migrating into the allograft during rejection. Similar and other factors seem to activate the LGL in situ and the differentiation of mononuclear phagocytes into macrophages. Activation of mononuclear phagocytes results in an enhanced synthesis of eicosanoids, where thromboxane A-2 is a major mediator of vasoconstriction and thrombocyte aggregation. Prostaglandins, particularly prostacyclin produced by the endothelial cells, countereffect these changes. Vasoconstriction increases renal vascular resistance and decreases renal blood flow. Platelet deposits are readily demonstrable in all kinds of allografts during rejection.

Acute and chronic rejection

One can assume that all these cascades operate both in acute and in chronic rejection, although their emphasis may be different in the two major rejection forms. Cellular infiltrates are demonstrated in both forms of rejection, as is presence of activated cell forms, but in acute rejection this results in parenchymal cell damage (where the microvascular endothelial cells are amongst the most sensitive ones) whereas in chronic rejection the primary consequence is intimal proliferation and, later, graft arteriosclerosis.

Until now, very little has been known about the cellular and molecular mechanisms of the arteriosclerotic response in chronically rejecting transplants. One reason has been that animal models to investigate this phenomenon have been scanty or mostly unavailable.

The group in Washington has transplanted heart allografts between random-bred rabbit strains, immunosuppressed with CsA (2, 3). A group in Pittsburgh have employed rat heart allografts exchanged between selected histocompatibility differences, mostly minor differences (4). Finally, a group in Uppsala has been transplanting rat heart allografts immunosuppressed briefly with anti-thymocyte globulin (5) or with cyclosporine (6).

We have recently developed a model in the inbred rat that very faithfully mimicks arteriosclerotic alterations in human allografts: DA thoracic aortas are transplanted heterotopically into WF recipients between the renal arteries and the bifurcation. These transplants undergo, without immunosuppression, an early inflammatory response, mainly in the allograft advantitia. In the early response activated cell forms dominate, like in acute allograft rejection but the grafts are not inversibly rejected. Later, 1—12 months after transplantation, the grafts undergo changes identical with chronically rejecting human allografts. There is a gradual loss of nuclei in the allograft media, indicating media necrosis. Concomitantly, the internal elastic lamina becomes perforated by occasional breaks, but gross integrity is preserved. Most prominent is the intimal response: there is a rapid accumulation of smooth muscle cells and occasional macrophages underneath the allograft endothelium, lacking in the syngeneic graft, which leads to an increase in the nuclear contents of the intima and an enormous intimal proliferative response. At the end of the first year, approximately one-third of the arterial lumen is occluded.

To our understanding, this is the first model in genetically defined background enabling a detailed investigation of arteriosclerotic process of chronically rejecting transplants.

References

1. Häyry, P.: Mechanisms of rejection. *Curr. Opin. Immunol.* **1**, 1230—1235 (1989).
2. Foegh, M.L., Khirabadi, B.S., Chambers, E. and Ramwell, P.W.: Peptide inhibition of acclerated transplant atherosclerosis. *Transplant. Proc.* **21**, 3674—3676 (1989).
3. Alonso, D.R., Starek, P.K. and Minick, C.R.: *Amer. J. Pathol.* **87**, 415 (1977).
4. Cramer, D.V., Qian, S., Harnaha, J., Chapman, F.A., Starzl, T.E. and Makowaka, L.: Accelerated graft arteriosclerosis is enhanced by sensitization of the recipient donor lymphocytes. *Transplant. Proc.* **21**, 3714—3715 (1989).
5. Claesson, K., Mjörnstedt, L., Klareskog, L., Larsson, E., Olausson, M. and Söderström, T.: Morphology of rat cardiac allografts with permanent survival induced by antithymocyte globulin. *Scand. J. Immunol.* **27**, 171—179 (1988).
6. Fellström, B., Dimeny, E., Larsson, E., Klareskog, L., Tufveson, G. and Rubin, K.: Importance of PDGF receptor expression in accelerated atherosclerosis-chronic rejection. *Transplant. Proc.* **21**, 3689—3691 (1989).

3. What does the alloreactive T cell see?

J.R. BATCHELOR, G. LOMBARDI and R.I. LECHLER

Introduction

The question posed by the title of this article is of fundamental importance to our understanding of immune responses to organ and tissue grafts. During the last two decades, a great deal has been learned about T cell responses to conventional antigens, often called nominal antigens. Such T cell responses are known to obey the rules of self-MHC restriction, that is, the T cell can only recognize the nominal antigen provided it is presented in association with self-MHC molecules. In contrast, T cells responding to allogeneic cells in culture apparently do not obey the rules of self-MHC restriction. Furthermore, strong primary responses against allogeneic-stimulating cells can be generated *in vitro*, whereas responses against nominal antigens are not seen under these conditions. The major reason for this difference in responsiveness is the high frequencies of precursor T cells capable of being activated by allogeneic cells (1); precursor frequencies of T cells specific for nominal antigens are very low in non-sensitized subjects.

Two hypotheses have been put forward to explain the uniquely strong primary immune responses to allogeneic cells, but only one will be discussed here (2, 3). This suggests that the MHC molecules on the allogeneic (stimulator) cell form binary complexes with an array of other molecules, both endogenous to the cell and exogenous. Thus a single allo-MHC polymorphism can form a series of different complexes, each of which can stimulate a separate population of T cells. In contrast, the response to nominal antigen is unlikely to be so polyclonal.

The three-dimensional structure of HLA molecules

Approximately three years ago the first X-ray crystallographic studies on HLA-A2 allowed the three-dimensional structure of that molecule to be solved (4, 5). Since then, the three-dimensional structure of another class I molecule, AW69, has been similarly established (6), and the structure of class II molecules has been predicted to be extremely similar (7). The extra cellular portion of both class I and II molecules consists of two immunoglobulin-like domains lying nearest to the cell membrane, surmounted by a platform of anti-parallel, beta-pleated sheets on which lie two alpha helices. It is generally thought that the cleft between the two alpha helices is the site in which nominal antigen, degraded during antigen processing to peptides of approximately 10—14 amino acids, lies, and it is consistent with this idea that electron dense material was found in the cleft during the crystallographic studies.

MHC—peptide complexes

Equilibrium dialysis experiments have demonstrated that the association—dissociation of peptide from MHC molecules is slow, with a half time of approximately 30 hours (8), suggesting that probably the majority of the peptide-binding clefts are occupied *in vivo*. In the case of class I molecules, recent evidence (9) implies that peptide association with the MHC molecule intracellularly is one of the important factors controlling assembly and expression of the MHC molecule—peptide complex at the cell surface.

As mentioned earlier, alloreactive T cell populations apparently exhibit rather different functional characteristics to those shown by T cells responding to nominal antigens. These differences might lead one to imagine that the T cell antigen receptor of an alloreactive cell 'sees' a different set of structures to those recognized by a T cell specific for nominal antigen. But there are at least two reasons for discarding that idea. The first is that genetic analyses show that nominal antigen specific T cells use the same T cell receptor (TcR) genes as those used by alloreactive T cells (10, 11). They also belong to the same T cell subpopulations. Second, T cell clones have been identified which (cross)react with both an allo-MHC molecule and self-MHC molecule plus nominal antigen (12).

Alloreactivity and MHC—peptide complexes

Our laboratory has been interested in the concept that alloreactive T cells may recognize precisely the same structures as nominal antigen-specific T cells, and that in both situations the TcR of the responder cell 'sees' a binary complex of MHC molecule with a peptide bound in the cleft (3, 13). Sequence data on a very large number of class I HLA genes have demonstrated that most of the variations between the different alleles are found to involve amino acid residues which are located either on the sides or floor of the peptide-binding groove (desetopic surface), or in positions on the top of the alpha helices (histotopic surface) which are predicted to interact directly with the TcR. The same generalization holds true for the variable residues of the class II molecules, assuming that the prediction of their three-dimensional structure based on similarities with class I molecules is correct.

What is the evidence that peptide bound in the groove of an MHC molecule contributes to allorecognition? One line of evidence is that T cell clones can discriminate between stimulator cells expressing MHC alleles which differ only at amino acid residues located in the floor or sides of the peptide-binding cleft (desetopic surface) and which would not make direct contact with the TcR of the responding T cell. For example, one of our alloreactive T cell clones, G8, proliferates strongly when stimulated by cells expressing DR4, Dw13, yet gives no response with DR4, DwKT2. These two alleles differ by a single amino acid residue at position 37, which is predicted to lie in the floor of the peptide-binding groove. Further examples of this sort are described in reference (3).

A second line of evidence is that T cell clones have been observed which can discriminate between the same HLA allele expressed on different types of cell (14). In our laboratory we generated T cell clones against HLA-DR1; certain of the clones will respond when stimulated with human cells expressing DR1, but do not respond when cultured with mouse fibroblasts transfected with DR1 and expressing high levels of the human allele. Other clones were identified with the opposite pattern of reactivity. We interpret these data to indicate that different peptides are bound by DR1 expressed on human and mouse cells, and that the peptides are significant moieties for recognition by the alloreactive T cell clones.

Table 1. Self-restricted recognition of *C. albicans* by anti-DR1 alloreactive T cell clones, G8 and G11.

		Thymidine incorporation by clone (cpm)[a]		
Stimulator cell	DR (Dw)	Ag[b]	G8	G11
ND	4(4), w13(19)	−	(56)	749 (14)
		+	48 167 (3)	7 674 (8)
RIL	w15(2), 4(4)	−	156 (14)	1 227 (8)
		+	58 756 (12)	763 (10)
CD	w15(2), w13(19)	−	168 (71)	674 (17)
		+	1 314 (15)	10 286 (3)
BH	w15(2), 7(−)	−	133 (41)	772 (5)
		+	456 (46)	589 (8)
NF	1(1), −	−	89 439 (3)	6 884 (2)

[a] Approximately 10^4 T clone cells were co-cultured with 10^5 X-irradiated blood mononuclear cells in the presence of *C. albicans* extract at 30 μg/ml. After 48 hours, cultures were pulsed with {^{3}H}thymidine and harvested 18 hours later. Numbers in parentheses are percentage error of the mean for triplicate cultures.

[b] Ag = antigen.

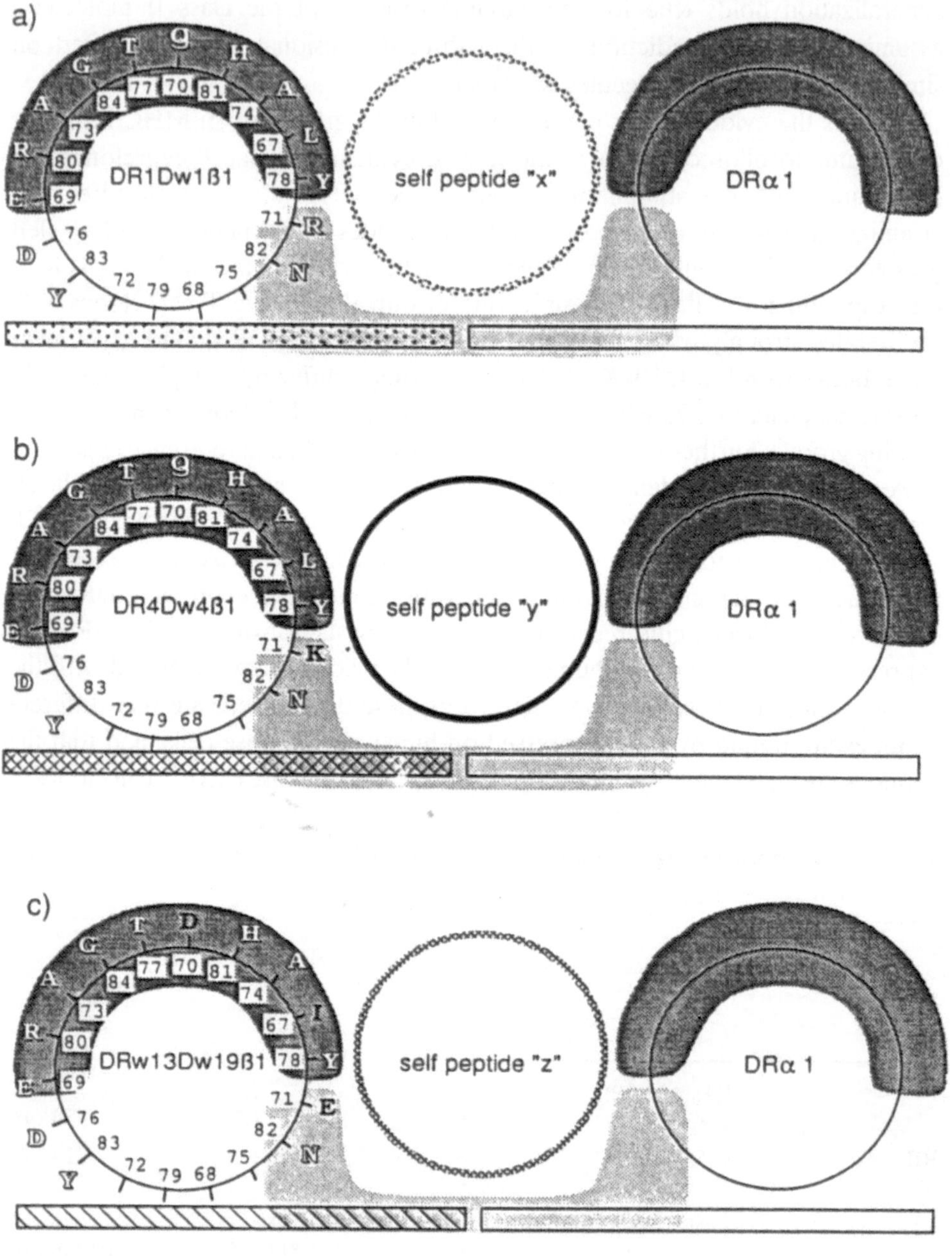

Fig. 1. Cross-section of the peptide binding grooves of (a) DR1Dw1, (b) DR4Dw4, (c) DRw13Dw19. See text for full explanation.

In further investigations of the T cell clones raised against DR1, some examples were found that (cross) reacted with *Candida albicans* extract when this was presented to the clones by autologous antigen-presenting cells (13). Data on two such clones are presented in Table 1. It can be seen that both clones, G8 and G11, respond to allogeneic stimulator cells bearing DR1 but they also respond when co-cultured with *C. albicans* and autologous antigen-presenting cells from subject ND (DR4, Dw4/DRw13, Dw19). By using antigen-presenting cells which expressed either DR4, Dw4 or DRw13, Dw19, it was found that the response of G8 *C. albicans* was restricted by DR4, Dw4 and that of G11 was restricted by DRw13, Dw19.

If the three-dimensional structures of the above DR molecules are compared with each other, some striking conclusions emerge. Figure 1 is a diagram illustrating cross-sections of the peptide-binding grooves of DR1, Dw1, of DR4, Dw4, and of DRw13, Dw19. The alpha helices which form the side walls of the groove have been compressed into a wheel. The positions of the amino acid residues, numbered according to sequence, are indicated according to the predictions based on the three-dimensional structure of class I molecules. Below each helical wheel are the beta-pleated sheets, part of which form the floor of the peptide-binding groove. Most of the amino acid differences between the molecules lie in these floors and this is shown by different patterns. The DR alpha chain does not vary in the different DR alleles.

Figure 1 shows that the histotopic surfaces, i.e. those predicted to make direct contact with the responding cell's TcR, are very similar for the three DR alleles. DR1, Dw1 and DR4, Dw4 have identical amino acid residues in the histotopic surfaces, and DRw13, Dw19 differs from the above alleles at positions 67 and 70 only. These similarities are a satisfying explanation of why self-restricted recognition of a *C. albicans* peptide plus DR4, Dw4, or DRw13, Dw19 mimics allorecognition of DR1, Dw1. Put another way, allorecognition of DR1 by DR4, Dw4 and by DRw13, Dw19 responder cells resembles self-restricted recognition of endogenous peptides capable of being bound by DR1.

Conclusion

If this view of allorecognition is correct, one would expect that responsiveness against allo-MHC molecules would depend on whether the responder and stimulator subjects happened to share alleles which were sufficiently similar that mimicry of self-restricted recognition would be possible. There is no doubt from clinical observations that there is considerable variation in the strength of alloimmune responses. The hypothesis described here may make it possible to predict which donor/recipient combinations are most likely to be associated with high alloresponses and thus allow them to be avoided.

References

1. Fischer-Lindahl, K. and Wilson, D.B.: *J. Exp. Med.* **145**, 500—507 (1977).
2. Matzinger, P. and Bevan, M.J.: *Cell. Immunol.* **29**, 1—5 (1977).
3. Lechler, R.I., Lombardi, G., Batchelor, J.R. *et al.*: *Immunol. Today* **11**, 83—88 (1990).
4. Bjorkman, P.J., Saper, M.A., Samraoui, B. *et al.*: *Nature* **329**, 506—511 (1987).
5. Bjorkman, P.J., Saper, M.A., Samraoui, B. *et al.*: *Nature* **329**, 512—518 (1987).
6. Garrett, T.P.J., Saper, M.A., Bjorkman, P.J. *et al.*: *Nature* **342**, 692—696 (1989).
7. Brown, J.H., Jardetzky, T., Saper, M.A. *et al.*: *Nature* **332**, 845—850 (1988).
8. Buus, S., Sette, A., Colon, S. *et al.*: *Cell* **47**, 1071—1077. (1986).
9. Townsend, A., Ohlen, C., Bastin, J. *et al.*: *Nature* **340**, 443—448 (1989).
10. Rupp, F., Brecher, J., Gielden, M.A. *et al.*: *Proc. Natl. Acad. Sci. USA* **84**, 219—222 (1987).
11. Matis, L.A., Sorger, S.B., McElligott, D.L. *et al.*: *Cell* **51**, 59—69 (1987).
12. Hunig, T. and Bevan, M.J.: *Nature* **294**, 460—462 (1981).
13. Lombardi, G., Sidhu, S., Batchelor, J.R. *et al.*: *Proc. Natl. Acad. Sci. USA* **86**, 4190—4194 (1989).
14. Lombardi, G., Sidhu, S., Lamb, J.R. *et al.*: *J. Immunol.* **142**, 753—754 (1989).

4. HLA matching and organ transplantation

DAVID W. GJERTSON and PAUL I. TERASAKI

Introduction

Controversy still surrounds the issue of whether or not HLA matching should be used for recipient selection. There is lingering doubt that HLA typing can select out such superior grafts from cadaver donors; even though, there is universal agreement that HLA can identify superior sibling — donor transplants (1).

Initial investigations (2, 3) regarding the benefit of HLA matching in kidney transplants from unrelated donors indicated that, although early graft rejection was not influenced by matching, long-term survival was marginally better in matched donor — recipient pairs (approximately a 10% increase in survival for matched versus non-matched transplants after the first year). These preliminary findings were based on few transplants and sparse numbers of class I, A- and B-locus, leukocyte antigens. The value of HLA matching for transplantation was further questioned in 1970 by Mickey *et al.* (4), who concluded that overall, a more suitable means for predicting successful transplants is required because a large number of patients do well in spite of HLA incompatibility.

Renewed interest in matching arose with the discovery of the DR locus. The first comprehensive report was by Opelz and Terasaki (5) and was based on 8th International Histocompatibility Workshop data, demonstrating that DR class II antigens were not 'the' transplantation markers because, as before, a significant number of transplants did well with one or two DR mismatches. However, the study did indicate that well-typed, well-matched DR transplants had enhanced early survival and BDR matching had an additive effect. These findings were confirmed by Opelz (6), in which a 20% difference in 1-year graft survival was noted between 0 BDR and 4 BDR mismatched transplants in patients treated with cyclosporine (CsA).

From our analyses over the past few years (7, 8), HLA matching continues to stand out as an important factor in transplantation despite strong center effects and improvements in immunosuppression. Analyses from other multi-center registries also demonstrate that HLA is a significant factor despite the introduction of CsA and identifying center (9). Further, Persijn *et al.* described the extensive experience of Eurotransplant, in which a 12% difference was noted at 3 years between the best and worst ABDR mismatches (10). Gore *et al.* have argued that beneficially matched transplants (i.e. 0 DR mismatches and, at most, 1 AB mismatch) have a 1-year graft survival rate which is about 15% higher than the highly mismatched transplants (11).

Many single center studies conclude that matching has no effect. In large single center studies from Najarian *et al.* (12) and Stratta *et al.* (13), no effect was noted. However, in their studies, the comparison was between degrees of poor mismatch grades, and not between excellent and poor matches. Since the recipients were selected on a random basis, almost no good matches were achieved. Transplants with high degrees of matching are available for comparison when single centers use HLA matching for selection. The Dyer *et al.* Manchester group who reported a strong BDR matching effect (14), and Cicciarelli *et al.* of Saint Vincent's who found AB and DR effects (15), are both excellent examples.

What follows is an update on the effect on survival of both first transplants and retransplants when antigens are mismatched at the A, B, DR and C loci. The C locus has received little attention thus far, despite the fact that these antigens are now being identified in transplant patients by more laboratories. It was especially interesting for us to follow up on Cook's findings of two years ago (16) that the AB and DR loci seem to have a different long-term impact on transplants. AB and DR mismatches may have a qualitatively different effect on transplants.

Materials and methods

The UCLA Registry contains data from 235 centers on 14 000 first cadaver adult kidney transplants and 2471 retransplants performed from 1985 to the present. HLA data available by locus (from the complete data set) follows:

Number (% of total) of transplants

Locus	*First grafts*	*Regrafts*
A	13 777 (99%)	2 462 (99%)
B	13 914 (99%)	2 461 (99%)
C	2 263 (16%)	373 (15%)
DR	12 951 (92%)	2 251 (91%)

Degree of matching was determined by counting the number of mismatched antigens per locus between recipient and donor pairs.

Actuarial statistics are product-limit estimates. Standard errors for cumulative survival functions were estimated by Greenwood's formula (17). Half-lives past 6 months and their standard errors were estimated according to previous published formulas (18). Tests of significance were done using the weighted chi-squared method (19). Estimated graft survival curves and their 6-month cumulative survival rates were used to gauge short-term effects; whereas half-lives beyond 6 months determined long-term effects.

Results

Results are shown in Figures 1—6. Figure 1 displays baseline cumulative graft survival for the 14 003 first graft recipients and the 2471 regraft recipients over a 4-year period. For first grafts, the 6-month survival rate was 81.7 ±0.3% and the estimated half-life past 6 months was 7.0 ± 0.2 years. A high baseline survival is attributable to CsA (over 90% of these transplants received some form of CsA therapy).

As in previous detailed analyses of regrafts (20), the major difference between first and retransplants is from early graft loss. The estimated 6-month survival rate dropped significantly to 71.1 ± 1.8%; whereas, half-life beyond 6 months decreased insignificantly to 5.8 ± 0.7 years. These baseline figures will be used for comparison with 6-month and half-life survival in Figures 2—6.

Single locus matching

Figures 2 and 3 display graft survivals by mismatches at the individual loci. In Figure 2, very little difference can be seen in the survival curves between 0, 1 and 2 mismatched A-locus antigens during the first 6 months. This is illustrated by observing no significant difference in survival rates between the three groups at 6 months (82.0 ± 0.8%, 82.2 ± 0.5%, 80.8 ± 0.6% for 0, 1 and 2 mismatches, respectively). However, for longer post-transplant periods, an

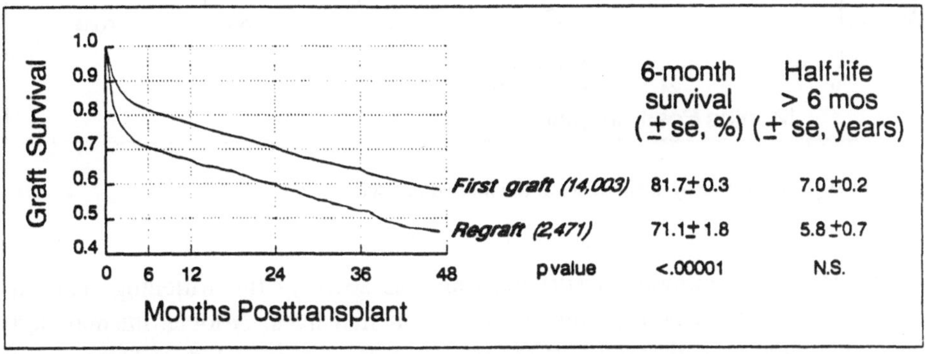

Fig. 1. Baseline cumulative graft survival for the 14 003 recipients of first cadaver transplants and the 2471 recipients of regrafted cadaver transplants over a 4-year period.

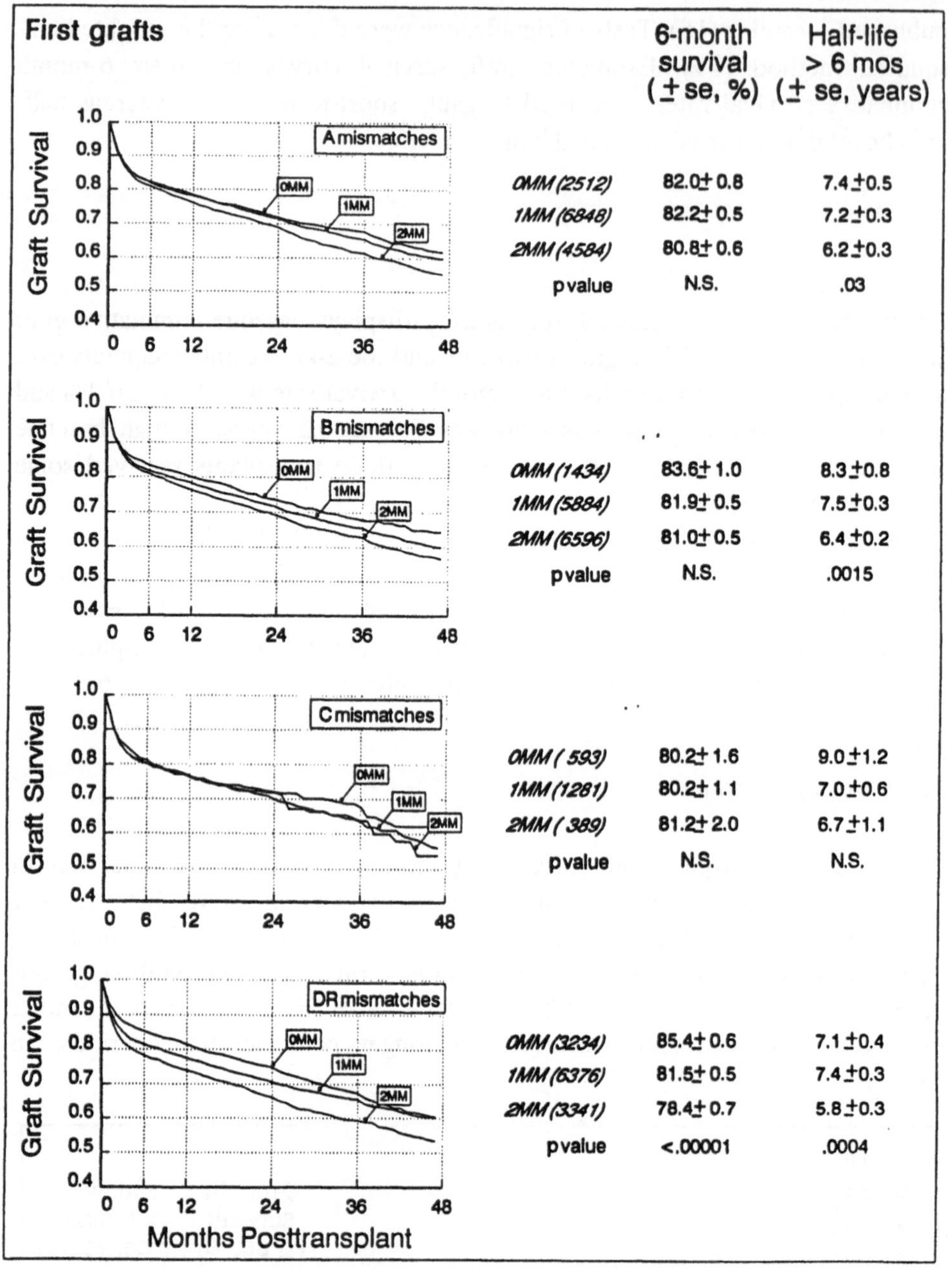

Fig. 2. First graft survival by mismatches at the individual loci.

A-locus mismatch influenced survival rates, as seen by the widening survival curves. This is confirmed by the difference in half-lives. A-locus mismatched transplants have an estimated half-life of 7.4 ± 0.5 years, 7.2 ± 0.3 years and 6.2 ± 0.3 years for 0, 1 and 2 mismatches, respectively.

The same pattern of no early effect and substantial latter effect is shown in

Figure 2 for B-locus mismatched antigens. Again, the survival curves nearly coincide for the first 6 months and estimated graft survival at 6 months is 83.6 ± 1.0%, 81.9 ± 0.5% and 81.0 ± 0.5% for 0, 1 and 2 mismatched B-locus antigens. Differential long-term effect is shown by the varying half-lives of 8.3 ± 0.8 years, 7.5 ± 0.3 years and 6.4 ± 0.2 years among the three groups.

Next, Figure 2 illustrates the effect of mismatch C-locus antigens. The C-locus mismatch shows no early or later effect, as evidenced by the overlapping survival curves. The failure to observe any trend in mismatches may be due to a dearth of complete data for the C locus. The following 6-month survivals and half-lives past 6 months were observed for mismatched C-locus antigens: 80.2 ± 1.6%, 80.2 ± 1.1% and 81.2 ± 2.0% graft survival for 0, 1 and 2 mismatches; 9.0 ± 1.2 years, 7.0 ± 0.6 years and 6.7 ± 1.1 years half-life for 0, 1 and 2 mismatches. No significant differences from baseline were observed.

The effect of mismatching DR antigens is nearly the opposite of that observed for the A and B antigens. The last graph in Figure 2 shows the results of DR mismatches on graft survival. Here the curves corresponding to the three categories of mismatch start to diverge very early post-transplantation. Six-month survival rates are significantly different among the three groups, with 0, 1 and 2 having survival rates of 85.4 ± 0.6%, 81.5 ± 0.5% and 78.4 ± 0.7%, respectively. Statistically significant differences in half-lives are observed among the three groups but the curves appear almost parallel beyond 6 months through 3 years.

In Figure 3, which shows regraft survivals by mismatches at the individual loci, regraft survival patterns at each loci are similar to the corresponding graphs in Figure 2. For example, no significant difference in survival is observed between 0, 1 and 2 mismatched A-, B- or C-locus antigens during the first 6 months; whereas, the effect on survival of mismatched DR antigens is obvious immediately post-transplant (6-month graft survival is 74.8 ± 1.8%, 71.8 ± 1.4% and 65.7 ± 2.0% for 0, 1 and 2 mismatched DR-locus antigens). In contrast to first grafts, significant differences in regraft half-lives among the mismatches were not found at any of the individual loci.

Joint locus matching

The divergences from baseline first graft survival were magnified when loci were studied in combination. Figure 4 shows the combined A and B locus results and the combined A, B and DR results for first grafts. Again for AB mismatches, there was no significant difference in their short-term survival rates (e.g. from 84.7 ± 1.4% survival rate for 0 mismatches to 80.8 ± 0.8% for 4 mismatches), but the long-term effects were strikingly different among the various degrees of mismatches (from a high of 10.1 ± 1.6 years for 0 AB

Regrafts

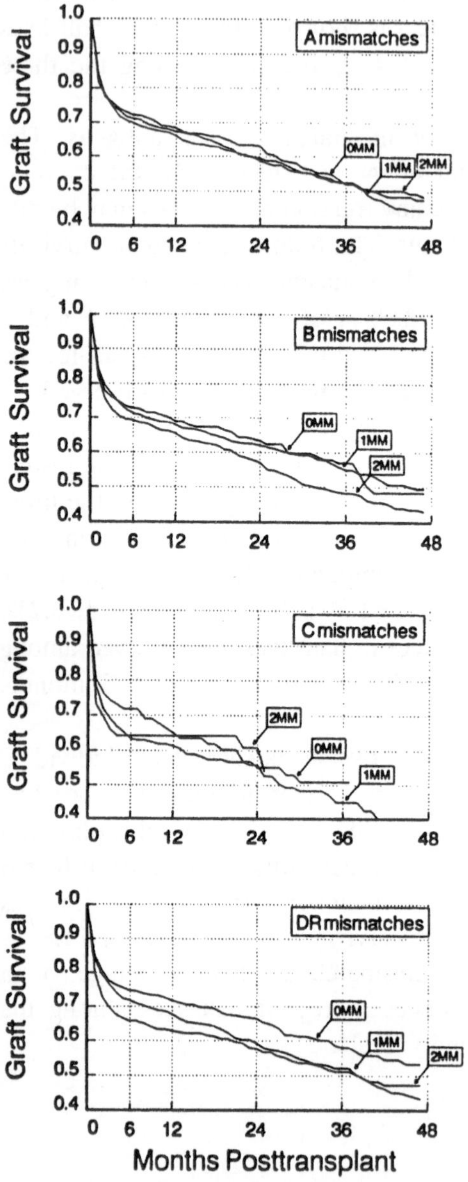

	6-month survival (± se, %)	Half-life > 6 mos (± se, years)
0MM (663)	71.1±1.8	5.8±0.7
1MM (1133)	69.8±1.4	5.8±0.5
2MM (666)	72.2±1.8	6.2±0.7
p value	N.S.	N.S.
0MM (392)	72.9±2.3	6.6±1.1
1MM (1039)	71.4±1.4	6.7±0.7
2MM (1030)	69.2±1.4	5.1±0.4
p value	N.S.	N.S.
0MM (97)	71.9±4.6	QNS
1MM (220)	63.4±3.3	5.4±1.1
2MM (56)	64.2±6.4	QNS
p value	N.S.	---
0MM (608)	74.8±1.8	7.3±1.0
1MM (1055)	71.8±1.4	5.2±0.5
2MM (588)	65.7±2.0	7.4±1.1
p value	.003	N.S.

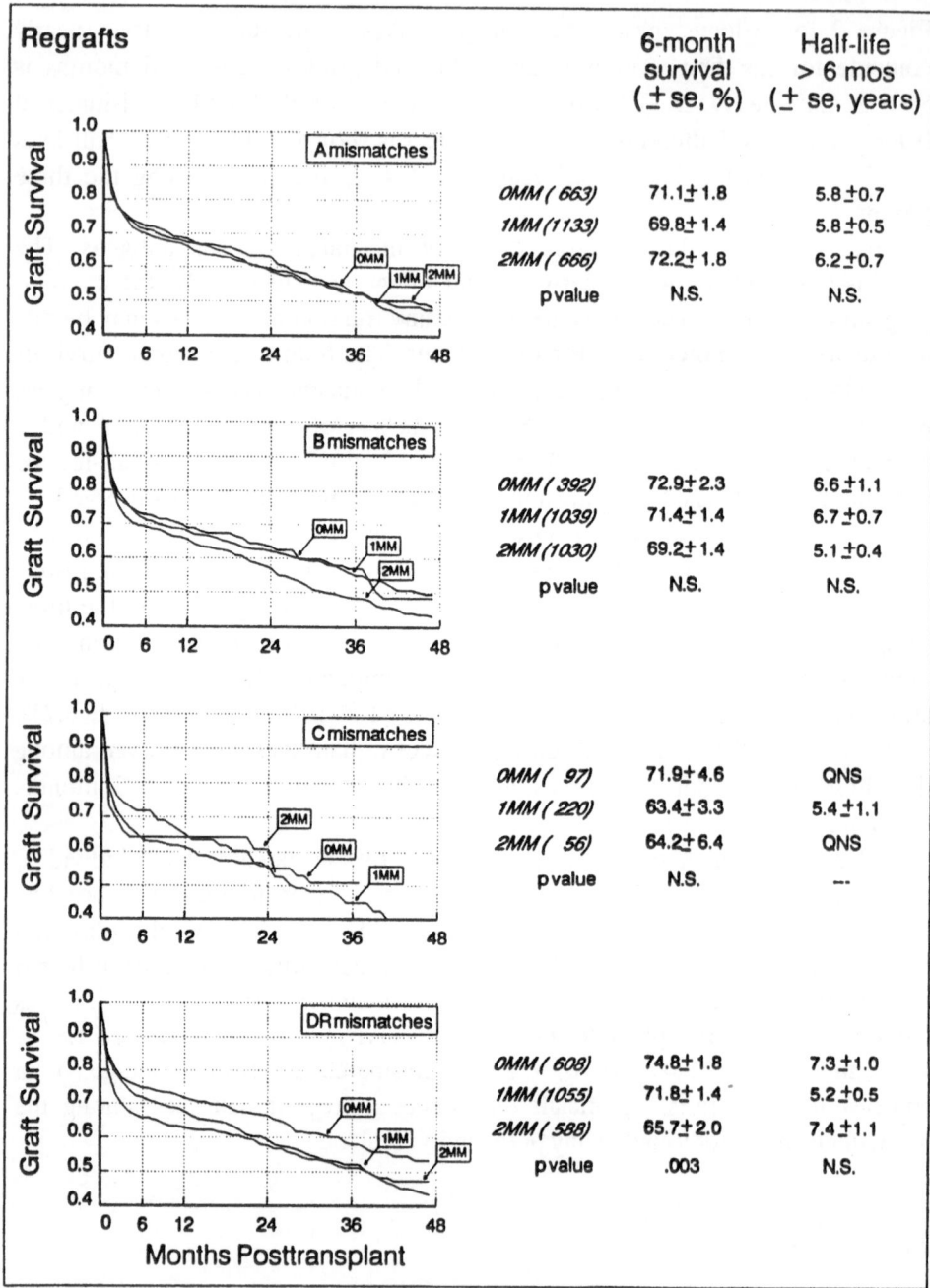

Fig. 3. Regraft survival by mismatches at the individual loci.

mismatches to a low of 6.2 ± 0.4 years for 4 AB mismatches). The long-term difference between best and worst mismatches for the combined results was approximately equal to the sum of the best/worst differences for A and B individually, implying an additive long-term effect.

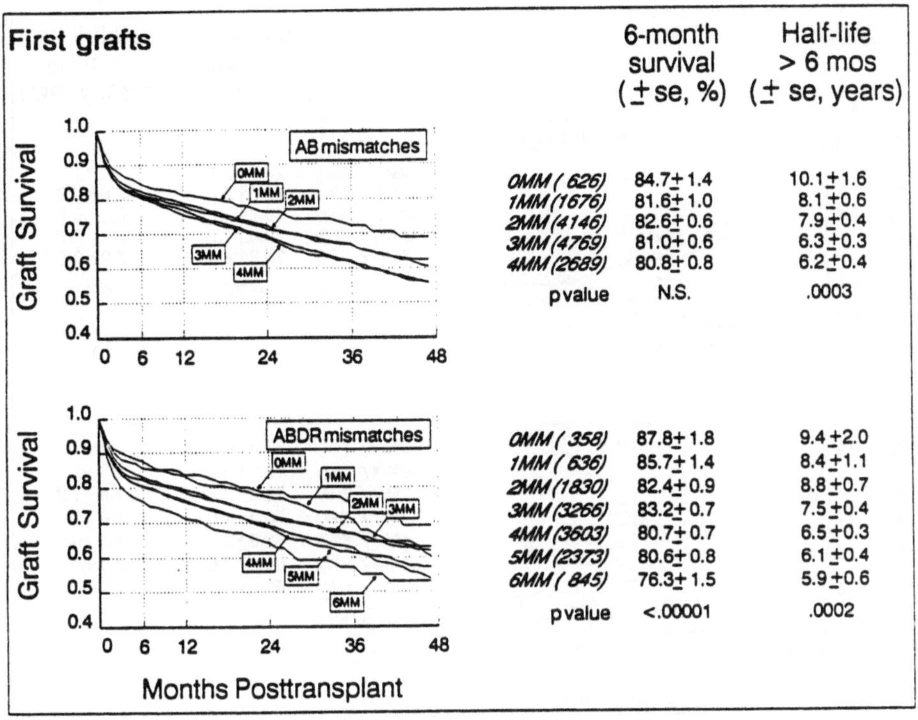

Fig. 4. First graft survival by AB and ABDR mismatches (combined loci).

Consistent with past findings, the most profound effect of matching on first graft survival is demonstrated when A, B and DR loci are combined. An overall difference of 11.5% among best to worst mismatch is seen at 6 months in the lower graph in Figure 4 while half-lives showed a steady decrease in mismatch from a high of 9.4 ± 2.0 years to a low of 5.9 ± 0.6 years.

For regrafts, joint locus comparisons (Figure 5) reveal survival patterns consistent with first graft outcomes, although they were not statistically significant owing to the small number of transplants. Half-lives tended to decrease with increasing AB mismatches as seen in the upper graph in Figure 5, and the earliest and largest diversification in regraft survival occurs when A, B and DR loci are combined (lower graph, Figure 5).

Figure 6 shows first graft and regraft survival rates for all 4 loci combined (i.e. A, B C and DR). Although the overall comparisons between graft survivals fell short of statistical significance (mainly due to small numbers), an additive effect appears when 2 C-locus antigens were mismatched, as opposed to 0 or 1 mismatch. A strong early drop in survival is noted when 8 antigens are mismatched. At 6 months for instance, first graft survival for 8 mismatches was 60.7 ± 9.2% and regraft survival was 20.0 ± 17.9% (not shown on actuarial plot).

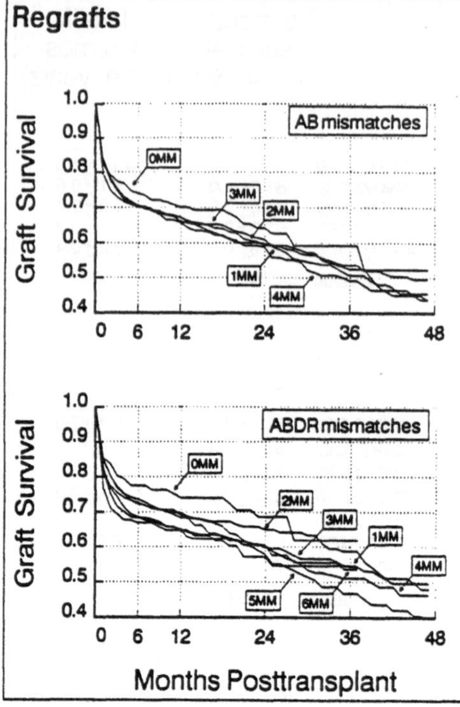

Regrafts	6-month survival (±se, %)	Half-life > 6 mos (±se, years)
0MM (203)	74.1±3.1	7.2±1.7
1MM (427)	70.2±2.2	5.8±0.8
2MM (734)	70.7±1.7	6.3±0.7
3MM (716)	70.6±1.7	5.8±0.7
4MM (379)	70.3±2.4	5.2±0.8
p value	N.S.	N.S.

0MM (117)	77.5±3.9	QNS
1MM (151)	72.6±3.6	QNS
2MM (406)	72.2±2.2	7.4±1.2
3MM (581)	73.6±1.8	5.6±0.7
4MM (502)	68.6±2.1	6.4±0.9
5MM (337)	68.4±2.6	5.0±0.8
6MM (121)	66.8±4.3	QNS
p value	N.S.	—

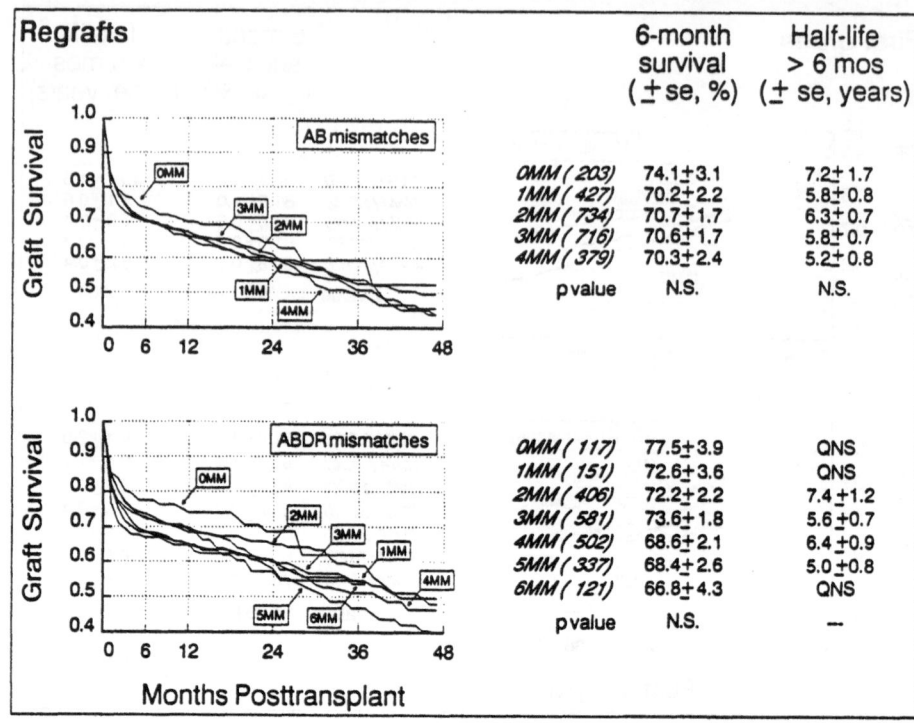

Fig. 5. Regraft survival by AB and ABDR mismatches (combined loci).

Discussion

An important aspect of HLA matching seen clearly in first graft data and suggested from regraft data is that the AB locus has a strong long-term effect after 1 year, whereas DR locus mismatches have their greatest influence in the first 6 months after transplantation. This effect was also noted in Cook's analysis in 1987 (16). Gore *et al.* also point out that the DR mismatch affects survival only in the first 5 months (11). These effects are completely independent of CsA therapy (16).

It is quite likely that early cellular immunity against a transplant is directed at the class II specificities, whereas the later humoral immunity is directed at class I specificities. Cytotoxic T cells are directed at HLA-D and DR differences which may be present directly on kidney cells. Failure of immunosuppression to control this attack may result in early transplant loss. The acute loss of transplants early in the first 3—6 months has a much steeper loss rate than the long-term loss rate which begins at about 6 months post-transplant. The loss of transplants in the later low-risk period (>6 months) results from chronic rejection, characterized by the gradual narrowing of blood vessels with deposition of fibrin in the internal lumen. Vascular endothelial cells have been shown to have class I antigens, but are conspicuously lacking in class II antigens (21).

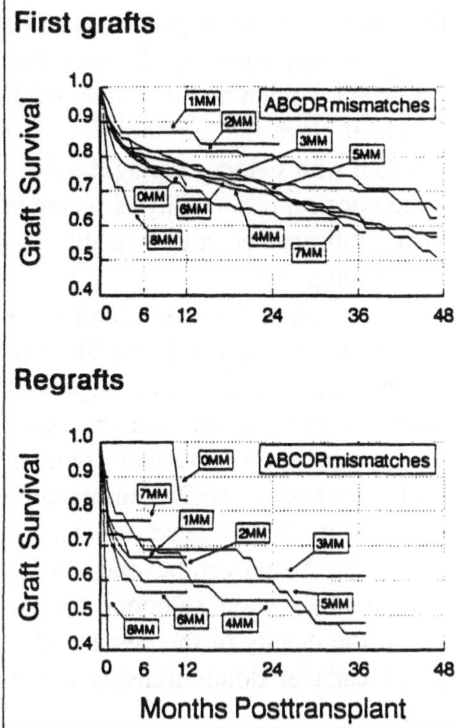

First grafts

	6-month survival (± se,%)	Half-life > 6 mos (± se, years)
0MM (34)	71.4±8.2	QNS
1MM (54)	87.0±4.6	QNS
2MM (154)	82.3±3.1	13.1±4.2
3MM (303)	80.7±2.3	10.1±2.0
4MM (476)	79.4±1.9	7.3±1.1
5MM (524)	82.6±1.7	6.1±0.8
6MM (382)	77.8±2.2	7.6±1.3
7MM (157)	75.6±3.4	6.0±1.5
8MM (31)	64.2±8.7	QNS
p value	N.S.	---

Regrafts

	6-month survival (± se,%)
0MM (8)	100
1MM (15)	66.7±12.2
2MM (29)	71.8±8.5
3MM (62)	69.0±5.9
4MM (84)	66.6±5.2
5MM (75)	59.6±5.7
6MM (53)	56.5±6.8
7MM (22)	77.3±8.9
8MM (8)	20.0±17.9
p value	N.S.

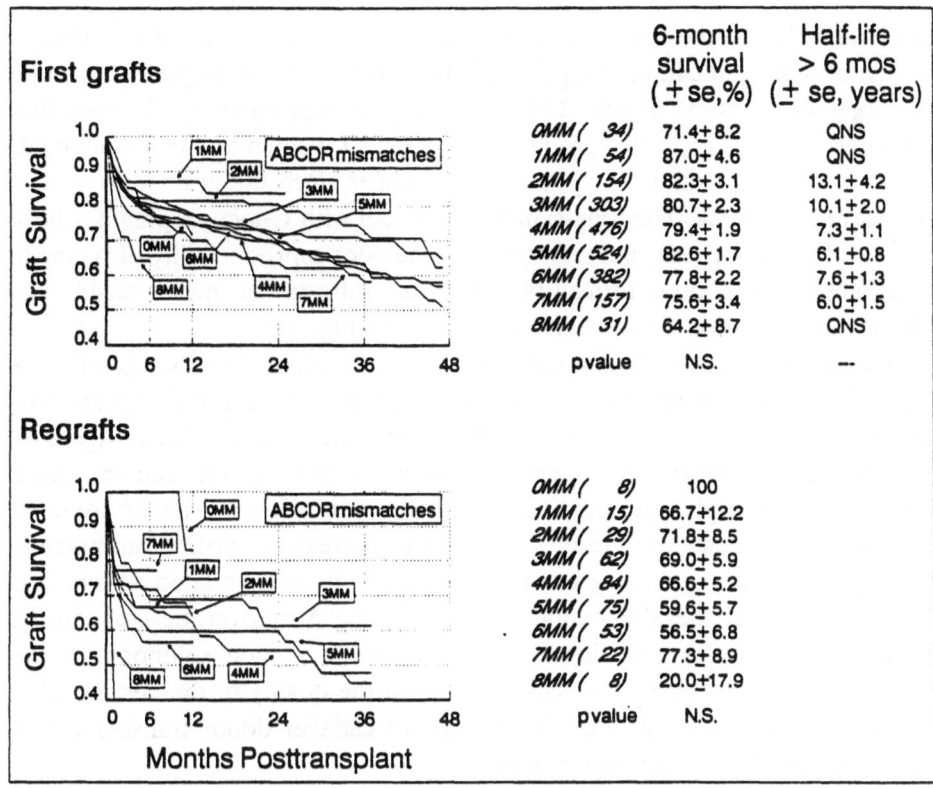

Fig. 6. Cumulative graft survival by ABCDR mismatches.

During chronic rejection, binding of class I antibodies to the endothelium initiates the cascade of events resulting in luminal obliteration (22). Thus, early acute rejection is most likely produced by cytotoxic T cells against class II antigens and late chronic rejection is produced by antibodies to class I differences on endothelial cells.

Although the acute and chronic phases are not clearly demarcated, there is a sharp inflection in survival curves at 3—6 months post-transplant. We assume that this is the time when the target of the immune response and the character of the response shifts. Interestingly, this inflection point in the older data was at 1 year for cadaver donor transplants (23), and has gradually become shorter in the newer data. For living-donor grafts, the change occurred at 3 months in the earlier and current data.

Data presented here shows that the A-locus and B-locus products are independent and additive. That is, increasing mismatches for the A or B locus adds to increase the rate of long-term loss. This may indicate that the products of these 2 loci exist separately on the endothelial cells and are subject to additive attack by antibodies. It appears that mismatches in the C locus may also be additive. As shown in Figure 6, 8 antigens of mismatch, which includes the C locus, led to the lowest survival rate in both first and regrafts. Although the numbers were small, the suggestion is that even the C locus product may be the target of humoral attack. This possibility is supported by the fact that antibodies to the C locus are produced by pregnant women and by alloimmunization. The C-locus antigens appear to be weaker since the antibodies against them have been weak. The long-standing problem with C-locus typing has been the lack of good antisera, and consequently the poor reproducibility of typing in the different typing laboratories (24). As better antisera becomes available, the C locus can be considered more seriously for matching.

Here, we show that with first cadaver donor transplants and the use of HLA typing, it is possible to alter the half-life from 5.9 years for 6 ABDR mismatched transplants to 9.4 years in 0 ABDR mismatched transplants (Figure 4). From a patient's viewpoint, the extra 3.5 years in half-life obtained through a matched transplant is certainly significant. Regrafts show a similar trend of decreasing short- and long-term survival with increasing ABDR mismatches. Although this effect is not as great as that achieved by using related donors, it is an effect which is achievable by today's tissue typing. Moreover, beyond starting out with a histocompatible donor, we have no other good solutions for the chronic rejection problem. As tissue typing and the quality of the best matches improve, we can anticipate that the half-life of cadaver donor transplants will begin to approach that seen with related donors.

References

1. Salvatierra, O.: Living related transplantation results. In: L.H. Toledo-Pereyra (ed.), *Kidney Transplantation*, p. 369. Davis, Philadelphia (1988).
2. Terasaki, P.I., Vredevoe, D.L. and Mickey, M.R.: Serotyping for homotransplantation. X. Survival of 196 grafted kidneys subsequent to typing. *Transplantation* **5**, 1057 (1967).
3. Patel, R., Mickey, M.R. and Terasaki, P.I.: Serotyping for homotransplantation. XVI. Analysis of kidney transplants from unrelated donors. *New Engl. J. Med.* **279**, 501 (1958).
4. Mickey, M.R., Kreisler, M., Albert, E.D. *et al.*: Analysis of HLA incompatibility in human renal transplants. *Tissue Antigens* **1**, 57 (1971).
5. Opelz, G. and Terasaki, P.I.: International histocompatibility workshop study on renal transplantation. In: P.T. Terasaki (ed.), *Histocompatibility Testing 1980*, p. 592. UCLA Tissue Typing Laboratory, Los Angeles (1980).
6. Opelz, G.: Correlation of HLA matching with kidney graft survival in patients with or without cyclosporine treatment. *Transplantation* **40**, 240 (1985).
7. Mickey, M.R.: HLA matching effects. In: P.I. Terasaki (ed.), *Clinical Transplants 1987*, p. 303. UCLA Tissue Typing Laboratory, Los Angeles (1987).
8. Cicciarelli, J. and Corcoran, S.: An update on HLA matching, including HLA 'epitope' matching: a new approach. In: P.I. Terasaki (ed.), *Clinical Transplants 1988*, p. 329. UCLA Tissue Typing Laboratory, Los Angeles (1988).
9. Sanfilippo, F., Vaughn, W.K., Alexander, J.W., LeFor, W.M., Lucas, B.A. and Pfaff, W.W.: Organ sharing for good HLA-A, B, and DR matching improves cadaver renal graft survival in SEOPF: retrospective and prospective studies considering delayed graft function, race, center effects, cyclosporine, and other factors. In: P.I. Terasaki (ed.), *Clinical Transplants 1988*, p. 211. UCLA Tissue Typing Laboratory, Los Angeles (1988).

10. Persijn, G.G., D'Amaro, J., de Lange, P. *et al.*: The effect of mismatching and sharing of HLA-A, -B, and -DR antigens on kidney graft survival in Eurotransplant 1982 to 1988. In: P.I. Terasaki (ed.), *Clinical Transplants 1988*, p. 237. UCLA Tissue Typing Laboratory, Los Angeles (1988).
11. Gore, S.M., Gilks, W.R. and Bradley, B.A.: Transplantation Statistics in the UK — and agenda for the next quinquennium. In: P.I. Terasaki (ed), *Clinical Transplants 1988*, p. 225. UCLA Tissue Typing Laboratory, Los Angeles (1988).
12. Najarian, J.S., Migliori, R.J., Simmons, R.L. *et al.*: Effects of HLA matching in cadaver renal transplants. *Transplant. Proc.* **20** (3), 249 (1988).
13. Stratta, R.J., Armbrust, M.J., Lorentzen, D.F. *et al.*: Cadaveric renal transplantation in the cyclosporine and OKT3 eras: the University of Wisconsin-Madison experience. In: P.I. Terasaki (ed.), *Clinical Transplants 1987*, p. 183. UCLA Tissue Typing Laboratory, Los Angeles (1987).
14. Dyer, P.A., Martin, S., Mallick, N.P. *et al.*: Kidney transplantation in the northwest region of England — experience of 1132 transplants in 21 years. In: P.I. Terasaki, (ed.), *Clinical Transplants 1987*, p. 201. UCLA Tissue Typing Laboratory, Los Angeles (1989).
15. Cicciarelli, J., Mendez, R., Mendez, R. *et al.*: The long term matching effect from a single large center. *Transplant. Proc.* (in press).
16. Cook, D.J.: Long-term survival of kidney allografts. In: P.I. Terasaki, (ed.), *Clinical Transplants 1987*, p. 277. UCLA Tissue Typing Laboratory, Los Angeles (1987).
17. Miller, R.G. Jr, Gong, G. and Munoz, A.: *Survival Analysis*, p. 51. Wiley, New York (1981).
18. Takiff, H., Mickey, M.R. and Terasaki, P.I.: Factors important in 10-year kidney transplant survival. In: P.I. Terasaki, (ed.), *Clinical Transplants 1986*, p. 157. UCLA Tissue Typing Laboratory, 1986.
19. Fleiss, J.L.: *Statistical Methods for Rates and Proportions*, p. 161. Wiley, New York (1973).
20. Imagawa, D.K. and Cecka J.M.: Renal regrafts. In: P.I. Terasaki (ed.), *Clinical Transplants 1988*, p. 387. UCLA Tissue Typing Laboratory, Los Angeles (1988).
21. Neppert, J., Nunez, G. and Stastny, P.: HLA-A, B, C; -DR; -MT, -MB, and SB antigens on unstimulated human endothelial cells. *Tissue Antigens* **24**, 40 (1990).
22. Porter, K.A.: Histopathology in clinical renal transplantation. *Transplant. Proc.* **6**, 79 (1974).
23. Terasaki, P.I. and Opelz, G.: Fifteen years of HL-A: what is the importance of HL-A compatibility for clinical outcome of renal transplantation? *Vox Sang.* **34**, 171 (1978).
24. Lau, M., Terasaki, P.I., Park, M.S. and Barbetti, A.: Fifteen-year overview of the international cell exchange. In: P.I. Terasaki (ed.), *Clinical Transplants 1989*, p. 447. UCLA Tissue Typing Laboratory, Los Angeles (1989).

5. An effective strategy for transplantation of highly sensitized patients

F.H.J. CLAAS, L.P. DE WAAL, J. BEELEN, P. REEKERS,
P. VAN DEN BERG-LOONEN, E. DE GAST, J. D'AMARO,
G.G. PERSIJN, F. ZANTVOORT and J.J. VAN ROOD

Introduction

Highly sensitized patients, who have developed alloantibodies against almost all foreign HLA antigens, are very difficult to transplant because the crossmatch with potential donors is often positive. The ideal donor for such patients is an HLA identical or compatible donor but due to the enormous polymorphism of the HLA complex, the chance to find such a donor is very low. Therefore, several approaches are used to increase the chance of finding a crossmatch negative kidney for these patients. We describe here the results of the acceptable mismatch program, which is based on careful laboratory analyses of the sera from such patients to detect those HLA-A and -B antigens toward which the patient did not develop antibodies.

Patients and methods

Patients

To be included in the acceptable mismatch program, patients had to meet the following criteria:

1. Sera of at least two different bleeding dates must show antibody reactivity against the lymphocytes of more than 85% of the panel donors (minimal panel size: 50 donors).
2. This antibody reactivity must be due to multispecific alloantibodies against HLA-class I antigens. The reactivity of autoantibodies should not contribute to this panel reactivity.

Patients waiting for a first transplant or for a regraft were included in the protocol.

Acceptable mismatch protocol

The protocol is based on data obtained within Eurotransplant, which show that HLA-A and -B mismatches are less important for graft survival in highly sensitized patients, whereas HLA-DR mismatches have a strong influence, especially in retransplantations (1). Therefore we decided to determine those HLA-A and B mismatches toward which the patient did not develop antibodies and to use this information in the donor selection. One can obtain this information in two ways:

1. By looking at the HLA types of the negative panel donors, in the screening, which is of course only possible when the patient has less than 100% panel reactivity.
2. By testing the sera from each individual patient against a panel of lymphocyte donors, selected in such a way that these donors have only one HLA-A or -B mismatch with the patient (Table 1).

Table 1. Determination of acceptable HLA-A and -B mismatches.

Patient: A1, A2, B7, B8				*Panel reactivity*: 100%
				Test sera from the patient against blood donors selected on the basis of only one HLA-A or -B antigen mismatch with the patient.
Donors				*Crossmatch*
A1	A2	B7	*B12*	–
A1	A2	B7	*B40*	+
A1	*A3*	B7	B8	+
A1	*A9*	B7	B8	–

Acceptable mismatches are B12 and A9.

The so-called acceptable class I mismatches are implemented in a computer together with the patients own HLA-A, -B and -DR antigens. Donor selection will take place by implementing the HLA-A, -B and -DR antigens of every potential donor in the computer, which will select crossmatch negative recipients on the basis of their own HLA-A, -B and -DR antigens in combination with the acceptable HLA-A and -B mismatches (2). In this way the donor is always optimally matched for HLA-DR, i.e. either identical of compatible but may have several HLA-A and -B mismatches.

Theoretically this approach should lead to an increased offer of potential crossmatch negative donors for these patients (Table 2). Acceptable mismatches are determined on the basis of non-reactivity of all sera from the patient (Table

Table 2. Consequences for donor selection.

Patients: A1, A2, B7, B8, DR2, DR3. 100% panel reactivity. Only HLA identical or compatible donors seem to be possible.

Acceptable mismatches: A9, B12.
Extra donors can be selected (until now HLA-DR compatible):

A1	A9	B7	B8	A2	A2	B12	B12	A9	A9	B12	B12
A2	A9	B7	B8	A2	A9	B7	B12	A9	A9	B7	B7
A9	A9	B7	B8	A2	A9	B8	B12	A9	A9	B8	B8
A1	A2	B7	B12	A1	A9	B7	B12	A1	A9	B12	B12
A1	A2	B8	B12	A1	A9	B8	B12	A1	A9	B7	B7
A1	A2	B12	B12	A9	A9	B7	B12	A1	A9	B8	B8
A1	A1	B12	B12	A9	A9	B8	B12	A2	A9	B12	B12
A2	A9	B8	B8	A2	A9	B7	B7.				

3) and the final crossmatches are performed in the tissue typing laboratory of the transplantation center, using both current and non-current sera.

Cooperative centers

The acceptable mismatch procedure has been started in Leiden. Next Amsterdam and, somewhat later, the other Dutch centers (Groningen, Maastricht, Nijmegen and Utrecht) joined the project. Recently, some centers from Belgium and Germany have started to participate. At December 31, 1989, 99 patients are currently waiting in this special Acceptable Mismatch Program.

Results

Determination of acceptable mismatches

Using the two approaches described it was possible to dermine acceptable mismatches for most of the patients tested. Especially the use of a patient specific panel composed of individuals mismatched for only one antigen with the patient leads to the detection of several HLA alloantigens toward which the patients did not develop antibodies. This is even the case for patients who have a 100% panel reactivity in repeated screenings. Altogether the laboratory in Leiden was able to detect acceptable mismatches in 69 of the 82 patients tested. Even high-frequency HLA antigens were found to be acceptable in some patients (Table 3). The problem with this approach is the amount of work for the laboratory and the need for a large amount of HLA-typed blood donors to compose the patient specific panels. However, recent data suggest that the HLA type of the mother of the patient may be very informative.

Table 3. All patient sera are tested for acceptable mismatches.

Patient N								
Serum	*Date*	*PRA*	*Acceptable mismatches*					
1	1985	89%	*A1*	A28	*A3*	B35		
2	1986	92%	*A1*		*A3*		B44	
3	1987	84%	*A1*		*A3*	B35		B60

Acceptable mismatches implemented: A1, A3.

Maternal HLA antigens are often acceptable mismatches

Although some of the acceptable mismatches were crossreactive antigens with patients own HLA antigens, also several non-crossreactive antigens were found to be acceptable. In a first study (3) we found that these antigens were often the non-inherited maternal HLA antigens, whereas this was hardly the case for the non-inherited paternal HLA antigens. These results could be confirmed in a second study (Table 4). These data suggest that in man a situation exists which may be similar to neonatal tolerance in the mouse. Preliminary studies of our group show that also donor-specific transfusions from mother to child give less sensitization than donor specific transfusions from father to child. Furthermore, looking at the cytotoxic T cell precursor frequency of children against their parental HLA class I antigens, it was found that in about 25% of children hardly any CTLp directed against the maternal HLA class I antigens could be found, whereas this was hardly the case for the CTLp frequency against the father (Zhang Li *et al.*, submitted). Thus careful analysis of the HLA-typings of the family, especially the mother, might be very helpful and rather easy to determine the acceptable mismatches.

Table 4. Leucocyte antibodies in highly sensitized patients are less likely to be directed against the NIMAs than the NIPAs.

Antibody	First study		Second study	
	NIMA	NIPA	NIMA	NIPA
Negative	21	2	17	6
Positive	24	23	14	21

$\chi^2 = 14.1$, $p < 0.001$.

Number of transplants performed and waiting time

By December 31, 1989, 89 patients had been transplanted on basis of this acceptable mismatch program (Figure 1). An increase in the number of patients reported to this program was observed since 1988 when the Dutch Kidney Foundation gave a special grant to the Dutch tissue typing centers to join this protocol. The current waiting list consists of 99 patients. Many of the patients who have been tranplanted were waiting for more than 5 years and some even more than 10 years. Once the acceptable mismatches are determined for a patient, the waiting time for the patients who have been transplanted is rather short (Figure 2).

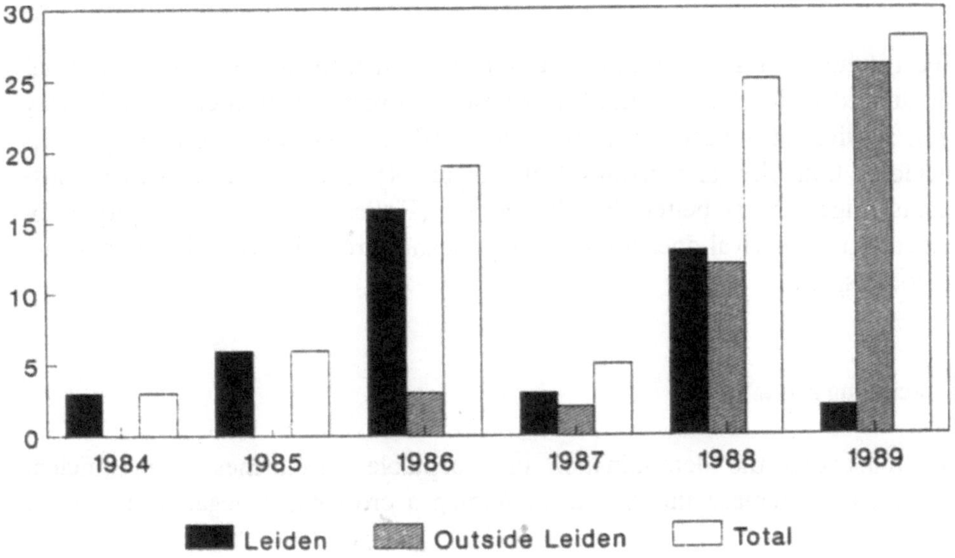

Fig. 1. Number of patients transplanted according to the acceptable mismatch protocol.

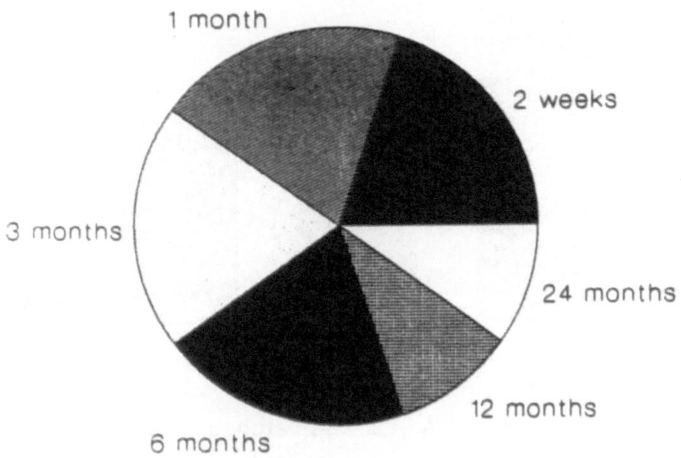

Fig. 2. Waiting time of patients transplanted via the acceptable mismatch protocol starting from the moment that the acceptable HLA-A and -B mismatches are implanted.

More than 80% of them are transplanted within 6 months after being implemented in the program and 40% even within 1 month. As donor selection is based on the combination of the patients own HLA antigens in combination with the acceptable HLA-A and -B mismatches, the kidney donors transplanted have between 0 and 4 acceptable HLA-A and/or -B mismatches (Figure 3). However, all donors are HLA-DR compatible.

Graft survival

The results of these transplants are not different from those obtained in non-immunized patients within the Eurotransplant organization after 1983. Kidney graft survival at 1 year being more than 80% for the total group of patients including both first and retransplants (Figure 4). Graft survival in first transplants (Figure 5) is better than in regrafts (Figure 6) but in both groups of patients graft survival does not differ significantly from the overall results within Eurotransplant.

Concluding remarks

We think that the determination of acceptable mismatches is an efficient approach to increase the chance of finding a crossmatch negative donor for

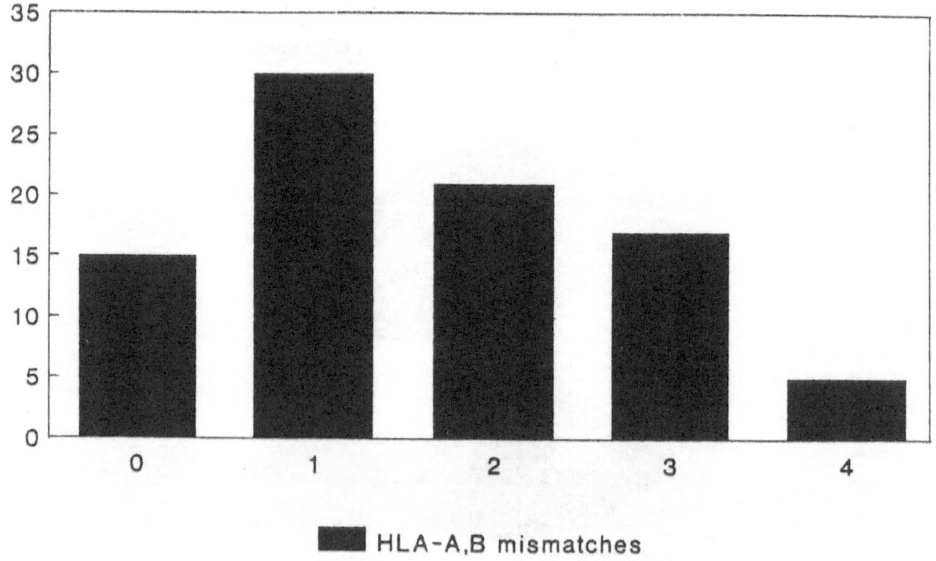

Fig. 3. Number of HLA-A and/or -B mismatches of the HLA-DR compatible kidney donors. Indicated on the *y*-axis the number of transplants in each category.

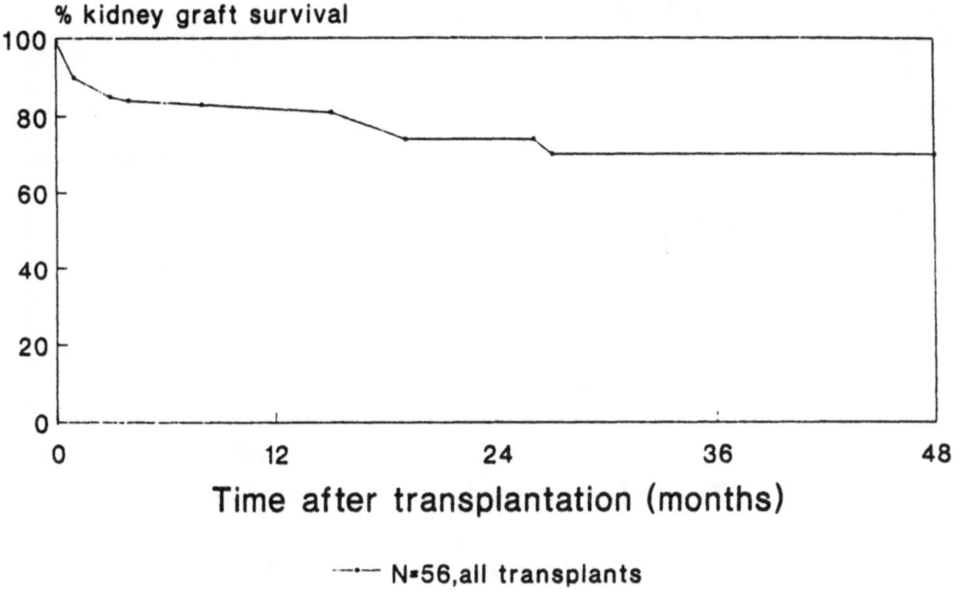

Fig. 4. Kidney graft survival in 56 patients transplanted according to the Acceptable Mismatch Program initiated in 1984. Kidney graft survival at 1 and 2 years is respectively 81% and 74%.

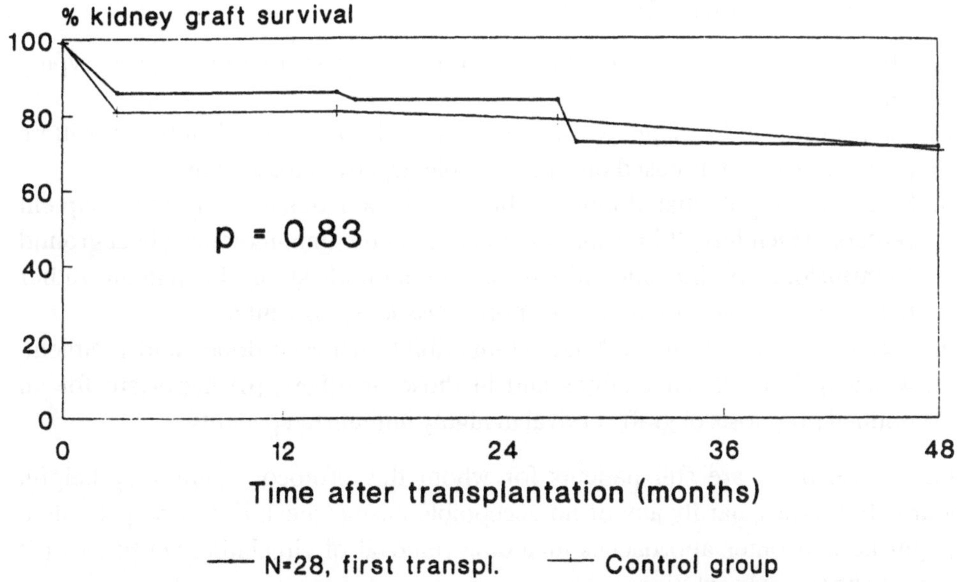

Fig. 5. Kidney graft survival in 28 patients who received a first transplant according to the Acceptable Mismatch Program (+) as compared to 9324 first transplant recipients, transplanted according to the standard Eurotransplant Program (—·—). Kidney graft survival at 1 year is respectively 86% versus 84% and at 2 years respectively 81% versus 79% (overall $p = 0.83$).

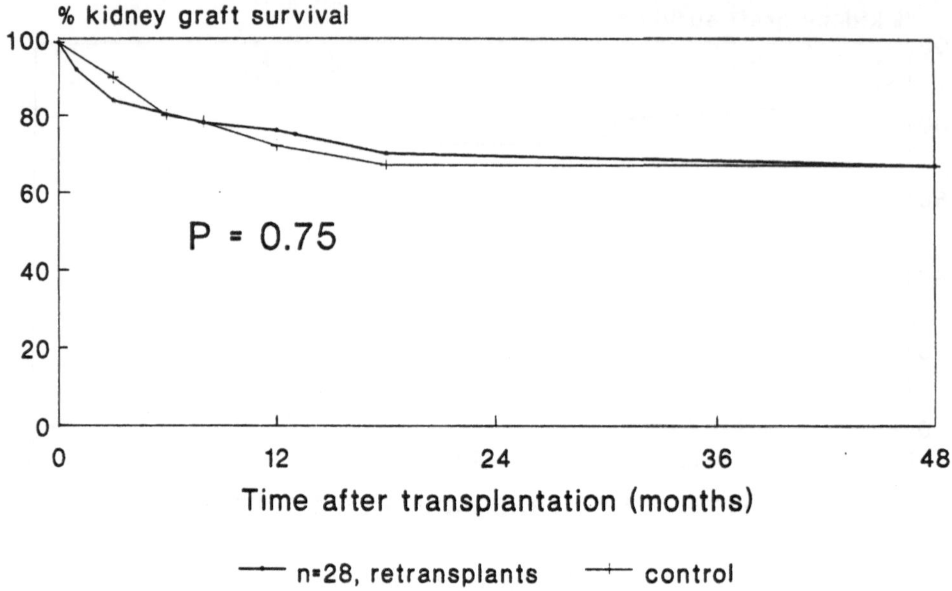

Fig. 6. Kidney graft survival of 28 patients receiving a retransplant according to the Acceptable Mismatch Program (+) versus 1648 Eurotransplant retransplant patients (— · —). Kidney graft survival at 1 year is respectively 75% versus 76% and at 2 years 67% versus 70% (overall p = 0.75).

highly sensitized patients. This approach has several advantages over other approaches described (4, 5) namely:

1. There is no need for distribution of patient sera to other tissue typing centers.
2. Rather than performing crossmatches with all donors, most of which will be positive, selection is based on a predictable negative crossmatch.
3. Selection of potential donors is based on data obtained by the recipient centers, which has all information concerning the immunological background (transfusion, specific alloantibodies, autoantibodies) of the patient rather than on a negative crossmatch in another tissue typing center.
4. Selection is based on HLA-DR compatibility between donor and recipient, which is, both in our analysis and in those of others, (6) important for an optimal prognosis of graft survival in highly immunized patients.

Of course, there are still patients for whom this protocol is not very helpful (rare HLA types, hardly any or no acceptable mismatches). For these patients it might be that other approaches including removal of circulating antibodies (7) seem to be the only solution.

Acknowledgement

This chapter was supported in part by the Dutch Foundation for Medical and

Health Research (MEDIGON), the J.A. Cohen Institute for Radiopathology and Radiation Protection (IRS), the Dutch Kidney Foundation and the Kuratorum fur Dialyse und Nierentransplantation.

The authors gratefully acknowledge all the physicians and their staff in the donor and transplant hospitals as well in the tissue typing laboratories participating in the Eurotransplant Organization.

References

1. Hendriks, G.F.J., De Lange, P, D'Amaro, J. *et al.*: Eurotransplant experience with highly immunized patients. *Scand. J. Urol. Nephrol.* **92**, 81 (1985).
2. Claas, F.H.J., Gijbels, Y., Van Veen, A. *et al.*: Selection of cross-match negative HLA-A and/ or -B mismatched donors for highly sensitized patients. *Transplant. Proc.* **21**, 665 (1989).
3. Claas, F.H.J. Gijbels, Y., van der Velden-de Munck and Van Rood, J.J.: Induction of B-cell unresponsiveness to non-inherited maternal HLA antigens during fetal life. *Science* **241**, 1815 (1988).
4. Bradley, B.A., Klouda, P.T., Ray, T.C. *et al.*: Negative cross-match selection of kidneys for highly sensitized patients. *Transplant. Proc.* **17**, 2465 (1985).
5. Schäfer, A.J., Hasert, K., Opelz, G.: Collaborative Transplant Study: cross-match and antibody project. *Transplant. Proc.* **17**, 2469 (1985).
6. Klouda, P.T., Ray, T.C., Kirckpatrick, J. *et al.*: Graft survival in highly sensitized patients. *Transplant. Proc.* **19**, 3744 (1987).
7. Palmer, A., Taube, D., Welsh, K. *et al.*: Extracorporeal immunoadsorption of anti-HLA antibodies: preliminary clinical experience. *Transplant. Proc.* **19**, 3750 (1987).

6. Rapid lymphocyte crossmatching for renal transplantation

A.G. WHITE, K.T. RAJU, M.S.A. KUMAR, E.M. PHILIPS and G.M. ABOUNA

Introduction

In Kuwait we have utilized imported cadaver kidneys which have prolonged cold ischaemia times frequently exceeding 50 hours (1). Such imported organs are crossmatched against local recipients on arrival in Kuwait and this may add an additional 4—4½ hours to the ischaemic interval when performed by conventional crossmatching techniques (2).

An attempt has been made to speed up the crossmatching procedure to enable a reduction in cold ischaemia time. We describe a modification of a previous described HLA typing technique (3) using the release of intracellular adenosine triphosphate (ATP) from lymphocytes, incubated with recipient serum and complement, as an indicator of cytotoxicity. ATP is quantitated using the luciferin/luciferase reaction and a luminometer to measure the light release.

Material and methods

Lymphocytes were most frequently isolated from lymph nodes transported with the kidney but occasionally spleen or peripheral blood had to be utilized. Lymphocytes were separated and washed using traditional laboratory methods. Lymphocyte crossmatching was then performed using the conventional and the ATP release technique in parallel.

Conventional cross-matching was performed using 1 μl of recipient serum at neat, 1/2, 1/4, 1/8 and 1/16 dilutions and 1 μl of lymphocytes at 2×10^6 ml. Appropriate autologous, AB and ALG controls were included. Incubation was at 22° C for 30 minutes, before addition of 5 μl of rabbit complement with further incubation for 120 min. The cells were stained with eosin and fixed with formalin and then read after a further 30 min. All reactions were performed on duplicate plates with triplicates on each plate for each reaction.

Cross-matching by ATP release

Twenty-five microlitres of lymphocytes at 2×10^6 ml and 25 μl of recipient serum were incubated for 30 min at room temperature in a luminometer cuvette. One hundred and twenty-five microlitres of rabbit complement are added, mixed and left for 15 minutes at room temperature, before the addition of 200 microlitres of ATP monitoring reagent. The light output is measured (baseline value) and then the lymphocytes lysed with a nucleotide releasing solution made from 1% Triton $\times$ 100 in tris EDTA buffer at pH 7.75. The integrated/peak light output is quantitated using an LKB 1215 luminometer (LKB Wallac, Turku, Finland) and interpretated in relation to the AB/ALG controls.

Results

The results are summarized in Table 1. There were no false positive or negative crossmatches when compared with conventional lymphocyte crossmatching. Furthermore, four kidneys were utilized on the basis of the ATP methods when cell viability did not permit interpretation of the conventional crossmatch.

Discussion

The measurement of ATP release as a measure of antibody and complement dependent cytotoxicity for crossmatching has several distinct advantages. The technique described here parallels conventional crossmatching in terms of proportions of volumes and incubation temperature. It simply estimates cytotoxicity early by quantitating a small molecule (ATP, MWT 551) that leaks from the lymphocyte within 4 min of complement addition rather than waiting for the death of the cell that is normally microscopically evaluated by dye exclusion/phase contrast. The technique measures the residual ATP in the

Table 1.

	Number of crossmatches	False positive	False negative
Conventional microtoxicity	42	—	—
ATP release[a]	41	0	0

[a] Kidneys were utilized on the basis of the ATP method. Cell viability did not permit interpretation of the conventional crossmatch.

lymphocyte after chemical lysis as ATP released into the medium during incubation breaks own rapidly and cannot be estimated accurately.

As described, the method parallels the sensitivity of conventional cross-matching but by adjustment of incubation temperature/time, it can be increased in sensitivity. Additionally it is not subject to observer error inherent in microscopical examination of reactions. Initial experiments using magnetic bead separated T lymphocytes and B lymphocytes indicate that it can be used for lymphocytes separated by these means.

The transplantation of four kidneys on the basis of the rapid crossmatch merits discussion. Frequently tissue accompanying the kidney for crossmatching purposes is preserved under suboptimal conditions. Tissue may not even be cold on arrival, it is not usually in a suitable preservation medium (often sent in saline) and sometimes even dry. A 55 h old spleen often yields cells of poor viability, possibly as a result of autolysis. The use of four kidneys which would have otherwise been discarded is a distinct advantage of the rapid technique.

Lastly, the ATP method may also be of value in organs which have much shorter preservation periods than kidneys and could have application in 'organ specific' crossmatching.

References

1. Kumar, M.S.A., Samhan, M., Philips, E.M. and Abouna, G.M.: Late function in 48 cadaver renal allografts preserved for 48 to 76 hours. *Transplant. Proc.* **20**, 940—941 (1988).
2. Amos, D.B.: (1974) Cytotoxicity testing. In: J.G. Ray, Jr, D.B. Hare, P.D. Pedersen and D.F. Kayhoe (eds), *Manual of Tissue Typing Techniques*, pp 23—26. Publication No. (N1H) 75-545. U.S. Dept. of Health, Education and Welfare, Washington, D.C.
3. Descamps, B.: Determination of intracellular adenosine triphosphate for detecting anti-HLA antibody mediated cytolysis. *Transplantation* **29**, 295—301 (1980).

7. Fifteen-year experience with fine needle aspiration biopsies at the University of Helsinki

PEKKA HÄYRY, EEVA VON WILLEBRAND and
IRMELI LAUTENSCHLAGER

Introduction

The first fine needle aspiration biopsies (FNAB) were performed by Abdul Casim, Physician to the Great Caliph of Cordova. Franzen applied the method to urogenital organs. At the beginning of the 1970s, Pasternack, Virolainen and Häyry performed experimental biopsies from dog renal allografts (1) and later from human renal transplant recipients (2). At that time we were unable to interpret the findings because of inadequate techniques in the preparation of the biopsies and incomplete knowledge of transplant aspiration cytology.

More information on the cytological structure of inflammation and concomitant cytological alterations in the transplant parenchymal cells in the rat was obtained by Soots, von Willebrand and Häyry (3—5) in the late 1970s. These experiments made it possible to interpret the cytological alterations also in human subjects (6). The aspiration cytology method was remodified and reapplied to human renal transplant recipients in 1978 (7), and subsequently to liver transplant recipients (8), on the basis of Lautenschlager's experimental findings (9, 10), in 1982.

At the present, we have performed more than 11 000 aspiration biopsies to human renal allografts, with only one notable complication: a spontaneously reversible episode of bleeding during the first 500 renal aspirations, and no graft losses. More than 1000 biopsies have been done from liver allografts and, in addition, more than 1000 bronchoalveolar lavations, deriving from transplant recipients, either from bone marrow transplant recipients during aGVHD or as a consequence of pulmonary complications of parenchymal organ transplants have been performed.

In parenchymal organ allografts, aspiration cytology makes it possible to adequately assess the inflammatory response of (acute) allograft rejection, to analyze concomitant alterations of graft parenchymal cells, to diagnose cyclosporine toxicity and to monitor the impact of treatment on these parameters. However, for complete evaluation of the transplant, particularly for the evaluation of vascular alterations, a needle biopsy must be performed.

This short overview summarizes our experience. The technical details have been reported previously (7) and more comprehensive information on this subject may be obtained from some recent reviews and textbook chapters (11–14). In addition, a comprehensive atlas on the aspiration cytology has recently been published by C. Hammer (15).

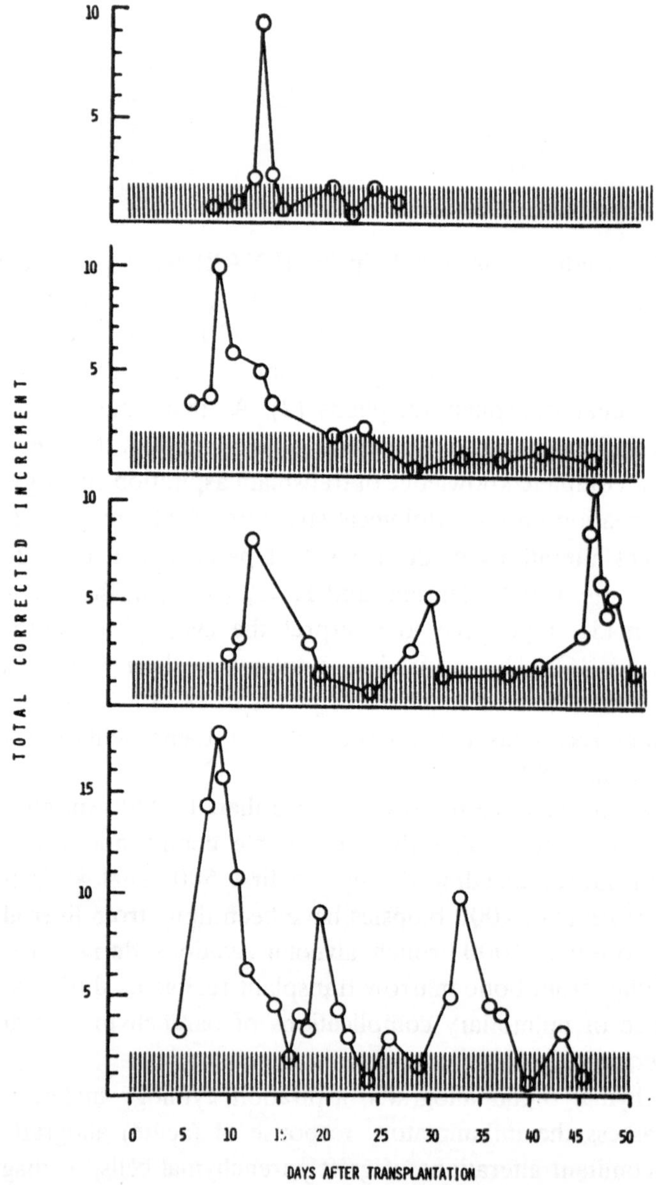

Fig. 1. Pattern of inflammation in renal allograft rejection. Shaded area represents background inflammation in clinically well-functioning transplants. (From Häyry and von Willebrand, *Transplantation and Clinical Immunology* XV, 1983; through the courtesy of Excerpta Medica, Amsterdam.)

Diagnostic efficacy of transplant aspiration cytology

Cytological specimens obtained by aspiration biopsies or by lavation may be used (i) for the monitoring of the graft, (ii) for the monitoring of inflammation and, what is very important, (iii) for the monitoring of the impact of treatment on these parameters.

Monitoring of the graft

Cytological diagnostics of the graft parenchymal components adequately differentiates the following disorders: acute tubular necrosis (ATN), cyclosporine toxicity and a necrotic graft. In addition the FNAB enables the quantitation of the major histocompatibility (MHC) antigens on the graft parenchymal cells, an important adjunct, for example, in the differential diagnostics of rejection vs infection.

In ATN, the graft tubular cells appear swollen; these changes disappear when graft resumes normal function.

In cyclosporine toxicity, the most characteristic change is fine 'isometric' vacuolization in the graft tubular cells. Concomitantly, cyclosporine or cross-reactive metabolites can be demonstrated by immunofluorescence or by immunoperoxidase methods in the tubular and, to a lesser extent, also in the endothelial cells. If all parenchymal cells of the graft appear necrotic in the specimens, this indicates that a vascular catastrophy has occurred in the transplant.

Normally human renal tubular and endothelial cells do not measurably express the class II MHC products. During rejection, class II products of the MHC are readily detectable on the surface of graft parenchymal cells as well as intracytoplasmically, as quantiated by *Staphylococcus aureus* rosette method of by ordinary immunoperoxidase stainings, respectively.

Quantitation of inflammation

Aspiration cytology methods enable a very precise quantitation of the inflammatory events associated with acute allograft rejection. The following inflammatory cell types may be adequately identified in the cytocentrifuged cell smears: lymphoblasts, plasmablasts and plasma cells, 'activated' lymphocytes, large granular lymphocytes, small lymphocytes, the various types of granulocytes, monoblasts, monocytes and tissue macrophages.

These different cell types are, however, not of equal value in the establishment of the diagnosis. Characteristic to *acute rejection* is the presence of lymphoblasts, plasmablasts, plasma cells and other activated cell forms, including monoblasts in the inflammatory infiltrate; in extended and irreversible rejections, there is a maturation of monocytes into tissue macrophages.

It should be noted, however, that acute rejection is not an on/off phenomenon. On all occasions there is a certain level of background inflammation in the graft. The actual inflammatory episodes may appear as a single peak, responding rapidly to intensified immunosuppressive treatment, or as several peaks, with several activations and remissions. Thus, to the contrary of a needle biopsy, which is not usually performed repeatedly, the FNAB gives, when properly used, a dynamic picture of rejection.

Considering the sequence of the inflammatory events in acute rejection, it may be stated that the CD4/CD8 ratio, usually over 1 in the blood and in the biopsy during periods of no inflammation, turns below 1 on most occasions during the inflammatory episodes. Blast cells are very early indicators of the activation of the inflammatory event; lymphoid blasts usually peak at the very beginning of rejection and precedes, for example, the transcription of the class II by 1—3 days.

A final 'cell type' present in the inflammatory infiltrate is the thrombocytes. Thrombocytes accumulate inside all rejecting allografts in all patterns of rejection. Mostly these aggregates are intravascular, and no attachment to graft endothelium appears (16). The episode of rejection is over when thrombocytes leave the graft. In contrast in irreversible rejections, there is a gradually increasing attachment of thrombocytes to the microvascular endothelium and, concomitantly, loss of the transplant is predicted (16).

Reproducibility

Several studies have been done to demonstrate the reproducibility of the FNAB in the monitoring of renal allografts. In our own study, we found a correlation coefficient of 0.945 between double biopsies, provided that both biopsies were representative (17).

In a worldwide quality control analysis (18), with more than 30 centres participating, sets of slides were circulated without any clinical background information. A diagnosis compatible with the Helsinki diagnosis, which was used as a standard, was obtained in the average in 80% of the readings. The disagreement on most occasions was only a minor one.

Thus the FNAB provides reproducible results provided that the biopsy is representative, and the readings in different trained laboratories are highly compatible.

Transplant aspiration cytology as a differential diagnostic tool

Use of transplant aspiration cytology as a diagnostic tool is summarized in

Table 1. Differential diagnosis between acute rejection and other complications of kidney transplants by FNAB. S-CREA = serum creatinine.

S-CREA	FNAB			Explanation
	Inflammation	Tubular cell changes	CyA deposits in graft	
Normal	–	±	±	A well-functioning graft
Elevated	–	++	–	ATN
Elevated	–	+++	+++	CyA toxicity
Elevated	+++	+	–	Rejection
Elevated	+++	+++	+++	Rejection and CyA toxicity

Table 1. In short, the following post-transplant complications may be adequately visualized by the FNAB: ATN, CyA toxicity, rejection or combination thereof.

Correlations between FNAB and needle core biopsy

It should be emphasized that the FNAB is not to replace ordinary needle biopsy (NB) in the evaluation of the transplant.

The correlations between the FNAB and NB are summarized in Table 2. In

Table 2. Differences between NB and FNAB.

	Needle core biopsy (NB)	Fine needle aspiration biopsy (FNAB)
Glomeruli	Transplant glomerulopathy, (recurrent) glomerulonephritis	–
Tubuli	Atrophy, vacuolation necrosis, calcification	Swelling, vacuolation, inclusions, necrosis of tubular cells
Blood vessels	Transplant vasculopathy, vasculitis	Number of endothelial cells activated endothelial cells
Interstitium	Edema, fibrosis	–
Inflammation	Density, expansion, distribution of the cellular infiltrate, immunohistochemistry	Quantification, state of activation, phenotypic differentiation of infiltrating cells, course of inflammation

Source: Hammer, C., personal communication.

short, the FNAB is good for frequent monitoring of the transplant particularly during the immediate post-transplant period when the complications are mostly those listed above. It should be clearly pointed out that it is not possible to obtain with the FNAB reliable information about the major parenchymal components of the graft, particularly of the graft glomeruli (unless special techniques are used) (19), of the graft vascular tree, particularly of chronic vascular changes and/or of the intensity of edema or fibrosis in the transplant. These alterations are particularly prominent in some less common early vascular rejection forms and in chronic rejection, and should be evaluated by needle biopsy.

FNAB in liver transplantation

The hallmark of acute liver allograft rejection is periportal inflammation. The FNAB technology was applied to human liver transplants via experimental studies in the pig. Comparison of pig needle biopsy histology and graft FNAB demonstrated that the inflammatory changes during acute rejection episodes, including the components of inflammation and the subsets of inflammatory cells, were virtually identical in both types of specimens.

By now, several liver transplant centers in North America and in Europe have taken the FNAB technology as their prime monitoring method for liver transplants. Inflammatory episodes in the liver may be adequately diagnosed by the FNAB and the rejection can usually be recorded approximately 1—3 days prior to any alteration in serum alkaline phosphatase or bilirubin are seen.

The differential diagnosis between acute rejection and other complications of liver transplants by the FNAB are summarized in Table 3.

Table 3. Differential diagnosis between acute rejection and other complications of liver transplants by FNAB. S-AFOS = Serum alkaline phosphatase, S-BIL = Serum bilirubin.

S-AFOS S-BIL	FNAB				Explanation
	Inflammation	Parenchymal changes	Bile droplets	CyA deposits	
Normal	–	±	–	–	A well-functioning graft
Elevated	+++	+++	++	–	Acute rejection
Elevated	–	+	+++	–	Cholestasis
Elevated	–	+++	–	+++	CyA toxicity
Elevated	+++	+++	++	+++	Acute rejection and CyA toxicity

Future aspects of transplant aspiration cytology

By now the method has been extended also to pancreas transplantation, and the first reports on experimental and human applications of the FNAB are being published.

Aspiration cytology methods have proven useful in lung transplantation, where the specimen is usually obtained by bronchoalveolar lavation, and in the monitoring of aGVHD from the FNAB of the liver and/or BAL of the lung (19, 20, 21).

References

1. Häyry, P., Lindström, B. L., Virolainen, M., Pasternack, V. and Lindfors, O.: Immunobiological diagnosis of rejection in dogs with renal allografts. *Surgery* **71**, 494—506 (1972).
2. Pasternack, V., Virolainen, M. and Häyry, P.: Fine needle aspiration biopsy in the diagnosis of human renal allograft rejection. *J. Urol.* **109**, 167—172 (1973).
3. Von Willebrand, E., Soots, A. and Häyry, P.: In situ effector mechanisms in rat kidney allograft rejection. I. Characterization of the host cellular infiltrate in rejecting allograft parenchyma. *Cell. Immunol.* **46**, 309—326 (1979).
4. Von Willebrand, E., Soots, A. and Häyry, P.: In situ effector mechanisms of rat kidney allograft rejection. II. Heterogenicity of the effector cells in the inflammatory infiltrate vs. that in the speen of the recipient rat. *Cell. Immunol.* **46**, 327—336 (1979).
5. Häyry, P., von Willebrand, E. and Soots, A.: In situ effector mechanisms in rat kidney allograft rejection. III. Kinetics of the inflammatory response and generation of donor-directed killer cells. *Scand. J. Immunol.* **10**, 95—108 (1979).
6. Von Willebrand, E. and Häyry, P.: Composition and in vitro cytotoxicity of cellular infiltrates in rejecting human kidney allografts. *Cell. Immunol.* **41**, 358—372 (1978).
7. Häyry, P. and von Willebrand, E.: Practical guidelines for fine needle aspiration biopsy of human renal allografts. *Ann. Clin. Res.* **13** 288—306 (1981).
8. Lautenschlager, I., Höckerstedt, K., Ahonen, J., Eklund, B., Isoniemi, H., Korsbäck, C., Pettersson, E., Salmela, K., Scheinin, T. M., von Willebrand, E. and Häyry, P.: Fine needle aspiration biopsy in the monitoring of liver allografts. II. Applications of human liver allografts. *Transplantation* **46**, 47—52 (1988).
9. Lautenschlager, I., Höckerstedt, K., Taskinen, E., Ahonen, J., Korsbäck, C., Salmela, K., Orko, R., Scheinin, B., Scheinin, T. M. and Häyry, P.: Fine needle aspiration cytology of liver allografts in the pig. *Transplantation* **38**, 330—334 (1984).
10 Lautenschlager, I., Höckerstedt, K., Taskinen, E., Korsbäck, C., Mäkisalo, H. and Häyry, P.: Fine needle aspiration biopsy in the monitoring of liver allografts. I. Correlation between aspiration biopsy and core biopsy in experimental pig liver allografts. *Transplantation* **46**, 41—46 (1988).
11. Häyry, P. and von Willebrand, E.: Transplant aspiration cytology. *Transplantation* **38**, 7—12 (1984).
12. Häyry, P. and von Willebrand, E.: Aspiration cytology in monitoring of human allografts. In: G.M. Williams, J.F. Burdick, and K. Solex (eds.), *Kidney Transplant Rejection, Diagnosis and Treatment*, pp. 247—262. Marcel Dekker, New York (1986).
13. Häyry, P., von Willebrand, E., Ahonen, J., Lautenschlager, I., and Leskinen, R.: Aspiration cytology in organ transplantation. *Transplant. Rev.* **1**, 133—137 (1987).
14. Häyry, P.: Fine needle aspiration biopsy in renal transplantation. *Nephrology Forum (Kidney Int.)* **36**, 130—141 (1989).
15. Hammer, C.: *Cytology in Transplantation.* Verlag R.S. Schulz (1989).

16. Von Willebrand, E., Zola, H. and Häyry, P.: Thrombocyte aggregates in renal allografts. Analysis by fine needle aspiration biopsy and monoclonal anti-thrombocyte antibodies. *Transplantation* **39**, 258—262 (1985).
17. Von Willebrand, E. and Häyry, P.: Reproducibility of the fine needle aspiration biopsy. Analysis of 93 double biopsies. *Transplantation* **38**, 314—316 (1984).
18. Häyry, P.: Transplant Aspiration Cytology. Quality Control Analysis. *Transplant. Proc.* **18**, 2100—2105 (1985).
19. Miller, S., Belitsky, P. and Gupta, R.: Kidney glomeruli collected by fine needle aspiration biopsy. *Transplant. Proc.* **21**, 3614—3617 (1989).
20. Leskinen, R., Volin, L., Taskinen, E., Renkonen, R., Ruutu, T. and Häyry, P.: Monitoring of bone marrow transplant recipient liver by fine needle aspiration biopsy. *Transplantation* **48**, 969—974 (1989).
21. Leskinen, R., Taskinen, E., Volin, L., Tukiainen, P., Ruutu, T. and Häyry, P.: Use of bronchoalveolar lavage cytology and determination of protein contents in pulmonary complications of bone marrow transplant recipients. *Bone Marrow Transplantation* (in press).

8. Study of antibody specificity in highly sensitized patients using human monoclonal antibody technology

IBRAHIM A. AL-MUZAIRAI, BARBRA K. WEBER and DAVID A. POWER

Introduction

Highly sensitized patients have lymphocytotoxic antibodies directed to either HLA and non-HLA antigens. Anti-HLA antibodies (alloantibodies) directed to private or public specificity have a deleterious effect on the graft, while cytotoxic antibodies to non-HLA antigens (mainly autoantibodies) may have beneficial effect on graft survival (1). It can be difficult to distinguish a positive crossmatch test due to autoantibodies from one caused by alloantibodies, particularly if the patient is highly sensitized and has both auto- and alloantibodies (2).

The antigenic target for autoantibodies found in sera from dialysis patients has not been well-defined. It had been suggested that they might be directed to IgM (3), whereas others (4) were able to correlate reactivity of these antibodies with cell surface expression of LFA-1. Moreover, there may be more than one antigenic target because autoantibodies can be specific for B lymphocytes alone or both B and T lymphocytes (2).

The tissue distribution of the antigen detected by such autoantibodies had been defined only in part. They were found to lyse K562 (5), an erythroid cell line, and could be removed by absorption with autologous lymphoblastoid B cells (5). Park and co-workers (6) reported that anti-B cell autoantibodies were removed by absorption with platelets, less effectively by splenocytes and very poorly by polymorphs, T cells and leukaemic cells.

These distinctive autoantibodies have been characterized, in previous studies, by the reactivity of whole sera which could contain antibodies directed to multiple specificities. We, therefore, attempted to produce oligoclonal Epstein—Barr virus transformed B cell lines secreting autoantibodies so as to study their binding characteristics and pattern of reactivity.

Patient and methods

We studied 10 highly sensitized patients with PRA >80% (group 1), 3 non-highly sensitized with PRA <10% (group 2), and 3 normal volunteers who never had received blood transfusions.

Establishment of EBV transformed lymphoblastoid cell lines

Peripheral blood lymphocytes from all individuals were transformed using Epstein—Barr virus (EBV) according to a standard method (7). After 4 weeks the supernatants were tested for antibody production by complement-dependent cytotoxicity assay against separated B and T lymphocytes from 12 unrelated individuals, autologous B and T lymphocytes, and against the K562 erythroid cell line. Five human oligoclonal EBV transformed cell lines were established from one patient by two sequential subculturing steps. These were tested against different cell lines to determine their specificity.

Complement dependent cytotoxicity assay (CDC)

The standard long incubation two-stage NIH microcytotoxic assay (8) was applied using separated B and T lymphocytes and different cell lines. B and T lymphocytes were isolated using the nylon wool column technique (9). Cell kill of 20% above background was considered positive. All incubations were carried out at 23°C, except where otherwise stated.

Maintenance of cell lines

All cell lines used were maintained in log-phase growth in medium comprising 10% fetal calf serum in RPMI 1640. They were obtained from American Type Culture Collection or the PHLS Centre, Porton Down, U.K. Nalm-6 was obtained from Prof. M. Greaves, Chester Beatty Cancer Institute, London, U.K.

Flow cytometry was performed against the cell line K562 using the method described elsewhere (10).

Enzyme-linked immunosorbent assay (ELISA) was used to determine immunoglobulin class and concentration.

Western blotting

This was performed by solubilizing 8×10^8 K562 cells in 2 ml of Triton X-100 0.5% in PBS with 1.5 mM phenoxymethylsulfonic acid and 100 μ/ml aprotinin as protease inhibitors. Nuclei were removed by centrifugation at 2500 g for 10 min, the supernatant was mixed with an equal volume of non-reducing SDS-

PAGE sample buffer and boiled for 5 min. The lysate was separated on a 10% SDS-PAGE gel and blotted onto nitrocellulose. Nitrocellulose strips were assayed after blocking by incubation with supernatant for 2 hours followed by addition of I^{125}-labelled antihuman IgM. Strips were developed by autoradiography.

Results

Production of oligoclonal B cell lines and reactivity against normal lymphocytes, autologous cells and K562 cell line

After 4 weeks, supernatants (S/N) were tested in CDC against a panel of B and T lymphocytes from six normal individuals, against autologous B and T cells and K562 cell line. In group 1; 10—100% of S/N from all patients were positive against peripheral lymphocytes from normal individuals, 49% reacted with B cells and 13% reacted with T cells. Reactivity of the S/N against autologous B cells in group 1 were found in three patients (14—27% of S/N were positive) while only one of these had activity against both T and B lymphocytes. Reactivity against K562 cells was found in seven patients (11—40% of S/N were positive). In group 2, two patients showed reactivity against the lymphocytes from normal individuals, compared with one patient in group 3 (32% of S/N). None of the S/N from group 2 was reactive against either autologus cells or K562 cells, while in group 3, S/N from two patients showed reactivity against autologous cells (29% and 5% S/N positive) and 19% and 5% S/N were positive against K562 cells. Activity against B lymphocytes was observed more frequently than against T lymphocytes.

One of these positive wells from a patient in group 1 was subcloned; five lines were derived and grown in culture to obtain large quantities of supernatant. Supernatants from these five lines were used in all subsequent studies.

Reactivity of the five oligoclonal cell lines against different cell lines

Four out of five S/N cell lines were positive with B lymphocytes from all members of the cell panel (*n*: 12) and all were positive against autologous B cells. Reactivity was less with peripheral T cells; none of the supernatants was positive against all members of the T cell panel. Titration of supernatants against autologous T and B lymphocytes confirmed lesser activity against T cells. This was also found with cells from an unrelated individual. There was also a marked reduction in antibody titre when the initial antibody incubation was performed at 37 °C, compared with 4 and 23 °C which were very similar.

Supernatants were also weakly positive against peripheral blood monocytes but negative against granulocytes (Table 1). Absorption with platelets removed antibody activity against B lymphocytes.

All supernatants reacted very similarly with neoplastic cell lines (Table 1). They were weakly positive with T cell lines (Molt 4 and Jurkat), the erythroid line K562 and Nalm 6, a pre-B cell line. All other cell lines were negative. These included B lymphoblastoid cell lines (Jestholm, WT49, BM15, BM16), Burkitt B cell lines (Daudi and Raji), RPMI 8226 (human myeloma) and myelomonocytic cell lines (U937 and HL-60). They were also negative against lymphocytes from eight patients with chronic lymphatic leukaemia (CLL) and myelocytes from two patients with chronic myelogenous leukaemia (CML).

Assay of the five supernatants by flow cytometry, Western blotting and ELISA

These antibodies bound K562 very weakly in flow cytometry with 6—12% of

Table 1. Reactivity of supernatants against cell lines (% cytotoxicity).

	Supernatants				
Cell line	2B4	1D3	1F6	1G2	1G4
Lymphoblastoid B cells					
Jestholm	0[a]	0	0	0	0
WT49	0	0	0	0	0
BM15	0	0	0	0	0
BM16	0	0	0	0	0
Burkitt B cells					
Daudi	0	0	0	0	0
Raji	0	0	0	0	0
Pre-B cell					
Nalm-6	20	40	50	60	40
Human myeloma					
RPMI 8226	0	0	0	0	0
Myelomonocytic cells					
U937	0	0	0	0	0
HL 60	0	0	0	0	0
Erythroid cell					
K562	10	30	30	30	30
T cell					
Molt 4	20	50	50	50	40
Jurkat	20	40	20	30	20
CLL cells ($n = 8$)	0	0	0	0	0
CML cells ($n = 2$)	0	0	0	0	0

[a] Cytotoxicity (%).

cells positive for the five different lines with a mean channel shift from 3 to 40 (data not shown). There was no reactivity with any surface protein by Western blotting. All were IgMκ but IgM concentrations varied widely in different supernatants. In general, antibody concentration correlated with titre and reactivity with T cells in particular.

Discussion

In this study, we monitored the reactivity of obligoclonal antibodies produced by EBV transformation from 10 highly sensitized patients and non-sensitized patients. Cytotoxic antibodies were detected in all patients and they were broadly reactive against both T and B lymphocytes. EBV supernatants were tested against a large panel of normal lymphocytes (*n*: 12), their reactivity with B cell was greater than with T cells (data shown). The data presented in this study suggests that the specificity of antibodies in highly sensitized patients is directed to both public HLA and/or non-HLA antigens (autoantibodies) but not private specificities (11). Reactivity against autologous B lymphocytes was found in 3/10 highly sensitized patients with one of these patients showing T cell reactivity as well. Reactivity against K562 cell line was found in 7/10 highly sensitized patients indicating that these are non-HLA antibodies and could be autoantibodies (1, 2). It is interesting to note that normal volunteers showed reactivity against both autologous cells and K562 cells which may indicate that some antibodies produced by normal individuals are autoantibodies. This study confirm that autoantibodies may appear spontaneously not related to an obvious antigenic challenge, although there is some evidence that autoantibodies may apear after viral infection (12, 13). The five cell lines obtained from one patient with B cell reactive autoantibodies in patient serum were tested for their tissue distribution. Their pattern of reactivity was predominantly with peripheral B and, less so, T lymphocytes. There was also lysis of peripheral blood monocytes and cell lines K562, Nalm 6, Molt 4 and Jurkat, although these were weak. There was no reactivity with CLL B lymphocytes, lymphoblastoid B cell lines or Burkitt B cells. Antibody activity was, however, removed by platelet absorption.

Previous studies have suggested that autoreactive antibodies may be directed to IgM (3, 14) or a molecule which is co-expressed with or identical to LEA-1 (8). These supernatants, however, did not lyse some cells which express surface IgM, such as CLL cells, and were reactive with non-B cells which do not express surface IgM. The distribution of reactivity is also inconsistent with that of LFA-1 (4). The reactivity of these cell lines is shown in Table 1: they were not compatible with the tissue distribution of any CD antigens.

Interestingly, these oligoclonal antibodies reacted with autologous T lymphocytes even though there was no such reactivity present in the patient's serum.

Since titres of the oligoclonal supernatants were higher against B than T lymphocytes when tested against either autologous or third-party cells, this data suggests that some autoantibodies reactive with B lymphocytes alone may be identical to those which lyse B and T cells, the difference being a higher antibody concentration or affinity in the latter. However, we do not know whether the oligoclonal autoantibodies we have produced are representative of all such antibodies directed against the cell surface in dialysis patients.

There was a profound effect of antibody incubation temperatures upon antibody titre, a finding also reported with studies using serum where some positive results at 4 and 23 °C are lost at 37 °C (1, 2). The binding kinetics of such antibodies are unknown but we were unable to produce strong positives by flow cytometry. These data suggest that these antibodies are of low affinity. Our inability to utilize binding assays creates a further problem in establishing the pattern of tissue reactivity, since different cells may not be equally susceptible to complement mediated lysis. For example, Naito *et al.* (15) reported that granulocytes could remove autoantibodies by absorption even though they were not lysed by such antibodies. Low affinity could also explain the rarity of autoantibodies directed against the cell surface in some studies performed in animals (16, 17). Immunohistology, too, may not detect these antibodies, particularly at higher incubation temperatures.

While autoantibodies remain a nuisance for those involved in transplantation, especially when it is necessary to separate positive crossmatches due to autoantibodies in patients who possess alloantibodies as well, there has been almost no information regarding the possible function of these antibodies. It has been reported by several groups that cold-reactive autoantibodies are associated with improved graft survival (1, 2). Moreover, Lobo showed that, although autoantibodies did not prevent sensitization (18), their presence was associated with reduced alloantibody titres, suggesting a regulatory role. Whether autoantibodies reactive with the cell surface have a function is unknown at the present time, but the availability of monoclonal or oligoclonal reagents of defined specificity should allow detailed study of their effect on *in vitro* cellular activity.

References

1. Ting, A.: The highly sensitised patients. In: G.R.D. Catto (ed.), *New Clinical Applications Nephrology: Transplantation*, pp. 39—58. Kluwer Academic Publishers, Dordrecht (1989).
2. Ting, A.: HLA matching and crossmatching in renal transplantation. In: P.J. Morris (ed.), *Kidney Transplantation*, p. 183. Grune and Stratton, New York (1988).
3. Cicciarelli, J.C., Chia, D, Terasaki, P.I. *et.al.*: S.7 Human IgM anti-IgM cytotoxin for B lymphocytes. *Tissue Antigens* **15**, 275 (1980).
4. Chapman, J.R., Taylor, C.J., Carter, N.P. and Morris, P.J.: Comparison of non-lineage antibodies with cytotoxic autoreactive antibodies in haemodialysis patients. In: A.J. Mc-

Michael (ed.), *Leucocyte Typing III. White Cell Differentiation Antigens*, p. 826. Oxford University Press, Oxford (1987).

5. Deierhoi, M.H., Ting, A. and Morris, P.J.: Reactivity of lymphocyte cytotoxic autoantibodies from renal patients with cell line K562. *Transplantation* **38**, 557 (1984).
6. Park, M.S., Terasaki, P.I. and Bernoco, D.: Autoantibody against B lymphocytes. *Lancet* **ii**, 465 (1977).
7. Roder, C.J., Cole, S.P.C., Atlaw, T. *et al.*: The Epstein-Barr Virus-Hybridoma Technique. In: Engleman, Foung, Larrick and Raubitschek (eds), *Human Hybridoma and Monoclonal Antibodies*, pp. 55–70. Plenum Press, New York (1985).
8. McIntosh, P.: HLA typing. In: R.A. Thomas (ed.), *Techniques in Clinical Immunology*, p. 203. Blackwell Scientific, Oxford (1981).
9. Stewart, K.N.: Separation of T and B lymphocytes by nylon fibre columns. *Med. Lab. Sc.* **38**, 123 (1981).
10. Goding, J.W.: *Monoclonal Antibodies: Principles and Practice*, Academic Press (1986).
11. Oldfather, J., Mora, A., Phelan, D. *et al.*: The occurrences of cross reactive 'public' antibodies in sera of highly sensitised patients. *Transplant. Proc.* **15**, 1212 (1983).
12. Jeannet, M. and Stalder, H.: Lymphocytotoxic antibodies in spontaneous cytomegalovirus infection. *Lancet* **1**, 509 (1978).
13. MacLeod, A.M., Kurtz, J., Chapman, J.R. *et al.*: Autolymphocytotoxins and virus infection in renal transplantation. *Transplant. Proc.* **19**, 901 (1987).
14. Ozturk, G. and Terasaki, P.I.: Cytotoxic antibodies against surface immunoglobulin. *Transplantation* **29**, 140 (1980).
15. Naito, S., Mickey, M.R., Hirata, A. and Terasaki, P.I.: Autolymphocytotoxins following immunization by pregnancy, transplantation, and disease. *Tissue Antigens* **1**, 219 (1971).
16. McHeyzer-Williams, M.G. and Nossal, G.J.V.: Clonal analysis of autoantibody-producing cell precursors in the preimmune B cell repertoire. *J. Immunol.* **141**, 4118 (1988).
17. Underwood, J.R., Pedersen, J.S., Chalmers, P.J. and Toh, B.H.: Hybrids from normal, germ free, nude and neonatal mice produce monoclonal autoantibodies to eight different intracellular structures. *Clin. Exp. Immunol.* **60**, 417 (1985).
18. Lobo, P.I.: Nature of autolymphocytotoxins present in renal hemodialysis patients. Their possible role in controlling alloantibody formation. *Transplantation* **32**, 233. (1981).

9. Idiotypic-antiidiotypic antibody interaction and renal transplant survival

I.A. AL-MUZAIRAI, A.A. MACLEOD, M. MACMILLAN,
K.N. STEWART and G.R.D. CATTO

Introduction

Lymphocytotoxic antibodies may develop following blood transfusions, pregnancies or failed allografts (1). The presence of such cytotoxic HLA antibodies in the pretransplant serum is almost always associated with rapid rejection of the kidney transplant.

We and others have shown previously, that the disappearance of such antibodies is associated with the development of antiidiotypic antibodies (Ab2) (2, 3). Moreover, the presence of antiidiotypic activity (Ab2) before transplantation is associated with improved renal allograft survival (4, 5). In one study, potentiating (Ab3) antibodies have been also detected in non-cytotoxic pretransplant sera in previously highly sensitized patients and their presence was associated with poor graft outcome (4). These studies supported previous work indicating that the humoral and cellular immune responses to HLA antigens are suppressed by antiidiotypic autoimmune reactions.

The aim of this study, was to determine the presence of either antiidiotypic antibodies (Ab2) or potentiating antibodies (Ab3) in pretransplant sera in patients who were not highly sensitized.

Patients

We studied pretransplant sera from 82 recipients of cadaver transplantation who were also given third-party blood transfusion prior to transplantation. Transplants were carried out when the crossmatch was negative using current and stored sera. The details of patients studied are shown in Table 1.

Materials and methods

The methods used for determination of antiidiotypic antibodies (Ab2) and

Table 1. The influence of clinical factors on transplant outcome.

	Group 1 Survival > 1 year	Group 2 Survival < 1 year
Overall	64 (78%)	18 (22%)
First graft[a]	58 (83%)	12 (17%)
Subsequent graft[a]	6 (50%)	6 (50%)
Therapy:		
Cyclosporine	36 (85%)	6 (14%)
Conventional	28 (70%)	12 (30%)
Mismatched antigens:		
A Locus	1.2 ± 0.8	1.5 ± 0.7
B Locus	1.4 ± 0.6	1.3 ± 0.6
DR Locus	0.7 ± 0.6	0.8 ± 0.7
Blood transfusion[b]:		
Overall	10.45 ± 9.52	16.66 ± 14.64
First graft	10.87 ± 8.87	16.08 ± 12.01
Subsequent graft	21.16 ± 13.52	25.06 ± 21.27

[a] $p < 0.05$ χ^2 test.
[b] Student 't' test: NS.

potentiating activity (Ab3) to cytotoxic HLA antibodies have been previously described (2, 6).

Results

Overall transplant survival at one year was 78% and the outcome was not influenced by the number of HLA antigens mismatched between donor and recipient (Table 1). In addition there was no significant correlation between allograft survival and the type of routine post-transplant immunosuppression or the number of transfusions administered before transplantation. Eighty-five percent of first grafts were functioning at one year compared with 50% of second or subsequent transplants; this difference was statistically significant ($p < 0.05$) (Table 1).

Eighty-two sera obtained before transplantation were tested for inhibitory (Ab2) or potentiating (Ab3) activity using the methods described previously.

Alloantibody activity

None of the 82 pretransplant sera possessed cytotoxic activity to any of the target cells tested. Sera from 17 (20.7%) patients showed alloantibody activity and these were excluded from further analysis.

Antiidiotypic antibody activity

Pretransplant sera from 65 patients were tested SAA for inhibitory (Ab2) or potentiating (Ab3) activity. Sera from 30 (36.5%) patients showed inhibitory activity against at least one of the target cells tested. Twenty-eight of the transplants were functioning one year later and 2 had failed (Table 2). Ab2 activity was shown to reside in the $F(ab')_2$ fragment of the IgG serum fraction prepared from two active sera.

Seventeen patients showed neither Ab2 nor Ab3 activity in their pretransplant sera in any of the sera/cell combinations tested. Eleven transplants from these patients survived one year and 6 failed. The difference in allograft survival between those with Ab2 activity and those with no antibody in their pretransplant serum was statistically significant ($p < 0.05$).

Potentiation of lymphocytotoxicity (Ab3 activity) was present in pretransplant sera from 18 patients. Since we had previously shown that several sera showing low grade lymphocytotoxicity detected only in the antihuman globulin CDC (AHG-CDC) assay could mimic potentiating activity (2, 6), all 18 sera were tested in AHG-CDC. Sera from 2 patients were positive and they were excluded from further analysis. Grafts in 11 of the 16 patients belonging to this group survived for one year and 5 failed. There was no significant difference in transplant survival between those showing potentiating activity and those in whom no antibodies were detected (Table 2). Furthermore, the immunosuppressive regime given to those showing Ab2 or Ab3 activity had no influence on allograft survival.

Table 2. The influence of antiidiotypic antibodies (Ab2) and potentiating activity (Ab3) on renal allograft survival rates.

	Survival		Total	Survivors (%)
	> 1 year	< 1 year		
Ab2 activity	28	2	30	93[a]
Ab3 activity	11	5	16	68[b]
No Ab activity	11	6	17	65

[a] $p < 0.05$ χ^2 test with Yates' correction.
[b] *p*: NS.

Discussion

This study shows that the presence of antiidiotypic activity in sera obtained before transplantation is associated with improved transplant outcome. Graft survival in patients showing antiidiotypic activity (Ab2) was significantly better than in those showing either potentiating activity (Ab3) or no antibody activity in their pretransplant serum. There was no difference in graft survival between those whose sera showed potentiating activity and those with no antibody activity at all in their pretransplant serum. This indicates that potentiating activity (Ab3) was not an independent predictor of transplant failure.

Although renal transplant survival has improved during the last 5 years around 20% of transplants fail in the first year largely because of immunological rejection. It has been extensively demonstrated in animal studies that blood transfusions given before grafting improve kidney transplant survival (7). Furthermore, the survival of a one haplotype mismatched transplant from a related donor is now equal to one matched for both haplotypes; this improvement has been achieved by giving transfusions of blood from the potential donor before transplantation (8). Third-party transfusion has also been shown to improve the survival of kidney transplants from cadaver donors (9). Overall transplant survival in the present study was 78% at one year and all patients had been transfused at least 5 units blood (mean = 10.49 ∝ units).

Why transfusions improve allograft survival is unclear but several mechanisms may be involved. We have already shown that non-cytotoxic Fc receptor blocking antibodies occur after third-party transfusion before cadaver donor transplantation and after donor specific transfusion (10, 11). The presence of such antibodies in pretransplant sera correlates with improved renal allograft survival particularly when recipients are less well matched for HLA antigens with their donors. Such antibodies however are not present in sera from all patients with successful graft outcome and hence we have sought the presence of antiidiotypic activity in pretransplant sera. We have previously shown that antiidiotypic activity can occur after donor specific transfusion in patients who go on to receive a successful one haplotype mismatched transplant from a living related donor (6).

In a further study we have found that non-cytotoxic sera obtained from transfused dialysis patients were able to decrease the cytotoxic activity of autologous sera obtained when the patients were highly sensitized (2). The development of antiidiotypic activity may explain why fluctuating titres of cytotoxic antibodies are found in sera from sensitized patients.

Reed and co-workers showed that, non-cytotoxic pretransplant serum could either inhibit or potentiate cytotoxicity present in stored serum. Where inhibition occurred the graft was successful, if potentiation occurred, it failed. They concluded therefore that antibodies of the idiotypic/antiidiotypic network predicted the ultimate outcome of transplants in these patients (4). The present study however shows that in the majority of renal patients whose sera have never shown cytotoxicity to donor HLA antigens inhibitory activity in the SAA also is associated with improved transplant outcome. Allograft survival in such patients was 93% at one year, and no additional beneficial effect of cyclopsporine A was found.

It is possible that non-cytotoxic alloantibodies or non-specific rheumatoid factors could block the activity of cytotoxic antibodies and thus mimic antiidiotypic activity. In this study therefore all sera were screened for alloantibody activity and any sera were positive for alloantibody were excluded from analysis. In the present study and in our previous work we have shown inhibitory activity to reside in the F $(ab)_2$ fragment of the IgG fraction of serum which makes non-specific inhibition by rheumatoid factors unlikely.

Antiidiotypic antibodies (Ab2) are believed to act by binding to determinants within the variable region of the combining site of HLA antibodies (Ab1). Ab2 can thus inhibit the binding of Ab1 to HLA antigens (12). Other immunosuppressive properties of Ab2 may be mediated by their ability to bind to the variable region of idiotypic receptors expressed on activated T lymphocytes producing Ab1 (12, 13).

The existence of Ab3 or 'anti-antiidiotypic' antibodies has been proposed by Jerne in his original network hypothesis (14). Reed and co-workers have proposed that non-cytotoxic sera might contain Ab3 which could mediate the release of Ab1 from Ab1—Ab2 complexes present in the Ab1-positive sera thus potentiating its cytotoxic activity (3). In the present study we were able to detect potentiating activity in sera from 16 patients and although graft survival in this group was worse than in those showing Ab2 activity it was not significantly different from those in whom no antibody activity was detected (Table 2). Furthermore, we have previously found potentiating activity in sera from patients who had received donor specific transfusion and all subsequent transplants from their specific living related donors were successful (6). Anti-antiidiotypic antibodies (Ab3) have been described previously as part of a network of antibody responses to transplantation antigens in animal studies (12, 13). Ab3 was shown to inhibit the binding of Ab2 to Ab1 rather than the release of Ab1 from Ab1—Ab2 complexes (12, 15). Furthermore, no rejection was observed in animals expressing high titre of Ab3 in their sera and who subsequently received skin transplant (15). The role of 'anti-antiidiotypic antibodies' (Ab3) in clinical transplantation therefore requires further investigation.

We conclude therefore that antiidiotypic antibodies can be determined before transplantation in patients who have not previously been sensitized to donor HLA antigens; the presence of antiidiotypic activity correlated with improved allograft survival whereas potentiating activity was not an indicator of poor transplant outcome.

References

1. Opelz, G., Graver, B., Mickey, R. and Terasaki, P.I.: Lymphocytotoxic antibody responses to transfusions in potential kidney transplant recipients. *Transplantation* **32**, 177—183 (1982).
2. Al-Muzairai, I.A., MacLeod, A.M., Innes, A. *et al.*: Antiidiotypic activity in sera from sensitised potential transplant recipients. *Nephrol. Dial. Transplant.* **3**, 803—808 (1988).

3. Reed, E., Hardy, M., Brensilver, J., Lattes, C., McCabe, I., D'gati, V., Reemtsma, K. and Suciu-Foca, N.: Anti-idiotypic antibodies to HLA and their influence on patient sensitisation. *Transplant. Proc.* **19**, 762—763 (1987).
4. Ree, E., Hardy, M., Benvenisty, A. *et al.*: Effect of antiidiotypic antibodies to HLA on graft survival in renal allograft recipients. *New Engl. J. Med.* **316**, 1450—1455 (1987).
5. Rodey G. and Phelan D.: Association of antiidiotypic antibody with successful second transplant of a kidney sharing HLA antigens with the previous hyperacutely rejected first kidney. *Transplantation* **48**, 54—57 (1989).
6. Al-Muzairai, I.A., Innes, A., Hillis, A. *et al.*: Renal transplantation: Cyclosporin A and antibody development after donor specific transfusion. *Kidney International* **34**, 1057—1063 (1989).
7. Fabre J.W. and Morris P.J.: The effect of donor strain blood pretreatment renal allograft rejection in rats. *Transplantation* **14**, 608—617 (1973).
8. Salvatierra O., Vincenti F. and Amend W. Deliberate donor specific transfusion prior to living related transplantation. *Ann. Surg.* **192**, 543—555 (1980).
9. Opelz G.: Current relevance of transfusion effect in renal transplantation. *Transplant. Proc.* **17**, 1015—1022 (1985).
10. MacLeod A.M., Power, D.A., Mason, R.J., *et al.*: Possible mechanism of action of transfusion effect in renal transplantation. *Lancet* **ii**, 468—470 (1982).
11. MacLeod A.M., Hillis, A., Mather, A., Bone, J.M. and Catto G.R.D.: Effect of cyclosporin, third party blood transfusion and pregnancy on antibody development after donor-specific transfusion before renal transplantation. *Lancet* **1**, 416—418 (1987).
12. Bluestone J.A., Leo, O., Epstein, S.L. and Sachs, D.H.: Idiotypic manipulation of the immune response to transplantation antigens. *Immunol. Rev.* **90**, 5—27 (1986).
13. Singal, D.P., Blajchman, M.A., Joseph, S. *et al.*: Production in vitro of antibodies directed against alloantigen-specific recognition sites on T cells and on lymphocytotoxic HLA antibodies. *Clin. Exp. Immunol.* **72**, 222—227 (1988).
14. Jerne, N.K.: Towards a network theory of the immune system. *Ann. Immunol. (Paris).* **125C**, 373—379 (1974).
15. Bluestone, J.A., Sharrow, S.O., Epstein, S.L., Ozato, L. and Sachs, D.H.: Induction of anti-H-2 antibodies in the absence of alloantigen exposure by in vivo administration of anti-idiotype. *Nature (London)* **291**, 233—234 (1981).

10. Transplantation and blood transfusion in 1990

ROBERT J. CORRY

In 1973, Gerhard Opelz demonstrated the favorable effect of preoperative blood transfusion in improving renal allograft survival by as much as 20% (1). He further showed that success was linearly related to the number of blood transfusions and graft survival rates of close to 80% could be achieved with ten or more units of transfusions administered prior to the operation (2). In retrospect, these data were even more striking in that it could be achieved in the pre-cyclosporine era using only azathioprine and prednisone. It was further noted that the effect was greater than could be accomplished by simply exclusion of those patients who were sensitized from the blood transfusions. Following this, a rash of papers were written showing a similar effect achieved by blood transfusion in animal models. In addition, a number of large centers looked at data retrospectively and showed the favorable effect by comparing their own patients who were transfused with those who had received no blood. Our own data in the mid-1970s showed a 50% success rate in patients who were not transfused, compared to a 70% rate of success in the transfused patients (3).

It will be the purpose of this manuscript to outline the history of the blood transfusion effect as well as provide some evidence that it may be related to suppressor cell induction. Most of this work has been presented elsewhere, and the following will represent a review of those data as well as some theoretical evidence supporting the concept of transfusion-induced suppressor cells as a possible mechanism for the transfusion effect.

Selected historical evidence

Prior to 1973, transfusions were avoided in patients awaiting transplantation because of the risk of sensitization. However, Opelz and Terasaki presented evidence at the International Congress of the Transplantation Society in San Francisco in 1972 that transfusions had a favorable, rather than unfavorable effect on graft outcome (1). In fact, there was a close to 35% spread in comparing patients who had no transfusions with those who received over ten transfusions. They further showed a few years later that the success rate was directly proportional to the number of units of blood, showing close to an 80% success rate with >20 units of blood compared to around 40% graft success rate in patients who were not transfused (2), a doubling of graft survival at one year in patients who were multiply transfused. This effect was substantially more than could be achieved by exclusion of the sensitized recipients, since only a small percent of those nulliparous patients became sensitized from transfusions.

Several single-center studies, including our own, showed that success was approximately 15—20% better in patients who had received prior transfusions, compared to those who were never transfused (3). We further showed by retrospective analysis that patients who were transfused only intraoperatively had approximately a 15% better success rate than those who were never transfused at all (4). Moreover, preoperative blood seemed to produce an intermediate effect between those who were given prior transfusions and those who were never transfused. For example, patients who were given prior transfusions had a 70% success rate compared with 60% survival of those who were transfused only during the operation, and those who were never transfused had a 45% success rate. Our center was also involved at this time in genotyping donor families and those patients who received single haplotype-matched kidneys as well as transfusions had a 30% better success rate than those who received poorly-matched kidneys and were never transfused (5). Other investigators were showing a beneficial effect of preoperative transfusion as well. The most significant work was performed by Williams and others at Oxford showing a 30% better graft success rate in patients who received intentional preoperative transfusions with those who were never transfused (6). Because of the beneficial effect of transfusions and the suggestion that preoperative transfusions might be effective, we elected to conduct a prospective randomized protocol to compare preoperative transfusions with intraoperative transfusions. Patients were randomized who had never received transfusions. In Group A, namely those receiving preoperative transfusions, were transfused with three units and became eligible for transplantation at one month. Group B patients were transfused only during the operation with 2—3 units of packed erythrocytes. Patients were excluded who were sensitized beyond 10% and those with low hematocrits. Fortuitously, 26 patients in each group were transplanted. Four of the transfused group had been sensitized, and were not transplanted. Patient survival was above 90% in both groups, but graft survival was 85% in the transfused group and only 64% in the group transfused during the operation (7). Therefore, this randomized study showed a substantial benefit in patients who were given prior transfusions, but did not support the thesis that intraoperative transfusions were effective.

We further showed prior to the cyclosporine era that the combined effect of HLA-A, B and DR matching with blood transfusions led to a surprising 87%

graft success rate in 38 patients who had been matched for three out of six antigens and were given prior transfusions (8, 9).

The benefit of donor transfusions in single haplotype-matched donor-recipient combinations was shown first by Salvatierra (10). His group showed a success rate approaching that of HLA-identical donor-recipient combinations, and Anderson later showed that the sensitization rate could be reduced to 7% by giving azathioprine during the transfusion (11).

Therefore, the effect of transfusion was clear. Graft success rates could be improved by almost 20%, and the combination of other factors, such as matching and transfusion, yielded even greater success rates. The stage was set for national sharing based on matching, and most centers were converted to using prior transfusions in a systematic fashion. The favorable effect of preoperative transfusion was thought to be not as strong as prior transfusion, but nevertheless had not been disproved totally. Frisk *et al.* hypothesized that there might be some beneficial effect in patients who had received kidneys from donors who had multiple transfusions (12). An analysis of our own data as well as others showed that this, in fact, could not be confirmed, and there was no difference between those patients who received kidneys from transfused donors versus those who received kidneys from non-transfused donors (13).

The mechanism of transfusion

Our group was attracted to the concept that while the beneficial effect may be due to multiple factors, suppressor cell induction certainly occurred. We used the mouse heart transplant model to show the beneficial effect of donor-specific transfusion (DST) given one week prior to the transplant (14). We also showed that when the spleen was removed one week prior to the donor-specific transfusion, the transfusion effect was totally abrogated (15). By performing adoptive transfer techniques, we were able to show that spleen cells removed from recipients who had been transfused and had prolonged survival of heart grafts were effective in prolonging graft survival in syngeneic recipients who were transplanted with the same donor strain graft (15). Spleen cells themselves could confer an immunosuppressive effect on syngeneic recipients receiving the same allogeneic heart graft. Thus, the fact that splenectomy one week before DST abrogates the transfusion effect in this animal model, and that spleen cells adoptively transferred can confer suppression, provided fairly conclusive evidence that some form of splenic suppressor cell existed.

We further showed that in certain donor–recipient strain combinations, suppressors cells were demonstrated to be non-specific (16). We concluded that although these suppressor cells were highly specific in most circumstances, they can confer suppression to third-party grafts when the grafts are not totally incompatible at H_2K, I, and D regions.

The cyclosporine era

Cyclosporine emerged in the early 1980s and became the universal immunosuppressive agent. At the International Congress of the Transplantation Society in Helsinki in 1986, Opelz, who originated the concept of the transfusion effect in clinical transplantation, showed evidence that the transfusion effect was reduced to $<10\%$ when comparing non-transfused patients with those who had received >20 units packed erythrocytes. It seemed clear that while there was a transfusion effect, cyclosporine was so effective in improving success rates that the effect was no longer as evident. We analyzed our own data and were unable to show an effect during the cyclosporine era. We were able to show, however, that those patients who received <3 transfusions compared to those who received $\geqslant 3$ had more rejection episodes and required more OKT3 (unpublished data).

In our laboratory, working with the spleen-pancreas transplant model in rats, Wakely was able to show that the combination of pretransplant donor-specific tranfusion and pancreas—spleen allotransplantation was able to totally eliminate a fatal graft-versus-host response that occurred when transfusions were not given prior to allogeneic pancreas—spleen transplantation. She further demonstrated that the combination of prior transfusions, pancreas—spleen transplantation, and a brief course of cyclosporine could not only eliminate graft-versus-host disease (GVHD), but confer permanent engraftment (17).

Summary

It is probably clear to all transplanters that, before the cyclosporine era, prior transfusion of the recipient was a very powerful means of improving graft survival. However, with the advent of cyclosporine, OKT3, and now perhaps 15-deoxyspergualin or FK-506, transfusion will probably not be worth the risk. In certain select situations, however, it may still prove to be effective, such as in eliminating graft-versus-host disease in combination with splenic allotransplantation, or in patients who are sensitized while receiving transfusions who later have declining antibody titers. These patients are clearly preferred recipients. Nevertheless, like most advances in technology, it appears that transfusion has served its purpose and will no longer be used, at least on the same widespread basis it was during the 1970s and the 1980s.

References

1. Opelz, G., Sengar, D.P.S., Mickey, M.R. and Terasaki, P.I.: Effect of blood transfusions on subsequent kidney transplants. *Transplant. Proc.* **5**, 253—259 (1973).

2. Opelz, G. and Terasaki, P.I.: Improvement of kidney graft survival with increased numbers of blood transfusions. *New Engl. J. Med.* **299**, 799—803 (1978).
3. Freeman, R.M. Thompson, J.S. and Corry, R.J.: Effect of RBC transfusion on cadaver renal allograft survival. *Trans. Amer. Soc. Artif. Intern. Organs* **23**, 437—441 (1977).
4. Corry, R.J., West, J.C., Hunsicker, L.G., Schanbacher, B.A. and Lachenbruch, P.A.: Effect of timing of administration and quantity of blood transfusion on cadaver renal transplant survival. *Transplantation* **30**, 425—428 (1980).
5. Oei, L.S., Thompson, J.S. and Corry, R.J.: Effect of blood transfusions on survival of cadaver and living related renal transplants. *Transplantation* **28**, 482—484 (1979).
6. Williams, K.A., Ting, A., French, M.E., Oliver, D. and Morris, P.J.: Preoperative blood transfusions improve cadaveric renal-allograft survival in non-transfused recipients. *Lancet* May, 1104—1106 (1980).
7. Corry, R.J. and Hunsicker, L.G.: Preoperative transfusions, *Transplant Proc.* **20**(6), 1079—1081 (1988).
8. Schulak, J.A., Goeken, N.E., Nghiem, D.D. and Corry, R.J.: Successful DR-incompatible cadaver kidney transplantation: combined effect of HLA-A and B matching and blood transfusion. *Transplantation* **38**(6), 649—653 (1984).
9. Corry, R.J., Schulak, J.A., Goeken, N.E. and Nghiem, D.D.: The effect of HLA-A, B and DR matching and blood transfusion status in first cadaver kidney transplantation. *Transplant. Proc.* **17**(1), 756—757 (1985).
10. Salvatierra, O., Vicenti, F., Amend, W., Garovoy, M., Iwaki, Y., Terasaki, P., Potter, D., Duca, R., Hopper, S., Slemmer, T. and Feduska, N.: Four-year experience with donor-specific blood transfusions. *Transplant Proc.* **15**(1), 924—931 (1983).
11. Anderson, C.B., Tyler, J.D., Rodey, G.E., Etheredge, E.E., Anderman, C.K., Flye, M.W., Jendrisak, M.D. and Sicard, G.A.: Preoperative immunomodulation of renal allograft recipients by concomitant immunosuppression and donor-specific transfusions. *Transplant Proc.* **19**(1), 1494—1497 (1987).
12. Frisk, B., Berglin, E. and Bryner, H.: Positive effect on graft survival of transfusions to the cadaveric kidney donor. *Transplantation* **32**, 252—255 (1981).
13. Berg, K.R., Nghiem, D.D. and Corry, R.J.: Effect of transfusion of donor on allograft survival. *Transplantation* **34**(6), 344—346 (1982).
14. Wakely, E., Shelby, J. and Corry, J.: The effect of peripheral blood components on allograft survival. *Transplantation* **40**(1), 113—114 (1985).
15. Shelby, J., Wakely, E. and Corry, R.J.: Suppressor cell induction in donor-specific transfused mouse heart recipients. *Surgery* **96**, 296—301 (1984).
16. Wakely, E., Cutkomp, J. and Corry, R.J.: Are DST/allograft-induced suppressor cells donor-specific? *Transplant Proc.* **21**(1), 488—489 (1989).
17. Wakely, E., Oberholser, J.H. and Corry, R.J.: Elimination of acute GVHD and prolongation of rat pancreas allograft survival with DST, cyclosporine, and spleen transplantation. *Transplantation* **49**, 241—245 (1990).

11. Quadruple-drug immunosuppressive induction treatments for immunological high-risk patients in cadaveric renal transplantation using poly- and monoclonal antibodies

H. SCHNEEBERGER, S. SCHLEIBNER, L. FRIEDL, M. SCHILLING, W.D. ILLNER, D. ABENDROTH and W. LAND

Introduction

The rates for graft survival in cadaveric renal transplantation became much better after the introduction of cyclosporine (CsA) into clinical immunosuppression. Although 1-year graft survival rates rose about 15% (1) with CsA as the main-immunosuppresant compared to azathioprine-immunosuppressed allograft-recipients, the same observation could not be made for immunological high-risk allograft-recipients. In our clinic these patients remained, even under CsA and triple drug immunosuppressive induction treatment, the group with poor and unsatisfying results. Therefore in 1985 we decided to apply an immunosuppressive induction treatment consisting of four drugs to those patients. In addition to the three 'traditional' drugs (CsA, azathioprine, steroids), we first applied one of the commercially available polyclonal antibodies during the first post-transplant week. Our intention was to reduce the capacity of immune response as early as possible after the patient had received his allograft. We expected from this potent immunosuppression in the very early phase after transplantation, a reduction of the frequency of untreatable rejection crises at no higher risk from dangerous infections. Later we used also monoclonal antibodies for this kind of immunosuppressive induction therapy. In 1986 we also started to give quadruple drug immunosuppressive induction in immunological non-risk patients, whose grafts were found to be initially non-functioning kidneys (Gr. 6). As the percentage of non- or late-detected rejection episodes is higher in patients with initially non-functioning grafts, we decided to give quadruple drug immunosuppressive induction therapy also to patients with this particular higher risk to reject the graft, when objective function parameters are still missing. This report includes most of the experience we made in quadruple drug immunosuppressive induction between 1985 to 1989.

Patients and methods

Immunological high-risk patients

Ninety-seven consecutive recipients of cadaveric renal transplants were considered to be immunological high-risk patients because they had either elevated levels of preformed cytotoxic antibodies (greater than 30%), or they were candidates for retransplantation and it was known that they had lost their former graft in an acute rejection crisis within 6 months after transplantation. Seventy-seven patients had panel reactivity of more than 30% (mean 66%) and 69 patients received a second or multiple graft (mean 2.2). Mean panel reactivity in all patients was 53% (range 0—99%) and the number of transplantations ranged from 1 to 4 (mean 1.9). There were 50 males (mean age 37 years (17—67 years)) and 47 females (mean age 40 years (19—72 years)) in this patient group. Prior to transplantation all of them were on hemodialysis treatment for 7.2 years on average (1.2—16.9 years). We defined four groups based on the different antibodies used as immunosuppressant: (Gr. 1) ALG group (n = 29), (Gr. 2) ATG group (n = 39), (Gr. 3) OKT_3 group (n = 20), (Gr. 4) BMA 031 group (n = 9). We compared the results in these groups to a historical group (Gr. 5) of recipients (n = 61), who were considered to be immunological high-risk patients following the same criteria as mentioned above.

The demographic and immunologic characteristics of the patient groups are listed in Table 1. The groups did not significantly differ in sex, age, panel reactivity, number of transplantations, number of mismatches and graft preser-

Table 1. Patient groups with immunological high-risk: demographics and immunologic characteristics.

	Triple drugs:	Quadruple drug induction			
	historical group (Gr. 5)	ALG group (Gr. 1)	ATG group (Gr. 2)	OKT_3 group (Gr. 3)	BMA 031 group (Gr. 4)
No. of patients	61	29	39	20	9
Sex and age:					
Male	41	12	24	9	5
Mean age (yr)	36	36	38	38	36
Female	20	17	15	11	4
Mean age (yr)	35	36	40	44	43
Duration of hemodialysis (yr)	4.2	7.0	7.8	5.9	5.8
Mean PRA (%)	47	57	59	40	60
Mean No. Tx	1.8	1.9	2.3	1.7	1.6
HLA mismatch:					
Median on A and B	1	2	2		2
Median on DR	0	1	1	0	0
Graft preservation:					
c.i.t. (h)	28	24	23	24	24
2w.i.t. (min)	33	30	28	28	30

vation times. Patients in quadruple groups (Grs. 1—4) were on average longer on hemodialysis treatment than the patients of the historic group (Gr. 5).

Basic immunosuppressive therapy. All quadruple drug groups received the same basic immunosuppression, which was a combination of CsA, azathioprine and methylprednisolone.

CsA was first applied post-transplant as a 24-hour infusion containing 1.5 mg CsA/kg/BW, followed by oral medication using a starting dose of 6 mg/kg/BW/day.

Azathioprine was first given intraoperatively as a injection of 2 mg/kg/BW and then daily for at least 21 days in the same amount until serum-creatinine was below 3 mg% and CsA trough-levels were at adequate range.

Methylprednisolone was given as 250 mg injection just before graft-reperfusion and then the following days in decreasing doses from 500 mg/day to a maintenance dose of 20 mg daily for the first 3 months. Then it was reduced to 10—5 mg/day or even withdrawn.

Antibody administration in the different immunosuppressive protocols (Grs. 1—5). (Gr. 1) ALG group (n = 29): 7 daily doses of ALG (Pressimmun^{R}) at 20 mg/kg/BW were given intravenously on postoperative day 1 to 7.

(Gr. 2) ATG group (n = 39): 7 day doses of ATG (Fresenius^{R}) at 4 mg/kg/BW were given intravenously on postoperative day 1 to 7.

(Gr. 3) OKT_3 group (n = 20): 7 daily does of OKT_3 (Orthoclone^{R}) at 5 mg each were given intravenously on postoperative day 1 to 7.

(Gr. 4) BMA 031 group (n = 9): 7 daily doses of BMA 031 (Behring AG, F.R.G.) at 5 mg each were given intravenously on postoperative day 1 to 7.

(Gr. 5) Historical group (n = 61): These patients had received triple-drug immunosuppressive induction and no prophylactic antibody application. The intravenous CsA infusion postoperatively contained 2 mg/kg/BW and the oral starting dose was 14—17 mg/kg/BW. Azathioprine and methylprednisolone were given according to the protocol mentioned above. But the methylprednisolone maintenance dose was 40 mg daily.

Patients with acute renal failure post-transplant delayed-ALG group (Gr. 6) and control group (Gr. 7)

Sixty recipients of cadaveric renal allografts (Gr. 6), whose kidney-graft function showed acute anuric or obliguric renal failure until the fifth day after transplantation are included in this studied series. There are 42 males (mean age 49 years (26—66 years)) and 18 females (mean age 44 years (23—64 years)) in this patient group. Pretransplant, all of them were on hemodialysis treatment for 4.2 years on average (0.9—13.4 years). As they were immunological normal-risk patients the mean panel reactivity was low at 2% and most of the patients received their first graft (mean No. Tx. 1.1). Cold-ischemia time (c.i.t.) was 28 h on average and 2.warm-ischemia time (2w.i.t.) was 34 min. (mean). All patients in this group received, in addition to the triple drug therapy, ALG (Pressimmun[R]) in a delayed form from day 5 to 12 after transplantation. We compared the results of this group to another control group of 218 patients (Gr. 7) who would have fullfilled the same inclusion criteria, but had not been treated with a fourth immunosuppressant. The demographic and immunological characteristics are in good agreement with those of the delayed-ALG group (Gr. 6). A detailed listing is presented in Table 2.

Table 2. Patient groups with acute renal failure post-transplant: demographics and immunologic characteristics.

	Triple drug: historical group (Gr. 7)	Quadruple drug induction: delayed-ALG group (Gr. 6)
No. of patients	218	60
Sex and age:		
Male	145	42
Mean age (yr)	46	49
Female	73	18
Mean age (yr)	45	44
Duration of hemodialysis (yr)	4.5	4.2
Mean PRA (%)	2	2
Mean No. Tx	1.0	1.1
HLA mismatch:		
Median on A and B	1	1
Median on DR	0	0
Graft preservation:		
c.i.t. (h)	27	28
2w.i.t. (min)	33	34

Basic immunosuppressive therapy delayed-ALG group (Gr. 6) and control group (Gr. 7). All patients in this series received the same basic immunosuppression, which was a combination of CsA, azathioprine and methylprednisolone.

CsA was first applied post-transplantationally as a 24 hour infusion containing 1.5 mg CsA/kg/BW, followed by oral medication using a starting dose of 6 mg/kg/BW/day.

Azathioprine was first given intraoperatively as a injection of 2 mg/kg/BW and then daily for at least 21 days in the same amount until serum-creatinine was below 3 mg% and CsA trough-levels were at an adequate range.

Methylprednisolone was given as 250 mg injection just before graft-reperfusion and then the following days in a maintenance dose of 20 mg daily for the first 3 months. Then it was reduced to 10—5 mg/day or even withdrawn.

Antibody application in the delayed-ALG group (Gr. 6). Sixty patients received the antibody ALG (Pressimmun[R]) from postoperative day 5 to 12 in a dose of 20 mg/kg/BW daily.

Results

Results in ALG group, ATG group, OKT_3 Group BMA 031 group and historical group (Grs. 1—5)

Graft and patient survival. The graft survival probability rate at 1 year is 79% in the ALG group, 74% in the ATG group, 63% in the OKT_3 group and 89% in the BMA 031 group. The graft survival probability rate at 2 years is 71% in the ALG group, 66% in the ATG group, 63% in the OKT_3 group and 78% in the BMA 031 group. The survival rates in the OKT_3 group are not significantly inferior to those in the ALG and ATG groups. The actuarial graft survival in the historical group was 55% for 1 year and 50% for 2 years (Table 3).

Table 3. Patient groups with immunological high-risk: graft outcome.

	Triple drugs:	Quadruple drug induction			
	historical group (Gr. 5)	ALG group (Gr. 1)	ATG group (Gr. 2)	OKT_3 group (Gr. 3)	BMA 031 group (Gr. 4)
No. of patients	61	29	39	20	9
Patients (*n*, %) with ATN	43 (70%)	17 (59%)	24 (62%)	12 (60%)	4 (44%)
Never functioning	9 (15%)	2 (7%)	3 (8%)	4 (20%)	0
Incidence of:					
no rejection	18 (30%)	13 (45%)	18 (46%)	14 (70%)	2 (22%)
steroid-sensitive rejection	21 (34%)	10 (34%)	13 (33%)	1 (5%)	0
steroid-resistant or antibody-resistant rejection	30 (49%)	6 (21%)	8 (21%)	5 (25%)	7 (78%)
Survival (%):					
1-year graft	55	79	74	63	89
2-year graft	50	71	66	63	78
1 year patient	93	96	97	100	100
2-year patient	92	96	95	100	100

The patient survival probability rate at 1 year is 96% in the ALG group, 97% in the ATG group, 100% in the OKT_3 group and 100% in the BMA 031 group. After 2 years it is 96% in the ALG group, 95% in the ATG group, 100% in the OKT_3 group and 100% in the BMA 031 group. In the ALG group 1 patient died during the first year. In the ALG group 1 patient died in the first and 1 in the second year. In the OKT_3 group and the BMA 031 group there have been no deaths so far. Although there have been 3 deaths in polyclonal antibody groups there is no significant difference between the groups. In the historical group there were 4 deaths in the first year (1 in the second year), so that actuarial patient survival is 93% for the first year and 92% for the second year. There is no significant difference between triple drug and quadruple drug groups (Table 3).

Incidence of acute renal failure. The incidence of acute renal failure (ATN) post-transplantations was 59% in the ALG group, 62% in the ATG group, 60% in the OKT3 group and 44% in the BMA 031 group. In the historical group the incidence of ATN was 70%. There is no significant difference in ATN incidence between the groups.

Incidence of never-functioning kidney grafts. The incidence of never-functioning grafts was 7% in the ALG group, 8% in the ATG group, 20% in the OKT_3 group and none in the BMA 031 group (15% in the historical group). There is no significant difference in the number of never-functioning kidney grafts between the groups.

Incidence of rejection. The percentage of patients who remained free of a rejection crisis were 45% in the ALG group, 46% in the ATG group, 70% in the OKT_3 group and 22% in the BMA 031 group. In the historical group 30% of patients had no rejection crisis. Results of the OKT_3 group are significantly ($p < 0.01$, χ^2) better compared to the historical group, but not to the other quadruple groups.

The incidence of steroid-sensitive rejections was 34% in the ALG group, 33% in the ATG group, 5% in the OKT_3 group and none in the BMA 031 group. In the historical group the incidence of steriod-sensitive rejection episodes was 34%. Only in the OKT_3 group is the incidence of steriod-sensitive rejection crises significantly ($p < 0.05$, χ^2) lower than in the historical group. In the quadruple drug groups there is no difference between the groups.

The incidence of steroid-resistant or antibody-resistant rejection crises were 21% in the ALG group, 21% in the ATG group, 25% in the OKT_3 group and 78% in the BMA 031 group. The historical group was 49%. The incidence of steroid-resistant or antibody-resistant is significantly ($p < 0.01$, χ^2) lower in the ALG and the ATG groups than in the historical group, not in the other groups. The high incidence in the BMA 031 group does not differ from the historical group, but is significantly ($p < 0.01$, χ^2) higher than in the polyclonal groups (Table 3).

Infections. Of all the patients, we only considered severe infections, such as pneumonia (legionella, pneumocystis or other), pyelonephritis, deep wound infections, complicated cytomegalovirus infections or severe herpes simplex infections. The rate of such infections was 24% in the ALG group, 31% in the ATG group, 30% in the OKT_3 group and 22% in the BMA 031 group. In the historical group the incidence of infection was 36%. The incidence of life-threatening infections was 7% in the ALG group, 8% in the ATG group, 5% in the OKT_3 group and none in the BMA 031 group. In the historical group 20% of the patients suffered from a dangerous infection. There are no differences in incidence of infections between the studied groups. A more detailed listing is presented in Table 4.

Table 4. Patient groups with immunological high-risk: infections.

	Triple drugs:	Quadruple drug induction			
	historical group (Gr. 5)	ALG group (Gr. 1)	ATG group (Gr. 2)	OKT_3 group (Gr. 3)	BMA 031 group (Gr. 4)
No. of patients	61	29	39	20	9
Incidence of:					
bacterial infection	12 (20%)	2 (7%)	6 (15%)	3 (15%)	1
CMV infection	6 (10%)	4 (14%)	4 (10%)	3 (15%)	1
herpes infection			1	1	
no infection	39 (64%)	22 (76%)	27 (69%)	14 (70%)	7 (78%)
life threatening infection	12 (20%)	2 (7%)	3 (8%)	1 (5%)	0

Results in the delayed-ALG group (Gr. 6) and the control group (Gr. 7)

Graft and patient survival. The graft survival probability rate at 1 year is 83% in the delayed-ALG group and 72% in the control group (Gr. 7). The 2 years rate is 71% in the delayed-ALG group and 67% in the control group (Gr. 7). The graft survival probability in the Delayed-ALG group does not differ significantly from the control group (Gr. 7) (Table 5).

The patient survival probability rate at 1 year is 96% in the delayed-ALG group and 97% in control group (Gr. 7). The 2 years patient survival probability rate is 93% in the delayed-ALG group and 94% in the control group. These rates are equal in both groups.

Table 5. Patient groups with acute renal failure post-transplant: graft outcome.

	Triple drug: historical group (Gr. 7)	Quadruple drug induction: delayed-ALG group (Gr. 6)
No. of patients	218	60
Never functioning	25 (11%)	5 (8%)
Incidence of:		
no rejection	126 (64%)	39 (58%)
steroid-sensitive rejection	74 (34%)	14 (23%)
steroid-resistant or antibody-resistant rejection	24 (12%)	7 (11%)
survival (%):		
1-year graft	72	83
2-year graft	67	71
1-year patient	97	96
2-year patient	94	93

Incidence of never-functioning kidney grafts. The incidence of never-functioning grafts was 8% in the delayed-ALG group and 11% in the control group (Gr. 7). There is no significant difference in number of never-functioning kidney grafts between the groups.

Incidence of rejection. The percentage of patients who remained free of a rejection crisis were 58% in the delayed-ALG group and 64% in the control group.

The incidence of steriod-sensitive rejections was 23% in the delayed-ALG group and 34% in the control group. There is no significant difference between the group.

The incidence of steroid-resistant or antibody-resistant rejection crises were 11% in the delayed-ALG group and 12% in the control group. (Table 5).

Infections. The incidence of infections were 23% in the delayed-ALG group and 21% in the control group. (Table 6).

Discussion

Immunologically high-risk patients

The studied patients and transplants are very comparable in demographic and immunological risk characteristics.

Table 6. Patient groups with acute renal failure post-transplant: infections.

	Triple drug: historical group (Gr. 7)	Quadruple drug induction: delayed-ALG group (Gr. 6)
No. of patients	218	60
Incidence of:		
bacterial infection	14 (6%)	9 (15%)
CMV infection	12 (6%)	4 (7%)
herpes infection	3 (1%)	0
fungal infection	1	0
no infection	172 (79%)	46 (77%)
life-threatening infection	12 (5%)	3 (6%)

The introduction of quadruple drug immunosuppressive induction therapy to immunological high-risk patients was effective to increase graft survival probability rates from 56 to 73% (on average through all quadruple drug groups) for 1 year, and from 50 to 66% for 2 years.

The kind of antibody used for quadruple drug immunosuppressive induction therapy appears to be secondary, because all studied groups showed better graft survival probability rates than the historical group.

Apparently, the results in the BMA 031 group are better than those of the other groups. But in the BMA 031 group, 7 out of 9 patients suffered from early and severe steroid-resistant rejection crisis. Therefore, 7 out of 9 patients received another polyclonal antibody anti-rejection therapy immediately after the BMA 031 induction therapy. One could call this immunosuppressive protocol almost a quintuple immunosuppressive induction. This fact, and the very small number of patients in that group, makes the comparison to the other groups difficult.

Except the BMA 031 group, all quadruple drug induction groups showed a higher percentage of patients who remained free from rejection crisis than the historical group; however, this fact could be proved by statistics only for the OKT_3 group. The same was found for the incidence of steriod-sensitive rejection episodes. Here also the OKT_3 group shows the best results, whereas in the other groups this incidence is the same as under triple drug induction therapy (2). The percentage of steriod-resistant or antibody-resistant rejections, what is in fact the frequency of antirejection therapies using another antibody, also appear lower in all quadruple drug immunosuppressive protocols, except the BMA 031 protocol, but could be proven by statistics only for the ATG group.

Even the patient survival probability rate seems to be higher when quadruple drug immunosuppressive induction therapy is used for immunologic high-risk patients than under 'traditional' triple-drug therapy (2).

To give an antibody in addition to the triple drug therapy does not change the incidence of initially non-functioning grafts, nor the incidence of never-functioning kidneys.

In regard to infections and life-threatening infections the data show a trend to even lower incidence of infections in all quadruple drug groups when they are compared to the historical group (2).

Patients with initially non-functioning grafts (Grs. 6, 7)

The graft survival probability rates first indicated a positive trend in favour to the quadruple drug treatment of the patients in the delayed-ALG group, but this initial advantage of 83 to 72% was not constant. The data of incidence of rejection episodes are similar in both groups. In this patient series we observed again no elevated risk for infections.

Conclusion

To administer a quadruple drug immunosuppressive induction therapy to immunological high-risk patients using antilymphocyte antibodies, provides better and fair results in graft survival probability. Actuarial annual graft survival rates of immunological high-risk patients became almost quite as high as those of normal-risk patients (Figure 1).

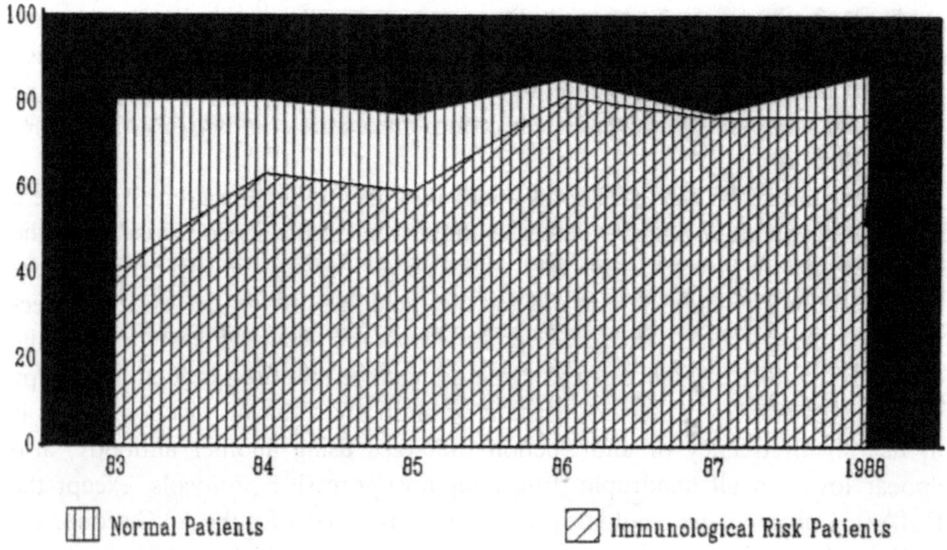

Fig. 1. One-year graft survival in immunological high- and normal-risk patients. *Source*: Transplantation Center, Munich, Germany.

There is no evidence that the incidence of infections is higher when quadruple drug immunosuppressive induction therapy is applied. On the contrary, it may be even lower.

It seems that quadruple drug induction therapy is able to reduce the frequency of rejection-episodes, especially the percentage of steroid-resistant rejection-episodes. Only in the BMA 031 group was the contrary observed, but after application of another antibody (most polyclonals) in sequence, 1-year graft survival showed the best result of all groups. Unfortunately we have the smallest number of patients in this interesting group.

The small numbers in each quadruple drug induction therapy group does not allow final evaluation of the biological agents used. We cannot determine from the present data if one antibody is superior to another, but we can see that polyclonal antibodies are not inferior to monoclonals.

There is no evidence that prophylactic quadruple drug induction therapy in immunological non-risk patients suffering from acute renal failure is superior to triple drug therapy.

References

1. European Multicentre Trial Group: Cyclosporin in cadaveric renal transplantation. One year follow-up of a multicentre trial. *Lancet* **ii**, 986—936 (1983).
2. Illner, W.D. *et al.*: Cyclosporine in combination with azathioprine and steroids in cadaveric renal transplantation. *Transplant. Proc.* **17** (1), 1181—1184 (1985).
3. Fries, D. *et al.*: A prospective study of a triple association: cyclosporine, corticosteriods, and azathioprine in immunologically high-risk renal transplantation. *Transplant. Proc.* **17** (1), 1231—1234 (1985).
4. Kupin, W. *et al.*: Use of cyclosporine and Minnesota antilymphoblast globolin in the early postoperative treatment of primary cadaveric renal transplant recipients. *Transplant. Proc.* **19** (1), 1882—1885 (1987).

12. Sequential combination immunotherapy for cadaveric renal transplantation: OKT3 versus rabbit ATG induction

M.P. POSNER, H.F. HENRIQUES, A.L. KING, Y. BERLATZKY, C. KLOSTERMAN, B.A.D. COOK and H.M. LEE

Introduction

In an effort to eliminate early cyclosporine (CyA) nephrotoxicity, and to avoid confusion of CyA toxicity with early rejection, interest in the use of combination drug protocols (1—5) and, more recently, 'sequential' combination drug protocols, has increased (6—11). In the induction phase of sequential combination immune suppression, antilymphocyte preparations are critical to ultimate success. Monoclonal antithymocyte preparations have obvious advantages: they are highly specific, uniform in quality (12, 13), and available in unlimited quantities. The theoretical advantages of polyclonal antilymphocyte induction therapy are twofold: first, it is more efficient in blunting the acute rejection response and inducing acquired immune tolerance because of its broad cellular and partial humoral specificities; second, its immunosuppressive effect may extend well beyond its administration period (11, 14).

Prophylactic monoclonal antibody use, specifically OKT3, is still somewhat experimental, but initial clinical studies show improved graft function without an increase in infection or rejection (6, 10, 16). Additionally, prophylactic induction use does not preclude later utilization in antirejection therapy (10, 15—18). Experience is more extensive and somewhat variable with anti-T cell polyclonal preparations (14). Recent studies of prophylactic antithymocyte globulin (ATG) suggest excellent graft function with diminished rejection and infection rates (9). Moreover, the reported tumorgenicity of ATG when used in conjunction with other immunosuppressive agents (19) has not been uniformly observed (9, 11, 20).

Although both prophylactic OKT3 or rabbit ATG sequential combination immunosuppressive protocols have been described, no group has compared these two preparations directly. Recently, Hanto *et al.* (20) have compared OKT3 and ALG with equivalent results. In this study, a sequential combination immunosuppressive regimen was used in patients receiving a cadaveric renal transplant, starting CyA as a maintenance immunosuppresant only when the graft was functioning well. Presented here is an 18 month experience with sequential combination immunotherapy using either ATG or OKT3, azathioprine (Aza), and prednisone (P) for induction, with delayed addition of CyA and triple drug therapy (Aza, P, CyA) for maintenance.

Patients and methods

Between January 1, 1986, and March 1, 1989, 108 consecutive cadaveric renal transplants were performed at the Medical College of Virginia (95 primary, 11 secondary, 2 tertiary). Twenty-five were excluded from this study: 10 (9.2%) for primary non-function and 15 (13.9%) for not meeting the criteria of either protocol group, leaving 83 patients for analysis. Patients were placed into groups in a sequential fashion based on availability of locally produced rabbit ATG (Table 1). Data was analyzed retrospectively. Fifty-six patients received ATG (Group 1), and 27 patients received OKT3 (Group 2) induction therapy (Figure 1). Follow-up was complete with a range of 2—27 months (mean 16.5 months). The two groups of patients were statistically similar in terms of age, race, sex, mean donor age, number of transfusions, number of primary transplants, preservation time, PRA, and ABDr match.

Immunosuppression protocols were broken into two phases — induction and maintenance. For induction, patients received either locally produced high potency rabbit ATG 100 mg/day for 5 days (Group 1, n = 56) or OKT3 (Ortho Pharmaceutical Inc., Raritan, N.J.) 5 mg/day for 7—14 days (Group 2, n = 27). Additionally, each group received P 1 mg/kg/day tapered every 3 days by 5mg to reach 20 mg/day by day 30, and Aza 3 mg/kg/day adjusted to keep

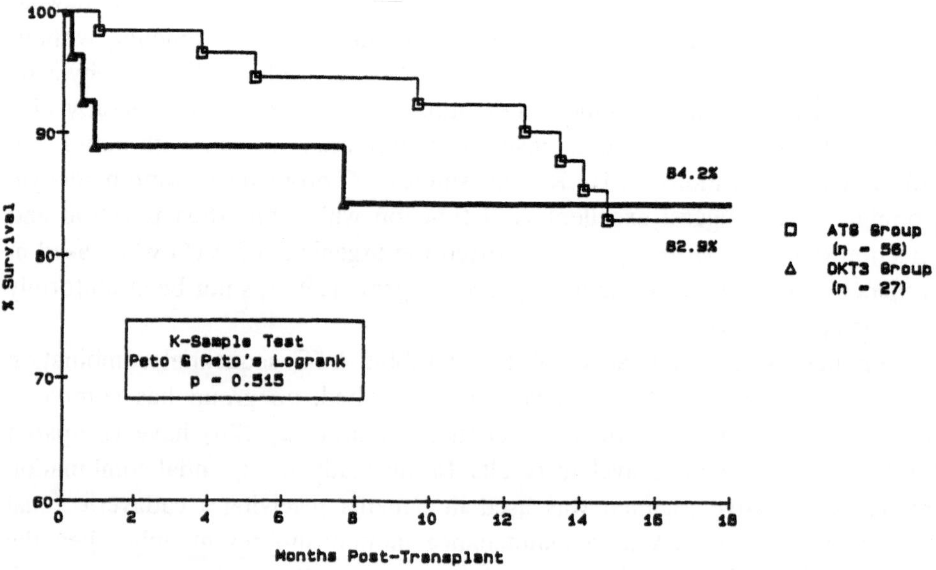

Fig. 1. Quadruple sequential immunotherapy protocol comparison graft survival.

Table 1. Patient demographics.

	Group 1 (ATG)	Group 2 (OKT3)	Statistics
$N =$	56	27	
Primary transplants (%)	87.3	88.9	N.S.
Primary non-function (%)	9.0	3.7	N.S.
Local donors (%)	43.6	85.2	$p < 0.05$
Mean donor age (yr)	27.2	32.5	N.S.
Mean recipient age (yr)	42.1	36.9	N.S.
Male (%)	75.0	55.6	N.S.
Diabetic (%)	8.9	11.0	N.S.
AB match (mean)	1.23	1.10	N.S.
DR match (mean)	1.72	0.74	N.S.
PRA (mean)	12.1	10.3	N.S.
Preservation time (mean, hrs)	17.0	12.9	N.S.
Prednisone dosage (mean, mg/kg)			
1 month	0.74	0.74	N.S.
6 months	0.28	0.22	N.S.
12 months	0.20	0.17	N.S.
Cyclosporine dosage (mean, mg/kg)			
1 month	5.9	5.8	N.S.
6 months	5.5	5.5	N.S.
12 months	4.4	4.2	N.S.

the total WBC > 4000. As maintenance, CyA was added when serum creatinine (SCr) was ⩽ 2.5 mg/dl at 6 mg/kg/day PO in divided doses and adjusted to maintain whole blood HPLC 24 hour trough levels between 150 and 250 ng/ml. Prednisone and azathioprine were maintained and tapered as described above.

In this study *delayed graft function* (DGF) was defined as the need for at least one dialysis treatment in the first 7 days following transplant (see Table 2); *serious infection* was considered as any viral, bacterial, or fungal infection that required in-hospital therapy. Rejection was diagnosed based on clinical criteria, supported by duplex sonography, nuclear imaging scans, and percutaneous core biopsy under sonographic guidance. Ninety-four percent of all rejections, and 100% of steroid-resistant rejections were biopsy proven.

Initial treatment of rejection consisted of pulse solumedrol at 1 g/day for 3—6 days. Steroid-resistant rejections were either treated with ATG 100 mg/kg/day for 5—7 days or OKT3 5/mg/day for 10—14 days, whichever agent was not used for induction.

Anti-OKT3 antibody measurements were performed by Ortho Pharmaceutical, Raritan, N.J. Samples were drawn on the second, third, and fourth weeks after cessation of OKT3 therapy. If patients had an anti-OKT3 titer of 1 : 100 or greater, samples were sent at 3 month intervals for follow-up.

Table 2. Graft function and complications.

	Group 1 (ATG)	Group 2 (OKT3)	Statistics
N =	56	27	
DGF (% patients)	23.2	11.0	N.S.
DGF (mean # days)	7.6	2.0	$p < 0.01$
SCR < 2.5 (% at 30 days)	94.6	88.0	$p < 0.05$
Graft survival (% at 1 year)	92.2	84.2	N.S.
Patient survival (% at 1 year)	98.1	96.3	N.S.
Serum creatinine (mean, mg%)			
1 month	1.9	2.1	N.S.
6 months	2.0	1.9	N.S.
12 months	2.4	1.7	N.S.
18 months	1.8	1.3	$p < 0.01$
Rejections (mean #/pt)			
0–1 month	0.12	0.30	$p < 0.05$
1–6 months	0.15	0.63	$p < 0.01$
6–12 months	0.12	0.07	N.S.
0–12 months	0.37	1.0	$p < 0.01$
Fatal infections	1	0	N.S.
Infections (mean #/pt)			
0–1 month	0.05	0.11	N.S.
1–6 months	0.20	0.26	N.S.
6–12 months	0.00	0.04	N.S.
0–12 months	0.25	0.41	N.S.

Statistical analysis for patient and graft survival was performed using Kaplan-Meler actuarial methods. Statistics generated from mean values or frequencies were done with either two-tailed Student's *t*-tests, non-parametric Wilcoxon's rank sum, or Dunnett's multiple comparison analysis of variance, whichever was appropriate.

Results

Eighteen-month patients and graft survivals were similar in both groups – 93.2%, 83% and 96.3%, 84.2% respectively for ATG and OKT3 (Figure 1). The percentage of patients receiving first transplants, and of those having primary non-function was statistically similar. The groups differed insignificantly in terms of percent of patients with DGF, which reflected the initial selection of patients for whom a sequential combination therapy was evolved. The percent of local donors significantly favored Group 2 ($p < 0.05$); however, total preservation times were statistically similar between the two groups. Because of the contingencies of local donor management and procurement, the 'center effect' might be presumed to have played a role in the decreased incidence of DGF in the OKT3 group despite equivalent preservation times.

Even though OKT3 statistically shortened the period of DGF ($p < 0.01$), renal function at 30 days, as measured by the percent of patients with SCr < 2.5 mg/dl, was better in the ATG group (94.6% vs 88% $p < 0.05$); see Table 2. SCr as an indication of graft function was not statistically different between the two groups in the interval between one month to one year, but was better in Group 2 at 18 months (1.8 vs 1.3 $p < 0.01$).

Significant differences were noted between the groups in terms of the overall incidence of rejection. These differences were most notable in the intermediate period after transplantation (1—6 months): the OKT3 group had a significantly higher rejection rate 0.63 versus 0.15 — $p < 0.01$. Late rejections (>12 months) were more common in the ATG group but did not reach statistical significance ($p = 0.12$). During the study period, 32% of the ATG group and 51% of the OKT3 group experienced at least one rejection episode; 54% and 53% respectively were steroid responsive (p = N.S.).

Infections were more common in the OKT3 group yet did not reach statistical significance. Only one fatal infection was noted during the study period, a herpes encephalitis in the OKT3 group. The infections were commonly viral — 78% and 83% in the ATG and OKT3 groups respectively. There was only one fungal infection during the study, which occurred in the ATG group.

Anti-OKT3 antibody was found in six patients (22%) at one month post-infusion. Five patients had titers of 1 : 100, and one patient had a titer of 1 : 1000.

Discussion

This study supports the thesis that, until good post-transplant renal function is obtained, combination immunotherapy with delayed administration of CyA is a safe and effective immunosuppressive regimen. Our data further suggest that the synergistic nephrotoxicity of CyA and preservation injury may be abrogated by delayed administration of CyA while maintaining effective induction immunosuppression with either OKT3 or ATG. These findings are in agreement with previous studies, which demonstrate excellent long-term renal allograft function with maintenance low dose, triple-drug immunotherapy (9, 10, 21, 23—25).

Rabbit ATG, used as an induction agent, has been shown to improve early graft function, shorten hospital stays, and improve long-term graft function without an increase in infection or rejection (9). As an induction agent, the immunosuppressive effect persists and can be measured for as long as 3 weeks after the last dose. This capability effectively allows a long therapeutic window during which renal function may be allowed to recover maximally before introduction of CyA with its attendant nephrotoxic potential. Induction OKT3 has been suggested to have equivalent effect; however, this study shows a higher rejection rate in OKT3-treated patients both overall, but especially in the 1 to 6 month period, using equivalent CyA doses. Because of the rapid depletion of OKT3 from the circulation at the close of therapy, effective overlap of adequate immunosuppression may not have persisted, resulting in an opportunity for breakthrough rejection to occur. In fact, a number of programs (21, 23, 24) institute CyA, and at higher doses, when diuresis occurs, rather than on the return of full renal function, to avoid an interval lapse of sufficient induction immune suppression.

Antilymphocyte preparations, either monoclonal or polyclonal, are potent immunosuppressive agents because they interrupt the exquisite productivity of immune response. Their effect may be allowing inefficient immune rejection to occur, permitting 'tolerance' to be induced without graft damage. The combination of CyA and adjuvant monoclonal or polyclonal antilymphocyte therapy has been suggested to be additive in the dampening of CD4 helper cells while sparing CD8 suppressor cells (26). The data presented in this study would support this contention: effective 'tolerance' is induced and maintained by sequential combination, low dose immune suppression.

At the 18 month interval, differences between the two groups are beginning to appear. Graft function in OKT3-treated patients is significantly better as measured by SCr, even though patient and graft survivals remain similar. The suggestion that lower SCr portends improved long-term graft survival has been shown by Terasaki (26).

The effectiveness of induction antilymphocyte preparations may be twofold: first, by delaying introduction of CyA, the synergistic nephrotoxicity of CyA with preservation injury may allow improved graft function and thus survival; second, interruption of focused immune rejection and dampening CD4 effects, possibly additively with CyA, may allow adaption to develop with minimal graft injury. The differences between OKT3 and ATG are subtle. ATG seems to offer the advantage of a shorter administration period and a longer therapeutic window. This advantage has resulted in fewer rejections and fewer subsequent infections. As suggested by Legendre *et al.* (27), and supported by this study, OKT3 may well offer improved induction of lasting 'tolerance'. Further long-term follow-up in carefully controlled trials will be necessary to completely elucidate these effects.

References

1. Deierhoi, M.H., Sollinger, H.W., Kalayoglu, M. and Belzer, F.O.: Quadruple therapy for cadaver renal transplantation. *Transplant. Proc.* **19**, 1917—1919 (1987).
2. Sommer, B.G. and Ferguson, R.M.: Three immediate postrenal transplant adjunct protocols combined with maintenance cyclosporine. *Transplant. Proc.* **17**, 1235—1238 (1985).
3. Jones, R.M., Murie, J.A., Allen, R.D., Ting, A. and Morris, P.J.: Triple therapy in cadaver renal transplantation. *Brit. J. Surg.* **75**, 4—8 (1988).

4. Delmonico, F.L., Auchincloss, H. Jr, Rubin, R.H. *et al.*: The selective use of antilymphocyte serum for cyclosporine treated patients with renal allograft dysfunction. *Ann. Surg.* **206**, 649—654 (1987).
5. Simons, R.L., Canafax, D.M., Strand, M. *et al.*: Management and prevention of cyclosporine nephrotoxicity after renal transplantation: use of low dose cyclosporine, azathioprine and prednisone. *Transplant. Proc.* **17** (Suppl. 1), 266—275 (1985).
6. Norman, D.J., Shield, C.F. III, Barry, J. *et al.*: Early use of OKT3 monoclonal antibody in renal transplantation to prevent rejection. *Amer. J. Kidney, Dis.* **11**, 107—110 (1988).
7. Sommer, B.G., Henry, M.L. and Ferguson, R.M.: Sequential conventional immunotherapy with maintenance cyclosporine following renal transplantation. *Transplant. Proc.* **18** (Suppl. 1), 69—75 (1986).
8. Matas, A.J., Tellis, V.A., Quinn, T.A., Glicklich, D., Soberman, R. and Veith, F.J.: Individualization of immediate posttransplant immunosuppression: the value of antilymphocyte globulin in patients with delayed graft function. *Transplantation* **45**, 406—409 (1988).
9. Posner, M.P., Mendez-Picon, G., King, A.L. *et al.*: Is sequential low dose immunotherapy the preferred treatment in cadaveric renal transplantation? *Transplant. Proc.* **21** (1), 1594—1597 (1989).
10. Shield, C.F., III, Hughes, J.D. and Lemon, J.A.: Prophylactic OKT3 and cadaveric renal transplantation at a single center. *Clin. Transplant.* **2** (4) 190—193 (1988).
11. Kupin, W.L., Venkatachalam, K.K., Oh, H.K., Dienst, S. and Levin, N.W.: Sequential use of Minnosota antilymphoblast globulin and cyclosporine in cadaveric renal transplantation. *Transplantation* **40** (6), 601—604 (1985).
12. Terasaki, P., Cats, S., Cicciarelli, J. *et al.*: Use of monoclonal antibodies for kidney transplant patients. *Transplant. Proc.* **17**, 1521—1525 (1985).
13. Herbert, J. and Roser, B.: Strategies of monoclonal antibody therapy that induce permanent tolerance of organ transplants. *Transplantation* **46** (Suppl. 2), S128—S134 (1988).
14. Thomas, F., Thomas, J., Flora, R., Mendez Picon, G., Peace, K. and Lee, H.M.: Effect of antilymphocyte-globulin potency on survival of cadaver renal transplants. *Lancet* **11** (67), 671—674 (1977).
15. Thistlethwaite, J.R. Jr, Stuart, J.K., Mayes, J.T., Gaber, A.O. *et al.*: Complications and monitoring of OKT3 therapy. *Amer. J. Kidney Dis.* **11**, 112—119 (1988).
16. Kreis, H., Chkoff, H., Vigeral, P., Chatenoud, L. *et al.*: Prophylactic treatment of allograft recipients with a monoclonal anti-T3 cell antibody. *Transplant. Proc.* **17**, 1315—1319 (1985).
17. Shield, C.F., III, Norman, D.J., Marlett, P., Fucello, A.J. and Goldstein, G.: Comparison of antimouse and antihorse antibody production during the treatment of allograft rejection with OKT3 or antithymocyte globulin. *Nephron.* **46** (Suppl. 1), 48—51 (1987).
18. Pennock, J.L., Reitz, B.A., Bieber, C.P. *et al.*: Cardiac allograft survival in cynomolgus monkeys treated with cyclosporine A in combination with conventional immune suppression. *Transplant. Proc.* **13**, 390—392 (1981).
19. Halloran, P., Ludwin, D., Aprile, M. and the Canadian Multicentre Transplant Study Group: Comparison of antilymphocyte globulin-cyclosporine therapy for cadaver renal transplantation. *Transplant. Proc.* **17**, 1201—1203 (1985).
20. Hanto, D.W., Jendvisak, M.D., McCullough, C.S., Flye, M.W., Phelan, D.L. and Mohanakumar, T.: A prospective randomized comparison of prophylactic OKT3 vs ALG in cadaver renal transplant recipients. Presented at Amer. Soc. Transplant Surg. (June 1989).
21. Thomas, J. and Hume, D.J.: A standardized ALG for use in man. *Transplant. Proc.* **4**, 477 (1972).
22. Shen, S.Y., Amin, A., Behrens, M.T., Weir, M.R., Klossen, D.K. and Couglin, E.E.: How beneficial is OKT3 as an immunosuppressive induction agent? *Amer. Soc. Transplant Phys. Abstract* #A12 (May 1989).
23. Banoenisty, A.I., Stegall, M.D., Cohen, D. and Hardy, M.A.: Improved results using OKT3 as induction immunosuppression in cadaveric renal allograft recipients with delayed graft function. Presented at Amer. Soc. Transplant Surg. (June 1989).
24. First, M.R., Schroeder, T.J., Mansour, M.E., Alexander, J.W. and Penn, I.: Prophylactic use

of OKT3 in immunological high risk cadaver renal transplant recipients. *Amer. Soc. Transplant Phys. Abstract* # A13 (May 1989).

25. Kahan, B.D., Didlake, R., Kim, E.E., Yosimura, N., Kondo, E. and Etepkowski, S. Important role of CyA for the induction of immunological tolerance in adult hosts. *Transplant. Proc.* **20** (Suppl. 3), 23–35 (1988).
26. Terasaki, P.I., Cecka, J.M., Takemoto, F. *et al.*: 'Overview', Chap. 42 in *Clinical Transplants* (ed. P. Terasaki). UCLA Tissue Typing Laboratory, Los Angeles (1988).
27. Legendre, C., Saltiel, C., Chkoff, N. and Kreis, H. 'Results of kidney transplantation of Necker Hospital', Chap. 12 in *Clinical Transplants* (ed. P. Terasaki). UCLA Tissue Typing Laboratory, Los Angeles (1988).

13. Multi-organ transplant experience with OKT3 and strategies for use at the University of Cincinnati Medical Center

TIMOTHY J. SCHROEDER, M. ROY FIRST and ISRAEL PENN

Orthoclone OKT3 is a murine monoclonal antibody to the CD3 (T3) antigen of human T cells (1). *In vitro*, OKT3 blocks the generation of functional effector T cells and inhibits the activity of mature cytotoxic effector lymphocytes (2). *In vivo*, OKT3 can act in three ways. It initially opsonizes circulating T cells, which are then removed by the reticuloendothelial system (3). OKT3 may also modulate the antigen recognition complex of circulating T cells (4). The drug is also able to block the function of sessile T cells on the allograft by coating these cells (3).

In the Multicenter Transplant Study Group, OKT3 was highly effective in reversing acute renal allograft rejection (5). Subsequent studies have further demonstrated the efficacy of OKT3 in the prevention and treatment of renal, hepatic and cardiac allograft rejection (6—10). This paper summarizes our use of Orthoclone OKT3 in renal, hepatic and cardiac transplant recipients at a single transplant center. Both adult and pediatric patients were treated, and the OKT3 was used as either prophylactic treatment, primary treatment, or secondary treatment (11—12). Our experience with OKT3 retreatment and immunologic monitoring is also described (13—14).

Materials and methods

Treatment of rejection

OKT3 was used on 155 occasions in 129 patients (Table 1). The drug was used for treatment of rejection 90 times in 99 renal allograft recipients. In all cases, rejection was confirmed histologically. Eight patients were treated during the multicenter study (5), and an additional 21 prior to release of OKT3 in July 1986. These patients were treated with azathioprine and prednisone maintenance. The remaining patients have all been treated with a pre-OKT3 triple-drug immunosuppressive therapy as detailed previously (15). Initially, all patients were maintained on triple-immunosuppressive therapy during OKT3 therapy; later, cyclosporine was discontinued at the start of OKT3 therapy and

Table 1. Use of OKT3 in solid organ transplantation.

Organ	Treatments	Patients
Kidney	117	101
Rejection	90	74
Prophylactic	27	27
Liver	20	14
Heart	13	10
Pancreas	5	4
Total	155	129

reintroduced during the last 3 days of treatment; more recently, the dose of cyclosporine was reduced for the first half of OKT3 thereapy. Azathioprine and prednisone were maintained at prerejection dose levels. The majority of the hepatic, cardiac, and pancreatic transplant recipients were kept on triple therapy throughout OKT3 treatment. Retreatment with OKT3 was performed in 16 kidney, 6 liver, 3 heart, and 1 pancreas transplant recipient.

Rejection prophylaxis

Twenty-seven patients receiving cadaver kidney transplants participated in this study. Patients were eligible to participate in the study if they met either of the following criteria: (a) retransplant (20 patients: 16 second transplants, 3 third transplants, and 1 fourth transplant), (b) peak or current PRA level greater than 50% before the first transplant (7 patients). Twelve patients met both criteria.

A sequential immunosuppressive protocol consisting of OKT3, prednisone, azathioprine, and cyclosporine was used in these patients. OKT3, 5 mg/day intravenous (i.v.), was administered intraoperatively and continued daily for a mean duration of 10 days. Duration of OKT3 therapy ranged from 2 days (in 3 patients with early graft loss) to 20 days (in 2 patients with prolonged acute tubular necosis [ATN]). OKT3 was discontinued only after therapeutic cyclosporine levels had been attained. In most patients, a 3—4-day overlap was required.

Immunologic monitoring

During therapy, OKT3 serum concentrations were determined daily using a double-antibody, solid-phase ELISA procedure (16). Serum murine IgG (OKT3) was bound to microtiter plates coated with affinity-purified goat antimouse IgG Fc fragment. Following this formation, the plate was washed, and conjugate (affinity-purified goat antimouse IgG alkaline phosphatase conjugate) was added. The conjugate reacted with the bound serum murine IgG (OKT3). The plate was washed, and a chromagen added, which caused a color change in direct proportion to the amount of OKT3 present. Comparison of a sample's absorbance values to known standards allowed for ng/ml quantitation of serum OKT3 levels.

Antimurine antibodies were measured 1, 2, 3 and 4 weeks after institution of OKT3 therapy and prior to a second course of therapy. Antimurine antibodies (IgG antibodies to OKT3) were detected by a double-antibody, solid-phase ELISA procedure (17). Serum IgG antibodies to OKT3 were bound by the OKT3 coated on the inner surface of the test wells. Alkaline phosphatase conjugated antihuman IgG was added; this reacted with the bound IgG. A chromagenic substrate for the alkaline phosphatase was then added. If IgG antibodies to OKT3 were present, there was a reaction that resulted in a yellow color.

During OKT3 therapy, lymphocyte subsets were obtained daily using the monoclonal antipan-T cell antibodies (18, 19). Absolute peripheral lymphocyte subgroups were determined by using CD2, CD3, CD4 and CD8 direct-labeled standard diagnostic reagents (Ortho Pharmaceutical Corp., Raritan, New Jersey). Whole blood samples were incubated with the appropriate reagent, red blood cells lysed, and samples were analyzed (19).

Results

Treatment of rejection

Ninety episodes of rejection in renal transplant recipients were treated with OKT3. It was used as either primary or secondary therapy for biopsy-proven rejection in both living related and cadaver renal transplant recipients. Reversal of rejection occurred in 73 of 90 (81%) patients with a 1-year graft survival of 67% (Table 2). Twenty-five patients (22 cadaver, 3 LRD) received OKT3 as primary therapy with 16 of 22 (73%) cadaver recipients and all 3 LRD recipients reversing their rejection episode. One-year graft survival was 59% and 100% respectively. Sixty-five patients (53 cadaver, 12 LRD) received OKT3 as secondary therapy; in 45 of 53 (85%) cadaver recipients and 9 of 12 (75%) LRD recipients rejection was reversed. One-year graft survival was 70% in the cadaver recipients and 58% in the LRD recipients. Overall results in renal transplant recipients revealed very similar rejection reversal rates and graft survival rates in cadaver transplant recipients and LRD transplant recipients (Table 2).

Sixty-five courses of OKT3 were given as secondary therapy (53 cadaver, 12 LRD receipients). In 36 cases OKT3 was given secondary to steroid therapy, in

Table 2. Results of OKT3 therapy in renal transplant recipients.

Treatment group	Reversal	1-year graft survival
Primary		
Cadaver	16/22 (73%)	13/22 (59%)
LRD	3/3 (100%)	3/3 (100%)
Secondary		
Cadaver	45/53 (85%)	37/53 (70%)
LRD	9/12 (75%)	7/12 (58%)
Combined		
Cadaver	61/75 (81%)	50/75 (67%)
LRD	12/15 (80%)	10/15 (67%)
Total	73/80 (81%)	60/90 (67%)

13 secondary to a polyclonal antilymphocyte preparation, and in 16 secondary to steroids and an antilymphocyte agent. Rejection was successfully reversed in 54 of the 65 cases (83%). Graft-function at 1 year or last follow-up was 68%. Reversal of rejection and graft survival were similar in the three groups receiving OKT3 as secondary antirejection therapy (Table 3).

Sixteen hepatic transplant recipients were treated with 20 courses of OKT3. In 18 instances (90%), OKT3 was successful in reversing the rejection (Table 4). One-year patient survival was 94%. One patient who received two courses of OKT3 developed a fatal B-cell lymphoma. Two patients required retransplantation for non-rejection related problems.

Ten cardiac transplant recipients were treated with 13 courses of OKT3. In 11 of 13 (85%) instances the rejection was successfully reversed; 4 of these patients subsequently died (Table 4).

Prophylaxis

Patient survival was 100% during a mean follow-up period of 13 months. One-

Table 3. Comparison of results of OKT3 used as secondary therapy.

Primary therapy	Reversal	1-year graft survival
Steroids	30/36 (83%)	25/36 (69%)
ATG/ATS	11/13 (85%)	8/13 (62%)
Steroids + ALG/ATS	13/16 (81%)	11/16 (69%)
Total	54/65 (83%)	44/65 (68%)

Table 4. Use of OKT3 in hepatic, cardiac and pancreatic transplant recipients.

HEPATIC	
Reversal of rejection	18/20 (90%)
1-year patient survival	15/16 (94%)
CARDIAC	
Reversal of rejection	11/13 (85%)
1-year patient survival	10/14 (71%)
PANCREATIC	
Reversal of rejection	1/5 (20%)
1-year patient survival	3/4 (75%)

year graft survival was 70% (19 of 27). Four grafts were lost as a result of hyperacute rejection or primary no-function. Two additional grafts were lost to acute rejection at 1 week and 1 month post-transplant. There were two technical losses, 6 and 42 days post-transplant. No grafts were lost after 6 weeks. Beyond the first month, single rejection episodes occurred in 4 patients and multiple rejection episodes occurred in 3 patients; all were successfully treated.

Serum creatinine level decreased steadily throughout OKT3 therapy from 822 μmol/l (9.3 mg/dl) on day 0 to 186 μmol/l (2.1 mg/dl) on day 15. It stabilized at 141 μ/l (1.6 mg/dl) 1 month post-transplant and remained at that level.

Retreatment

Twenty-six patients were retreated with OKT3 (Table 5). Reversal of rejection was the same in patients with no antimurine antibodies (15/18 = 83%), as in

Table 5. Results of OKT3 retreatment.

Organ	Antibody titer			Total
	Negative	Low (1 : 100)	High (≥ 1 : 1000)	
Kidney	11	4	1	16
Liver	5	1	0	6
Heart	2	1	0	3
Pancreas	0	0	1	1
Total	18	6	2	26
Reversal	15 (83%)	5 (83%)	0	20 (77%)

patients with a low antibody titer (5/6 = 83%) but was not successful in the 2 patients with a high-titer antimurine antibody.

Immunology monitoring

Administration of OKT3 for the first time caused the level of all lymphocyte markets to fall to less than 100/mm3 by the third day of therapy, regardless of transplant organ type. However, only the CD3+ cells remained modulated (<20/mm^3) throughout therapy (Figure 1). Trough serum OKT3 concentrations rose to greater than 800 ngml by the third day of treatment and remained above this level for the duration of therapy (Figure 2).

In the prophylaxis group, OKT3 levels slowly increased to 800 ng/ml by the fourth day of therapy. Similarly, CD3+ lymphocytes were depleted by the third day post-transplant and remained below 20/mm^3 throughout therapy in all patients, including 3 receiving up to 20 days of monoclonal antibody therapy. Five of 27 (22%) patients developed an antimurine antibody during or after OKT3 therapy. Only one of these patients developed a high titer antibody ($\gtrsim$1: 1000). Antibody formation occurred during therapy in 1 patient and 1–6 weeks later in the remaining 4 patients.

Retreatment with OKT3 in patients with no anti-OKT3 antibody present resulted in depletion of CD3+ cells from the peripheral blood, but it took

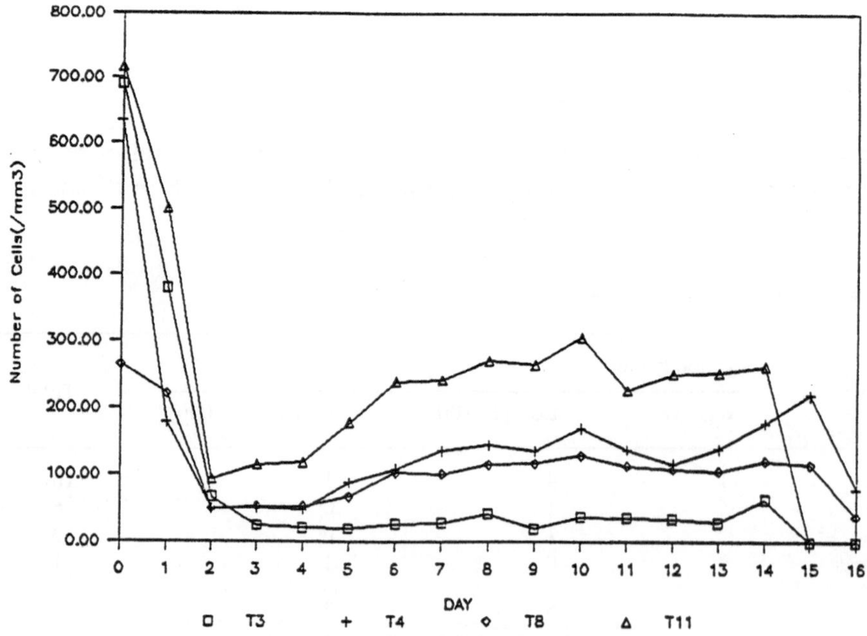

Fig. 1. Lymphocyte subsets vs days: First treatment (all).

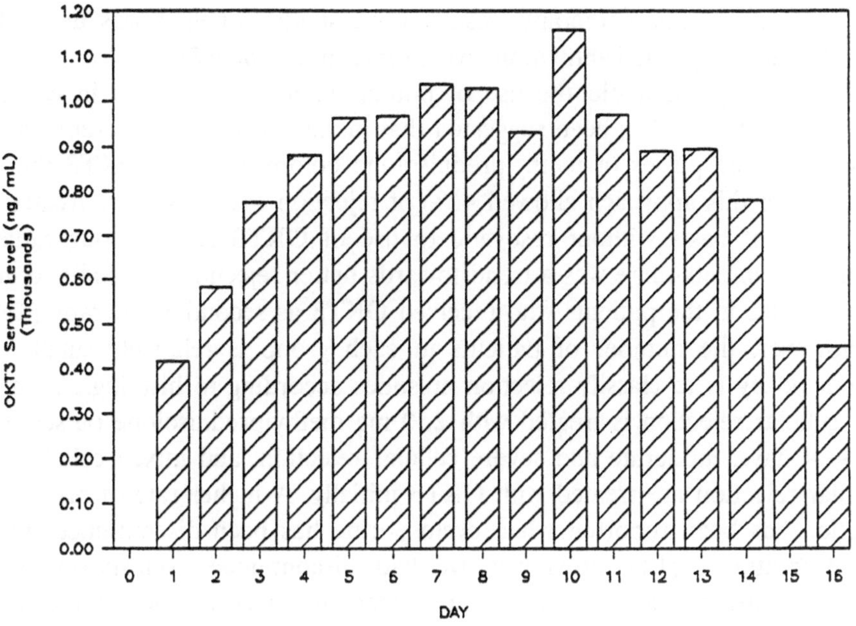

Fig. 2. Mean OKT3 levels vs days: First treatment (all).

longer than in patients being treated with OKT3 for the first time. In retreating patients with a low-titer antimurine antibody, removal of CD3+ cells from the peripheral circulation was accomplished in most cases by the fourth day of therapy. However, to achieve this it was necessary to double or triple the dose of OKT3 in some patients. In both groups of retreated patients (with and without anti-OKT3 antibodies), the serum OKT3 levels rose more slowly and did not exceed 800 ng/ml until the seventh day of treatment. De novo antimurine antibody developed in 4 of 18 (22%) patients on re-exposure to OKT3.

Discussion

Orthoclone OKT3 was shown to be effective in reversing acute cellular rejection in the initial multicenter study in renal transplant recipients (5). Since that study, discussions have centered on the best way to optimize OKT3 therapy. This study involves the use of OKT3 as primary, secondary, or prophylactic therapy on 155 occasions in 129 patients.

In this study OKT3 was equally effective in reversing rejection in both living related and cadaver renal allograft transplant recipients with equivalent 1-year graft survival rates. Reversal of rejection and 1-year graft survival was similar when OKT3 was used a primary or secondary therapy (Table 2). When OKT3 was used as secondary therapy, results were similar when it was used after steroids and a polyclonal antilymphocyte preparation (Table 3).

In an attempt to avoid the use of potent immunosuppression in cases of minimal rejection, it has been suggested that initial antirejection therapy should consist of three pulses of methylprednisolone before initiating OKT3 therapy (20). Use of this approach allowed 46% of rejection episodes to be treated on an outpatient basis without resorting to use of OKT3 (20). In our cadaver allograft recipients there was a trend towards better rejection reversal and graft survival rates in the patients who received OKT3 as secondary therapy (Table 2); however, the number of patients in each group is relatively small. Our current policy is to classify rejection episodes according to histologic severity; mild cellular rejection is treated with 250 mg methylprednisolone pulses daily for 3—4 days; moderate and severe cellular rejection, and mixed cellular and vascular rejection are treated with OKT3 initially. A higher rate of reversal of rejection has been reported when cyclosporine has been discontinued during OKT3 treatment (14); previously we had discontinued cyclosporine when OKT3 therapy was started, and reintroduced the cyclosporine for the last 3 days of OKT3 therapy; currently, we are reducing the dose of cyclosporine during the first half of OKT3 therapy, then returning to the prerejection dose. This approach has resulted in a lower incidence of anti-OKT3 antibody production (21).

Use of OKT3 in hepatic transplant recipients resulted in a 90% rejection reversal rate and a 94% patient survival (Table 4). These results are slightly better than those previously reported with OKT3 in liver transplant recipients and are far superior to those previously reported with other immunosuppressive agents (22—24).

Reversal of rejection was accomplished in 85% of cardiac transplant (Table 4). This resulted in a 1-year graft survival of 71%. Excellent results had been obtained when OKT3 was used to prevent and to treat cardiac allograft rejection.

Transplantation in immunologic high-risk recipients has generally met with poor results. A poorer outcome has been associated with higher PRA levels. Specific protocols for these individuals generally have not been developed. We studied the effect of having a specific immunosuppressive regimen for patients classified as high-risk immunologic recipients. Prophylactic use of OKT3 in this patient population was well tolerated and resulted in superior graft survival when compared with a similar group of patients treated at our center who did not receive prophylactic OKT3. No grafts were lost after the first 6 weeks, and renal function has remained stable throughout the follow-up period.

We have demonstrated that retreatment with OKT3 can be successfully accomplished in the majority of patients but should not be attempted without immune monitoring. Knowledge of the patient's antibody status after the first course of OKT3 is essential. Successful retreatment appears to depend upon the patient's peak antimurine antibody titer after the first treatment. Patients who do not develop antibodies after a first course of treatment have rejection reversal rates on retreatment equivalent to those with primary therapy. Results of retreatment in patients with low-titer antimurine antibodies are similar to those with retreatment in patients with no antimurine antibodies. However, both groups of retreated patients tend to have a slower clearance of CD3+ cells from the peripheral circulation and a slower rise in the serum OKT3 levels. In patients with low-titer antibodies it may be necessary to increase the dose of OKT3 in order to overcome the antibody and to achieve depletion of all CD3+ cells. Reappearance of CD3+ cells and a fall in the circulating OKT3 level during OKT3 therapy have been shown to be associated with antimurine antibody formation. This is an indication that the dose of OKT3 should be increased, or an alternative antirejection therapy should be instituted. Patients with high-titer antimurine antibody levels have extremely low rejection reversal rates upon retreatment with OKT3, and other forms of antirejection therapy should be employed in this patient population.

References

1. Goldstein, G.: Monoclonal antibody specificity: Orthoclone OKT3 T-cell blocker. *Nephron* **46** (Suppl. 1), 5 (1987).
2. Goldstein, G.: Overview of the development of Orthoclone OKT3 monoclonal antibody for therapeutic use in transplantation. *Transplant. Proc.* **19** (Suppl. 2), 1 (1987).
3. Miller, R.A., Maloney, D.G., McKillop, J. *et al.* In vivo effects of murine hybridoma monoclonal antibody in a patient with T-cell leukemia. *Blood* **58**, 78 (1981).
4. Chatenoud, L., Bandrihage, M., Kreis, H. *et al.*: Human in vivo antigenic modulation induced by anti-T cell OKT3 monoclonal antibody. *Eur. J. Immunol.* **12**, 979 (1982).
5. Ortho Multicenter Transplant Study Group: A randomized clinical trial of OKT3 monoclonal antibody for acute rejection of cadaveric renal transplants. *New Engl. J. Med.* **313**, 337 (1985).
6. Norman, D.J., Shield, C.F., Barry, J. *et al.*: A U.S. clinical study of Orthoclone OKT3 in renal transplantation. *Transplant. Proc.* **19** (Suppl. 2), 21 (1987).
7. Thistlewaite, J.R., Gaber, A.O., Haag, B.W. *et al.*: OKT3 treatment of steroid-resistant renal allograft rejection. *Transplantation*, **43**, 176 (1987).
8. Fung, J.J., Markus, B.H., Gordon, R.D. *et al.*: Impact of Orthoclone OKT3 on liver transplantation. *Transplant. Proc.* **19** (Suppl. 2), 37 (1987).
9. Bristow, M.R., Gilbert, E.M., Renlund, D.G. *et al.*: Use of OKT3 monoclonal antibody in heart transplantation: Review of the initial experience. *J. Heart Transplant.* **7**, 1 (1988).
10. Millis, J.M., McDiarmid, S.V., Hiatt, J.R. *et al.*: Randomized prospective trial of OKT3 for early prophylaxis of rejection after liver transplantation. *Transplantation* **47**, 82 (1989).
11. First, M.R., Schroeder, T.J., Melvin, D.B. *et al.*: OKT3 therapy in kidney, liver, heart, and pancreas transplantation. *Clin. Transplant.* **2**, 185 (1988).
12. First, M.R., Schroeder, T.J., Hurtubise, P.E. *et al.*: Successful retreatment of allograft rejection with OKT3. *Transplantation* **47**, 88 (1989).
13. Schroeder, T.J., First, M.R., Hurtubise, P.E. *et al.*: Immunologic monitoring with Orthoclone OKT3 therapy. *J. Heart Transplant.* **8**, 371 (1989).
14. Schroeder, T.J., First, M.R., Mansour, M.E., Alexander, J.W. and Penn, I.: Prophylactic use of OKT3 in immunological high risk renal transplant recipients. *Amer. J. Kidney Dis.* **14** (Suppl. 2), 14 (1989).

15. First, M.R., Alexander, J.W., Wadhwa, N.K. *et al.*: The use of low doses of cyclosporine, azathioprine, and prednisone in renal transplantation. *Transplant. Proc.* **18** (Suppl. 1), 132 (1986).
16. Goldstein, G., Fuccello, A.J., Norman, D.J. *et al.*: OKT3 monoclonal antibody levels during therapy and the subsequent development of host antibodies to OKT3. *Transplantation* **42**, 507 (1986).
17. Schroeder, T.J., First, M.R., Mansour, M.E. *et al.*: Antimurine antibody formation following OKT3 therapy. *Transplantation* **49**, 48 (1990).
18. Cosimi, A.B., Colvin, R., Burton, R.C. *et al.*: Use of monoclonal antibodies to T cell subsets for immunologic monitoring and treatment in recipients of renal allografts. *New Engl. J. Med.* **305**, 308 (1981).
19. Shield, C.F., Marlett, P., Smith, A. *et al.*: Stability of human lymphocyte differentiation antigens when stored at room temperature. *J. Immunol. Methods* **62**, 347 (1983).
20. Thistlethwaite, J.R., Stuart, J.K., Mayes, J.T., Gaber, A.O. and Stuart, F.P.: Use of brief steroid traial before initiating OKT3 therapy for renal allograft rejection. *Amer. J. Kidney Dis.* **11**, 94 (1988).
21. Hricik, P.R., Zarconi, J. and Schulak, J.A.: Influence of low-dose cyclosporine on the outcome of treatment with OKT3 for acute renal allograft rejection. *Transplantation* **47**, 272 (1989).
22. Kremer, A.B., Barnes, L., Hirsch, R.L. *et al.*: Orthoclone OKT3 monoclonal antibody reversal of hepatic and cardiac allograft rejection unresponsive to conventional immunosuppressive threapy. *Transplant. Proc.* **19** (Suppl. 2), 54 (1987).
23. Goldstein, R.D., Kremer, A. B., Barnes, L. *et al.*: OKT3 monoclonal antibody reversal of renal and hepatic rejection in pediatric patients. *J. Pediatr.* **111**, 1046 (1987).
24. Gordon, R.D., Tzakis, A.G., Iwatsuki, S. *et al.*: Experience with Orthclone OKT3 in liver transplantation. *Amer. J. Kidney Dis.* **11**, 141 (1988).

14. Cyclosporine withdrawal in renal transplant recipients maintained on azathioprine, prednisone and cyclosporine

M. KALAWI, N.A. AL-SABAWI, M. SAMHAN, D. PANJWANI,
M.S.A. KUMAR, E.M. PHILIPS and G.M. ABOUNA

Introduction

The introduction of cyclosporine as an immunosuppressant in clinical organ transplantation has improved the results with respect to patient and graft survival (1, 2, 3). However, its long-term renal toxicity and other wide-ranging adverse reactions are its limiting factors. In the Kuwait renal transplantation programme cyclosporine (CsA) was introduced in cadaver renal transplantation in 1983 and in HLA mismatched living donor transplantation in 1988 as one of the constituents of triple drug prophylactic immunosuppressive therapy, together with azathioprine and prednisone. Despite the small maintenance doses of CsA, many of our patients developed serious side effects such as nephrotoxicity, hypertension, hirsutism, tremors, gingival hypertrophy and hepatoxicity, which in turn contributed to non-compliance with regard to cyclosporine intake. This observation together with previous reports on cyclosporine withdrawal prompted us to carry out a randomized prospective clinical trial of cyclosporine withdrawal in renal transplant recipients with stable graft function on triple therapy for at least 1—2 years after transplantation. The aim of this study was to determine the effect of cyclosporine withdrawal on renal graft function and the possible benefit of ameliorating the toxic effects after withdrawal of the drug. Additionally the method of CsA withdrawal, either gradual over a period of few weeks or abrupt discontinuation, was also assessed.

Patients and methods

During the 11-year period, March 1979 to May 1990, more than 540 renal transplants have been carried out at the Kuwait Transplant Centre of which 375 are from living related donors, 110 from cadavers and 55 from genetically unrelated but emotionally related donors, such as spouses and distant relatives. The post-transplant follow-up and care is provided by the same transplant team. Additionally another 82 recipients who had received living unrelated kidneys abroad are also followed up at our center.

In living donor transplantation, donor selection is according to our previously described protocol based on strict and rigorous medical, ethical and legal criteria in accordance with the guidelines of the Transplantation Society (4, 5).

Cadaveric kidneys were usually obtained from centers in North America and Europe and in few cases from local cadavers. Imported cadaveric kidneys were preserved for prolonged periods of 30—80 hours and many had additional risk factors (6). Maintenance immunosuppression was with triple therapy consisting of azathioprine, prednisone and cyclosporine. At the time of initiation of this study in May 1989 there were 162 recipients of either living donor or cadaveric kidneys maintained on triple therapy.

According to our protocol, cyclosporine withdrawal was carried out after an informed consent by the recipients/guardians provided (1) they were aged 12 years or more, (2) had stable graft function with serum creatinine of <200 minol/l for 1 year or more in recipients of living related donor kidneys and for 2 years or more in living unrelated donor and cadaveric kidneys. Prior to withdrawal, the daily maintenance dose of CsA was 3—5 mg/kg, azathioprine 0.75 to 1 mg/kg and prednisone 0.05—0.1 mg/kg body weight. The dose of CsA being adjusted to maintain levels in the therapeutic range of 150—300 ng/ml of whole blood. Forty-three recipients fulfilled this protocol and agreed to enter the study. They were randomized into two groups: in one group withdrawal of cyclosporine was gradual over a 4-week period (group 1) at the rate of 1 mg/kg week while in another group CsA was abruptly discontinued (group 2). There were 22 recipients in group 1, and 21 in group 2. On the day of CsA withdrawal, in both groups, the daily dose of azathioprine was increased to 2.5 mg and that of prednisolone to 0.3 mg/kg body weight and maintained for 3 months after which they were reduced gradually over a period of 1 month to pre-withdrawal levels. Following CsA withdrawal the recipients were monitored as outpatients twice weekly for 3 months, once weekly for 3—6 months, once every 2 weeks for 6 months and then once monthly. Monitoring included measurements of body weight, blood pressure, blood count, renal profile (serum creatinine and blood urea) and liver profile (serum albumen, bilirubin, ALT, AST and alkaline phosphatase). The diagnosis of acute rejection was made when the serum creatinine became persistently elevated by 25% or more compared to the pre-withdrawal levels and was confirmed by radionuclide renogram and by biopsy of the transplant kidney. Acute rejections were promptly treated by pulse doses of intravenous methylprednisolone 1 g daily for 3 to 5 days. In steroid-resistant rejections intravenous infusion of ATG (Fresenius ®) 2.5 mg/kg body weight or intravenous OKT3 5 mg daily for 10—14 days were used. Recipients with acute rejection resistant to both methylprednisolone and ATG/OKT3, were converted back to triple therapy by the addition of cyclosporine. All recipients have been followed up for a minimum period of 1 year after CsA withdrawal. The results were statistically analyzed using the chi-square and student's '*t*' test.

Results

Patient and graft survival

After a follow-up period of 12—15 months after CsA withdrawal, the overall patient and graft survival in all the 43 recipients in the study is 100% at 1 year. One recipient of cadaver kidney who refused surgical treatment for a duodenal ulcer, died of massive bleeding and sepsis at 13 months after CsA withdrawal, with normal renal function at the time of his death.

Rejections

Six (15%) of the 43 recipients developed acute rejections. Of these one was in group 1 (5%), which was easily reversed by steroid therapy. Five recipients were in group 2 (24%), of which 4 were reversed by steroid therapy, while the remaining recipient who received a kidney from his mother, failed to respond to steroid, ATG or OKT3 therapy and has since been converted back to triple therapy by the addition of cyclosporine. He also developed salmonella septicemia during antirejection therapy which resolved with appropriate treatment (Table 1). When the incidence of rejection was analyzed according to graft source, this was higher when the graft was from unrelated or cadaver donor in both study groups (Table 2).

Renal function

In all the 6 recipients who developed acute rejections, there was a rise in the mean serum creatinine levels from 141.5 ± 34.8 μmol/l before CsA withdrawal to 224.3 ± 115 μmol/l after CsA withdrawal. However, in the remaining 37 (85%) of recipients without rejection episodes, the mean serum creatinine decreased from 141 ± 45 μmol/l before CsA withdrawal to 131.6

Table 1. Incidence of rejection.

	Group 1: Gradual CsA withdrawal	Group 2: Abrupt cessation of CsA
No. of recipients	22	21
No. of recipients with acute rejection	1	5
No. of acute rejections reversed with steriod/ATG/OKT3	1	4
No. of recipients reconverted to CsA therapy	none	1

Table 2. Source of donors and incidence of rejection.

	Living related		Cadaver and living unrelated	
	No.	Rejection	No.	Rejection
Group 1	12	0	9	1 (11%)
Group 2	11	2 (18.2%)	11	3 (27%)
Total	23	2 (8.6%)	20	4 (20%)

± 42 μmol/l after cyclosporine withdrawal. However, the difference in the mean serum creatinine levels was not statistically significant (Table 3).

Table 3. Effect of cyclosporine withdrawal of renal function.

	Group 1 $N = 22$	Group 2 $N = 21$	Total
No. of recipients without rejection	21	16	37
Serum creatinine (μmol/l):			
Before CsA withdrawal	134 ± 29	140 ± 47	141 ± 45
After CsA withdrawal	111 ± 30	128 ± 37	131 ± 42
No. of recipients with acute rejection	1	5	6
Serum creatinine (μmol/l):			
Before CsA withdrawal	120	141 ± 34	141 ± 34
After CsA withdrawal	150	224 ± 115	224 ± 113

Hypertension

Thirty-two (74%) of the 43 recipients in this study had hypertension prior to CsA withdrawal. In 15 recipients hypertension had been controlled with single drug therapy, while in the remaining 17 antihypertension therapy consisted of 2 to 4 drugs. One year after CsA withdrawal only 20 recipients (46%) remained hypertensive, of which 11 are controlled with a single drug and only 9 with 2 to 3 drugs, $p = 0.05$ (Table 4).

Other toxic effects

Gingival hypertrophy, tremors and hirsutism were assessed both subjectively by the patients and objectively by the transplant team. Gingival hypertrophy was seen in 18 recipients (41%) and in 6 it was severe causing bad oral hygiene and

Table 4. Effects of cyclosporine withdrawal on toxicity and side effects ($N = 43$).

	Before CsA withdrawal	After CsA withdrawal	*p*
Hypertension	32 (74%)	20 (46%)	NS
Antihypertensive medication:			
Monontherapy	15	11	NS
Multitherapy	17	9	0.05
Gingival hypertrophy	18 (41%)	2 (9%)	0.01
Tremors	23 (53%)	5 (11.6%)	0.01
Hirsutism	19 (44%)	8 (18.6%)	0.01

bleeding from the gums. After CsA withdrawal, mild gingival hypertrophy persists in only 2 recipients (9%), ($p = 0.01$). Tremors were seen in 23 recipients (53%) and were severe and disabling in 4. Following CsA withdrawal tremors disappeared in 18 and persisted in only 5 (11.6%), ($p = 0.01$). Nineteen recipients (44%) had hirsutism during CsA therapy which persisted only in 8 (18.6%) after CsA withdrawal ($p = 0.01$).

Discussion

Cyclosporine is a valuable immunosuppressant but has a wide variety of toxic effects and especially nephrotoxicity. Several investigators have tried to overcome the nephrotoxicity of CsA by conversion from CsA/prednisolone to either Aza/prednisolone prophylaxis or to triple therapy with azathioprine, prednisolone and low dose CsA (7, 8, 9). These investigators reported that discontinuation or reduction of CsA dose resulted in improved renal function. However complete CsA withdrawal resulted in 5—10% of patients developing acute rejection episodes, most of which were successfully treated (10).

CsA was initiated in Kuwait renal transplantation programme in June 1983 and to date over 200 recipients have been treated with the drug as combination therapy with azathioprine and prednisolone. Although many of these recipients were maintained on small doses of CsA (3—4 mg/kg/day), they developed side effects. A prospective randomized trial of CsA withdrawal was therefore carried out not only to reduce the nephroxicity, but also the other side effects of CsA such as hypertension, hirsutism, gingival hypertrophy and tremors. In clinical practice the immunosuppressive action of CsA is always associated with varying degrees of nephrotoxicity: measurement of nephrotoxicity by serum creatinine and 24-hour creatinine clearance is not always reliable as these parameters may remain normal despite toxic pathological changes in the kidney (11). Since most of the cadaveric kidneys transplanted in Kuwait were obtained from North

America or Europe with prolonged cold ischaemia time of 30—80 h, the incidence of chronic CsA nephrotoxicity in these is much higher compared to that in living donor transplantation (12). Thirty-seven recipients suffered no acute rejections. In these there was an improvement in renal function, following CsA withdrawal which continued for up to 3 months. The rapid improvement of graft function may be due to improvement of renal blood flow or reduction in renal tubular toxicity (13, 14).

A significant number of recipients had hypertension, which improved following cyclosporine withdrawal. This may also be atrributed to improved renal blood flow (13). The requirement for antihypertensive medications in patients with residual hypertension was also reduced significantly after CsA withdrawal. Tremors, hirsutism and gingival hypertrophy are not uncommon in cyclosporine-treated patients. In this series, these side effects were seen in 40—50% of the recipients. Although many of these are not considered to be very serious, they contributed to non-compliance with regard to cyclosporine intake, especially in adolescent young female. Many recipients with such side effects were relieved of them following CsA withdrawal.

However, CsA withdrawal is not without problems especially with regard to graft rejection and graft dysfunction. Acute rejection episodes were seen in 6 or 14% (8.6% in LRD and 20% in cadaver grafts) although in all but one, these were easily reversed by pulsed steroid therapy. Reconversion to cyclosporine in our series was necessary in only one patient (3%).

In conclusion, CsA withdrawl in renal transplant recipients with stable graft function at 1—2 years after transplantation, results in improvement in graft function, relief from many side effects of CsA such as hypertension, hirsutism, tremors and gingival hypertrophy in the majority of the recipients. However acute rejection episodes may occur in 14% of the recipients following CsA withdrawal and a much smaller number of recipients (<3%) may develop permanent graft dysfunction following uncontrolled acute rejection. However, before CsA withdrawal can be recommended as a routine procedure, further long-term observation on graft function are required.

References

1. European Multicentre Trial Group: Cyclosporin in cadaveric renal transplantation: One year follow up of a multicentre trial. *Lancet* **2**, 986—989 (1983).
2. The Canadian Multicentre Transplantation Study Group: A randomized clinical trial of Cyclosporine in cadaveric renal transplantation: Analysis at three years. *New Engl. J. Med.* **314**, 1219—1225 (1986).
3. Calne, R.Y., Rolles, D., White, D.J.G. *et al.*: Cyclosporine-A initially as the only immunosuppressant in 34 recipients of cadaveric organs: 32 kidneys, 2 pancreases and 2 livers. *Lancet* **2**, 1033—1036 (1979).
4. The Council of the Transplantation Society: *Transplantation* **419**, 1—3 (1986).
5. Abouna, G.M., Kumar, M.S.A., Samhan, M., Dadah, S.K. and Sabawi, N.M.: Commercializa-

tion in organ transplantation — a Middle Eastern perspective. *Transplant. Proc.* **22**, 918–921 (1990).

6. Kumar, M.S.A., Samhan, M., Philips, E.M. and Abouna, G.M.: Late function in 48-cadaver renal allografts preserved for 48—76 hours. *Transplant. Proc.* **20**(5), 940—941 (1988).
7. Canafax, D.M., Martel, E.J., Ascher, N.L., Payne, W.D., Sutherland, D.E.R., Simmons, R.L. and Najarian, J.S.: Two methods of managing cyclosporine nephrotoxicity: conversion to azathioprine, prednisolone or cyclosporine, azathioprine and prednisolone. *Transplant. Proc.* **17**(1), 1176—1177 (1985).
8. Hall, B.M., Tiller, D.J., Hardie, I., Mahony, J., Mathew, T., Thatcher, G., Miach, P. and Thompson, N.: Comparision of three immunosuppressive regimens in cadaver renal transplantation: long-term cyclosporine, short-term cyclosporine followed by azathioprine and prednisolone and azathioprine and prednisolone without cyclosporine. *New Engl. J. Med.* **318**, 1499—1507 (1988).
9. Speilberger, M., Aigner, E., Schmid, T., Bosmuller, C., Konigstrainer, A. and Margreiter, R.: Long-term results of cadaveric renal transplantation after conversion from cyclosporine to azathioprine: a controlled randomized trial. *Transplant. Proc.* **20**, 169—170 (1988).
10. Garcia, R., Zschaek, D., Ogeerally, J., Dominguez, J. and Rodgriguez-Itarbe, B.: Discontinuation of cyclosporin with low incidence of rejection in human renal transplantation (letter), *Clin. Nephrol.* **32**(1), 46—47 (1989).
11. Kumar, M.S.A., White, A.G., Alex, G., Antos, M.S., Philips, E.M. and Abouna, G.M.: Correlation of blood levels and tissue levels of cyclosporine with histologic features of cyclosporine toxicity. *Transplant. Proc.* **20**(2), 344—353 (1988).
12. Kumar, M.S.A., Samhan, M., John, P., Al-Adnani, M.S. and Abouna, G.M.: Chronic cyclosporine nephrotoxicity in renal transplantation. Is it the effect of preservation? *Transplant. Proc.* **21**, 1552—1553 (1989).
13. Curtis, J.J., Luke, R.G., Dubovsky, E., Diethelm, A.g., Whelchel, J.D. and Jones, P.: Cyclosporine in therapeutic doses increases renal allograft vascular resistance. *Lancet* **2**, 477—479 (1986).
14. Chapman, J.R., Grifiths, D., Hardin, N.G.L. and Morris, P.J.: Reversibility of cyclosporin nephrotoxicity after three months' treatment. *Lancet* **1**, 128—130 (1985).

15. Early experience with FK 506 in liver transplantation

ROBERT D. GORDON, SATORU TODO, JOHN J. FUNG, ANDREAS G. TZAKIS, NORIKO MURASE, ASHOK JAIN, MARIO ALESSIANI and THOMAS E. STARZL

Since the introduction of cyclosporine-steroid therapy in 1980 for liver transplantation, 1 year clinical survival rates have approached 70% for most of the common indications for liver replacement and 5 year survival rates are better than 60%. Nevertheless, allograft rejection continues to be a significant cause of retransplantation or death. Clinical rejection occurs in 70% of liver allograft recipients on cyclosporine-steroid therapy. Many patients require treatment with polyclonal or monoclonal antibody preparations to control acute cellular rejection. An increased risk of opportunistic infection, especially from cytomegalovirus, is associated with such therapy.

Nephrotoxicity is a principal and dose limiting side effect of cyclosporine. Chronic renal damage and functional impairment has been shown to occur in many liver transplant patients. Hypertension (secondary to direct renal effects of cyclosporine) requiring antihypertensive therapy is required in over half of these patients. Reduction of cyclosporine dose and/or combination therapy including lower dose cyclosproine, steroids and other agents, usually azathioprine, have been resorted to in order to maintain adequate immunosuppression while reducing intolerable side effects of cyclosporine.

FK 506, a macrolide antibiotic produced from *Streptomyces tsukubaensis*, is produced by the Fujisawa Pharmaceutical Company, Ltd of Japan and is a new immunosuppressive agent which is at least 100 times more potent than cyclosporine.

Animal models

FK 506 was shown to be immunosuppressive *in vitro* by Kino *et al.* (1) and in rats by Inamura *et al.* (2) It has demonstrated a remarkable ability to prolong allograft survival in a number of experimental animal models including renal, liver, and heart allografts (2—11). In studies conducted in Pittsburgh by Todo and co-workers in rats, dogs, and subhuman primates, no evidence of prohibitive toxicity was found. In contrast, studies by Thiru *et al.* reported serious toxicity consisting of widespread arteritis in dogs and baboons (12). However, studies by Todo *et al.* and Ochiai *et al.* (13) have shown such vascular lesions to be present in non-immunosuppressed dogs after whole organ transplantation or in dogs treated with other agents including cyclosporine. Arteritis has not been seen in baboons treated with FK 506 or in other toxicology studies (10, 11).

Mechanism of action

FK 506 has shown synergism with cyclosporine in experimental systems. The mechanism of action of FK 506, like that of cyclosporine, is not completely understood, but both agents, which are chemically unrelated, show similarities in their effects on T cells.

In studies of the *in vitro* effects of FK 506 on cloned T cell activations, Sawada *et al.* have shown that FK 506 inhibits the response of cloned T cells to concanavalin A and to murine spleen cells in a dose-dependent manner at 40- to 200-fold lower concentrations than cyclosporine. Allo-cytolytic T cell lymphocyte induction from murine thymocytes was inhibited, but not the ability of sensitized T cells to lyse specific target cells. Interleukin-2 (IL2) driven proliferation of activated cloned T cells was not inhibited. However, FK 506 inhibited IL2 secretion and IL2 receptor expression on cloned T cells after stimulation by specific antigen. Cyclosporine has been shown to affect T cell activation in a similar manner but at far higher dosages.

Yoshimura *et al.* (15) have demonstrated FK 506 dose dependent inhibition of IL-2 and gamma-interferon secretion by peripheral human bone marrow cells (PBMC) stimulated with phytohemaglutinin (PHA). FK 506 failed to inhibit B cell stimulating factor 2 (BSF-2) production by PBMC. Both cloned B and T cells, once activated, were not significantly affected by FK 506. Lymphocytes from primary MLR cultured in the presence of FK 506 did not allow for expression of alloantigen activated suppressor cells when used in a dose sufficient to inhibit CTL generation (16). Furthermore, there is evidence that both cyclosporine and FK 506 inhibit transcription of the IL-2 gene and that FK 506, like cyclosporine, acts on an early event in T cell activation (17).

Phase I clinical trials of FK 506 were begun at the University of Pittsburgh with the approval of the Institutional Review Board and the USFDA, in 1989. The initial experience was reported at a special symposium held in Barcelona, Spain, in October 1989 (see *Transplant. Proc.* vol. 22, no. 2, February 1990). The following discussion will summarize the experience reported at that meeting.

Rescue therapy with FK 506

Our experience with the first 40 patients in which FK 506 was used for rescue of patients with intractible rejection or cyclosporine intolerance has been reported by Fung *et al.* (18) These are among the first human patients to be given FK 506. All patients entered into the study were treated with cyclosporine and prednisone prior to conversion to FK 506. Although some patients were switched to FK 506 purely because of cyclosporine intolerance, most were converted for uncontrolled liver allograft rejection despite maximal therapy with CsA and prednisone and many of these patients also had complications related to cyclosporine including renal dysfunction or hypertension. One patient was withdrawn from FK 506 therapy after 3 days when it was recognized that the patient had recurrent acute hepatitis rather than acute severe graft rejection. The remaining 39 patients were therefore considered treatment failures of conventional immunosuppression.

There were 19 females and 21 males, ranging in age from 5 to 74 years. Liver biopsies were performed in all but 3 patients prior to entry and confirmed the diagnosis of cell mediated rejection. In 6 patients, it was the clinical impression that the biopsy findings underestimated the severity of rejection and in these patients the decision to rescue with FK 506 was based on clinical biochemical parameters. One patient was entered into the trial because of severe steroid intolerance.

Thirty-nine allografts were studied definitively for at least one month or more and all but 8 of these were successfully rescued as judged by histopathologic criteria and liver biochemistry studies. In each case, significant improvement was observed in protocol liver biopsies obtained 2 weeks after the start of treatment with FK 506. Of particular interest was the apparent reversibility under FK 506 of the vanishing bile duct syndrome in those patients with some ducts still remaining in the portal triads. This lesion is usually refractory to treatment with conventional immunosuppression.

Abnormalities in liver function tests also showed significant improvement. An early decline in the cannulicular enzymes (alkaline phosphatase and gamma-GTP) was again of special interest since this correlated with the striking histological improvement seen in patients with vanishing bile duct syndrome. Similar improvements in hepatocellular enzymes (AST and ALT) were also observed in patients with histological improvement seen on protocol biopsies.

One patient subsequently required retransplantation after successful reversal of rejection of his fifth liver graft by FK 506 because of hepatic artery thrombosis resulting from a technical flaw (a local anastomotic stricture). Pathological examination of the resected allograft showed no evidence of residual cell mediated rejection. The patient was given a sixth graft and has since been successfully sustained with this graft under continued immunosupression with FK 506.

Renal function

Preexisting renal dysfunction was noted in approximately 70% of the patients entered in this trial. Two patients had prior renal transplants and, in biopsies of both patients, cellular rejection and chronic fibrosis were seen, suggesting that both acute and chronic rejection of the kidney allograft was occurring. Cyclosporine nephrotoxicity was present in most of the other patients treated.

The heterogeneity of the kidneys in patients in this study made it difficult to assess the nephrotoxicity of FK 506. Nine patients had such severe renal dysfunction at the time of switchover to FK 506, including hyperkalemia, that effective cyclosporine therapy was not possible.

Evidence was observed that the effect of FK 506 on renal function is related to an interaction with cyclosporine and that FK 506 augmented cyclosporine nephrotoxicity. With the eventual elimination of cyclosporine after discontinuance of this agent, a reduction in the BUN and Cr was eventually observed in most cases, in spite of therapeutic levels of FK 506. Two of the five patients who required hemodialysis recovered renal function. One patient required institution of hemodialysis, after bilateral renal vein thrombosis was discovered, shortly after institution of FK 506 therapy. Three patients required cadaveric renal transplantation for persistent renal failure during the course of FK 506 therapy.

Primary therapy with FK 506

A phase 1 primary treatment study was begun in the latter half of 1989 and the initial 20 patients were reported by Todo (19). The following is a summary of 33 adult conventional liver transplant recipients who had entered the protocol as of October 15, 1989. In addition, follow-up 3 patients, whose graft rejection could not reversed with the FK 506 'rescue' protocol and who therefore required retransplantation under FK 506, are also included. These are the first human patients to be given FK 506, along with low dose steroids, as their primary immunosuppressive baseline regimen. The results show the remarkably potent immunosuppressive qualities of FK 506 and its relative lack of toxicity in the first several months after transplantation.

A biostatistical survival analysis (Kaplan-Meier) has been performed on the entire series of 33 patients with at lease one month of follow-up and a computer selected group of 81 CsA treated controls matched for age, sex, diagnosis, and clinical urgency (UNOS score). The FK 506 and CsA control patients were well matched for age, sex, and liver disease, but there was a higher proportion of critically ill patients (UNOS score 4) in the FK 506 treated patients than in the CsA treated controls.

A subgroup of the first 20 these 33 patients, for whom follow-up for at least 60 days is available, and a matched group of 20 CsA treated patients were compared for several outcome variables including measures of liver and renal function, gastrointestinal toxicity, hypertension, the incidence and severity of rejection, and the incidence and severity of major infections.

FK 506, along with low dose steroid therapy, was used for all FK treated patients receiving primary liver allografts, as well as in the three surviving patients initially entered in the 'rescue' protocol and retransplanted under FK 506. FK 506 therapy was initiated following liver transplantation, using a traditional steroid taper over 5 days. (In subsequent phases of the trial the initial high dose steroid taper has been eliminated and the patients simply started on prednisolone at 20 mg per day.) Doses of FK 506 were standardized to 0.15 mg/kg/day as initial intravenous therapy, with conversion to oral FK 506 at ranges of 0.075 mg/kg/day to 0.30 mg/kg/day, based upon blood trough levels and observed side effects. A median of 6 days of intravenous FK 506 was given, before conversion to oral therapy.

Patient survival: Only 2 patients in the initial primary series died. One patient, with primary pulmonary hypertension and unsuspected advanced atherosclerotic heart disease, prior to transplantation, died on postoperative day 15, from heart failure with good liver function and histology. Another patient, who was critically ill (UNOS score 4) at the time of transplantation, developed thrombocytopenia after transplantation and died at 5 days of a hemorrhagic stroke, a well-known complication after liver transplantation, especially in critically ill patients.

Figure 1 presents Kaplan-Meier plots comparing survival of the 33 patients receiving their first liver graft under FK 506 compared to patient survival for the 81 CsA treated and matched historical controls. Thirty-day patient survival for the FK treated patients is 93.9% compared to 87.6% for the CsA treated controls. At a minimum we can say that FK 506 has not had any deleterious

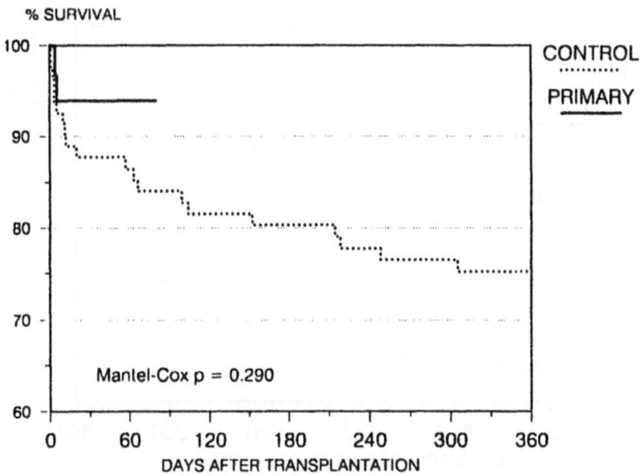

Fig. 1. Patient survival (Kaplan-Meier plot) for primary liver transplantation under FK 506 compared to cyclosporine-steroid treated matched historical controls.

effect on early patient survival. Moreover, although the plots were not yet different at a level of statistical significance, the trend suggested 50% improvement for patients treated with FK 506 compared to those treated with CsA. These early observations have been confirmed and achieved statistical significance in our extended experience recently reported by Todo *et al.* (20).

Liver allograft function

Of the 36 liver allografts analyzed in the protocol (including the 3 retransplantations), all functioned immediately, and no patient required retransplantation for primary graft non-function.

Figure 2 presents Kaplan-Meier plots comparing primary graft survival of the FK 506 treated patients to primary graft survival for 81 grafts in the CsA treated controls. In the FK 506 group, 30 of the 33 grafts are surviving 28 to 80 days after transplantation. Actuarial survival at 30 days is 93.9% For the CsA treated, matched controls, 30 day actuarial survival is 80.0%. The differences in survival had not yet reached statistical significance but the trend suggests a 65% improvement in early graft survival in the FK 506 treated patients. Again, subsequent longer follow-up and a larger case experience recently reported by Todo have confirmed the significance of these observations (20).

Graft function after transplantation was also assessed by serial biochemical measurements. Bilirubin fell to normal levels much more rapidly in FK 506 treated patients than in CsA treated controls (Figure 3). The pattern of hepatocellular enzymes were similar in both groups of patients (Figure 4). Although

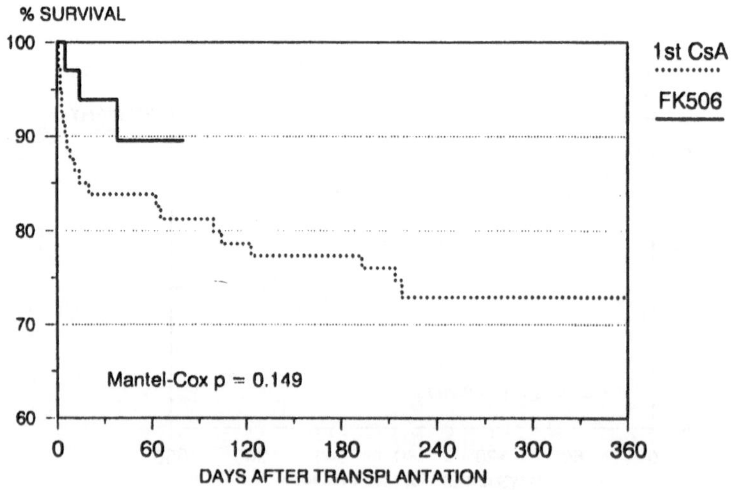

Fig. 2. Graft survival (Kaplan-Meier plot) for primary liver transplantation under FK 506 compared to cyclosporine-steroid treated matched historical controls.

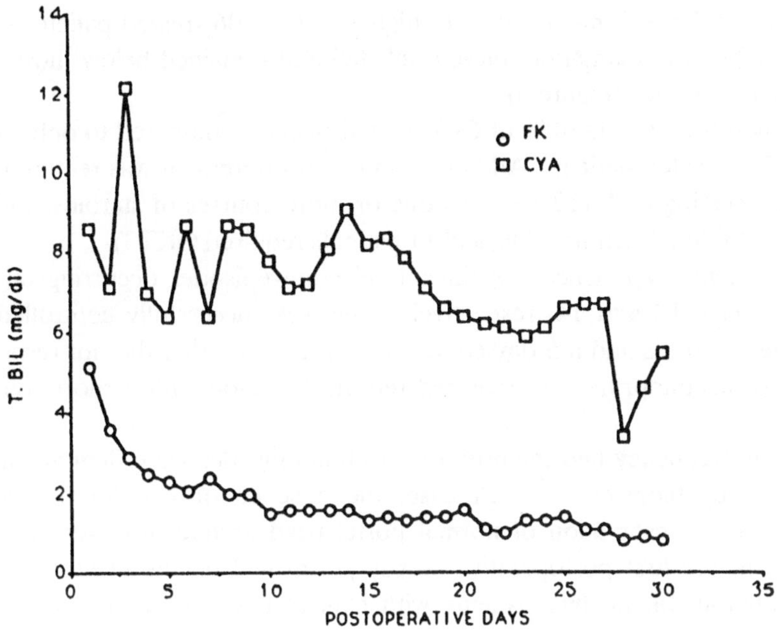

Fig. 3. Postoperative bilirubin for primary recipients of liver grafts treated with FK 506 compared to CsA treated controls (from reference (19)).

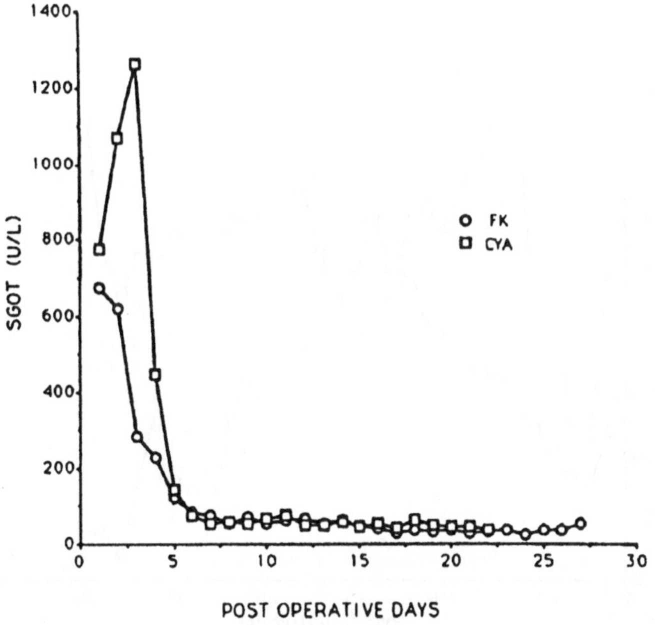

Fig. 4. Postoperative SGOT (AST) for primary recipients of liver grafts treated with FK 506 compared to CsA treated controls (from reference (19)).

initial canalicular enzyme levels were higher in FK 506 treated patients, within 2 weeks after transplantation, these levels fell and remained below those in the CsA treated controls (Figure 5).

Rejection was seen in 60% of CsA treated patients compared to only 10% of the FK 506 treated patients. Additional immunosuppression was required in 18 patients receiving CsA (17 received one or more courses of steroids, while 18 received additional azathioprine, and 11 patients required OKT3).

Two patients experienced significant rejection episodes occurring on post-operative days 12 and 14, respectively. One was successfully controlled with augmented steroids and a 5 day course of OKT3. The other did not respond to steroids or azathioprine, and required retransplantation with a short course of OKT3.

The low frequency and intensity of rejection episodes were demonstrable in protocol liver biopsies. In each case, the absence of lymphocytic cellular infiltrates and preservation of normal portal triad architecture were routinely observed in the first postoperative biopsy performed on the twelfth day after transplantation. In the two patients with clinical rejection, typical findings of cellular rejection were present.

Steroid requirements

The requirement for steroids in patients treated with FK 506 has been less than

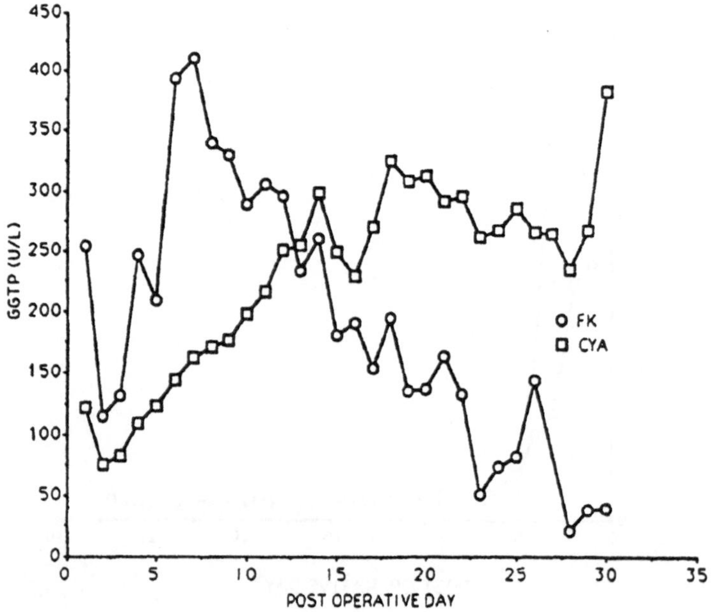

Fig. 5. Postoperative canalicular enzymes (gGTP) for primary recipients of liver grafts treated with FK 506 compared to CsA treated controls (from reference (19)).

that for patients treated with CsA. The mean daily steroid dose in the FK 506 patients was 9 mg/day at one month compared to 19 mg/day for the CsA control group.

Renal function

FK 506 is not a classic nephrotoxin such as the aminoglycosides and does not produce renal cell death and acute renal failure. FK 506 does affect renal function but there are differences from the effects seen with CsA. Elevations in postoperative renal function are not uniform, and promptly decline during the first week following transplantation. We have found a poor correlation (r = 0.45) between FK 506 drug level and serum creatinine (SCr) compared to the strong correlation (r = 0.88) seen between CsA levels and SCr (r = 0.88). Thus, changes in changes in SCr, a dependable indicator of CsA toxicity, is not such a reliable indicator of FK 506 toxicity.

Among the 33 patients treated with FK 506 for their first graft, only one patient, who was on hemodialysis prior to transplantation, required dialysis after transplantation. This pateint, who eventually recovered, was in hepatorenal failure and was on dialysis prior to transplantation. This patient eventually recovered renal function and serum creatinine returned to normal levels while the patient was continued on FK 506. Three patients in the CsA historical control group required hemodialysis during their initial hospital stay.

FK 506 and CsA treated patients were not matched for renal function and serum creatinine (SCr) was higher in the CsA treated controls compared to FK 506 treated patients at all time points, including prior to transplantation. Seventeen FK 506 treated patients and 12 CsA control patients had a SCr less than 1.5 mg/dl prior to transplantation. In this subgroup, pretransplant SCr was less in the CsA treated patients (0.62 ± 0.24 mg/dl) than in the FK 506 treated patients (0.74 ± 0.04 mg/dl). However, SCr was greater in the SsA treated subgroup thereafter.

The acute rises in serum creatinine seen in the first patients treated for graft rescue with FK 506 were alarming. However, this is now believed to be a result of the combined severe nephrotoxicity of CsA combined with the milder nephrotoxicity of FK 506. Prior exposure to CsA and its resulting nephrotoxicity leads to a predictable deterioration in renal function, but fortunately this improves after several weeks. FK 506 appears to have much less of a nephrotoxic effect in patients not previously treated with CsA. Thus, patients being converted from CsA to FK 506 are at higher risk of renal dysfunction than patients being treated primarily with FK 506. In patients not suffering from chronic CsA nephrotoxicity, renal function is well preserved.

Hyperkalemia was frequently seen both in CsA and FK 506 treated patients.

Previous studies in CsA treated patients have usually found hyporeninemic hypoaldosteronism and this is also seen in patients treated with FK 506. In addition, there is an association between an increase in SCr and hyperkalemia, suggesting that a reduction in GFR also contributes to the retention of potassium. The hyperkalemia observed was moderate and responded in all cases to fludrocortisone acetate.

Hypertension

Hypertension is the second most troublesome side effect of treatment with CsA. No patient in the primary FK 506 group required addition of antihypertensive medication during the postoperative observation period. One patient with renal artery stenosis had some antihypertensive medications continued, although at a lower level than prior to transplantation.

Gastrointestinal/metabolic effects

The serum cholesterol level was statistically lower in the FK 506 treated group, as compared to the CsA group. Uric acid levels remained in the normal range in patients receiving FK 506. No differences in fasting blood sugar or pancreatic amylase were seen in FK 506 patients compared to CsA treated patients and no significant changes in the appearance of the pancreas have been seen on postoperative CT scans.

Adverse reactions

Unlike the patient population described for CsA to FK 506 conversion, this population of patients receiving FK 506 as primary therapy, had a much lower incidence of side effects. Side effects were assessed by careful interview of the patients by a trained nurse clinician. Although it can be difficult to determine whether subjective patient complaints are attributable to surgery itself or a side effect of medication, there were distinct differences in the incidence of side effects reported by patients taking oral FK 506 when compared to those reported by patients receiving intravenous drug. Eighty-seven percent of patients reported no significant side effects while taking oral FK 506 compared to 42% of patients on intravenous treatment.

The most common side effect of primary intravenous FK 506 administration was headache. The headaches were usually described as mild and required narcotic analgesia in only 2 patients. The headaches responded to symptomatic treatment and did not require reduction in dosages. Switching to oral administration relieved the headache in all but 1 patient.

The next most frequent side effects of intravenous therapy were gastroenterologic, especially nausea. Treatment consisted of antiemetics, and spontaneous resolution of these symptons occurred in all patients following conversion to oral therapy. With intravenous therapy, mild anorexia was sometimes associated with nausea. Oral intake was adequate in all patients.

No adverse hemodynamic reactions, such as hypotension or other alterations in cardiac performance, were noted during the oral or intravenous administration of FK 506. Detailed cardiovascular profiles were developed during the initial intravenous infusion with FK 506. No patient required augmented antihypertensive medications as an outpatient.

Other side effects seen with intravenous FK 506 were a feeling of warmth and flushing. Less frequent side effects were rash, chest pain (without EKG changes), anxiety, abdominal cramping, night sweats, fatigue, photophobia, and blurred vision. These symptom complexes were also markedly reduced following conversion from intravenous to oral FK 506.

Infection

The incidence of serious infections (defined as life-threatening infections), was not increased with the use of FK 506 when compared to CsA. In fact, the incidence of bacterial infections was low, occurring in only 4 patients in each group. Transient bacteremia from an indwelling intravenous catheter was seen in 1 patient on FK 506 and resolved with removal of the catheter. Two wound infections were seen, one mild and the other extending into subfascial planes which required drainage. One patient, treated for staphylococcal endocarditis prior to transplantation, developed spontaneous staphylococcal peritonitis while on FK 506. Viral infections, in particular cytomegalovirus (CMV) infections, were seen in 2 patients in the initial 20 FK 506 treated primary patients, as compared to 5 patients on CsA. These CMV infections were clinically mild and responded to treatment with gancyclovir.

Charges and hospital stay

An additional measure of the relative effectiveness and safety of FK 506 has been its impact on the length of hospital stay and related hospital charges after liver transplantation when compared to similar measures for CsA treated patients. The findings are even more striking when it is remembered that there was a significantly higher proportion of critically ill (UNOS class 3 and 4) patients in the FK 506 treated group than in the CsA treated control group. Patients treated with CsA tended to stay in the hospital twice as long and accrued total bed charges almost three times greater than FK 506 patients (21).

Pharmacologic monitoring

Because of the possibility that FK 506 and cyclosporine would be used together, pharmacokinetic studies were performed with each drug individually, and then in combination, with both the intravenous and oral administration (22). Pharmacolinetic data of FK 506 suggests that the metabolism is primarily hepatic in nature. Peak levels in the 5—10 ng/ml range could be detected 1—2 hours after intravenous administration. The terminal blood half-life appears to be 12 hours after a redistribution phase following an intravenous dose. The nature of absorption, peak levels and possibily the terminal half-life seem somewhat different following an oral dose. A relatively flat peak is generally seen, and the absorption of the oral dose is estimated at 30%.

Both polyclonal and monoclonal immunoassay techniques have been perfected to monitor both blood and tissue levels of this drug and its metabolites.

Conclusion

FK 506 is an extraordinary immunosuppressive agent that has shown great promise in the early clinical trials in liver transplantation. It is much more potent than cyclosporine and, although it has a similar spectrum of side effects, it nevertheless appears to be much better tolerated than CsA. In particular, nephrotoxicity appears to be much milder with FK 506. Equally impressive is the ability of FK 506 to arrest the vanishing bile duct syndrome of chronic liver rejection at a later stage than with any previously available agent. Finally, the drug is much more effective than CsA in preventing acute rejection early after transplantation which permits early reduction in steroid dosage, avoids the need for use of antibody therapy and the penalties associated with the use such agents, and permits earlier discharge from the hospital after transplantation.

Acknowledgement

This work was supported by research grants from the Veterans Administration and Project Grant No. DK 29961 from the National Institutes of Health, Bethesda, MD.

References

1. Kino, T., Hatanaka, H., Inamura, N. *et al.*: FK 506, a novel immunosuppressant isolated from Streptomyces. II. Immunosuppressive effect of FK 506 *in vitro*. *Transplant. Proc.* **19** (Suppl. 6), 64—67 (1987).
2. Inamural, N., Nakahara, K., Kino T. *et al.*: Prolongation of skin allograft survival in rats by a novel immunosuppressive agent, FK 506. *Transplantation* **45**, 206—209 (1988).
3. Gudas, V.M., Carmichael, P.G. and Morries, R.E.: Comparison of the immunosuppressive and toxic effects of FK 506 and cyclosporine in xenograft recipients. *Transplant. Proc.* **21** (1 Pt 1), 1072—1073 (1989).
4. Ochiai, T., Nakajima, K., Nagata, M. *et al.*: Effect of a new immunosuppressive agent, FK 506 on heterotopic allotransplantation in the rat. *Transplant. Proc.* **19**, 1284—1286 (1987).
5. Ochiai, T., Nagata, M., Suzuki, T. *et al.*: Studies of the effects of FK 506 on renal allografting in the beagle dog. *Transplantation* **44**, 729—733 (1987).
6. Ochiai, T., Nakajima, K., Nagata, M. *et al.*: Studies of the induction and maintenance of long term graft acceptance by treatment with FK 506 in heterotopic cardiac allotransplantation in rats. *Transplantation* **44**, 734—738 (1987).
7. Lim, S.L.M., Thiru, S. and White, D.J.G.: Heterotopic heart transplantation in the rat receiving FK 506. *Transplant. Proc.* **19** (Suppl. 6), 68 (1987).
8. Todo, S., Demetris, A.J., Ueda, Y. *et al.*: Canine kidney transplantation with FK 506 alone or in combination with cyclosporine and steroids. *Transplant. Proc.* **19** (Suppl. 6), 57—62 (1987).
9. Todo, S., Podesta, L., Chapchap, P. *et al.*: Orthotopic liver transplantation in dogs receiving FK 506. *Transplant. Proc.* **19** (Suppl. 6), 64—67 (1987).
10. Todo, S., Ueda, Y., Demetris, A.J. *et al.*: Immunosuppression of canine, monkey, and baboon allografts by FK 506 with special reference to synergism with other drugs, and to tolerance induction. *Surgery* **104**, 239—249 (1988).
11. Todo, S., Demitrsi, A., Ueda, Y. *et al.*: Renal transplantation in baboons under FK 506. *Surgery* **106**, 444—451 (1989).
12. Thiru, S., Collier, D. St J. and Calne, R.: Pathologic studies in canine and baboon renal allograft recipients immunosuppressed with FK 506. *Transplant. Proc.* **19** (Suppl. 6), 98—99 (1987).
13. Ochiai, T., Sakamoto, K., Gunji, Y. *et al.*: Effects of combination treatment with FK 506 and cyclosporine on survival time and vascular changes in renal-allograft-recipient dogs. *Transplantation* **48**, 193—197 (1989).
14. Sawada, S., Suzuki, G., Kawase, Y. and Takaku, F.: Novel immunosuppressive agent, FK 506. In vitro effects on cloned T cell activation. *J. Immunol.* **139**, 1797—1803 (1987).
15. Yoshimura, N., Matsui, S., Hamashima, T. and Oka, T.: Effect of a new immunosuppressive agent, FK 506, on human lymphocyte responses in vitro. II. Inhibition of the production of IL2 and gamma-IFN, but not B cell-stimulating factor 2. *Transplantation* **47**, 351—359 (1989).
16. Yoshimura, N., Matsui, S., Hamashima, T. and Oka, T.: Effect of a new immunosuppressive agent, FK 506, on human lymphocyte responses in vitro. II. Inhibition of expression of alloantigen-activated suppressor cells, as well as induction of alloreactivity. *Transplantation* **47**, 351—356 (1989).
17. Tocci, M.J., Matkovich, D.A., Collier, K.A. *et al.*: The immunosuppressant FK 506 selectively inhibits expression of early T cell activation genes. *J. Immunol.* **143**, 718—726 (1989).
18. Fung, J.J., Todo, S., Jain, A. *et al.*: Conversion from cyclosporine to FK 506 in liver allograft recipients with cyclosporine-related complications. *Transplant. Proc.* **22** (Suppl. 1) 6—12 (1990).
19. Todo, S., Fung, J.J., Demtris, A.J., *et al.*: Early trials with FK 506 as primary treatment in liver transplantation. *Transplant. Proc.* **22** (1 Suppl. 1), 13—16 (1990).

20. Todo, S., Fung, J.J., Starzl, T.E. *et al.*: Liver, kidney, and thoracic organ transplantation under FK 506. *Ann. Surg.* (in press).
21. Staschak, S., Wagner, S., Block, G. *et al.*: A cost comparison of liver transplantation with FK 06 or CyA as the primary immunosuppressive agent. *Transplant. Proc.* **22**, 47—49 (1990).
22. Venkataramanan, Jain, A., Cadoff, E. *et al.*: Pharmacokinestics of FK 506: Preclinical and clinical studies. *Transplant. Proc.* **22**, 52—56 (1990).

16. Deoxyspergualin. A novel immunosuppressant: experimental and clinical studies

H. AMEMIYA, S. SUZUKI, K. OTA, K. TAKAHASHI, T. SONODA, M. ISHIBASHI, R. OMOTO, I. KOYAMA, K. DOHI, Y. FUKUDA and K. FUKAO

Deoxyspergualin (DSG) is an analogue of an antibiotic having antitumor effect, spergualin (1), which was isolated from the culture filtrate of *Bacillus laterosporus* in 1981. In 1985, it was reported that DSG had immunosuppressive effect (2, 3), and thereafter the characteristics of the agent as an immunosuppressant against rejection has been examined in detail. Figure 1 shows the chemical structure of DSG, which has a molecular weight of 496.91, occurs as white powder, and is very soluble in water and stable for a long period at 15 °C and below.

The mechanism that DSG suppresses immunological response has not been elucidated completely. Nemoto *et al.* (4) reported that DSG did not suppress the production of IL-1 by macrophages nor that of IL-2 by helper T cells. DSG suppresses proliferation and differentiation of bone marrow cells (BMc), leaving easy response of BKc to IL-3 or macrophage-CSF. From the above results, it is assumed that DSG does not damage BMc but suppresses differentiation of BMc into mature cells, which would be the immunosuppressive mechanism of DSG, being quite different from that of cyclosporine (5).

Figure 2 shows the immunosuppressive effect of DSG on rejection, when used prophylactically. The dosage of DSG was limited because the agent strongly induced gastrointestinal disturbance in dog species, but the intravenous dose employed of 0.6 mg/kg/day, could suppress the rejection for 28 days (6). This fact clearly shows that DSG also has the immunosuppressive effect and can maintain the immunosuppressive state in big animals. Another characteristic of

$$(\pm)$$

$$H_2N\underset{\underset{NH}{\|}}{C}NH(CH_2)_6CONH\underset{\underset{OH}{|}}{C}HCONH(CH_2)_4NH(CH_2)_3NH_2 . 3HCl$$

M.W. 496.91

Fig. 1. Chemical structure of deoxyspergualin.

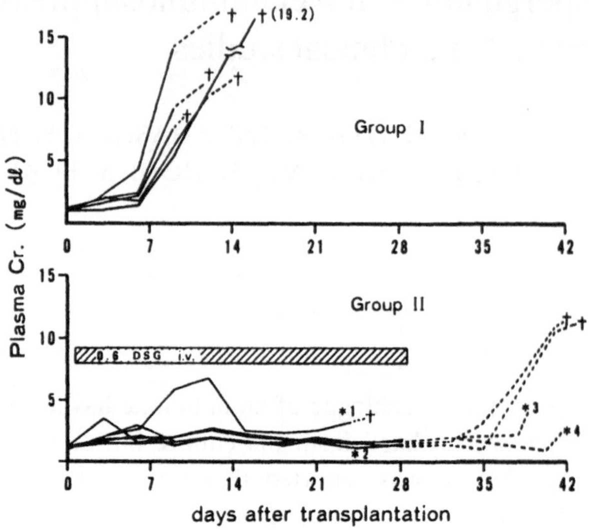

Fig. 2. Immunosuppressive effect of deoxyspergualin in dog renal allografting. Group I: Non-treated. Group II: Treated with 0.6 mg/kg DSG. *1: Death with functioning graft *2: Sacrificed 29 days after grafting for histological study *3 and *4: In these two dogs, used afterwards for another experiment on rescue use of DSG, plasma Cr level increased due to rejection.

DSG as an immunosuppressant is effectiveness against on-going rejection. To the rejection developing in the dog renal allograft model, DSG could remit eight cases out of nine of rejection at intravenous doses of 4.8, 2.4 and 1.2 mg/kg/day for consecutive 2, 2 and 3 days, respectively (7).

Data that DSG could be used for treatment of on-going rejection were also obtained in the rat heart allograft model (8). Furthermore, it is more interesting that, as shown in Figure 3, immunological unresponsiveness becomes more easily obtained when DSG administration is started on the appearance of the rejection sign on ^{31}P-NMR 3—4 days after grafting than on the day of grafting. The immunologically unresponsive state could be transferred by spleen cells of a recipient who had acquired the immunological unresponsiveness. That is, it is assumed that clones expanded by allografting were eliminated by DSG and that at the same time suppressor cell clones which were not affected by DSG expanded with time leading to formation of immunologically unresponsive state. The fact suggests that DSG is effective not only as an immunosuppressive maintenance drug or a pulse-therapy drug against on-going rejection but also as a drug used in the induction phase of organ transplant.

From September 1988 to March 1989, a multicentral clinical trial to examine the effectiveness of DSG was performed in 35 kidney transplant patients developing 41 episodes of rejection. Clinical types of rejection were 8 accelerated acute rejections, 26 acute rejections, and 7 chronic rejections. Every case suffered from rejection was maintained mainly by cyclosporine. Overall

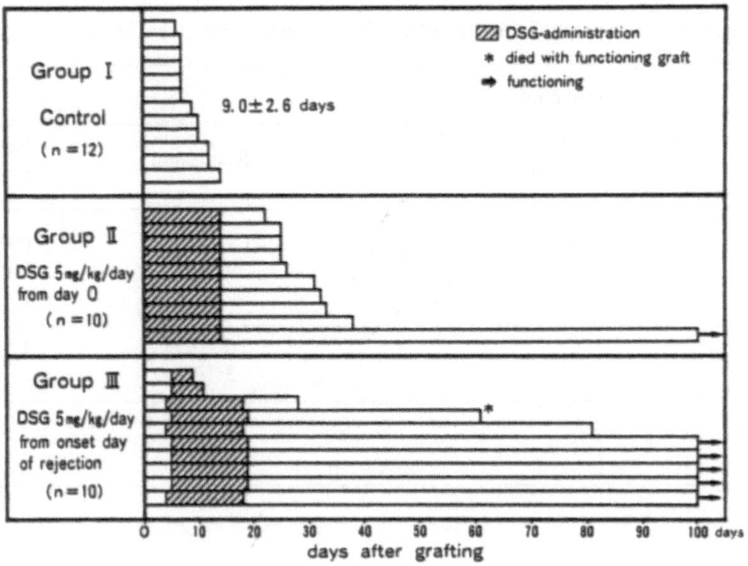

Fig. 3. Immunosuppressive effect of deoxyspergualin on on-going rejection and tolerance induction in rat heart allografting.

results are shown in Table 1. Out of 41 episodes, 32 or 78% revealed remission of rejection. The graft survival rate at 6 months after DSG treatment was 96% in the cases showing remission by DSG, while 56% in those showing no remission by DSG. Table 2 gives the effect of DSG by patterns of treatment. There are three patterns of DSG treatment, DSG alone, rescue DSG, and combined use (mainly with methylprednisolone), and overall, they seem to be effective against acute rejection within six months after grafting. In the cases receiving DSG as a rescue drug, the preceding drug for bolus therapy was mainly methylprednisolone, but OKT3 or ALG in three cases each. Main adverse reactions by DSG pulse therapy were leukocytopenia less than $4 \times 10^3/mm^3$ in 51% of the cases, and thrombocytopenia less than $10 \times 10^4/mm^3$ in 37%. In addition, 24% of the patients complained of facial numbness and 12%

Table 1. Overall results of deoxyspergualin pulse therapy on rejection in clinical renal recipients.

Rejection			Graft survival after DSG			
			Remitted		Non-remitted	
No.	Remission	Recurrence in 0—2 w	1 Mo	6 Mo	1 Mo	6 Mo
	(%)	(%)	(%)	(%)	(%)	(%)
41	32 (78)	8 (25)	100	96	100	56

Table 2. Pattern of deoxyspergualin treatment and its immunosuppressive effect on rejection.

Pattern of treatment	Rejection			
	Post-Tx duration	No.	Remission	Recurrence in 0—2 w
	Mo		(%)	(%)
DSG alone	<6	4	4 (100)	0 (0)
	>7	7	2 (29)	0 (0)
Rescue DSG	<6	11	10 (91)	1 (10)
	>7	4	3 (75)	0 (0)
Combined use	<6	8	6 (75)	3 (50)
	>7	7	7 (100)	4 (57)

did of anorexia. But none of the adverse reations was serious and there was no need to discontinue the DSG administration.

Our studies indicate that DSG has a new mechanism of action completely different from that of conventional immunosuppressants including cyclosporine, and is a very useful drug from a viewpoint of its immunosuppressive effects.

In summary, we conclude that deoxyspergualin (DSG) has a marked immunosuppressive effect in the rat heart allograft model and dog renal allograft model. In addition, DSG has noteworthy characteristics that it is effective against on-going rejection and can induce immunological unresponsiveness. The multicentral clinical trial of DSG revealed that DSG was significantly effective against acute rejection and could be used not only as a primary drug of the pulse therapy but also as a rescue drug which allows repeated use safely.

Acknowledgements

Supported in part by the Japanese Ministry of Education Grant 63870049 and the Japanese Ministry of Health and Welfare (Research grant for organ replacement technology 63SHI05, 63SH12). Clinical trial was performed by the Japanese Collaborative Transplant Study on Deoxyspergualin.

References

1. Takeuchi, T., Iinuma, H., Kunimoto, K. *et al.*: A new antitumor antibiotic, Spergualin: Isolation and antitumor activity. *J. Antibiot.* **34**, 1619 (1981).
2. Dickneite, G., Walter, P., Schorlemmer, H.U. *et al.*: The immunosuppressive properties of

15-deoxyspergualin and its effects on experimental skin and islet cells transplantation. In: Ishigami (ed.), *Recent Advances in Chemotherapy.* Univ. Tokyo Press, Tokyo (1985), 949 pp.

3. Umezawa, H., Ishizuka, M., Takeuchi, T. *et al.*: Suppression of tissue graft rejection by spergualin. *J. Antibiot.* **38**, 283 (1985).
4. Nemoto, K., Abe, F., Nakamura, T. *et al.*: Blastogenic responses and the release of interleukins 1 and 2 by spleen cells obtained from rat skin allograft recipients administered with 15-deoxyspergualin. *J. Antibiot.* **40**, 1062 (1987).
5. Nishimura, K. and Tokunaga, T.: Effect of 15-deoxyspergualin on the induction of cytotoxic T lymphocytes and bone marrow suppression. *Transplant. Proc.* **21**, 1104 (1989).
6. Amemiya, H., Suzuki, S., Niiya, S. *et al.*: A new immunosuppressive agent, 15-deoxyspergualin, in dog renal allografting. *Transplant. Proc.* **21**, 3468 (1989).
7. Itoh, J., Takeuchi, T., Suzuki, S. *et al.*: Reversal of acute rejection episodes by deoxyspergualin (NKT-01) in dogs receiving renal allografts. *J. Antibiot.* **41**, 1503 (1988).
8. Suzuki, S., Kanashiro, M., Watanabe, H. *et al.*: Therapeutic effect of 15-deoxyspergualin on acute graft rejection defected by ^{31}P nuclear magnetic resonance spectrography, and its effect on rat heart transplantation. *Transplantation* **46** (1988).

17. Preliminary results with FK 506 in pancreas grafting in a non-human primate model

G. KOOTSTRA, B.G. ERICZON, R. WIJNEN, T. TIEBOSCH, K. KUBOTA and C.-G. GROTH

FK 506 is a new drug with strong immunosuppressive properties. It is a macrolide, produced by *Streptomyces tsukubaensis*. The immunosuppressive activity was investigated *in vitro* by Kino *et al.* (1). As with cyclosporine A(2), FK 506 (3) specifically inhibits the T-cell response. Ochiai (4) performed studies in the rat and the strong immunosuppressive effect was confirmed by other groups (5) and in other species (6, 7). Calne and co-workers (8) observed a severe arteritis when FK 506 was used in the allotransplanted model in the dog, but not in the baboon. In the latter animal however, hyperglycemia was observed. Thus toxicity might be species dependent. We had an opportunity to study FK 506 in the non-human primate, the cynomolgus monkey. We have previously found that while FK 506 given i.m. is highly toxic in the cynomolgus monkey, oral administration of the drug is well tolerated (9). We report here our preliminary results with this drug in a pancreatic allotransplantation model in the cynomolgus monkey.

Materials and methods

Healthy adult cynomolgus monkeys weighing between 1.7 and 9.3 kg (mean 3.3 kg) were provided by two different institutions, and care was taken to perform transplants between animals from these different colonies. Although there are no preformed antibodies for the ABO system, red cell crossmatches were performed.

The animals were kept in a temperature-controlled room in separate cages. They had unrestricted access to water. Food consisting of pallets (Hope Farms primate diet, Woerden, The Netherlands) and fresh fruit was provided twice a day. In the preoperative work up an intravenous glucose tolerance test (IVGTT) was performed in all donors to exclude preexisting diabetic disease.

Pre- and postoperative care, anesthesia, medicaments

The fasted animals received 1 mg/kg Ketalar i.m. for induction of anesthesia.

Anesthesia was maintained with nitrous oxide, fluothane and oxygen with artificial ventilation. Ampicillin and Claforan were given i.v. for 3 days in a dose of 2 × 500 mg. Preoperative fluid replacement consisted of Ringer's Lactate. Blood gasses, pH and blood sugars were monitored at regular intervals and corrected if needed with adjustment of the ventilation and addition of glucose. The operating room was heated to 25 °C, the animals were placed on a heated water mattress and the rectal temperature was kept between 35 and 37 °C.

Surgical procedure

The recipients were rendered diabetic by total pancreatectomy according to the technique described by Gray and Leon (personal communication). In short, a total pancreatectomy with preservation of the spleen and of the arcades supplying the duodenum is performed. This meticulous procedure takes 3 to 4 hours and needs the application of magnification glasses. The allotransplant consists of a segment of duodenum, the whole pancreas and temporarily the spleen. A Carrel patch of the aorta including the coeliac artery and the superior mesenteric artery is sutured end to side to the distal aorta and the portal vein is connected end to side to the distal caval vein of the recipient. Exocrine drainage is guaranteed by a side to side anastomosis of the closed segment of duodenum to the recipient jejunum. The sequence of the procedure was donorpancreatectomy on a separate operating table, preparing of the recipient with a central venous and an arterial line, then transplantation of the graft, recipient pancreatectomy and afterwards graftsplenectomy. The donor pancreas was cold stored in Ringer's Lactate at 4 °C. Cold ischemia time did not exceed 1 hour.

Immunosuppressive protocol

Our immunosuppressive protocol has been described elsewhere (11). Briefly, immunosuppression was induced with a single gift of 1 mg/kg body weight/day. FK 506 intramuscular during the first 4 days postoperative. Therafter FK 506 was given orally in a single dose of 10 mg/kg body weight/day. When weight loss exceeded 10%, to oral dose was reduced to 5 mg/kg/day. FK 506 was given as monotherapy.

Plasma levels of FK 506 were determined afterwards and no dose adjustments were made according to plasma levels. When the fasted blood glucose levels increased, rejection was supposed to exist and the animals received for 3 consecutive days FK 506 intramuscular in a dose of 1 mg/kg body weight.

The animals were sacrificed by intravenous high dose barbiturates when the blood sugar exceeded 40 mmol/1 or at the end of the study period, which was set at 3 months.

Currently, 5 animals are included in the treatment arm and 3 in the control arm, which implies no immunosuppressive therapy. The animals were randomly selected to either arm.

Results

The 3 animals in the control group had a blood sugar over 10 mmol/l between day 7 and 17 and remained thereafter hyperglycemic (Figure 1). Two died on day 15 and 28, and one was sacrificed after 61 days when blood glucose was 40 mmol/l. At the time of autopsy all had rejected their pancreas graft.

Of the 5 animals in the treatment arm, 3 have reached the end point of the study, which was set at 3 months (Figure 2). The remaining 2 animals are now two and a half month post-transplantation, and both seem to be able to complete the period of the study. All 5 animals tolerated the oral dose of the drug well. Weight loss necessitated a dose reduction in 3 animals.

Two monkeys do have completely normal blood sugars. One of them has been sacrificed and no signs of rejection were observed at histology. The other animal is still in the study.

Three monkeys were presented with elevated blood sugars, 2 at the end of the first month, 1 at the end of the second month. All received FK 506 for 3 days i.m. In one improvement of the blood sugars was observed, but in the 2 others no improvement was noticed. Two have been sacrificed at 3 months. At histologic examination one graft showed signs of rejection, the other showed

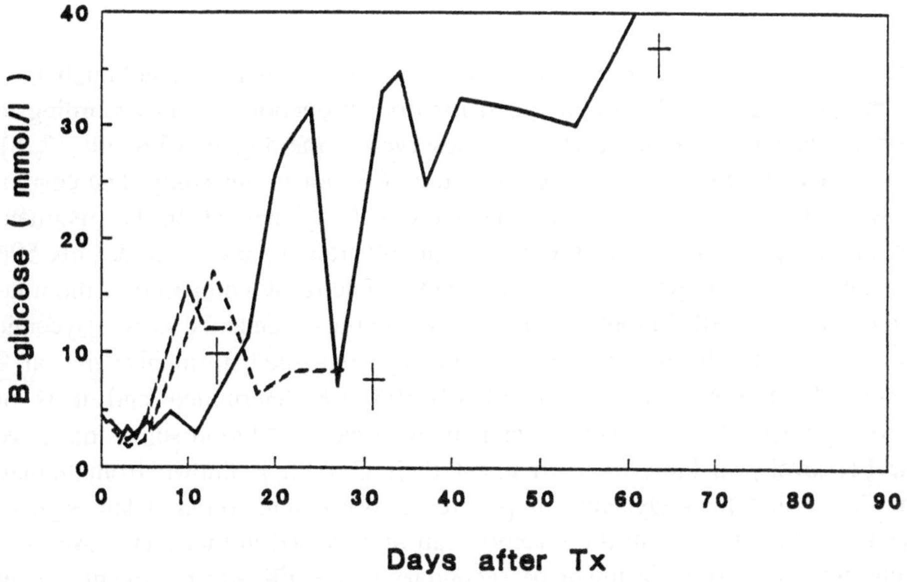

Fig. 1. Blood glucose concentration in the control monkeys, no immunosuppression ($n = 3$).

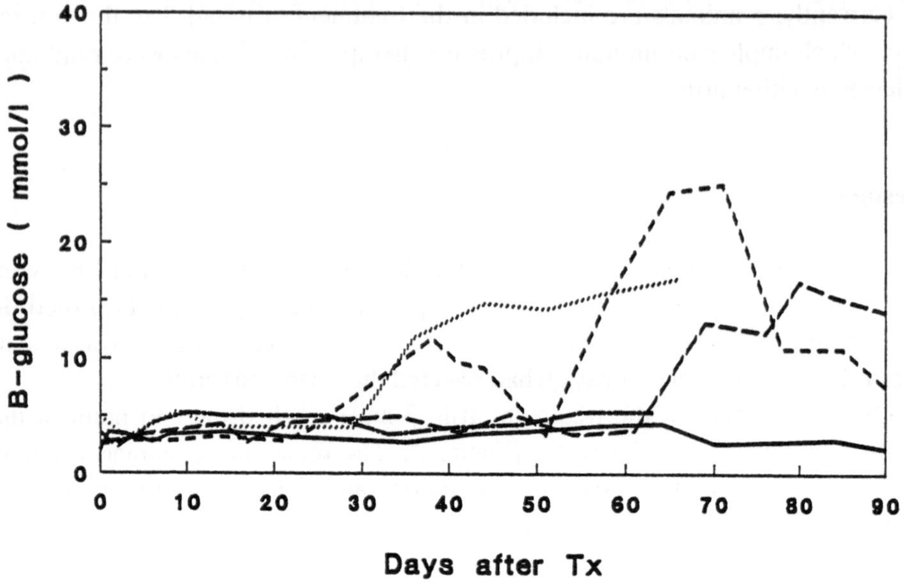

Fig. 2. Blood glucose concentration in the monkeys treated with FK 506 ($n = 5$).

some inflammation, but no signs of rejection. This animal responded initially to the i.m. FK 506. The third animal with elevated blood sugars is currently alive and still in the study.

Discussion

Oral FK 506 was well tolerated by the cynomolgus monkeys, although in 3 weight loss exceeded 10% and called for dose reduction to half according to protocol. Emanciation and arteritis as observed in the dog with FK 506 (7, 8), was neither observed in our toxicology study (9), nor in this study. The current study has not yet ended, but it is very likely that all 5 animals in the treatment arm are going to survive for 60 days with an allografted pancreas under FK 506 as a sole immunosuppressant. This is a remarkable result compared to the non-treated controls. All 5 monkeys in the treatment arm remained normoglycemic for the first month, and 3 of the 5 monkeys remained normoglycemic at 2 months. Currently plasma levels of FK 506 are determined and it is of importance to detect whether the animals with elevated blood sugars did have low FK levels, enabling them to reject their graft. It is known from human experience that hyperglycemia in pancreatic transplantation is a late sign of rejection and very seldom the rejection can be reversed in that phase. Alternatively, the hyperglycemia might be secondary to the FK 506 treatment and in this case these animals might indeed have elevated drug levels.

References

1. Kino, T., Hatanaka, H., Miyata, S., Inamura, N., Nishiyama, M., Yajima, T., Goto, T., Okuhara, M., Kohsaka, M., Aoki, H. and Ochiai, T.: FK 506 a novel immunosuppressant isolated from streptomyces. II. Immunosuppressive effect of FK 506 in vitro. *J. Antibiot. (Tokyo)* **40**, 1256—1265 (1987).
2. Borel, J.F.: The history of cyclosporine A and its significance. In: D.J.G. White (ed.), *Cyclosporine A: Proceedings of an International Conference on Cyclosporine A*, pp. 5—17. Elsevier Biomedical Press (1982).
3. Goto, T., Kino, T., Hatanaka, H., Nishiyama, M., Okuhara, M., Kohsaka, M., Aoki, H. and Imanaka, H.: Discovery of FK 506, a novel immunosuppressant isolated from *Streptomyces tsukubaensis. Transplant. Proc.* **19**, 4—8 (1987).
4. Ochiai, T., Nakajima, K., Nagata, M., Suzuki, T., Asano, T., Uematsu, T., Goto, T., Hozi, S., Kenmochi, T., Nakagoori, T. and Isono, K.: Effect of a new immunmosuppressive agent, FK 506, on heterotopic allotransplantation in the rat. *Transplant. Proc.* **19**, 1284—1286 (1987).
5. Murase, N., Todo, S., Lee, P.-H., Lai, H.-S., Chapman, F., Nalesnik, M., Makowka, L. and Starzl, T.E.: Heterotopic heart transplantation in the rat receiving FK 506 alone or with cyclosporine. *Transplant. Proc.* **19**, 71—75 (1987).
6. Todo, S., Podesta, L., Chap, P., Kahn, D., Pan, L.-E., Ueda, Y., Okuda, K., Imventurza, O., Casavilla, A., Demetris, A.J., Makowka, L. and Starzl, T.E.: Orthotopic liver transplantation in dogs receiving FK 506. *Transplant. Proc.* **19**, 64—67 (1987).
7. Todo, S., Ueda, Y., Demetris, A.J., Imventarza, O., Nalesnik, M., Venkataramanan, R., Makowka, L. and Starzl, T.E.: Immunosuppression of canine, monkey, and baboon allografts by FK 506, with special reference to synergism with other drugs and to tolerance induction. *Surgery* **104**, 239—249 (1988).
8. Thiru, S., Collier, D., St. J. and Calne, R.: Pathologic studies in canine and baboon renal allograft recipients immunosuppressed with FK 506. *Transplant. Proc.* **19**, 98—99 (1987).
9. Tiebosch, T., Wijnen, R., Ericzon, B.G., Arends, J.W., Groth, C.G. and Kootstra, G.: Side effects of FK 506 in Cynomolgus monkeys: a pathological study. *Transplant. Proc.* (in press).

18. The effect of DST on graft outcome – the Turkish experience

S. SERT, H. GULAY, M. KOÇ and M. HABERAL

Introduction

Blood transfusions are probably the simplest, safest and most cost effective treatment improving the graft outcome in renal transplant patients. The most attractive aspect of transfusions is to improve the graft survival without suppressing the immune response. The first report by Opelz and co-workers (8) showed that non-specific blood transfusions have considerably beneficial effects on renal allograft survival and then Salvatierra and his co-workers initiated the donor specific blood transfusion prior to renal transplantation (6). DST effect is thought to have beneficial effect on graft survival due to: (i) anti-idiotypic antibodies; (ii) suppressor T cells; (iii) selection of donor; and (iv) enhancement of immunogenic unresponsiveness. Cellular immunity is depressed by transfusions providing it is less than five units of blood (4, 5, 6).

Sensitization due to DST is a major handicap and the sensitization rate may be up to 40%. Most authors have found that azathioprine does not decrease the sensitization rate of DST and this drug also has side effects such as liver toxicity and leukopenia (4). In this study, we will present long-term results between DST and non-DST groups in respect to graft and patient survival, rejection rate, complications rate, HLA mismatch and immunosuppressive therapy.

Materials and methods

Between October 16, 1985 and October 1, 1989, 415 kidney transplants have been performed in 410 patients: 316 patients received living related grafts, 80 living unrelated and 19 cadaveric (18 of living related and one of living unrelated transplants were ABO incompatible).

Patients were evaluated in two groups. In the DST group there were 233 patients: 55 females, 178 males with mean ages of 34.4 and 9.3, and a female/male ratio of 0.30. In the non-DST group there were 90 patients: 17 females, 73 males with mean ages of 30.9 and 9.6 and a female/male ratio of 0.23.

Donor specific blood was of one unit (450 ml) and was divided into three parts (150 ml each). These were stored in the Blood Bank and were administered to patients at 10-day intervals. No azathioprine was used during DST treatment. There was no significant differences according to HLA mismatches in the two groups (Table 1).

All patients were administered the same immunosuppressive regimen of low dose triple drug therapy: cyclosporine-A 5 mg/kg/day, azathioprine 2 mg/kg/day, prednisone 1 mg/kg/day. Prednisone dose was tapered to 20 mg/day before leaving hospital and to 15 mg at the third month, 10 mg at the fourth month as the maintenance dose. Cyclosporine-A dose was regulated to its blood level using fluorescence polarization immunoassay (FPIA) technique (Td-x, Abbot). Rejection episodes were treated by bolus methylprednisolone 0.5 intravenously for three consecutive days. If necessary, this regimen was repeated once more. Patients were followed with blood biochemical values and radionuclide imaging technique. When rejection episode persisted and became steroid resistant as confirmed by fine needle aspiration biopsy (FNAB), OKT3 and plasmaphoresis combination therapy was used for 10 days.

Table 1. HLA mismatches of DST and non-DST groups.

HLA mismatches	DST group	Non-DST group
0	33 (14.1%)	11 (12.1%)
1	83 (35.6%)	32 (35.5%)
2	75 (32.1%)	37 (41.1%)
3	42 (18%)	10 (11.1%)
Total	233	90

Results

Patients were followed for 10—48 months (mean 22 months). Our sensitization rate was 14.7% after DST. In DST group, 7 patients died (3%), 4 due to sepsis, 1 to hepatic failure, 1 to gastrointestinal bleeding and 1 from renal artery rupture. Seventeen patients lost their grafts with rejection (7.2%). Totally, 165 rejection episodes were observed (70.8%). Mean rejection episode per patient was 1.18. Mean creatinine value was 1.21 ± 0.8 mg%. In the non-DST group, 8 patients died (8.8%, 4 from sepsis, 2 from hepatic failure, 1 from gastrointestinal bleeding and 1 from duodenal ulcer perforation). Twenty patients lost their kidneys through rejection (22.2%). Totally, 68 rejection episodes were observed (75.5%). Mean rejection episode per patient was 1.8 and mean creatinine value was 1.19 ± 0.55 (Table 2).

Table 2. Comparison of the results of DST and non-DST groups.

	DST group (*n*: 233)	Non-DST group (*n*: 90)
Deaths	7 (3%)	8 8.8%)
Graft lost	17 (7.2%)	20 (22.2%)
Rejection episode	165 (70.8%)	68 (75.5%)
Mean rejection episode per patient	1.18	1.8
Mean Cr value	(1.21 ± 0.8) mg%	(1.19 ± 05.5) mg%
PS and GS overall	PS 97% GS 89.7%	PS 91.2% GS 69%

Complication rate was nearly similar in the two groups. Overall patient survival and graft survival was 97 and 89% respectively in the DST group versus 91.2 and 69% in the non-DST group (Figures 1 and 2).

Discussion

The major handicap in DST treatment is sensitization. Various authors have found different sensitization rates of 21—40% (1, 2, 5, 6) and they reported that azathioprine decreased the sensitization rate. However, azathioprine did not decrease the sensitization rate in our previous study and we observed high rates of side effects such as liver toxicity and leukopenia (4). The sensitization rate was at a low level of 14.7% in this study. We are unable to explain our low sensitization rate but it may be due to using stored blood and to a limited number of transfusions. There is considerable difference in our patient and graft

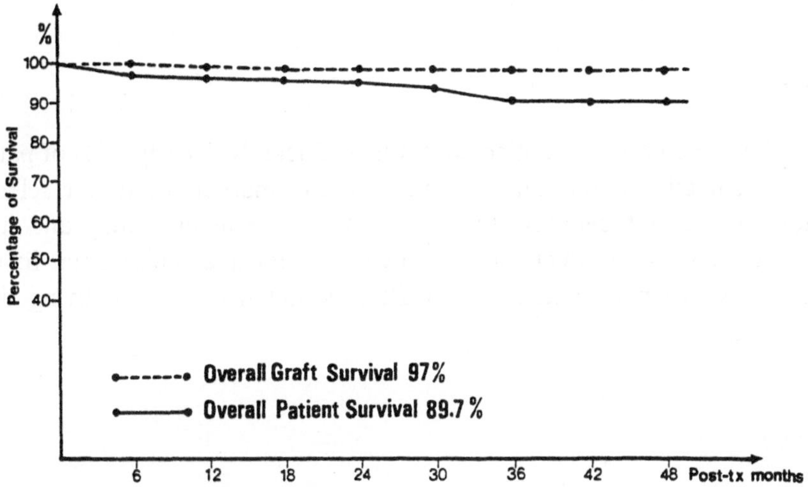

Fig. 1. Overall patients and graft survival patients with donor specific blood transfusions.

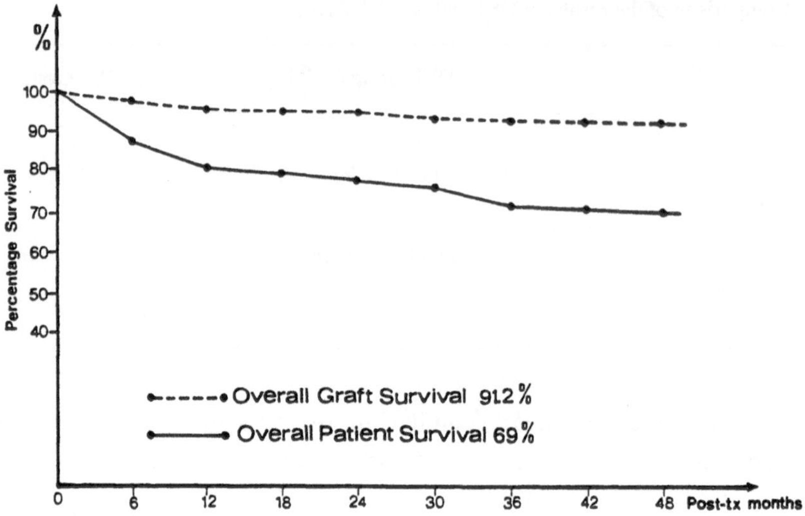

Fig. 2. Overall patients and graft survival patients received non-donor specific blood transfusions.

survival in DST and non-DST groups. Salvatierra *et al.* (6) reported 10—15% better results with DST. We found 5.8% better results in patient survival and 20.7% in graft survival with DST. Probably, DST produces better results because of antiidiotypic antibodies selection of donor, supressor T cells and immunogenic unresponsiveness. With DST over-immunosuppression is avoided and this leads to a high rate of patient and graft survival. In the DST group, the mean rejection episode per patient was 1.18 versus 1.8 in the non-DST group and this supported our view that cellular immunity was being depressed by transfusions providing this was less than five units of blood.

Summary

DST can improve graft and patient survival significantly. Nearly 15% of patients became sensitized and this may provide a useful marker for donor selection. Azathioprine did not decrease the sensitization rate in our study and it was observed to have side effects such as liver toxicity and leukopenia. In these circumstances, we may conclude that DST is still necessary in living donor kidney transplantation.

References

1. Anderson, C.B., Sicard, A.G. and Etheredge, E.E.: Pre-treatment of renal allograft recipients with azathioprine and donor specific blood products. *Surgery*, Aug., 319—321 (1982).

2. Glass, N.R., Miller, D.T., Sollinger, H.W. and Belzer, F.O.: Comparative analysis of the DST and Immuran-plus DST protocols for live donor renal transplantation. *Transplantation* **36**(6), 636—641 (1983).
3. Haberal, M., Öner, Z., Koç, M. and Bilgin, N.: The effect of one unit of DST on graft outcome. *Transplant. Proc.* **18**(5), 1445—1447, (1986).
4. Haberal, M., Sert, Ş., Aybasti, N. *et al.*: The effect of azathioprine on sensitization due to DST. *Transplant. Proc.* **20**(1), 300—301 (1988).
5. Moorhead, J.F., Chan, K.M., Malik, E.F., Raferty, M. *et al.*: Blood transfusion for renal transplantation: benefit and risks. *Kidney Int.* **23**(14), 20—23 (1983).
6. Salvatierra, O., Vincent, F., Amend, W.J.C., Garovay, M.D. *et al.*: The role of blood transfusion in renal transplantation. *Urol. Clin. N. Amer.* **10**(2), 243—251 (May 1983).
7. Salvatierra, O., Melzer, J.J., Patter, D., Garonovoy, M. *et al.*: A seven year experience with donor specific blood transfusion. *Transplantation* **40**, 654—659 (1985).
8. Opelz, G., Senger, D.P.S., Mickey, M.R. *et al.*: Effect of blood transfusion subsequent kidney transplants. *Transplant. Proc.* **5**, 253 (1973).

19. Induction of specific unresponsiveness (tolerance) to experimental and clinical allografts using polyclonal antilymphocyte serum and donor-specific bone marrow

ANTHONY P. MONACO

Introduction

In their classic studies, Medawar and colleagues (1) first demonstrated that donor-specific antigen itself could be used to attenuate or eliminate the allograft rejection reaction. They injected living-replicating lymphoid cells *in utero* or into neonatal recipients — a time when the recipients were naturally immunosuppressed by virtue of their underdeveloped immune system — and demonstrated that such recipients were rendered specifically unresponsive to donor grafts as adults. They termed this phenomenon actively acquired immunological tolerance, and noted that tolerant adults were lymphoid cell chimeras, that they rejected third-party grafts, and could reject donor-specific grafts if their immune system was reconstituted with adult syngeneic lymphoid cells that had not been exposed *in utero* to the donor antigens. Although the exact immunological basis for this observation is still not completely defined, this experiment has served as a persistent goal to induce specific non-reactivity to tissue allografts without the use of chronically administered non-specific immunosuppression. All attempts to translate Medawar's experiment to adult animals have been more or less based on the assumption that it would be done in immunologically mature, adult animals. Thus, most attempts to use donor-specific antigen to modulate the allograft response have utilized an initial period of transient non-specific immunosuppression (to mimic the neonatal state) during which exposure to donor-specific antigen is superimposed.

Early studies utilized total body irradiation or chemotherapeutic drugs followed by various forms of donor antigen prior to or after a donor-specific test allograft, usually a skin graft. These early studies gave only minimal, augmented specific prolongation, most likely due to the fact that the degree of transient immunosuppression was not very profound. With the advent of antilymphocyte serum or globulin (ALS, ALG) as an experimental immunosuppressive agent, the ease with which specific unresponsiveness could be induced experimentally was greatly increased (see review, (2)).

The term *specific unresponsiveness to allografts* (tolerance) is now generally used in experiments on immunologically competent adult animals to describe specific non-reactivity to allografts rather than *actively acquired immunological tolerance to allografts* since the latter refers to a phenomenon obtained by a defined experimental protocol in neonatal animals. Specific unresponsiveness to tissue allografts may be defined as suppression of the immune response to donor specific alloantigens without suppression of the immune responses to other antigens (bacterial, viral, other alloantigens of a different donor graft, etc.) leading to prolonged survival of the given specific allograft while retaining the ability to reject a different (third-party) allograft and to make normal immune responses to other antigens. Conversely, non-specific suppression of allograft rejection involves generalized suppression of the immune response, usually with methods selected for effectiveness against the allograft rejection mechanism but invariably suppressing other immune responses to other allografts (third-party) as well as to bacterial, viral, etc., antigens to varying degrees. The ideal system for inducing unresponsiveness for clinical cadaveric organ transplantation would involve use of donor antigen *after* organ grafting since it would be unlikely that adequate amounts of donor antigen would be available for significant periods prior to organ availability *unless* better methods of long-term organ preservation become available.

ALS-bone marrow tolerance studies in mice

The studies below describe in detail the use of one form of transient immunosuppression, antilymphocyte serum or antilymphocyte globulin, and predominantly one form of donor antigen, bone marrow harvested from adult animals to induce unresponsiveness. In the broadest sense, specific unresponsiveness in these studies refers to the specific prolonged allograft survival achieved in animals given transient, non-specific immunosuppression with antilymphocyte serum and donor antigen over allograft survival seen in animals giving only transient immunosuppression.

Early studies clearly suggested that ALG would be unusually effective in inducing specific unresponsiveness. ALG is an extraordinarily potent immunosuppressive agent for prolongation of allografts (3). Furthermore, when adult animals are thymectomized and given ALG, the induced immunosuppression is markedly potentiated (4). Monaco *et al.* (5) very early showed that if adult-thymectomized ALS-treated mice are infused with F1 hybrid lymphoid cells, specific immunological unresponsiveness to the donor strain resulted which was similar in every way to the actively acquired tolerance produced by Medawar and colleagues (1). This observation served as the basis for extensive study of ALG to prepare adult animals for induction of unresponsiveness. Since F1 hybrid lymphoid cells would never be available for cadaveric organ transplant studies, the first attempts involved infusion of homozygous donor-specific lymphoid cells in adult-thymectomized, ALG-treated recipients. As might be expected, severe graft-versus-host reactions were induced and no clinically effective unresponsiveness was obtained. Attempts to use non-replicating, immunologically incompetent cells, i.e. epidermal kidney and hepatic cells failed to induce any unresponsiveness (5). Use of cell-free antigen preparations gave some specific prolongation but it was not long-lasting (6). Subsequently, Medawar and Lance (7) showed that specific unresponsiveness in adult mice, treated with ALG but not thymectomized, could be produced with injections of low doses of F1 hybrid cells. Monaco and colleagues (5, 8) systematically studied the use of low doses of non-F1 hybrid, homozygous allogeneic lymphoid cells for efficacy in inducing specific unresponsiveness. In the typical experiment recipient mice receive ALS (ALG) on day −1 and +2 relative to skin allografting on day 0 followed by infusion of donor-specific antigen on day +8, i.e. after transplantation. Lymphoid cells (25×10^6 cells/mouse) from lymph nodes, spleen, thymus bone marrow were compared as the tolerance conferring innoculum in this standard protocol. At this dose, lymph node lymphocytes, splenocytes, or thymus induced very little augmented graft survival over ALS alone. In contrast, bone marrow cells induced significant specific augmented survival, some ALG-BM treated mice bearing grafts for over 100 days, while retaining the capacity to reject third-party grafts. Also, donor-specific BM cells failed to prolong third-party grafts.

When 50×10^6 lymphoid cells were used in the standard protocol, there was little effect using lymph node cells or thymus cells, while bone marrow cells were more effective than a 25×10^6 cell dose, splenocytes were as effective as bone marrow at the 50×10^6 cell dose. At 100×10^6 cell dose, lymph node lymphocytes curtailed graft survival (i.e. sensitized animals), thymocytes prolonged grafts slightly, but marrow still was the superior tolerogen, although splenocytes were almost as effective. In all studies there was no suggestion of clinical graft-versus-host reactions. The effect of progressive doses of BM cells from 1×10^4 to $\times 10^8$ in the standard model was also studied. 1×10^4 cells failed to induce tolerance, while 1×10^5 and $\times 10^6$ gave slight prolongation (9). No apparent sensitization (shortened graft survival) was induced by these doses. Doses of 10, 25, 50×50^6 and 100×10^6 were clearly tolerogenic, with 50×10^6 being most tolerogenic. Most important, there was a clear decrease in tolerogenic effect at 100×10^6 dose, but no obvious sensitization. An important consideration for future clinical application is that the tolerogenic effect of BM does not increase progressively with increased dose. Above a maximal effective level, decreased effectiveness and possible sensitization may follow BM infusion in ALG-treated animals.

Timing of BM cell infusion is important (9). When a standard dose of donor specific BM cells (25×10^6) was injected iv into ALS-treated recipients (days −1 and +2 relative to test skin allografting on day 0) on days +1, +2, +3, +4 +8 (the standard protocol), +16, *or* +23 profoundly different results were obtained. Infusions on day +8 as well as +4 were highly tolerogenic, while BM given on day +3 (24 hours post-ALS injection) were significantly tolerogenic but less than BM given on day +4 or +8. Cells given on day +2 failed to induce any specific unresponsiveness, and in fact occasionally sensitizes some recipients. One of the most striking effects was the marrow given on day +1 had a sensitizing effect. This is probably due to an effect of subsequent ALS on day +2 on the marrow cells. Recent studies have shown that BM given shortly after ALS is effective as long as ALS treatment is not repeated shortly thereafter (10). Infusion on day +16 or +23 failed to induce any significant unresponsiveness. Thus, for eventual clinical application, not only would the dose of BM be important, but so would the timing of marrow infusion relative to ALG administration.

The unresponsiveness induced with ALS and marrow in adult immunologically competent mice differs in a number of respects from the classical actively acquired immunological tolerance described by Medawar and colleagues. The iv route is not obligatory; in certain instances donor marrow given by i.p. or even intraorgan injection (intrasplenic, intrahepatic, etc.) induced long-lived specific unresponsiveness (11). Also, *in vitro* treatment of recipients with various bacterial adjuvants dramatically alters the unresponsiveness induced (12). Administration of the adjuvants *Bordetella pertussis, Bacillus Calmette Guerin* (BCG), *or Corynebacterium parvum* abrogated tolerance when given 5 days after grafting but only *B. pertussis* produced a striking increase in tolerance when given 7 days before skin grafting with ALS and subsequent marrow injection. *B. pertussis* may exert this unique effect by the extraordinary changes it produces in regional and systemic lymphatics. Another interesting observation was the differential effect produced by cyclophosphamide administration. If cyclophosphamide is given before marrow in the standard protocol, i.e. on day +4 or +6, the specific graft prolonging effect of marrow was clearly abrogated, but if cyclophosphamide was given within one week after marrow, the graft prolonging effect of marrow was definitely potentiated. Subsequent experiments suggested that the effects of adjuvants and cyclophosphamide were mediated through modification in the generation of suppressor cells.

In early studies, it was clearly shown that unresponsive ALS-treated mice were not gross lymphoid cell chimeras after marrow infusion as determined by the Mitchison Chimera assay. However, Liegeois *et al.* (13) subsequently showed by elegant chromosonal analysis studies using the T6T6 system that ALS-treated marrow-injected mice retained donor lymphoid cells at least to 146 days in their spleens in very low numbers (<1.5%). The term microchimerism was used to describe this phenomenon. It should be noted that unresponsiveness could never be transferred with serum from unresponsive mice. Subsequently, Wood and Monaco (14) studied the capacity of spleen cells from unresponsive ALS-treated marrow-infused mice to transfer specific unresponsiveness (i.e. for the presence of suppressor cells) to syngeneic recipients.

Suppressor cell transfer assays of spleen cells from ALS-treated bone marrow-infused tolerant mice showed that administration of ALS and a skin graft with or without donor specific bone marrow resulted in the production of suppressor-type cells by day 12 post-grafting. However, when suppressor cell transfer assays were performed utilizing splenocytes from mice taken on day +42, suppressor cells were identified only in the ALS-treated donor group that had received both a graft and marrow, i.e. the donor group bearing enhanced grafts. Spleen cells from donors that had received a graft alone transferred immunity, while graft survival in the recipients injected with cells from donors treated with marrow alone or ALS alone was similar to controls. The ability of spleen cells from mice bearing enhanced grafts to transfer suppression to syngeneic recipients decreased by day +56. Significant prolongation of graft survival was achieved in only 20% of the recipients injected with spleen cells removed from mice bearing enhanced grafts on day 56, although all of the donors bore skin grafts in perfect condition grossly at the time their spleens were removed.

In these studies, the ability of antitheta serum-treated spleen cells from ALS-treated BM-infused tolerant mice to transfer unresponsiveness was totally abrogated, confirming that the cellular mechanism of unresponsiveness was most likely a T suppressor cell. Furthermore, specificity of the suppression transferred with syngeneic spleen cells from ALS-treated marrow-infused mice was demonstrated in that spleen cells from $B6AF_1$ ALS-treated C3H/He marrow-infused mice transferred unresponsiveness only to C3H/He skin grafts in the suppressor assay, but not to DBA/2 skin grafts.

The nature of the response that marrow elicits in an ALS-treated animal to enhance graft survival beyond the time of ALS immunosuppression is not clear. Spleen cells from ALS-treated mice injected with marrow alone do not show strong suppressive activity after transfer. Possibly, marrow injected into skin-grafted mice initiates a 'second' suppressive response. There is a proliferation of donor strain cells 7 days after the injection of marrow in the spleens of ALS-treated mice bearing skin grafts (13). This proliferation does not occur after marrow injection in ALS-treated mice that have not been grafted. This proliferation of donor cells could be an added antigenic stimulus for activation of suppressor cells. The injection of marrow could also elicit an antibody response, which might in turn stimulate generation of suppressor cells.

Precursors of suppressor cells are sensitive to cyclophosphamide and certain immune responses are increased in cyclosphosphamide-treated animals. Prolongation of graft survival is decreased in ALS-treated mice given cyclophosphamide before marrow, whereas cyclophosphamide has no effect on graft survival in ALS-treated mice not given marrow. Cyclophosphamide possibly removes a population of (? suppressor) cells whose response to marrow results in enhancement of the graft. Enhanced proliferation of suppressor cells after marrow could protect the graft by delaying sensitization of the host. Suppressor cells are most efficient in suppressing the early stages of differentiation of cytotoxic cells into mature cells, while cytotoxic cells that have differentiated beyond a certain stage can no longer be suppressed.

The presence of suppressor cells in other lymphoid tissues of unresponsive mice in the ALS-marrow model has been confirmed (15). Suppressor cells could only be found in the spleen of ALS-treated marrow-injected mice on day +13, but not in the other lymphatic tissues. By day +42 suppressor cells were still present in the spleen, but then appeared in the lymph nodes emphasizing that the suppressor cells in this model were not restricted to just the spleen. The role of the spleen in the induction and maintenance of unresponsiveness to skin allografts and in the generation of suppressor cells has been studied in ALS-treated $B6AF_1$ mice grafted with C3H/He skin and injected with C3H/He marrow (16). These results indicate that the spleen is not necessary for the induction or maintenance of unresponsiveness to skin allografts in ALS-treated marrow-injected mice. In addition, suppressor cells can be generated in the lymph nodes of unresponsive mice in the absence of the spleen, although the production of suppressor cells appears to be less effective in splenectomized mice than in mice with intact spleens.

Since bone marrow contains many cell types, experiments were undertaken to determine if marrow could be fractionated and an active unresponsiveness producing fraction isolated. Gozzo *et al.* (17) showed that whole murine marrow could be fractionated into four distinct fractions in a $1 \times g$ velocity sedimentation chamber utilizing a linear bovine serum albumin density gradient. Groups of $B6AF_1$ mice treated with ALS (day −1 and +2) and grafted with C3H/He skin (day 0) were infused on day +7 with 25×10^6 whole marrow cells or the cells of each fraction isolated from 25×10^6 whole marrow. One fraction (so-called fraction 3) was as effective as whole marrow in inducing specific unresponsiveness even though only 1.38×10^6 cells were injected. When the dose of fraction 3 was increased, marked graft prolongation over that in mice given 25×10^6 whole marrow cell was achieved. Fraction 3 was found to be 93% small lymphocytes when examined by Wright's stain smears.

The phenotypic characteristics of active bone marrow cells necessary for induction of unresponsiveness has been studied by exposing whole marrow cells to various specific antisera prior to infusion in the standard protocol (18). Thus, active marrow cells that prolong skin graft survival in ALS-treated mice appear to be Ia^-, Th-1^-, largely complement receptor negative and Ig^-, but are largely positive for Fc receptors. Active cells in marrow co-fractionated during sedimentation in Ficoll at unit gravity with populations that were reduced in Ia^+, Ig^+ and Thy-1^+ cells but had modest percentages of Fc R^+ cells. The active bone marrow cells may be a natural suppressor or natural regulatory cell or 'veto' cell.

The fractionation of active marrow has also been extended using velocity sedimentation in Ficoll (9). Nucleated marrow cells were loaded into a sedimentation chamber in a stabilizing gradient of 2 to 4% Ficoll. Individual nucleated cell fractions were combined to four pooled fractions (a through d) with separation monitored by morphological and cell diameter analysis. Cell fractions were analyzed for cell surface receptors. This method permitted resolution of previously active fraction 3 into fractions c and d. When fractions c and d were injected into ALS-treated mice only fraction c induced considerable specific graft survival. Fraction c contained small percentages of Ia^+ cells (10%) and moderate percentages of EA^+ and EAC^+ cells (15%). Small numbers (3%) of Thy.1 2+ cells were in c.

Although velocity sedimentation at unit gravity can be used for active marrow fractions, it is not useful where large volumes of cells are required. A rapid high-capacity method is required. Therefore, density gradient fractionation with Percoll has been successfully applied to the fractionation of large volumes of marrow cells. Using variable density gradients, the density of a major portion of the cells active in graft prolongation was estimated as being in a range of 1.061—1.066 g/l and to produce one fraction with superior graft-prolonging activity (20). This fraction which constituted only 10% of the recovered cells, was enriched for small to medium lymphocytes, Ia^+, $Thy-1^+$ and IgM^+ cells, and contained cells bearing a marker known to be present on active cells, (Fc R). Percoll gradient cell separation presents significant advantages for potential clinical application. These are increased cell capacity, improved cell recovery (85% for Percoll, 50% for Ficoll), speed (the Percoll process takes one-fourth the time of Ficoll separation) and the final separation-collection step is much easier.

The effect of the donor marrow age and various storage and freezing parameters on BMC effectiveness in this model has been studied in detail. Donor marrow from adult as well as juvenile animals is equally effective in inducing unresponsiveness in ALS-treated recipients (21). BMC retained their graft-prolonging effect if stored at 4 °C in 10% fetal calf serum for 18 hours prior to infusion, but not if maintained for 18 hours at 37 °C under standard lymphocyte culture conditions. BMC retain their unresponsiveness inducing property after freezing and thawing or overnight refrigeration (22). Thus, the model could be applied clinically to cadaver grafts using frozen, stored marrow.

The use of spleen or other tissue as a source for the active tolerance-inducing cell could be attractive since harvesting of marrow from cadavers or living-donors is a time-consuming procedure. Kapnick *et al.* (23) were able to induce modest degrees of unresponsiveness to skin allografts in ALS-treated mice using blood platelets, although they had to be injected later (usually 2 weeks post-grafting) and in association with adjuvants. De Fazio and associates also showed that infusion of peripheral blood lymphocytes (PBLS) after ALS treatment and grafting in the standard protocol extended graft survival beyond that noted for control mice given ALS alone. The PBLS active in graft prolongation are Thy-1 negative and display a density in Percoll gradients similar to that of previously demonstrated active marrow cells. When PBLS were injected in combination with bone marrow cells, the length of graft survival was shortened in comparison to that produced by marrow alone. The cells associated with abrogation appear to be mature T cells. This abrogation cannot be produced by PBLS treated with anti-Thy-1 plus complement or by thymocytes, but it is a property of lymph node cells enriched for T cells by nylon wool fractionation. Thus, it would appear that peripheral blood lymphocytes, although they specifically prolong graft survival in ALS-treated mice, contain mature T cells which can also abrogate this effect. The density gradient fractionation method which was found effective (above) in preparing active graft prolonging fractions from whole bone marrow simultaneously removes those PBLS deleterious to graft survival. These studies show that if whole marrow is used clinically, the degree of contamination with blood should be minimized.

The *in vitro* analysis of the immune responses in this model emphasize that the mechanism of unresponsiveness is mediated by suppressor cells and the generation of suppressor cells is achieved in several steps (24). Mice treated with ALS, bone marrow and specific allografts have significant alterations in their immune responses. Responses to mitogens in standard protocol animals and controls was first studied. To evaluate the functional properties of T cells and B cells, spleen cells (SPC) obtained at various times from three groups of $B6AF_1$ mice, i.e. ALS, ALS-Graft, and ALS-Graft-BM groups, were stimulated by optimal concentrations of PHA, Con A, and LPS. The proliferative response to T cell mitogens was markedly suppressed in all the groups given ALS treatment. Although an initial suppression (approximately 10% of normal $B6AF_1$ SPC) of Con A response was seen immediately followed by gradual recovery in the ALS and ALS-graft groups, more prolonged suppression of Con A responsiveness was observed in the ALS-Graft-BM group. The PHA responsiveness remained low in all three groups; less than 50% of normal reactivity was observed as late as day 42. In the ALS-Graft group, which rejected C3H skin grafts at day 28, no significant change in responsiveness to either PHA or Con A was observed at the time of rejection. By day 56, reactivity to PHA and Con A returned to normal levels in all groups. On the other hand, reactivity to the B cell mitogen, LPS, was minimally suppressed in all the groups throughout the time course studied.

Direct lymphocyte-mediated cytotoxicity (LMC) is also modified in these animals. Lymphocytes obtained from the ALS-Graft group exhibited high LMC against donor specific target cells at day 21 before any grafts showed macroscopic signs of rejection. On the other hand, the LMC in the ALS-Graft-BM group remained low until the time of allograft rejection. No significant cytotoxicity was obtained against third-party target cells at a wide range of lymphocyte to target cell ratios throughout the time course studied. A similar analysis of proliferative responses and generation of CML (cell mediated lymphocytotoxicity) in the MLC was performed. SPC taken from the ALS-

Graft-BM group showed prolonged inability to respond proliferatively to C3H alloantigens. SPC obtained from the ALS-Graft group exhibited suppressed proliferative response (MLR) for 3 weeks, followed by a high 'secondary type' response on day 28 when the skin grafts were rejected. A secondary type MLR of SPC obtained from the Graft-only group was seen by day 7, peaked at day 14, and returned to the 'primary type' level by day 42. In contrast, the SPC of the ALS-Graft-BM group exhibited a markedly prolonged suppression of the MLR. Even at the time of rejection, the stimulation index rose only moderately.

SPC of both ALS-Graft and ALS-Graft-BM groups were capable of differentiating into highly cytotoxic effector cells upon resensitization to the donor antigens, despite the absence of the proliferative response. In the ALS-Graft group, a rapid increase in the CML was observed after day 7, reaching a high secondary type response (65% specific lysis) by day 21. In the ALS-Graft-BM group, a low CML was initially observed for 2 weeks, followed by a progressive increase in reactivity similar to that seen in the ALS-Graft group. SPC of the ALS-Graft-BM group exhibited high CML (approximately 50% specific lysis) as early as day 21, when their MLR was still markedly suppressed. High CML in all three groups was mediated by T cells, since anti-Thy-1.2 serum + C treatment of the effector cells abrogated their cytotoxicity.

Although ALS treatment induced non-specific impairment of T cell reactivity as evidenced by a low proliferative response to PHA and Con A and by the initial low MLR and CML to C3H and DBA/2 alloantigens, ALS treatment alone failed to inhibit the eventual generation of cytotoxic reactivity against donor alloantigen, i.e. SPC obtained at day 21 from the ALS-Graft group already exhibited high LMC and CML despite continued low MLR against C3H stimulators. In contrast, donor marrow-injection in the ALS-Graft-BM group led to the further inhibition of generation of effector activity as illustrated by prolonged low LMC in this group. However, when co-cultured with C3H stimulator cells in a standard MLC, the SPC obtained as early as day 21 exhibited 'secondary-type' CML, while they continued to exhibit depressed MLR to C3H alloantigens. Thus, despite low MLR and LMC, SPC of the ALS-Graft-BM group contained a cell population that was sensitized to C3H alloantigens and that was capable of differentiating into highly reactive cytotoxic lymphocytes upon resensitization. This result indicates that the specific unresponsiveness induced in ALS-treated marrow-injected mice is not due to the classical actively acquired tolerance by clonal deletion.

Initially, the administration of ALS alone probably results in the production of ALS-induced antigen non-specific suppressor cells. Thus, Maki *et al.* (25) have shown that mere administration of rabbit anti-mouse lymphocyte serum results in the development of suppressor cells which can be detected by coculture mixed lymphocyte culture experiments. The putative suppressor cells inhibit non-specifically the proliferative response as well as generation of cytotoxicity of normal responder cells. Subsequently, additional antigenic stimulation by skin allografting in ALS-treated mice shifts the specificity of suppressor cells from non-specific to specific for the skin donor alloantigen. ALS-induced suppressor cells are Lyt-1^+2^- T cells while suppressor cells present in ALS-treated, skin allograft-bearing mice are Lyt-1^-2^+ T cells. The exact mechanism of induction of suppressor cells by ALS is not known. ALS may stimulate a subset of T cells to differentiate into suppressor cells, as has been shown in the case of concanavalin A induced suppressor cells. ALS may contain various anti-T cell receptor antibodies which may trigger induction of polyclonal suppressor cells. Finally, ALS which is cytotoxic to some subpopulation(s) of T cells may spare suppressor cells or suppressor cell precursors. In similar experiments Maki *et al.* (24) compared the suppressor cell activity in vitro of spleen cells (SPC) removed from $B6AF_1$ mice given ALS and a C3H skin graft versus those from $B6AF_1$ mice given ALS and C3H marrow and skin grafts. They showed that SPC from the ALS-Graft group were capable of inhibiting the anti-C3H MLR of normal $B6AF_1$ responders early after grafting (day 14) but they lost suppressive activity when grafts showed signs of rejection (day 35). On the other hand SPC obtained either at day 14 or 42 from mice of the ALS-Graft-BM group bearing intact skin graft exhibited marked suppression of anti-C3H MLR. By complex genetic analysis, they were able to show that specific suppressor cells were derived at least in part from the donor marrow.

In view of the present findings, the following hypothesis concerning the induction and maintenance of the unresponsiveness in the ALS-treated, C3H marrow-injected $B6AF_1$ mice is suggested. ALS treatment depresses the activity of immunocompetent T cells, while possibly sparing the suppressor cell precursors. Subsequent antigenic stimulation by C3H skin allografting may lead to the generation of suppressor cells of host $B6AF_1$ origin. These suppressor cells are most efficient in suppressing the early recognition phase of reaction, thus limiting the expansion of cytotoxic T lymphocytes. In addition, the presence of donor antigen specific and/or non-specific suppressor cells at the time of C3H marrow injection would prevent the rejection of donor marrow and allow its proliferation in the recipient's thymic and/or splenic environment. By yet unknown mechanisms, the generation of marrow-derived GVH responsive cells is hampered and the marrow cells give rise to suppressor T cells. The C3H marrow-derived suppressor cells are specific for self-(C3H) antigens, thus further limiting the host ($B6AF_1$) response to the skin grafts as well as to the surviving marrow cells that bear C3H alloantigens. Skin grafts are rejected after the balance between the suppressor cell activity and cytotoxic activity shifts toward the latter.

Several recent experiments in our laboratory are of great importance. Since cyclosporine A is so effective in clinical transplantation, it will be very difficult to try a tolerance-inducing protocol clinically which does not incorporate cyclosporine initially and for a significant portion of time post transplantation.

Experiments in the standard ALS-BM protocol in mice show that the addition of a brief course of cyclosporine after bone marrow infusion markedly enhances the number of animals rendered tolerant as well as the duration of tolerance (26). This is presumably secondary to the enhancing effect cyclosporine has on suppressor cell development. Thus, use of ALS-bone marrow protocols can easily and ethically be incorporated in clinical protocols currently using cyclosporine. Another important recent theoretical observation has been made using artificial donor-specific urethane sponge grafts which are coated with donor-specific MHC antigens by a brief period of intraperitoneal residence in donor strain animals. Such grafts can be removed at various times from tolerant animals and their cell content analyzed. Recent experiments have shown that such sponge allografts collect suppressor cells with donor specificity. This finding introduces the concept of a local-form of tolerance and is in keeping with important observations in the rhesus monkey adaptation of the ALS-BM model (see below).

Also, the possibility of altering the supply and quality of donor-specific bone marrow has been studied. The fraction of bone marrow cells effective in inducing tolerance has been isolated as described above (19). Clones of cells which are IL-3 dependent have been derived from this active fraction of whole bone marrow. Clones of these IL-3 dependent cells have been successfully utilized as a substitute for whole bone marrow in this rodent model. In a second series of studies, we have studied the use of hematopoietic growth factors that promote the differentiation and maturation of various stem cell lines in the marrow. Two factors, granulocyte-macrophage colony stimulating factor (GM-CSF) and IL-3 stimulate the differentiation and proliferation of early multi-linage precursor cells. GM-CSF administered to bone marrow donors for 2 weeks prior to bone marrow harvest clearly increased the tolerance-inducing capacity of the donor specific marrow in our rodent model (Wood, M.L., Gottschalk, R. and Monaco, A.P.: Effect of granulocyte macrophage colony stimulating factor (GM-CSF) on the induction of unresponsiveness by lymphoid cells. Submitted for publication). Furthermore, additional fractionation studies have shown that the spleen and bone marrow contain active tolerance inducing cells which are very similar with similar surface markers (Monaco, A.P., Wood, M.L., Gottschalk, R. *et al.* Characterization of spleen and lymph node cells capable of inducing unresponsiveness to skin allografts in ALS-treated mice. Submitted for publication).

The bone marrow, ALS model in dogs

The studies that have been completed in dogs have shown that the marrow—ALS model is totally applicable to whole organ immediately vascularized grafts in large species. The early canine experiments were designed as follows:

immunosuppressive regimens and timing of bone marrow infusion were chosen in order to reproduce in dogs the critical timing which had been demonstrated in mice, i.e. injection of bone marrow 2—5 days following completion of ALS treatment (27). For each experiment two groups of dogs were treated with the same pool of rabbit anti-dog lymphocyte serum (RADLS), and one group was subsequently injected with donor-specific bone marrow. RADLS was given daily at various doses (1 ml/kg, 2 ml/kg) from day −7 to +7 relative to placement on day 0 of a canine renal allograft. Kidney donor bone marrow was harvested from resected ribs and infused intravenously on day +10 (3 days after completion of RADLS treatment) in doses varying from $2–4 \times 10^8$ cells/kg. In one experiment a second bone marrow infusion was given on day +20. In two control groups bone marrow was given on day +2 or +5. In these very early experiments using ALS and donor-specific bone marrow with canine renal allografting, a definite augmented survival of renal allografts was achieved in bone marrow-infused ALS-treated groups only (27). Successful augmented survival after BM infusion was only found in those dogs given adequate ALS to produce significant initial immunosuppression.

It is obvious that for the marrow model to be applied clinically to cadaver transplantation, marrow would have to be harvested and stored for various times to be infused post-grafting. Thus, it was important to establish the efficacy of stored marrow in a large animal, whole organ allograft model. Hartner and colleagues (28) demonstrated the effectiveness of fractionated and frozen-stored canine bone marrow cells in prolonging renal allograft survival in ALS-treated dogs.

Renal allografts were performed in histoincompatible outbred dogs treated daily with rabbit or horse anti-dog ALS from day −6 to +7 relative to kidney allografting on day 0. Fresh, whole, unfractionated donor-specific bone marrow (BMC) or a bone marrow fraction (BMFr3) produced by centrifugation in a discontinuous Percoll density gradient was infused intravenously into recipients on days +13 or +14. Alternatively, frozen /thawed (F/Th) BM or BMFr3 was infused after storage at −80 °C for 2 weeks. BMFr3 and unfractionated BM significantly ($p < 0.005$) prolonged the median allograft function time (MST) beyond the controls treated only with ALS (46 and 35 day vs. 18 days). One in 5 dogs given ALS and BM survived over 1 year with essentially normal renal function. The longer MST with BMFr3 was achieved with 20—40% of the unfractionated BM cell dose. Also, BMFr3-treated dogs which did not have long-term graft survival still exhibited slower rates of loss of kidney function. F/Th marrow was as effective as fresh BM in prolonging graft survival. Reduced MLR responses to the specific donor and third-party cells, and markedly reduced responsiveness to ConA, PHA and pokeweed mitogens at 30 and 45 days post-transplant suggested that animals were non-specifically immunosuppressed at this time. However, by 60 days post-transplant 2 dogs treated with BMFr3 showed normal MLR responses to third-party cells but not to specific donor cells and the responses to mitogens had also returned to pre-ALS treatment values. Thus, *in vitro* studies in 2 animals suggested long-term specific immunosuppression was induced by fractionated bone marrow. Furthermore, *in vivo* confirmation of this specific unresponsiveness suggested by *in vitro* studies was achieved when third-party renal allografts placed in the neck of dogs with well-tolerated renal allografts after ALS and marrow treatment were rejected while the original marrow donor graft remained unrejected. This suggests that application of this model to human transplantation may be effective using fresh or frozen-thawed BM fractions obtained from living-related or cadaver donors. Unfortunately, the number of dogs rendered unresponsive for a long-term (> 300 days) with ALS and BM is only about 20%. Recent observations in our laboratory have shown that addition of a short course of cyclosporine after ALS and BM treatment also increases the number of tolerized animals and duration of tolerance in the canine renal allograft model as it does in rodents. As many as 35% of dogs given ALS and BM followed by a short course of cyclosporine showed specific, long-term unresponsiveness. Other recent experiments in our laboratory have shown that BM can be given shortly after ALS treatment and grafting with excellent effectiveness so that the need for long-term storage of BM may be eliminated. This would make further clinical application of the ALS-BM model. Nevertheless, it should be emphasized that in the canine model, the median survival time for all canine allografts given ALS and BM is superior to that in dogs in given only ALS; however, only 30—40% of animals show long-term tolerance and these long-term survivors have varying degrees of chronic rejection reflected in slightly elevated creatinines and abnormal biopsies. Thus, not all long-term canine renal allograft recipients are completely tolerant in this model.

The ALS—marrow model in primates

The use of the ALS bone marrow model has been applied with great success to renal allografts in primates by F. and J.M. Thomas and colleagues (29, 30, 31). These investigators enhanced skin allograft survival in rhesus monkeys with ATG and donor lymphoid cells over that achieved with ATG alone. Encouraged by these results, they extended their studies to renal allografts in highly incompatible outbred rhesus monkeys (*Macacca mulatta*). Four groups of recipients received either no treatment, ATG only (50 mg × 5 days post-transplant), ATG plus donor marrow on day 12 (0.7×10^6 cell/kg), or ATG plus donor marrow on day +12 and +20. Monkeys received no other immunosuppression. Untreated monkeys rejected kidneys in 6—14 days, and ATG only monkeys in 28—42 days. Recipients receiving ATG plus one infusion of marrow did not reject grafts from 140 to 400 days at the time of reporting with normal serum creatinines (a single monkey died of trauma with normal creatinine and histology). Monkeys given ATG and two marrow injections showed a bimodal survival curve; one-half had survival equivalent to ATG alone, while one-half had extended survival from 73 to 127 days. Monkeys given ATG and a single marrow infusion were initially non-specifically unresponsive to polyclonal mitogens and allogeneic cell stimulation. Eventually the MLR to allogeneic cell stimulation reversed to normal, but the MLR to the specific donor was consistently negative as the kidneys remained unrejected. Co-culture experiments of lymphocytes from non-specific donors with normal allogeneic cells and donor stimulating cells gave reduced MLR reactions; if stimulating cells came from indifferent donors, MLR suppression was not found. These extraordinary observations strongly suggested that a state of donor-specific unresponsiveness in the MLR was related to the present of antigen-specific suppressor cells. They have also shown that long-term surviving rhesus renal allografts after RATG and DBM are infiltrated with nodular collections of lymphocytes. A significant portion of these lymphoid cells have donor specificities and suppressor cell phenotypes. Thus, a local suppressor cell effect (local tolerance) is also suggested as part of the unresponsive mechanism in the rhesus monkey. They have shown that along with the dramatic prolongation of median survival time following RATG and DBM treatment, there is a dramatic reduction in incidence of anti-donor lymphocyte mediated cytotoxicity (LMC) but a preservation of capacity to exert anti-donor antibody-dependent cellular cytotoxicity (ADCC) reactions. They also studied the effect of adjunctive immunosuppression in this model. Azathioprine decreased the observed MSTs and increased anti-donor MLC responses. In contrast, low dose cyclosporine and prednisone increased MSTs by 50% and prevented detectable LMC. However, cyclosporine and prednisone appeared to increase the humoral alloimmune response increasing the incidence of recipients with anti-donor ADCC. Long-term survival in this group was limited by chronic rejection and cyclosporine toxicity. In their most recent studies (Thomas, J.K., Carver, M., Cunningham, P. *et al.* Kidney allograft tolerance in primates without chronic immunosuppression: The role of veto cells. Submitted for publication), these investigators presented evidence that long-term survival of renal allografts in the ALS-BM primate model was induced by donor bone marrow cells which express veto activity. They speculated that the effective cell was a minor population of donor BM cells of the NK (natural killer) or LAK linage. Their findings point out additional evidence (as implied by the rodent studies above) that success in tolerance induction will not be an all or none phenomenon. They also emphasized that improved success in this system will require adjunctive immunosuppression that is directed to the humoral alloimmune response.

The ALS—marrow model in man

The ALS—BM model has been effective in producing various degrees of unresponsiveness in all species tested (both large and small) and in both non-immediately and immediately vascularized allografts. Monaco *et al.* (32) did an initial trial of BM infusion in living related, MLC positive combinations in the pre-cyclosporine era. This was an uncontrolled trial and although the results were encouraging (only two acute rejections in the first 100 patient months) they were also inconclusive and evidence for chronic rejection in long-term survivors was present. Barber *et al.* (33) initiated a controlled trial in primary cadaver transplantation in which the control patient received quadruple therapy (ATG, cyclosporine, prednisone, Imuran) versus the experimental group given quadruple therapy plus donor specific bone marrow infusion. The initial results were encouraging and recent analysis suggest a definite improvement in allograft survival at 12 and 18 months (Barber, W.H., Mankin, J.A., Laskow, D.A. *et al.* Long-term results of a controlled prospective study with transfusion of donor-specific bone marrow in 50 cadaveric renal allograft recipients. Submitted for publication) in the bone marrow group.

Future considerations

Donor bone marrow is the ideal donor cellular antigen for widespread trials in clinical organ allografting. Multi-organ donors can have their organs harvested and then donor ribs could subsequently be removed to be used as the bone marrow source. In the original clinical trials above, aspiration of iliac crests was done. In the case of multi-organ donor cadavers prolonged harvesting from iliac crests can lead to hemodynamic instability and could lead to loss of some potentially harvestable organs. Use of donor ribs (after all harvests are completed) is simple and does not interfere with the technical aspects of harvesting. BM derived from ribs could be fractionated to its active fraction which could be frozen and preserved for infusion a week or two later depending on the timing of BM infusion. Isolated, preserved donor-specific marrow could be distributed to recipients from a central processing laboratory. Furthermore, it is possible that in the future prospective cadaver donors might be prepared for donor-specific bone marrow harvest by injection with a granulocyte stimulating factor (or some related lymphokine or monokine) to improve the tolerance inducing capacity of the BM.

The lack of availability and/or reproducibility of current polyclonal ALS preparations may be a problem. Experiments are now being done in our laboratory to determine if current monoclonal anti-T cell antibodies (OKT3 for example) can be used to replace the polyclonal sera tested experimentally. As noted above, a simple standard protocol of grafting, post-transplantation ALS treatment, along with prednisone and Imuran followed by BM infusion and addition of cyclosporine treatment would be easy to incorporate into current immunosuppressive protocols. Many units use polyclonal ALS, prednisone, Imuran, for 7—14 days and then cycle in cyclosporine. Donor BM infusion could be just a simple addition to these protocols for both renal and extrarenal organs. Also, as noted above, infusion of BM shortly after ALS treatment may obviate the necessity for preservation of the bone marrow.

Although the ALS-BM protocol would be easy to incorporate into current multi-drug immunosuppressive programs, interpretation of a salutary effect attributable to BM infusion might be difficult. All of the above experiments suggest that pure tolerance as an all or none phenomenon will not be produced. Rather, some type of partial tolerance will be achieved. Thus, BM-infused patients in a multi-drug program might do better in patient and graft survival over similarly treated multi-drug patients not given BM. Also, differences could be measured by the ease with which various drugs in the maintenance programs of bone marrow and control groups can be subtracted, decreased or totally eliminated, hopefully demonstrating that BM-infused patients could be maintained with less drugs and with less rejection reactions. The likely drug to be subtracted initially is steroids. If steroids can be successfully subtracted, another drug could then be removed. It is important to emphasize that complete removal of all immunosuppressive drug therapy, although a commendable and worthy goal, is not likely to be achieved rapidly. Furthermore, as noted above, as drugs are subtracted, one can not necessarily rely on persistent normal function. Indeed, periodic biopsy surveillance of organ allografts subjected to tolerance inducing programs will have to be added to the monitoring program until a non-invasive *in vitro* or *in vivo* assay for clinical tolerance (i.e. the absence of anti-graft alloreactivity) is forthcoming.

References

1. Billingham, R.E., Brent, L. and Medawar, P.B.: Acquired immunological tolerance. *Nature (London)* **172**, 603, (1953).
2. Monaco, A.P.: Antilymphocyte serum and other methods of lymphocyte depletion. In: J.S. Najarian, R.L. Simmons (eds), *Transplantation*, Chap. 6, Section IV, pp 222–251. Lea & Febiger, Philadelphia (1972).
3. Monaco, A.P., Wood, M.L., Gary, J.G. *et al.*: Studies on heterologous antilymphocyte serum in mice. II. Effect on the immune response. *J. Immunol.* **96**, 229 (1966).
4. Monaco, A.P., Wood, M.L. and Russell, P.S.: Adult thymectomy: Effect on recovery from immune depression in mice. *Science* **149**, 432 (1965).
5. Monaco, A.P. and Wood, M.L.: Studies on heterologous antilymphocyte serum in mice. VII. Optimal cellular antigen for induction of immunologic tolerance with antilymphocyte serum. *Transplant. Proc.* **2**, 489–496 (1970).
6. Abbott, W.M., Monaco, A.P. and Russell, P.S.: Antilymphocyte serum and cell-free antigen loading. *Transplantation* **7**, 291 (1969).
7. Lance, E.M. and Medawar, P.B.: Quantitative studies in tissue transplantation immunity. IX. Induction of tolerance with antilymphocyte serum. *Proc. Roy. Soc. B* **173**, 447 (1969).
8. Wood, M.L., Monaco, A.P., Gozzo, J.J. *et al.*: Use of homozygous allogeneic bone marrow for induction of tolerance with antilymphocyte serum: Dose and timing. *Transplant. Proc.* **3**, 676 (1971).
9. Wood, M.L., Monaco, A.P., Gozzo, J.J. *et al.*: Use of homozygous allogeneic bone marrow

for induction of tolerance with antilymphocyte serum: Dose and Timing. *Transplant. Proc.* **3**, 676—679 (1971).
10. Hartner, W.C., Monaco, A.P. and Gozzo, J.J.: Effect of timing of bone marrow injection on the prolongation of skin grafts in ALS-treated mice. *Transplant. Proc.* **21**, 242 (1989).
11. Monaco, A.P., Gozzo, J.J., Wood, M.L. *et al.*: Use of low doses of homozygous allogeneic bone marrow cells to induce tolerance with antilymphocyte serum (ALS): Tolerance by intraorgan injection. *Transplant. Proc.* **3**, 680—683 (1971).
12. Clark, A.W., Monaco, A.P.: The effect of bacterial adjuvants on allograft survival after antilymphocyte serum (ALS) and donor bone marrow. *Immunology (British)* **27**, 887—893 (1974).
13. Liegeois, A., Escourrow, J., Ouvre, E. *et al.*: Microchimerism: A state of low ratio proliferation of allogeneic bone marrow. *Transplant. Proc.* **9**, 272 (1977).
14. Wood, M.L. and Monaco, A.P.: Adoptive transfer of specific unresponsiveness to skin allografts by spleen cells from ALS-treated, marrow-injected mice. *Transplant. Proc.* **11**, 1023—1027 (1979).
15. Wood, M.L. and Monaco, A.P.: Suppressor cells in specific unresponsiveness to skin allografts in ALS-treated, marrow-injected mice. *Transplantation* **29**, 196 (1980).
16. Wood, M.L., Gottschalk, R. and Monaco, A.P.: Effect of splenectomy on specific unresponsiveness to skin allografts induced in ALS-treated, marrow injected mice. *Transplantation* **29**, 320 (1980).
17. Gozzo, J.J., Litvin, D.A., Monaco, A.P. *et al.*: Fractionated bone marrow: Use of lymphocyte containing fraction for skin prolongation in antilymphocyte serum (ALS) treated mice. *Transplant. Proc.* **13**, 592 (1981).
18. De Fazio, S.R., Hartner, W.C., Monaco, A.P. *et al.*: Mouse skin graft prolongation with donor strain bone marrow of the active bone marrow cells. *J. Immunol.* **135**, 3040 (1985).
19. De Fazio, S.R., Hartner, W.C., Monaco, A.P. *et al.*: Prolongation of graft survival in ALS-treated mice by donor-specific bone marrow: Density gradient fractionation of the active bone marrow cells. *Transplantation* **43**, 564 (1987).
20. De Fazio, S.R., Kowlenko, M. and Gozzo, J.J.: Isolation by continuous density gradient centrifugation and characterization of bone marrow cells active in prolonging allograft survival in antilymphocyte serum-treated mice. *Transplant. Proc.* **19**, 547 (1987).
21. De Fazio, S.R., Hartner, W.C., Monaco, A.P. *et al.*: Mouse skin graft prolongation with donor strain bone marrow and antilymphocyte serum. Effect of donor age. *Transplantation* **40**, 563 (1985).
22. De Fazio, S.R., Hartner, W.C., Monaco, A.P. *et al.*: Mouse skin graft prolongation with donor strain bone marrow and antilymphocyte serum: Effect of bone marrow cell storage. *Transplantation* **41**, 26 (1986).
23. Kapnick, S.J. and Monaco, A.P.: Induction of unresponsiveness to skin allografts with donor strain platelets in antilymphocyte serum-treated mice. *Transplant. Proc.* **11**, 982—985 (1979).
24. Maki, T., Gottschalk, R., Wood, M.L. *et al.*: Specific unresponsiveness to skin allografts in antilymphocyte serum-treated, marrow-injected mice: Participation of donor marrow-derived suppressor cells. *J. Immunol.* **127**, 1433—1438 (1981).
25. Maki, T., Simpson, M., Monaco, A.P.: Development of suppressor T cells by antilymphocyte serum treatment in mice. *Transplantation* **34**, 376—381 (1982).
26. Wood, M.L., Gottschalk, R., Monaco, A.P.: The effect of cyclosporine on the induction of unresponsiveness in ALS-treated, marrow-injected mice. *Transplantation* **46**, 449 (1988).
27. Caridis, T., Liegeois, A., Barrett, I. *et al.*: Enhanced survival of canine renal allografts of ALS-treated dogs given bone marrow. *Transplant. Proc.* **5**, 671—674 (1973).
28. Hartner, W.C., De Fazio, S.R., Maki *et al.*: Prolongation of renal allograft survival in antilymphocyte serum-treated dogs by post-operative injection of density gradient-fractionated donor bone marrow. *Transplantation* **42**, 593 (1986).
29. Thomas, F., Carver, F.M., Foil, M.B. *et al.*: Long-term incompatible kidney survival in outbred higher primates without chronic immunosuppression. *Ann. Surg.* **198**, 370 (1983).
30. Thomas, J.M., Carver, F.M., Foil, M.B. *et al.*: Renal allograft tolerance induced with ATG and donor bone marrow in outbred rhesus monkeys. *Transplantation* **36**, 104 (1983).

31. Thomas, J.M., Carver, F.M., Cunningham, P. *et al.*: Promotion of incompatible allograft acceptance in rhesus monkeys given post-transplant antithymocyte globulin and donor bone marrow. I. In vivo parameters and immunohistologic evidence suggesting microchimerism. *Transplantation* **43**, 332 (1987).
32. Monaco, A.P., Wood, M.L., Maki, T. *et al.*: Attempt to induce unresponsiveness to human renal allografts with antilymphocyte globulin and donor-specific bone marrow. *Transplant. Proc.* **17**, 1312–1314 (1985).
33. Barber, W.H., Diethelm, A.G., Laskow, D.A. *et al.*: Use of cryopreserved donor bone marrow in cadaver kidney allograft recipients. *Transplantation* **47**, 66 (1989).

20. Comparison of cyclosporine assays using radioimmunoassay, fluorescent polarization immunoassay and high-performance liquid chromatography

A.G. WHITE, D. PANJWANI, M. ANGELO KHATTAR, A.S. EL-DEEN, M.S.A. KUMAR, E.M. PHILIPS and G.M. ABOUNA

Introduction

We have investigated three different methods for the assay of blood levels of cyclosporine to compare the results obtained by the different assays and to see which assay is the most suitable for routine use in our laboratory.

Material and methods

The following commercially prepared kits were used.

1. Sandimun cyclosporine radioimmunoassay using a monoclonal antibody that specifically measures parent cyclosporine (SP. RIA).
2. Sandimmun cyclosporine radioimmunoassay using a monoclonal antibody that measures both parent drug and metabolites (non-SP. RIA).
3. ABBOT TDX fluorescent polarization immunoassay (FPIA) that measures parent cyclosporine and its metabolites.
4. A local modified high-performance liquid chromatography assay (HPLC) using solid phase extraction that measures parent cyclosporine.

Peripheral blood was collected from 50 patients attending our outpatient clinic in one day to measure the trough levels of cyclosporine. The commercially available cyclosporine assay kits were used in accordance with the manufacturer's instructions.

The HPLC assay is summarized as follows: 4 ml of acetonitrile (ACN), methanol and 10% zinc sulphate solution is added to a spiked blood sample and the denatured proteins separated by centrifugation. The supernatant is diluted with deionized water and the mixture added to a 6 ml c-18 bond elute cartridge. The cartridge is washed with 50% acetonitrile in water and the cyclosporine eluted with 2 ml of ethanol into a clean tube. The eluent is evaporated to dryness under nitrogen at 45 °C and then the reisdue reconstituted with 180 μl of ACN, methanol and water. The samples are injected into a

C-1-Reverse phase column at 58 °C with a flowrate of 1 ml/min. The column eluents are monitored at 214 nm using a detector.

The assays were compared by calculating the correlation coefficient and plotting a linear regression line.

Results

Figures 1 and 2 summarize the comparison between Sandimmun specific and

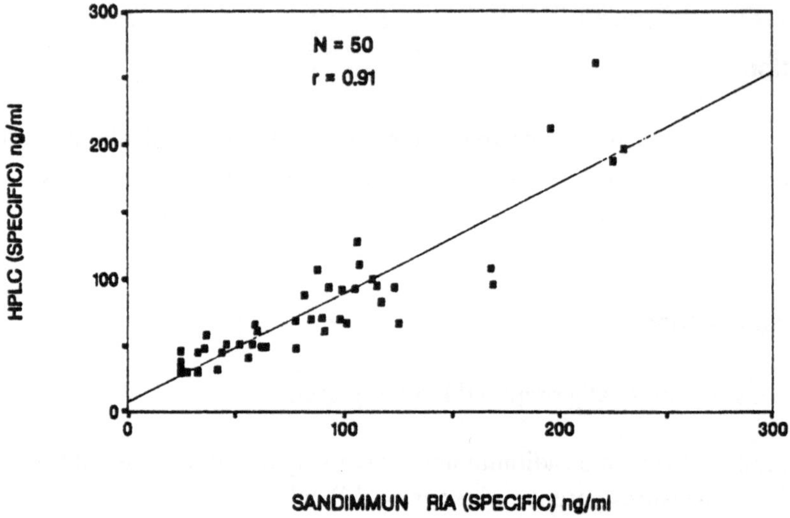

Fig. 1. Assay of cyclosporine: HPLC vs Sandimmun RIA (specific).

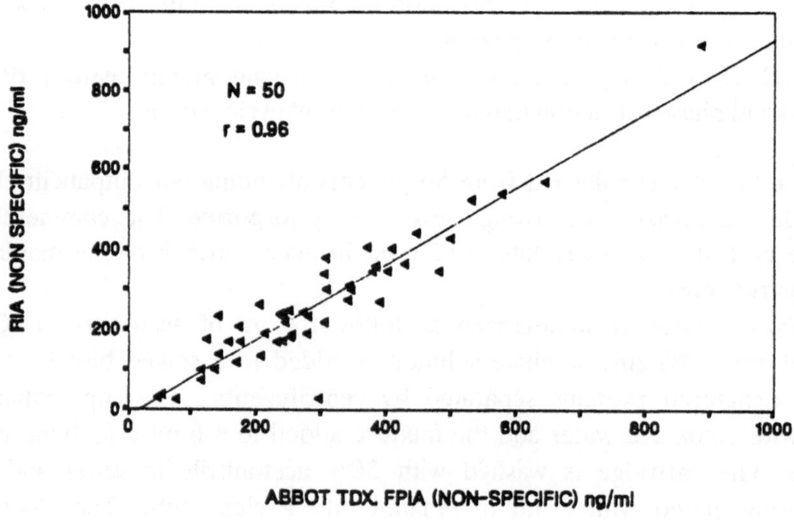

Fig. 2. Asssay of cyclosporine: Sandimmun RIA (non-specific) vs Abbot TDX. FPIA (non-specific).

HPLC and Sandimmun non-specific and Abbot FPIA respectively. The best correlation ($r = 0.96$) was obtained between the Sandimmun non-specific RIA and the Abbot TDX FPIA, although the specific cyclosporine assays were also highly correlated ($r = 0.91$).

Table 1 gives the mean values obtained for each of the assays, the HPLC giving slightly higher values than the Sandimmun specific assay and the Abbot TDX FPIA slightly higher than the Sandimmun non-specific RIA. The differences between the values obtained between the specific assays and between the non-specific assays were not significant (T test for paired samples). Comparisons were not made between the assays for parent cyclosporine and parent cyclosporine plus metabolites because of the wide range or metabolism of cyclosporine between patients (4.1 ± 1.52; range 1.6—9.2).

Table 1. Mean values obtained in 50 samples using various cyclosporine assays.

	$\bar{x}$ ng/ml	
HPLC	93	$r = 0.91$
Sandimmun specific RIA	81	
Sandimmun non-specific RIA	263	$r = 0.96$
Abbot TDX FPIA	294	

Discussion

The results obtained between the specific assays for cyclosporine and for the assays measuring cyclosporine and metabolites were comparable. The choice of assay for routine laboratory use therefore depends on the rapidity and ease of operation in addition to what data the physicians require. Without doubt the easiest and most rapid assay is the FPIA using the Abbot TDX system but our physicians prefer measurement of the parent drug rather than the parent drug + metabolites. The reasons given are that they prefer the narrower range of the specific assay and that in general most of the toxicity and immunosuppressive activity, is believed to be associated with the parent molecule.

The metabolism of cyclosporine by individual patients merits comment. It is possible that in the early stages of patient monitoring that assays of the parent drug and also its metabolites should be made. Individual calculations can then be made on the dosage for each patient based on the metabolic profile. We would therefore consider using the Sandimmun specific RIA in concert with the Abbot TDX FPIA in the initial phase after transplantation.

Our findings compare favorably with those reported by other investigators. Lindholm and Henricsson (1) compared Sandimmun specific and HPLC finding a correlation coefficient of 0.98 compared with our value of 0.96. Joyce and Bacchus (2) compared Incstar non-specific RIA with Abbot TDX FPIA finding a correlation coefficient of 0.96, our comparison of Sandimmun non-specific RIA with Abbot TDX FPIA gave a coefficient of 0.91.

The anticipated development of an FPIA for measurement of the parent drug would be a distinct advantage.

References

1. Lindholm, A. and Henricsson, S.: Simultaneous monitoring of cyclosporin in blood and plasma with four analytical methods: A clinical evaluation. *Transplant. Proc.* **21**, 1472–1474 (1989).
2. Joyce, B.G. and Bacchus, R.: Cyclosporine monitoring by fluroscent polarisation immunoassay of whole blood. *Ann. Saudi Medicine* **9**, 52–54 (1989).

21. Long-term outcome in renal transplantation

H. BRYNGER

The renal transplant programme in Göteborg, Sweden, has been active for 25 years, with a total number of more than 2300 renal transplants performed up to now. The organizational part has been uniform over the years, with a main policy to continue regular follow-up of patients even on a long-term basis. Between 250 and 300 patients with renal grafts and chronic immunosuppression for more than 10 years are currently having their regular check-up in our unit.

From this group of patients, 172 were investigated regarding long-term mortality, morbidity and rehabilitation during the second decade after transplantation (study A).

Another group of 52 patients, 10—22 years after transplantation and on chronic conventional immunosuppression, were studied regarding long-term effects of immunosuppression by investigating lymphocyte subpopulation counts, lymphocyte stimulation indices, immunoglobuline levels and by correlating the immunological profiles with the occurrence of infectious or dysplastic (i.e. malignant and premalignant) skin disease as one detectable sign of depressed immunocompetence (study B).

Results

Study A

The patient survival was calculated by setting 10 years as 100%. Actuarial patient survival was 80% and 69% at 15 and 20 years, respectively, implying 3% annual mortality rate throughout the second decade. The causes of death are listed in Table 1. Fifty percent of the deaths were caused by vascular disasters. Three patients died of liver failure, all secondary to chronic B-hepatitis. Forty-two of the 172 patients were hepatitis B surface antigen carriers, at least since the time of transplantation.

In 72 patients surviving 15 years, morbidity was studied during the 10 and 15 year period after transplantation (Table 2). It should be noted that the same

Table 1. Cause of death during the second decade post-renal transplantation.

	No. of deaths	No of deaths with functioning grafts
Cardiocerebrovascular disease	17	13
Bacterial infection	6	3
Liver failure	3	3
Malignancy	5	4
Pancreatitis	1	1
Cause unknown	2	–
Total	34	24

Table 2. Morbidity between 10 and 15 years post-transplant (*n*-72).

	No. of patients
Cardiocerebrovascular disease	13
Infection	9
Malignancy	10
Non-melanoma skin cancer	8
Squamous cell carcinoma of the vulva	1
Carcinoma of the cervix	1
Liver dysfunction	4
Others	2

patient might occur in more than one disease group. In about 50% of the patients no morbidity was registered during the 5-year period.

Of the patients, 78% and 70% were in a good physical condition at 10 and 15 years, respectively, and had no or only a minor degree of physical disability. Severely disabling disorders were found in 4% and 8% at 10 and 15 years. However, no patient was bedridden.

Study B

Fifteen patients (29%) had no immunosuppression related skin lesions. In 28 patients (54%) infectious skin lesions were found of which 25 had viral warts, 6 had fungal or bacterial lesions. Nineteen patients (37%) had dysplastic skin lesions at the time of the investigation or previously during the post-transplant period. They were defined as basaliomas (8), squamous cell carcinomas (3), sweat gland carcinoma (1), Bowen's disease and/or actinic keratoses (11).

The immunological profiles were analysed according to the presence or absence of infectious skin lesions and dysplastic skin lesions, as accounted for in

Table 3. A significantly depressed CD4/CD8 ratio was found in patients with infectious skin lesions.

Table 3. Immunological profiles analyzed in the presence or absence of skin lesions.

	Infectious skin lesions			Dysplastic skin lesions		
	Yes ($n = 28$)		No ($n = 24$)	Yes ($n = 19$)		No ($n = 33$)
CD4[a]	781 ± 65	b	1090 ± 100	869 ± 99	NS	955 ± 78
CD8[a]	707 ± 57	NS	599 ± 52	634 ± 66	NS	670 ± 50
Other subpopulations		NS			NS	
CD4/CD8 ratio	1.19 ± 0.09	c	1.93 ± 0.17	1.59 ± 0.23	NS	1.50 ± 0.10
Con-A—PHA		NS			NS	
IgA, IgM, IgG 1—4		NS			NS	

[a] = $\times 10^6$ cells/l, mean ± SE.
[b] = $p < 0.01$.
[c] = $p < 0.001$.
NS = not statistically significant (*t*-test, 2-tailed).

Comments

In study A, the majority of patients had a high level of medical and social rehabilitation. There is, however, some risk for morbidity and mortality mainly from cardiocerebrovascular disease and from causes probably associated with chronical immunosuppressive therapy: One-third of the mortality and about one-half of the morbidity was due to malignancy or infection. Chronic liver disease was a less frequent cause of death despite a high number of chronically HBsAg positive patients.

In study B, patients with infectious skin lesions were found to have depressed CD4/CD8 ratio obviously not needed for the maintenance of the renal transplant function. This might indicate overimmunosuppression and might therefore serve as an impetus to reduce drug dosages.

In our experience, the vast majority of patients with long-term function of renal transplants and on chronic conventional immunosuppression are in excellent health. However, a number of patients might suffer from overimmunosuppression that might lead to increased morbidity and possibly also mortality. Further investigations are needed to elucidate the role of long-term immunosuppression in this rather quickly growing cohort of patients.

22. Ten-year experience with 500 renal transplants

G.M. ABOUNA, M.S.A. KUMAR, A.G. WHITE, M. SAMHAN, O.S.G. SILVA, I.H. AL-ABDULLAH, M. KALAWI, S. AL-DADAH, N. AL-SABAWI, P. JOHN and E.M. PHILIPS

Introduction

Renal transplantation at the Kuwait University Medical Center began in 1979. Since that time, the program has rapidly developed to become one of the largest single multi-organ transplant centers in the Middle East. By May 1990, some 560 renal transplants and several pancreas and bone marrow grafts were carried out at the Center. With the development of the transplant activity a large self-contained and purposely built transplant center — The Hamed Al-Essa Organ Transplant Center, with 36 beds and all laboratory and other support facilities — was opened in 1988. All current transplant activity takes place at this center which is also a major referral center for many patients from neighboring Arab countries for renal transplantation which are performed free, as part of the health aid given by the Government of Kuwait to the less privileged Arab countries.

Although Kuwait recently enacted an advanced law for cadaver organ transplantation, there has been marked scarcity of such organs locally, which is largely due to social and cultural factors. As a result of this, most of the renal transplants carried out to date have been from living related donors, a small number from genetically unrelated but emotionally related donors. Also, because of this factor, the Kuwait Transplant Program has accepted a large number of cadaver grafts from the United States (UNOS), and Europe (Eurotransplant), many of which have problems with the kidney or with the donor and all have long preservation times. At our Center, as in other major transplant centers, immunosuppressive protocols both prophylactic and therapeutic have evolved during the decade, as have the criteria for donor and recipient selection.

This study analyzes our overall experience in the first 500 renal allografts performed at this Center over a decade, with regard to indications for transplantation, the overall long-term outcome, the effect on graft function, of original disease, donor type, tissue matching and the duration of cold preservation. The study also outlines the causes of patient and graft loss, the type of complications, the effect of changing immunosuppressive therapy on the results, the economic benefits of successful renal transplantation on the overall cost of the renal failure program in the country and the future importance of recent legislation on organ transplantation from cadavers.

Patients and methods

Between March 1979 and December 1989, 486 recipients aged 1 to 68 years were given 501 renal allografts. The indications for transplantation were a variety of causes of terminal renal failure, as shown in Table 1. The male to female ratio was 2.1 and 52 patients or 11% were children, 1—16 years of age. The graft source was living related donor (LRD) in 349 (70%), living unrelated (LUD) in 51 (10%) and cadavers in 101 (20%). In the LRD transplants, 217 were siblings, 68 were child to parent and 64 parent to child. Of the LUD transplants, 27 were spouses, 13 were distant relatives and 11 were friends and well-wishers. In living donor transplantation, donor age was 18—75 years and, before acceptance, a vigorous medical, social and immunological protocol of donor evaluation was employed as previously reported (1, 2, 3, 4). Standard ABO, HLA-A and B, DR typing and lymphocyte crossmatch were carried out. More recently, further refinement of the crossmatch technique has been employed for both the T and the B lymphocytes and when the latter was positive, it was further analyzed with regard to the IgG or IgM class. While every attempt was made to select the best possible donor with regard to class I and class II HLA antigens, no medically suitable donor was rejected because of poor histocompatibility matching (4, 5). In the LUD transplantation, extraordinary effort was made with regard to the ethical, moral and legal aspects in the selection of the donor and in conformity with the guidelines of the Transplantation Society. These donors were interviewed by an institutional committee consisting of nephrologists, surgeon, social worker, psychiatrist and a legal counsel and only when the committee was satisfied that donation was

Table 1. Indications for renal transplantation in 501 recipients.

Cause of renal failure	No.
Chronic glomerulonephritis	248
Chronic pyelonephritis	117
Diabetic nephropathy	13
Hypertensive nephrosclerosis	14
Focal segmental glomerulosclerosis	8
Congenital polycystic kidney disease	15
Others (congenital medullary cystic disease, dysplasia, hypoplasia, etc.)	86
Total	501

Table 2. Risk factors present in cadaver kidneys imported from U.S.A. and Europe.[a]

Problems	Number
Technical problems in the grafts:	
Multiple vessels	14
Injured ureters	2
Pediatric grafts	26
Medical problems in the donors:	
Diabetes	2
Hypertension	10
Atherosclerosis	8
Prolonged ischemia time > 48 hours	58

[a] Some grafts had more than one risk factor present.

being made for altruistic reason and not for any commercial or material gain, was the donor accepted and the transplant carried out (6, 7, 8). In the LUD and the cadaver grafts, there were at least 2 or more HLA antigen mismatches between donor and recipient. In the group of cadaver donors, 14 kidneys were harvested locally and 87 were imported from U.S.A. and Europe. The mean ischemia time in the imported grafts was 48 ± 15 hours (30—80 hours), while in the locally harvested group it was only 12 ± 3 (6—20 hours). Between 1980 and 1985, preservation and transportation of imported kidneys was carried out either by pulsatile perfusion or by simple cooling using Eurocollin's solution (9, 10). Since 1985, all such kidneys were preserved by simple cooling with Eurocollin's solution and more recently with the UW solution. In addition to long ischaemia times most of the kidneys shipped to our Center from U.S.A. and Europe were suboptimal because of several risk factors in the donor and/or in the grafts (Table 2), while in 26 cases the kidneys came from pediatric donors < 5 years of age (10, 11, 12).

During this decade of experience, several protocols of prophylactic immunosuppression were introduced and tested (Table 3). In the LRD group, conventional immunosuppression with azathioprine and prednisone was routinely employed until December 1988. Since that time, cyclosporine (CsA) was added as part of a triple immunosuppression except in recipients of HLA-identical grafts. In the LUD and the cadaver grafts, conventional immunosuppression was used until 1982. After that time, ATG (Fresenius) or ALG (Institute Merieux) were added to the conventional induction therapy from one day of transplantation until adequate graft function became established when CsA was added (10, 13). In all cases, CsA was used at 8 mg/kg initially and later adjusted according to the whole-blood level as determined by monoclonal RIA, polyclonal RIA or the TDX technique. Antirejection therapy with pulse doses of methylprednisolone and local graft irradiation was used until 1981 (Table 4).

Table 3. Prophylactic immunosuppression protocols used during the 10-year period.

Living related transplantation:	
1979—1988	Azathioprine/prednisone
1989 onwards[a]	Azathioprine/prednisone/cyclosporine
Cadaveric and living unrelated transplantation:	
1979—1982	Azathioprine/prednisone
1983—1984	Cyclosporine/prednisone
1985 onwards[b]	Azathioprine/prednisone/cyclosporine

[a] Recipients from abroad are maintained on azathioprine/prednisone.
[b] In cadaver kidney recipients sequential triple therapy is used. Initially AZA/ATG/P which was converted to AZA/CsA/P after resumption of graft function.

Table 4. Evolution in antirejection therapy during the period of the study.

Period	Dose
1979—1981	Pulse doses of i.v. methylprednisolone
1981—1986	Pulse doses of i.v. methylprednisolone; i.v. infusion of ALG/ATG
1986—onwards	Pulse doses of i.v. methylprednisolone; i.v. infusion of ALG/ATG; i.v. OKT3

Plasmaphoresis and graft irradiation have also been used in few cases.

Since that time, ATG/ALG has been used in our Center as antirejection therapy in all steroid-resistant rejections (14). In 1986, OKT3 was introduced as an alternative to ATG therapy or in cases when ATG failed to reverse the rejection. In several patients we used high dose cyclosporine (15) and sometimes repeated plasmaphoresis, especially when renal biopsy indicated vascular rather than cellular type rejection. Random blood transfusion was given to all patients while donor-specific transfusion (DST) was used in some patients as part of a randomized control trial (16).

Besides renal failure, many patients had additional medical problems including past history of tuberculosis in about 3%, sero-positive HbsAg antigen in about 8%, type 1 and type 2 diabetes mellitus in 6% and cardiovascular disease with coronary artery bypass surgery in some cases (17, 18). Most patients with history of tuberculosis were placed on antituberculosis therapy for 6—12 months. All diabetic patients and all other patients with a history of ischemic heart disease underwent full cardiac assessment including coronary angiography. Patients with dialysis-resistant hypertension (about 10%) underwent unilateral native nephrectomy at the time of transplantation as part of a study to control post-transplant hypertension (19).

In most adult recipients of adult kidneys, a standard surgical technique was used with the kidney placed in the lower quadrant extraperitoneally with an antireflux uretero-neocystostomy. In pediatric recipients [< 5 years] of adult kidneys, the graft was placed intraperitoneally after removal of one or both native kidneys. In the case of small pediatric cadaver kidneys and particularly when multiple vessels were present, a variety of surgical procedures were used. Sixteen pediatric kidneys were transplanted as single grafts in adult recipients, two as single grafts in pediatric recipients and two as en-bloc grafts into an adult recipient.

All patients were managed in a highly specialized and purposely built organ transplant center with trained nursing, medical and laboratory staff and all post-transplant care was carried out by the same transplant team of surgeons, nephrologists and other medical personnel for monitoring of graft function, adjustment or immunosuppression and identification and management of complications. In addition to our own patients, another 70 recipients who, contrary to our advice, had gone to India, Egypt, Iraq and elsewhere and purchased their kidney from paid unrelated living donors, were followed by our team, but these are not included in this study (20). As a regional referral center for transplantation, about 30% of the patients transplanted in Kuwait came from different parts of the Middle East with their living related donors and after a period of 2 to 3 months, of post-transplant care at our Center, they return home for long-term follow-up by their referring physicians but were periodically seen in Kuwait or were followed-up by correspondence with their local physicians. Graft and patient survival were calculated by the actuarial method and appropriate comparisons were made using the chi-squared analysis and the student's '*t*' test.

As a result of persisting efforts by members of the transplant team, several events took place which had an important impact on cadaveric organ donation in Kuwait and the Islamic Middle East. In 1979, a milestone religious ruling was issued by the Islamic Fatwa Committee of Kuwait which declared for the first time, that 'If the donor is dead, it is permissible to take his organs whether or not he had so willed, providing there is dire necessity . . .' (21). Based on this declaration, the Government of Kuwait enacted Law No. 7 in 1984 which made it possible to remove kidneys from cadavers for transplantation and, in 1987, a new and more comprehensive legislation, Law No. 55, made it possible to remove all organs from cadavers after diagnosis of brain death, if they had a signed donor card or their relatives gave permission.

Results

The annual transplant output

Transplantation activity at the Kuwait Transplant Center has been rising, reaching 74 transplants in 1989, while in the first half of 1990, 60 renal transplants were already performed. This increase is largely due to better patient and public education and especially to the increase in the number of cadaveric grafts both imported to Kuwait from Europe and the U.S.A. and also harvested locally following the introduction of the new Kuwait Transplant Law No. 55 for 1987 (Figure 1).

Patient survival

The actuarial 2-, 5- and 10-year patient survival in recipients of LRD grafts is 97, 93 and 87%. In the LUD grafts it is 91, 91 and 80% respectively while in the cadaver grafts it is 84, 80 and 78%, although some of the original recipients with failed cadaveric grafts were retransplanted from living related or unrelated donor graft (Figures 2, 3, 4). A total of 38 patients were lost during the entire period due to several causes, the commonest of which were cardiovascular and

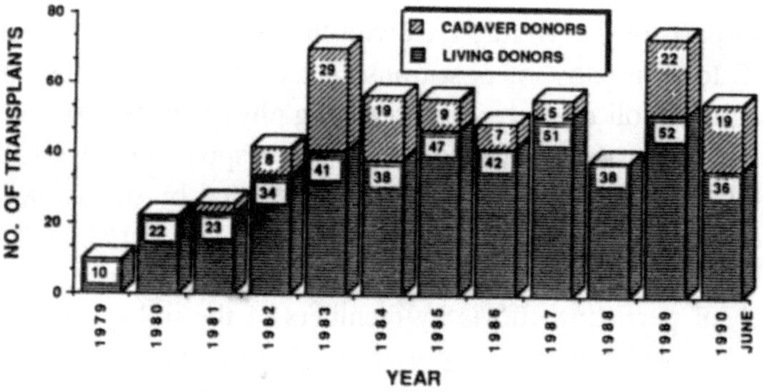

Fig. 1. Annual renal transplant output, 1979—1990.

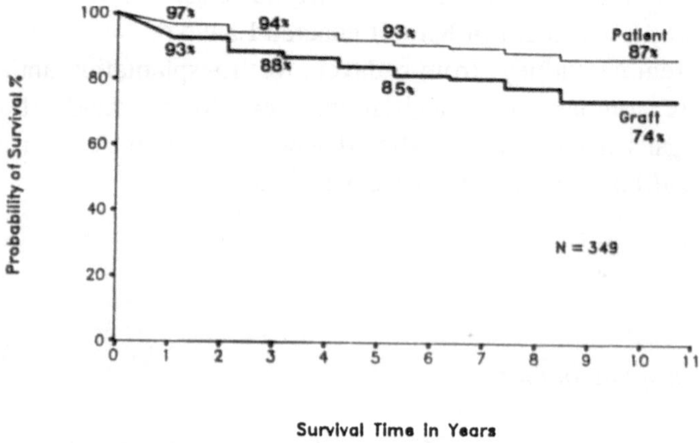

Fig. 2. Actuarial patient and graft survival rates for living related donor transplantation.

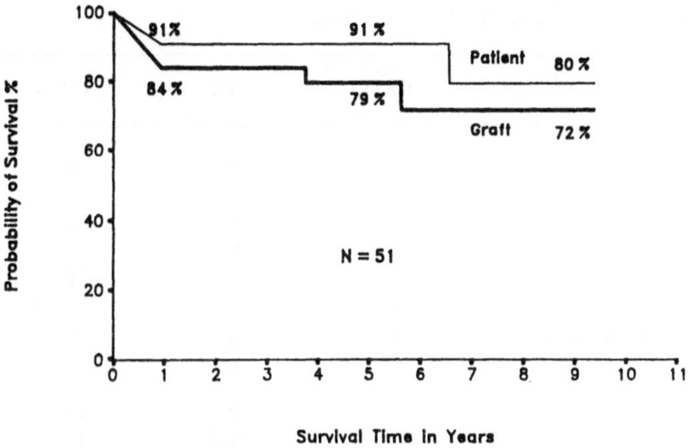

Fig. 3. Actuarial patient and graft survival rates for living unrelated donor transplantation.

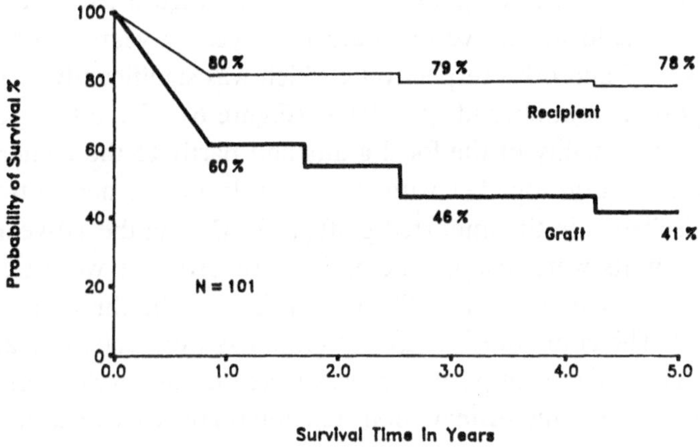

Fig. 4. Actuarial patient and graft survival for cadaver renal transplantation.

infections. The lowest rate of patient loss was in the LRD transplants and the highest in the cadaver grafts (Table 5).

Graft survival

The 2-, 5- and 10-year graft survival in the LRD group is 93, 85 and 74% respectively (Figure 2). In the LUD group, it is 84, 79 and 72% respectively (Figure 3), while in the cadaveric group the overall survival at 1, 3 and 5 years is 60, 46 and 41% (Figure 4).

When the period of cold ischemia was considered, the graft survival rate in kidneys preserved longer than 48 hours was significantly inferior to that of

Table 5. Causes of recipient death after transplantation.

Causes	LRD	LUD	CAD	Total
Cardiovascular	7	4	3	14
Infections	7	2	4	13
GI bleeding	1	0	2	3
AZA hepatotoxicity	2	0	1	3
ATG pneumonitis	2	0	0	2
Viral hepatitis	1	0	0	1
Cessation of immunosuppression	1	0	0	1
Malignancy	0	0	1	1
Total	21	6	11	38
(%)	6.3	11.7	12	7.6

kidneys preserved for shorter periods ($p = 0.05$) (Figure 5). Likewise, in the small number of the locally harvested grafts the 1 year, 3 years and 5 years graft survival was 87, 65 and 60% respectively, which was significantly higher than in the grafts imported from abroad ($p = 0.04$) (Figure 6). This difference is partly the result of better quality of the local grafts and partly to the higher incidence of primary non-function together with greater cyclosporine nephrotroxicity due to prolonged ischemia in the imported grafts (13). During the 10-year period of the study, 113 grafts were lost. Of these, 51 were LRD, 11 were LUD and 51 were cadaveric or 14.6, 19.6 and 50% within each of the three groups respectively (Table 6). The commonest causes of graft loss were patient death, chronic and acute rejection. Other important causes were chronic cyclosporine toxicity, patient non-compliance and primary non-function (in the cadaveric groups).

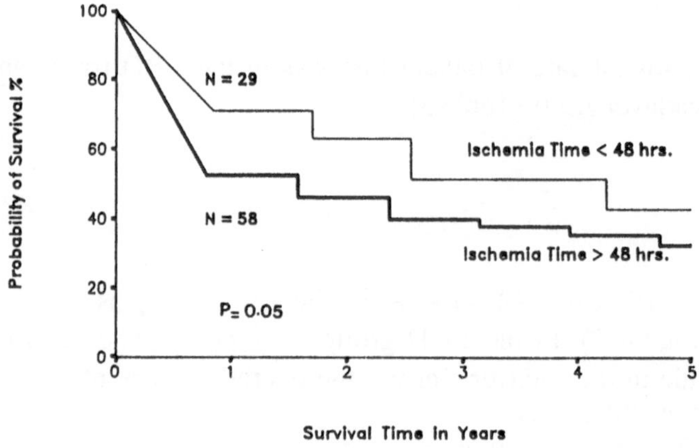

Fig. 5. Actuarial graft survival for imported cadaver kidneys according to cold ischemia times.

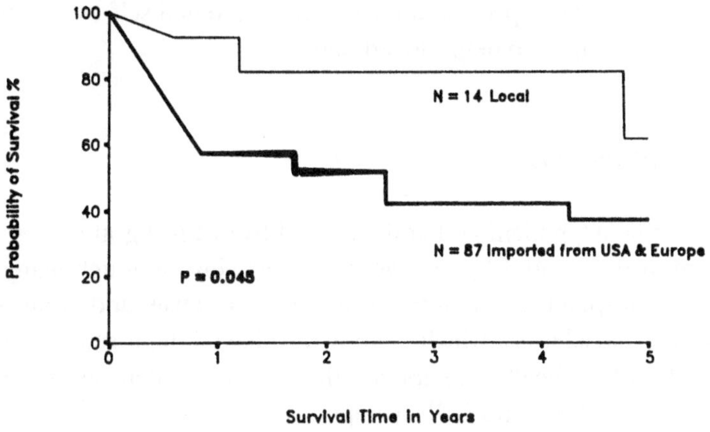

Fig. 6. Actuarial graft survival for locally harvested and imported cadaver kidneys.

Table 6. Causes of graft loss after transplantation.

Cause	LRD	LUD	CAD
Hyperacute rejection	2	0	2
Acute rejection	7	4	8
Chronic rejection	15	1	8
Patient's death	17	4	12
Chronic CsA nephrotoxicity	0	0	5
Diabetic nephropathy	1	1	1
Surgical	0	0	1
Non-compliance	3	1	1
Cessation of immunosuppression	0	0	4
Primary non-function	0	0	7
Renal artery stenosis	2	0	1
Renal artery thrombosis	1	0	1
Recurrence of primary renal disease	3	0	0
Total	51	11	51

The living donors

All living donors are alive and well and most were able to return to their former occupations and activities within 2 to 3 weeks after donation. There was only minor and temporary morbidity seen in this large series of living donors which included atelectasis, superficial wound infections and occasional wound pain. There have been no deterioration of renal function or the development of hypertension in any of these donors during the period of study. In addition, most of the donors have expressed a feeling of heightened self-esteem and pride for having the opportunity to help a loved one.

Recipient age and outcome

In pediatric recipients, patient and graft survival from LRD grafts ($n = 42$) have been excellent at 90% and 70% at 5 years respectively, although many of these children were transplanted for upper urinary tract sepsis and some for focal segmental glomerulosclerosis which is known to have a high rate of recurrence. Likewise, in the older healthy recipients there was excellent graft and patient survival, especially in LRD and LUD groups.

Pre-existing medical problems and outcome

There was a marked reduction in the incidence of post-transplant hypertension when unilateral nephrectomy was carried out simultaneously with renal transplantation. Many patients became normotensive or required very little anti-hypertension medications after transplantation (19).

Patients with positive hepatitis B surface antigen did have decreased patient and graft survival but in our experience, patient loss was not due to hepatic dysfunction but to greater susceptibility of this group to other infectious complications (18). The results obtained in diabetic patients were similar to the non-diabetic in the LRD and LUD groups. Patients with previous history of tuberculosis had equally good survival rate providing they had been pretreated with antituberculosis therapy prior to transplantation (17).

An important finding was that in those patients who had a low left ventricular ejection fraction (VEF) before transplantation but without coronary artery disease, their VEF improved significantly following successful renal transplantation most probably due to improvement in pre-existing uremic myocarditis (22).

HLA matching and outcome

The effect of histocompatibility on graft survival was investigated in this series and had been partly reported previously (4, 5). In the LRD series 69 (20%) were HLA identical, 105 (30%) were complete mismatches and the remainder were hepalo-identical. The HLA-identical grafts had considerably better graft survival rate even with conventional immunosuppression than mismatched grafts but the differences were just short of being statistically significant (Figure 7). However, the rate of rejection was significantly less and the amount of

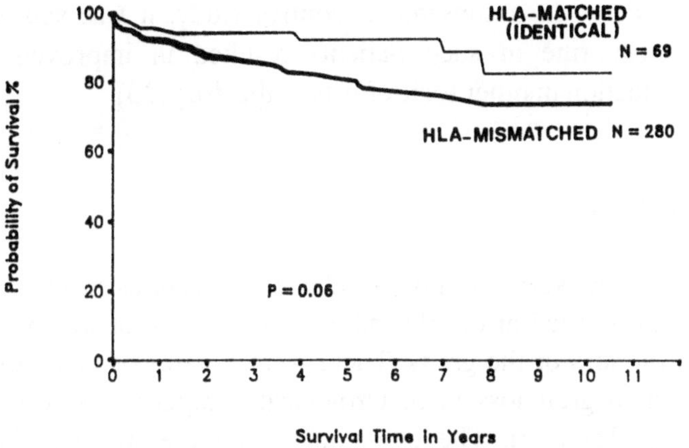

Fig. 7. Actuarial graft survival for HLA-identical and mismatched living related donor kidneys.

immunosuppression required was much smaller in recipients of HLA-identical grafts.

Type of immunosuppression regimen

In living related donor transplantation the results obtained with conventional immunosuppression were not significantly different than when cyclosporine was used although the prednisone dose was smaller and the frequency of rejection appeared to be reduced (Figure 8). Triple therapy with sequentially added cyclosporine did produce a marked improvement in early graft survival in LUD and cadaver transplantation but later many patients developed problems with

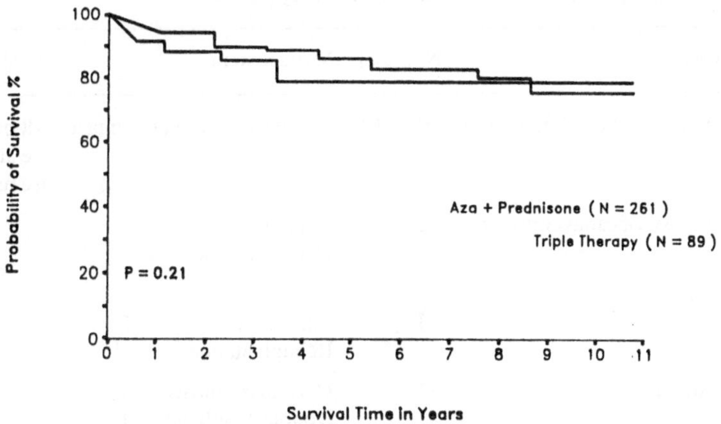

Fig. 8. Actuarial graft survival in living related donor kidneys according to immunosuppression protocol.

cyclosporine toxicity. In a subsequent control study, it was shown that withdrawal of cyclosporine in such patients resulted in improvement in graft function and reduction in other toxic effects of the drug (23).

Major complications

There were very few surgical and vascular complications in this series. These included 3 cases of renal artery thrombosis (0.6%), one of which was technical and all led to the loss of the grafts. There were 5 cases of renal artery stenosis (1%) which led to graft loss in 3. Urological complications were seen in 16 patients (3.2%) (Table 7). The commonest of these was lymphocele which caused ureteric obstruction. Ischemic necrosis of the ureter in 2 imported cadaveric kidneys were other important complications. However, all these were managed successfully and no patients or grafts were lost as a result.

Infections of bacterial, viral and fungal origin were the most common complications seen. In 13 instances, these were the principle cause of patient loss and were major contributing factors of graft loss in 32. There were several unusual bacterial infections in this series including salmonella and/or listeria septicemia in 12 patients and acute tuberculosis in 8. These were fatal in 50% of cases despite intensive antimicrobial therapy.

Herpes simplex, herpes zoster and CMV were common viral infections which often responded to specific antiviral therapy such as acyclovir or the use of hyperimmune globulin (Cytotec, Biotest) together with reduction or cessation of immunosuppression.

Denovo malignant neoplasms were seen in 5 patients, including 3 cases of Kaposi sarcoma, 1 lymphoma and 1 GI cancer.

Table 7. Urological complications seen during the study period.

Complications	No.	(%)	Management		Final outcome
Lymphocele with ureteric obstruction	9	(1.8)	Internal or external drainage		All patients are alive; all grafts are functioning
Ischemic necrosis of cadaver ureters	2		Repairs U/U anastomosis		
Vesical leakage:					
Ureteric	3		Bladder repair Reimplantation	2 1	
Ureteric stenosis	2		U/U anastomosis Double-J-catheter	1 1	
Total	16	(3.2)			

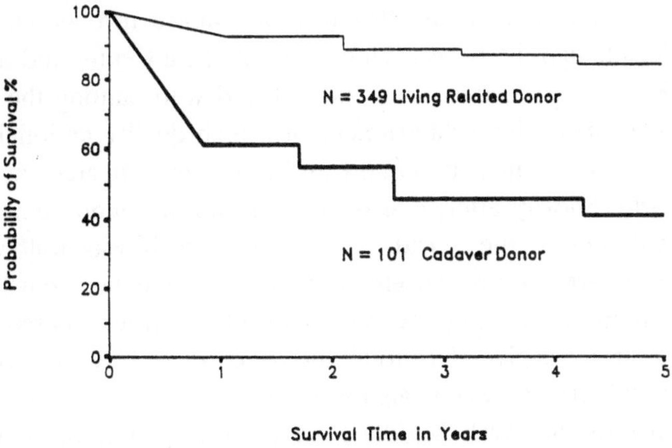

Fig. 9. Graft survival after living related donor versus cadaveric transplantation.

Rehabilitation and quality of life

Following successful renal transplantation the quality of life was far superior than any other form of therapy. Four of the 12 patients currently alive and well for more than 10 years after transplantation were medical colleagues and are practising their profession quite normally. Twelve female recipients have gone through one or more successful pregnancies and delivered normal infants and in one case normal mature twins. All the patients with successful grafts are back to their formal occupation and all the children are back at school in full-time education.

The cost benefit ratio

An analysis of the cost of transplantation in our Center was carried out recently. Renal transplantation surgery including 10—14 days' stay in hospital costs approximately Kuwaiti Dinar (KD) 4500 or US$ 15 000. The cost of medication, hospital readmission, etc., per patient per year is about KD 1500 or US$ 5000, making the total cost of a successful renal transplant per patient per 5 years about US$ 40 000. On the other hand, the cost of dialysis in Kuwait is KD 8000 or US$ 27 000 per patient per year, making the cost of maintenance dialysis per patient per 5 years about KD 40 000 or US$ 136 000.

Discussion

Renal transplantation is now accepted as the preferred and the most cost-effective method of treatment of chronic renal failure throughout the world. More than a decade ago the Kuwait University Medical Center and the Ministry of Health of Kuwait appreciated this concept and were among the first in the Middle East to support the establishment of a high-quality national transplant program which soon became the largest and most sophisticated facility in that area of the world. Shortly after, one of the first full academic departments of organ transplantation in the world was created which was followed by the establishment of a large and purposely built and self-contained transplant center with over 100 medical, nursing, technical and administrative personnel. While transplantation service is given free to all the residents of Kuwait, it is significant to mention that this free service is also extended to all the recipients who come from many parts of the Arab Middle East for transplantation at the Kuwait Transplant Center, who at the present time comprise 30% of the total transplant recipients of the center.

As a result of this support and of the enthusiasm of the transplant team, the annual renal transplant output increased rapidly over the years, reaching 74 transplants in 1989 and 60 transplants in the first 6 months of 1990. Initially, only living related donor transplantation could be performed due to the non-acceptance of removing organs from cadavers. However, in view of the high incidence of terminal renal failure in that part of the world, about 75 persons per million population or about 130 new patients per year, for a local population of 1.8 million, it was necessary to look for other sources of donors in order to meet the local need. The transplantation team began to solve this major problem in three ways: (a) by accepting unused cadaveric kidneys from centers in Europe and the United States, which were 'suboptimal' and had long preservation times; (b) by embarking on the use of genetically unrelated but emotionally related living donors under strict ethical and legal protocols; (c) by working tirelessly to bring about religious, social and legal acceptance of cadaveric organs and the concept of brain death locally. These efforts proved successful: the first LUD interspouse transplant was carried out in 1980 and, by 1989, 51 such transplants or 10% of the total output were carried out. The imported cadaveric program began in 1982 and, by 1989, 87 such grafts or 18% of the total output were carried out. The local cadaveric program began slowly after the introduction of the first transplantation law of Kuwait in 1984, but more rapidly following the introduction of a more comprehensive and advanced law in 1987. A total of 22 renal and 2 pancreatic grafts were harvested and used by June 1990. Excluding the patients referred to our Center from other Middle Eastern countries, the average annual transplant output for Kuwaiti residents has been about 40 kidneys per year or 22 per million population which is below the rate in Europe and North America. Although this rate has increased to about 31 per million per year during the period of 1989–1990, it still does not meet the local needs. Of the 230 patients currently on dialysis, 101 (44%) are on the transplant waiting list, and unless more cadaveric kidneys become available locally, many of these patients will be deprived of the benefits of transplantation while many others will be pushed to go to countries like India, Egypt, Iraq and the Philippines to buy kidneys in the marketplace — a practice which our Center has vigorously opposed because of the many negative medical, moral and logistic effects which such a practice has on any transplant program as well as on the practice of medicine generally (20). This important topic is dealt with in another chapter of this book. We believe that with the introduction of the new transplant law No. 55 for 1987, the acceptance of brain death and the creation of a local organ procurement organization, there is real hope that renal and extrarenal organs will become available locally to meet the need, especially since Kuwait has one of the highest death rates from traffic accidents in the world of about 360 cases a year, or nearly 200 per million of the population.

The overall 10-year patient and graft survival of LRD renal transplantation of 87 and 74% respectively in our Center is comparable to, and even better than, many major transplant centers in Europe and North America. When HLA-identical LRD donors are considered, patient and graft survival rates are even better (94 and 83%), the post-transplant complications fewer and the level of immunosuppression required much smaller. These excellent results may be partly due to the 'center effect' and partly to the smaller number of type I diabetics in our series.

The results of transplantation from living genetically unrelated but emotionally related donors using triple immunosuppression are also excellent in our experience. Our first patient, who received a kidney from her newly wedded husband in 1980, has continued to enjoy good renal function and has delivered two healthy children during the past 10 years. Other centers have recently reported similar successful series using LUD transplants, both in the European and the North American continent (24, 25, 26), however, it is important to emphasize that great care has to be taken at the institutional level to ensure that unrelated living donor transplantation is practised within the moral and ethical guidelines of the Transplantation Society (8, 20) and that this viable source of donor organs does not become 'rewarded gifting' as is being practised in some centers in the Indian subcontinent (27).

The overall results of our cadaveric transplantation, as expected, are inferior to those currently obtained in other major transplant centers for two main reasons: (a) The use of 'suboptimal' kidneys with many technical problems in the grafts and/or medical problems with the donor and (b) the prolonged ischemia times of up to 80 hours. Despite these problems, it was possible with extra care and effort to get many of these kidneys to function giving one-year graft survival of 60%. It was noted from the study that when only one of these factors was present, the graft survival was comparable to that in other centers in Europe and North America. For example, when the cold ischemia time was less than 48 hours, the one-year graft survival was nearly 70%. We also noted that while some pathologic changes in the kidneys resulting from medical conditions in the donor, such as very early diabetic nephropathy, were reversible when such kidneys are transplanted in non-diabetic recipients (11), other changes such as hyptertensive nephrosclerosis, especially when associated with prolonged ischemia times almost always resulted in failure. From this observation, we no longer recommend the use of kidneys from donors who die from complications of hypertension, when there is histological evidence of hypertensive changes in the kidney and when the cold ischemia time is > 48 hours.

Our findings in this series confirm those of other centers (28, 29), that excellent patient survival is possible, especially with LRD transplants, regardless of recipient age. The 5-year patient and graft survival in 42 pediatric recipients was 90% and 70% respectively. This is extremely important for this age group in terms of rehabilitation and quality of life particularly since they do not tolerate chronic dialysis therapy easily because of several adverse medical and emotional consequences. In the older patients (< 55 years) our findings also show that excellent outcome is also possible providing that they are free from serious cardiovascular disease at the time of transplantation.

Other pre-existing medical conditions in the recipient which in former years were regarded as contra-indications to transplantation are no longer the case at the present time, such as patients with positive hepatitis B antigen status without liver disease, chronic tuberculous infections, renal diseases due to chronic Mediterranean fever and diabetic patients. Most of these patients can be successfully rehabilitated by transplantation providing a complete preoperative evaluation is carried out and/or appropriate prophylactic support measures taken. Our observation that patients with patent coronary arteries but with severely depressed myocardial function could be considerably improved after transplantation. is significant. In the past. many such patients were considered to be high risk and were rejected. Our observations provide the evidence that many uremic patients develop myocardial dysfunction which can be corrected through successful renal transplantation. Indeed, some of our patients were transplanted with an ejection fraction of less than 25% and within a few weeks after transplantation, this increased to within the normal range.

The effect of HLA matching on patients and graft survival has been a controversial problem for many years. Our current results indicate that long-term patients and graft survival is far superior when the graft comes from HLA-identical living related donors even under conventional immunosuppression. Other degrees of histocompatibility matching, while they do not seem to influence long-term survival, influence the frequency of rejection.

The type of immunosuppression regimen used in our series did not seem to have any significant effect on the long-term survival in living related donor transplantation confirming the earlier observations of Sutherland and colleagues that azathioprine and prednisone with short-course of ALG is as successful as triple immunosuppression with cyclosporine (30). However, in the LUD and particularly in cadaveric transplantation, triple therapy with cyclosporine is definitely important. In the cadaveric kidneys with prolonged ischemia time, as we have reported previously (10, 13), early administration of cyclosporine is detrimental and is associated with higher rate of primary non-function. However, if cyclosporine is used sequentially, following a period of induction with prednisone, azathioprine and antilymphocyte globulin or OKT3, then it is effective and is associated with improved graft survival. However, chronic cyclosporine toxicity remains an important cause of morbidity in the long term. Our own observations and those of others indicate that when graft function is stable at 1—2 years after transplantation, cyclosporine can be safely withdrawn with a small risk of controlable rejection (23, 31, 32, 33).

In this as in other large series, the major causes of patient loss were cardiovascular and infections. In this area of the world, protozoal infections such as pneumocystis was not seen. However, other unusual infections like salmonella, listeria and acute tuberculosis were commonly seen and are important causes of both patient and graft loss. CMV was the most important viral infection causing morbidity and mortality, although we were able to reduce this by the judicious use of hyperimmune globulin (Cytotec), and more recently with the therapeutic use of Gancyclovir. There is considerable recent evidence that prophylactic administration of combinations of low dose Acyclovir and hyperimmune globulin or Gancyclovir can reduce the incidence and severity of CMV in high-risk CMV-negative recipients of CMV-positive donors (34, 35). Another unusual finding in our series was the fact that de novo malignancy was seen in only 5 patients or 1%, which is considerably lower than that reported in other series (29) and by Penn (Chapter 64 of this book).

Our observations confirm previous reports that patient rehabilitation and quality of life following successful renal transplantation are far superior to any form of dialysis therapy (36—39). Many of our patients are leading a normal and productive life. Many female patients have gone through several successful pregnancies which they could not have done had they remained on dialysis. Four of the 12 patients who were transplanted longer than 10 years ago are physicians in a full medical practice. One of these former patients recently became the recipient of the Kuwait Prize in Science for 1990, nearly 11 years after renal transplantation from his sister. Besides better quality of life, renal transplantation, particularly from LRD grafts, confers a better prospect of long-term patient survival than dialysis. Although it is often difficult to compare transplant and dialysis population of patients, in our series of 350 LRD transplants, the over 10-year patient survival rate of 87% is far superior to the rate of 58.8 ± 3.5% amongst dialysis patients in Europe in the age group 35—44 years, as reported by Brynger and his colleagues from the EDTA Registry (39).

While cadaveric transplantation is being actively sought throughout the world due to the shortage of organ for the ever-increasing number of patients now on dialysis, there is clear and unequivocal evidence that, in spite of cyclosporine, the long-term graft survival at 5 and 10 years after cadaveric transplantation is significantly inferior to that obtained with LRD transplants (29, 40). In our series, the 5- and 10-year graft survival was 90 and 83% for HLA-identical and 82 and 73% respectively for mismatched LRD grafts. The 5-year graft survival in our best, locally obtained, cadaveric kidneys was 60% and for the entire cadaveric series, only 40%, in spite of triple therapy with cyclosporine. In the multicenter Transplant Registry, Terasaki has reported a 5-year graft survival of 78% for HLA-identical LRD grafts, 60% for parent to child grafts and only 40% for cadaveric grafts under cyclosporine therapy (40). At the present time, the same multicenter Transplant Registry gives a 5-year cadaveric graft survival of 54% and a projected 10-year survival of only 35% (41). In our own series of LUD transplants, the actuarial 5- and 10-year graft survival is similar to that of mismatched LRD grafts and were better than our locally harvested cadaveric grafts. Similar excellent results with LUD grafts have been reported from other centers (24—26). The reasons for this unexpected finding are most likely due to better quality of LUD grafts, absence of ischemia time and, consequently, very low incidence of primary non-function and reduced nephrotoxicity from cyclosporine.

Based on these observations, we and others (24, 25, 37, 40, 42, 43) believe that living related donor and, in specific circumstances, living unrelated inter-spouse donors should be sought as an important and successful source of kidneys for transplantation and that the families of all renal failure patients should be evaluated and encouraged regarding the possibility of donating a kidney before placing the potential transplant recipient on a cadaver transplant program. In this way, the waiting period is reduced, a much better outcome can be assured for the recipient and the current and increasing shortage of kidneys for transplantation can be partially met. In a recent editorial, Flatmark *et al.* rightly point out that the volunteer living related and spouse donors should be used whenever possible, since, by doing this, many family members will not be denied the opportunity to improve the quality of life for their next of kin and scarce health care resources will be better utilized (42).

The usual objection put forward against the use of live donors is the possible health risk to the donor. Starzl (44) has put forward a strong arguement that living donation is not completely safe and he refers to at least 20 postoperative deaths, most of which have never been published. While such a theoretical risk to the donor cannot be denied, death or serious injury is extremely unlikely especially if donor nephrectomy is carried out under optimum conditions and by a skilled team. In our present series of more than 400 LRD and LUD donors, there was only minor and temporary morbidity following donor nephrectomy. All donors are alive and well and were able to return to their former occupation and activities within 2 to 3 weeks after surgery. In a previous study of 100 donors, it was shown that none of them developed hypertension or impairment of renal function (45). Similar excellent results with no mortality and very low morbidity have been reported in a much larger series of donors from Scandinavia (42, 46). Furthermore, in our opinion, organ donation is not entirely without benefit to the donor. Our observations and the studies of Simmons (37, 38) clearly show that most of the donors gain a major emotional benefit, a heightened self-esteem and a feeling of pride for being able to save the life of, or help, a loved relative. One of our donors who had successfully donated a kidney to his diabetic brother one year earlier, insisted on helping his brother further by donating part of his pancreas which was duly carried out and transplanted to his brother successfully. This donor, who continues to enjoy a normal renal and pancreatic function, is one of the proudest and most contented donors in our series. Another healthy father, anxious to help his 40-year-old son, 'made-up' convincing evidence that he was under 60 years of ago so that he would not be refused. However, after an uneventful and successful transplant operation and upon his discharge from the hospital, he proudly admitted that his real age was 75 years. Indeed, news of this case brought an influx of many young family donors to our Center who had been reluctant previously.

Besides improved survival and better quality of life, renal transplantation has a major impact on the cost of any national chronic renal failure program. In our center, the cost of successful renal transplantation over a 5-year period was less than one-third of the cost of maintaining a patient on dialysis for the same period. Measured in monetary terms, it costs the country more than US$ 6 million to maintain a pool of 240 patients on dialysis every year or some US$ 30 million over 5 years. With successful renal transplantation, two-thirds of this enormous financial burden can be saved and gainfully used for other important health care services. Similar observations on the cost to benefit ratio of renal transplantation have been reported from Europe and more recently from the United States by P.G. Eggers from the Health Care Financing Administration (47).

References

1. Abouna, G.M., Kumar, M.S.A., White, A.G., Dadah, S., John, P., Samhan, M., Omar, O.F. and Kusma, G.: Experience with 130 consecutive renal transplants in the Middle East with special reference to histocompatibility matching, antirejection therapy with antilymphocyte globulin (ALG) and prolonged preservation of imported cadaveric grafts. *Transplant. Proc.* **16**(4), 1114–1117 (1984).
2. Abouna, G.M., White, A.G., Kumar, M.S.A., Dadah, S.K. and Samhan, M.: The development of renal transplantation program in Kuwait and the results in the first 142 grafts. In G.M. Abouna (ed.), *Current Status of Clinical Organ Transplantation*, pp. 193–207, Martinus Nijhoff, The Hague (1984).
3. Abouna, G.M., Kumar, M.S.A., White, A.G., Samhan, M., Dadah, S., Silva, O.S.G. and John, P.: Renal transplantation in the Middle East – experience with 250 transplants. *Dialysis Transplant.* **16**(2), 81–84 (1987).
4. White, A.G., Kumar, M.S.A. and Abouna, G.M.: HLA, MLR, P and Lewis antigens in living donor renal transplantation in a single center in the Middle East. *Tissue Antigens* **27**, 279–284 (1986).

5. Abouna, G.M., White, A.G., Abdullah, I., Kumar, M.S.A., Panjwani, D. and Philips, E.M.: The late results of living related donor renal transplantation — the effect of HLA, MLR and ABO antigen matching. *Clin. Transplant.* **2**, 15—20 (1988).
6. Abouna, G.M., Kumar, M.S.A., White, A.G. and Silva, O.S.G.: Transplantation in Kuwait — a Middle Eastern and North African perspective. *Transplant. Proc.* **19**(2), 21—26 (1987).
7. Abouna, G.M., Panjwani, D., Kumar, M.S.A., White, A.G., Al-Abdullah, I.H., Silva, O.S.G. and Samhan, W.: The living unrelated donor — a viable alternative for renal transplantation. *Transplant. Proc.* **20**(5), 940—941 (1988).
8. The Council of the Transplantation Society: *Transplantation* **41**, 1 (1986).
9. Abouna, G.M., Kumar, M.S.A., White, A.G., Dadah, S.K., Omar, O.F., Samhan, W., Kusma, G. and John, P.: Experience with imported human cadaveric kidneys having unusual problems and transplanted after 30—60 hours of preservation. *Transplant. Proc.* **16**, 61 (1984).
10. Abouna, G.M., Samhan, W., Kumar, M.S.A., White, A.G. and Silva, O.S.G.: Limiting factors in successful preservation of cadaveric kidneys with ischemia times exceeding 50 hours. *Transplant. Proc.* **19**(1), 2051—2055 (1987).
11. Abouna, G.M., Al-Adnani, M.S., Kremer, G.D. *et al.*: Reversal of diabetic nephropathy in human cadaveric kidneys after transplantation in nondiabetic recipients. *Lancet* **2**, 1274—1276 (1983).
12. Abouna, G.M., John, P., Samhan, M. and Kumar M.S.A.: Transplantation of single pediatric cadaveric kidneys into adult recipients after prolonged preservation. *Transplant. Proc.* **22**(2), 407 (1990).
13. Kumar, M.S.A., Samhan, W., John, P. and Abouna, G.M.: Chronic cyclosporine nephrotoxicity in renal transplantation: is it the effect of preservation? *Transplant. Proc.* **21**(1), 1552—1553 (1989).
14. Kumar, M.S.A., White, A.G., John, P. and Abouna, G.M.: Antilymphocyte globulin infusion in the treatment of acute allograft rejection — a prospective study. In: G.M. Abouna (ed.), *Current Status of Clinical Organ Transplantation*, pp. 49—56. Martinus Nijhoff, The Hague (1984).
15. Kumar, M.S.A., White, A.G., Samhan, W. and Abouna, G.M.: Cyclosporin in the treatment of acute renal allograft rejection. *Proc. Int. on Cyclosporine in Clinical Transplantation; Excerpta Med.*, 162—166 (1987).
16. Kumar, M.S.A., White, A.G., Samhan, W., Johnny, K.V., Kusma, G., Silva, O.S.G. and Abouna, G.M.: Donor specific transfusion in renal transplantation. Is it worth it? *Transplant. Proc.* **17**(1), 1069—1071 (1985).
17. Samhan, W., Panjwani, S., Dadah, S.K., Kumar, M.S.A., Araj, G. and Abouna, G.M.: Tuberculosis: Is it a contraindication for renal transplantation? *Transplant. Proc.* **21**(1), 2036—2038 (1989).
18. White, A.G., Kumar, M.S.A., Strannegard, O. and Abouna, G.M.: Renal transplantation in hepatitis B surface antigen positive patients. *Transplant. Proc.* **19**(1), 2150—2152 (1987).
19. Abouna, G.M., Samhan, W. and Kumar, M.S.A.: Unilateral native nephrectomy at time of renal transplantation is effective in the treatment of resistant hypertension. *Transplant. Proc.* **21**(1), 2028—2030 (1989).
20. Abouna, G.M., Kumar, M.S.A., Samhan, M., Dadah, S.K. and Sabawi, N.M.: Commercialization in human organs — a Middle Eastern perspective. *Transplant. Proc.* **22**, 918—921 (1990).
21. Islamic Fatwa Committee: In: G.M. Abouna (ed.), *Current Status of Clinical Organ Transplantation.* Martinus Nijhoff, The Hague (1984). [Muslim position on organ donation as expressed by the Islamic Fatwa Committee assembled by the Ministry of Islamic Affairs in Kuwait on December 31, 1979.]
22. Silva, O.S.G., Shuwaikeh, I., Shafei, E., Hasan, I.M., Panjwani, D., Kumar, M.S.A. and Abouna, G.M.: Poor myocardial function in uremic patients improves significantly after renal transplantation. *First Int. Congress of the Middle East Society for Organ Transplantation (MESOT), Ankara, Turkey.* (Abstract), November 2—4 (1988).
23. Abouna, G.M., Kumar, M.S.A., White, A.G., Samhan, M., Kalawi, M. and Al-Sabawi, N.: Cyclosporine withdrawal in renal transplantation recipients maintained on triple therapy. *Transplant. Proc.* (1991; in press).

24. Squifflet, J.P., Pirson, Y., Poncelet, P. and Alexandre, G.P.J.: Unrelated living donor kidney transplantation. *Transplant. Int.* **3**(1), 26 (1990).
25. Pirsch, J.D., Sollinger, H.W., Kolayoglu, M., Belzer, F.O. *et al.*: Living unrelated renal transplantation: Results in 40 patients. *Amer. J. Kidney Dis.* **12**, 499 (1988).
26. Cortisini, R., Berloco, A., Famalari, E. *et al.*: Long-term results in recipients of mismatched related and unrelated living kidneys in the Cyclosporine age. *Transplant. Proc.* **20** (Supp. 2), 41 (1988).
27. Reddy, C.M., Thiagarajan, D., Shunnugasundaran, R. *et al.*: Unconventional renal transplantation in India. *Transplant. Proc.* **22**(3), 910 (1990).
28. Howard, R.J., Pfoff, W.W., Scornik, J.C., Salomon, P.R., Peterson, J.C. and Bumson, M.E.: Kidney transplantation in older patients. *Clin. Transplant* **4**, 181 (1990).
29. Fabrega, A., Matas, A.J., Payne, W.D., Fryd, D.S., Damm, D.L., Sutherland, D.E.R. and Najarian, J.S.: Ten to 20 year follow-up of 123 consecutive HLA identical living related kidney transplants from the pre-Cyclosporine era. *Clin. Transplant.* **4**, 145 (1990).
30. Sutherland, E.R., Strand, M., Fryd, D.S., Ferguson, R.M., Simmons, R.L., Archer, N.L., Najarian, J.S.: Comparison of azathioprine — antilymphocyte globulin versus cyclosporine in renal transplantation. *Amer. J. Kidney Dis.* **3**(6), 456 (1984).
31. Spieberger, M., Aigner, F., Schmid, T., Bosmuller, C., Konigsrainer, A. and Margreiter, R.: Long-term results of cadaveric renal transplantation after conversion from cyclosporine to azathioprine — a controlled randomized trial. *Transplant. Proc.* **20**(3), 169 (1988).
32. Jacobson, J.E., Pontin, A., Van Zyl-Smit, M., Pascol, M., Cassidy, M.J.D. and Swanepoel, C.R.: Results of conversion of immunosuppression in 143 cadavers and 42 living related donor renal allografts. *Transplant. Proc.* **20**(3), Suppl. 3, 155 (1988).
33. Sweny, P., Lui, F.F., Scobie, J.E., Varghese, Z., Fernando, O.N. and Moorehead, J.F.: Conversion of stable renal allografts at one year from cyclosporine to azathioprine — a randomized controlled study. *Transplant. Int.* **3**(1), 19 (1990).
34. Snydman, D.: Cytomegalovirus infections in solid organ transplantation: prospects for prevention. *Transplant. Rev.* **4**(1), 59 (1990).
35. MacDonald, A., Belitsky, P., Lee, S. and Cohen, A.: Prevention of CMV disease in kidney transplant recipients with Acyclovir and CMV hyperimmune globulin. *Transpl. Proc.* **23**(1), 1355 (1991).
36. Simmons, R.G., Anderson, C.R., Koustra, L.K. *et al.*: Quality of life and alternate end-stage renal disease therapies. *Transplant. Proc.* **17**, 1577 (1985).
37. Simmons, R.G., Marine, S.K. and Simmons, R.L.: Living related donors: counts and gains. In: *Gift of Life*. Transaction Books, New Brunswick (1987).
38. Evans, R.W.: Quality of life assessment and the treatment of end-stage renal disease. *Transplant. Rev.* **4**(1), 28 (1990).
39. Brynger, H., Frubbern, F.P. and Wing, A.G.: In B.H.B. Robinson and J.B. Hawkings (eds), *Proceedings of the European Dialysis and Transplant Association*, Vol. 17. Pitman Medical (1979).
40. Terasaki, P., Toyotome, N., Mickey, M.R. *et al.*: Patient, graft and functional survival rate. In: P. Terasaki (ed.), *An Overview in Clinical Kidney Transplantation 1985*, pp. 1—26. UCLA Typing Laboratory (1985).
41. Terasaki, P.I.: Personal communication (September 1990).
42. Flatmark, A., Bryer, H. and Groth, C.C.: Kidney transplantation from living donors: the neglected opportunity. *Transplant. Int.* **3**(1), 50 (1990).
43. Monaco, A.P.: Problems in transplantation: ethics, education and expansion. *Transplantation* **43**, 4 (1987).
44. Starzl, T.E.: Living donors. *Transplant. Proc.* **19**, 174 (1987).
45. John, P., Kumar, M.S.A., Samhan, M. and Abouna, G.M.: The living donor for kidney transplantation: a review of 100 consecutive donors. In: G.M. Abouna (ed.), *Current Status of Clinical Organ Transplantation*, p. 163. Martinus Nijhoff, The Hague (1984).
46 Talseth, T., Fauchald, P., Skeds, S. *et al.*: Long-term blood pressure and renal function in kidney donors. *Kidney Int.* **29**, 1072 (1980).
47. Eggers, P.: Effect of transplantation on the Medicare end-stage renal disease programs. *New Engl. J. Med.* **318**, 223 (1988).

24. Squifflet, J.P., Pirson, Y., Gianello, P. and Alexandre, G.P.J.: Unrelated living donor kidney transplantation. Transplant Int. 3: [illegible] (1990).
25. [illegible], Sollinger, H.W., [illegible], M., Belzer, F.O. et al.: Living unrelated renal transplantation: Results in [illegible] patients. Amer. J. Kidney Dis. 12: 489 (1988).
26. [illegible], [illegible], A., [illegible] et al.: [illegible] mismatched related and unrelated living donor [illegible] cyclosporine and [illegible] ([illegible]).
27. [illegible] [illegible] transplantation. [illegible]
28. [illegible] [illegible] [illegible], J.C. and [illegible], M.R.: [illegible]
29. [illegible], A., [illegible] W.D., [illegible], [illegible] D., Sutherland, D.E.R. and [illegible]: [illegible] HLA [illegible] living related [illegible] transplant [illegible] 4: 145 (1990).
30. [illegible]
[illegible]: Comparison of [illegible] [illegible] ([illegible]).
31. [illegible]
[illegible]
[illegible] (1990).
32. [illegible] [illegible] 20 (3 Suppl. 1) 183 (1988).
33. [illegible], [illegible], [illegible] and [illegible]: Comparison of [illegible] one year [illegible] cyclosporine [illegible] controlled study. [illegible] 311: [illegible] (1984).
34. [illegible]: [illegible] in [illegible] transplantation [illegible]. Transplant. [illegible] (1990).
35. [illegible] and [illegible]: [illegible]
[illegible]
36. [illegible] [illegible] 17: [illegible] (1985).
37. [illegible] [illegible]
38. [illegible]
39. [illegible] In: [illegible] Transplant [illegible] Vol. 12 [illegible]
40. [illegible] [illegible] In: [illegible]
[illegible]
41. [illegible] (1970).
42. [illegible], [illegible] and [illegible]: Kidney transplantation from living donors [illegible].
43. [illegible]: [illegible] in transplantation [illegible]. [illegible] 45: 1 [illegible].
44. [illegible]. Transplantation 19: [illegible] (1975).
45. [illegible], M.A., [illegible] and [illegible], G.M.: The living donor for kidney transplantation: [illegible]. [illegible] Ciba Foundation Symposium. [illegible] The Hague (1968).
46. [illegible]
[illegible]
47. [illegible]: [illegible] transplantation on the [illegible] and [illegible] New [illegible] 7 [illegible] (1969).

23. Long-term results in recipients of cadaveric renal allografts under cyclosporine therapy

S. SCHLEIBNER, H. SCHNEEBERGER and W. LAND

When cyclosporine (CsA) was first given to renal transplant patients, at the Transplantation Centre Munich in 1980, it was used as a sole immunosuppressant according to the protocol of the European Multicentre Study Group on cyclosporine (1).

In February 1982, CsA had become the routine immunosuppressive agent in renal transplantation in Munich. At that time, first reports on the beneficial effect of combined immunosuppressive therapy using CsA in combination with steroids had been published (2), and therefore a combination of CsA and low-dose steroids was chosen as an induction treatment for all renal transplant patients.

In this report, the long-term results of renal allotransplants performed between February 1982 and March 1984 will be presented. All patients transplanted within this period have a minimal follow-up of 6 years, thus enabling us to present the actual 6-year results concerning grafts and patients.

From February 1982 to March 1984, a total of 282 renal transplantations were carried out. Nine living related donor transplants are not included in this report as well as 17 combined renal and pancreatic transplantations. The remaining 256 cadaveric renal transplants are composed of 206 primary transplantations and 50 regraftings (46 second transplantations, 4 third transplantations). A total of 27 patients (16 primary transplantation candidates, 11 retransplant candidates) showed sensitization to alloantigens in terms of panel reactivity of 30% or more in the last test performed prior to transplantation. Further demographic data are given on Table 1.

Immunosuppressive protocol

Cyclosporine

All patients received CsA from the day of transplantation. A 24-hour period of intravenous CsA (3—4 mg/kg BW) was followed by oral CsA therapy, starting

Table 1. Patients treated with cadaveric renal transplantation between 1/1982 and 3/1984.

			Mean age ± s.d.
Males ($n = 159$)			30.5 ± 14.2 years
Females ($n = 97$)			37.1 ± 13.8 years
Total ($n = 256$)			32.9 ± 14.1 years
Mean duration of dialysis: 54 months ± 11.8 (s.e.m.)			
Underlying diseases:	Glomerulonephritis		$n = 139$
	Pyelonephritis		$n = 53$
	Polycystic kidneys		$n = 11$
	Interstitial nephritis		$n = 10$
	Nephro/uro-dysplasia		$n = 10$
	Other		$n = 11$

dose 14—17 mg/kg BW. In the further course, oral CsS dose was gradually decreased to a maintenance dose of 6 mg/kg BW.

Steroids

A single bolus of 250 mg given intravenously during surgery was followed by oral administration of low-dose (8—32 mg) methylprednisolone for a scheduled period of 6 months. From the seventh month after transplantation, withdrawal of steroids was attempted in all patients considered to be 'immunologically stable'.

Protocol for 'immunologic risk' patients

From 7/82, retransplant patients (with a history of immunologic graft loss) and sensitized transplant candidates (30% or more panel reactivity) were treated according to the following protocol: CsA, as mentioned above, in combination with high-dose steroids and Azathioprine (1—2 mg/kg BW) for the first 7 days.

Antirejection treatment

A first rejection crisis was treated with three intravenous bolus injections of 500 mg methylprednisolone. Further histologically confirmed rejection crises were treated by application of a 7 day course of either ALG (20 mg/kg BW) or ATG (4 mg/kg BW).

ALG/ATG treatment was limited to a total of 21 doses; methylprednisolone was cut to a total dose of 3.5 g. In any further rejection, conversion to conventional immunosuppression (azathioprine/steroids) was considered.

Drug monitoring

Measurement of CsA trough levels was first attempted in late 1982 with serum levels of 100—300 ng/ml (RIA) considered to be normal.

In early 1983, a RIA test kit for measurement of whole blood trough levels became available; the 'therapeutic window' was thought to be 300—900 ng/ml (RIA).

Results

Graft and patient survival 6 years after transplantation.

1. *Graft survival*

Six years after transplantation, 46.1% of the renal allografts are currently functioning (Figure 1). The highest incidence of graft losses ($n = 62$) was seen — as

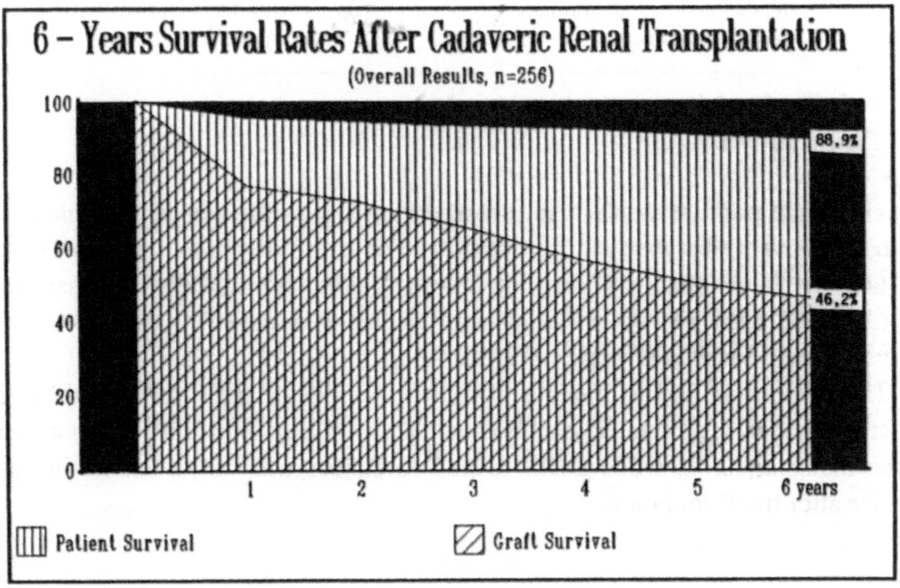

Fig. 1. Six-year graft and patient survival rates after cadaveric renal transplantation. (Overall results, $n = 256$.)

expected — in the first year post-transplant, when acute and early chronic rejection as well as technical problems contributed to the number of unsuccessful transplantations.

Acute humoral/vascular rejection (n = 22) and early chronic rejection (n = 23) were the major reasons of transplant loss; patients' death (with functioning graft, n = 10), technical failure (n = 6), never-functioning kidneys (n = 6) and hemolytic-uremic syndrome in one case also contributed to the total number of 62 transplant losses in the first year.

In the following years, chronic progressive renal dysfunction became the most important reason for loss of the renal allograft. Renal biopsies from patients with progressive chronic renal dysfunction almost always showed a 'mixed pattern' of histopathological changes. Interstitial fibrosis and obliterative transplant vasculopathy are the most common features of renal allografts lost in the years 2 to 6 after transplantation (Table 2).

Table 2. Histopathological changes in chronic graft loses (n = 42). Patients transplanted between 1982 and 1984.

Predominant findings:		
Transplant-vasculopathy	n = 13	(30%)
Interstitial fibrosis	n = 16	(38%)
Glomerulonephritis	n = 3	(7%)
Arteriolopathy	n = 4	(10%)
Pyelonephritis	n = 1	(2%)
Hemolytic-uremic syndrome	n = 1	(2%)
Transplant glomerulopathy	n = 4	(10%)

2. *Patient survival*

Twenty-eight patients died within the observation period either with functioning transplants or within the first 3 months after return to dialysis. It seems justified to take the latter ones into account, since it cannot be excluded that patients' death in the early period following graft failure is in any way associated with transplantation and/or immunosuppression.

The reasons of death in renal transplant recipients are shown in Table 3. Bacterial sepsis is the most common lethal complication within the first year after transplantation, while death related to cancer was only seen in the late course after transplantation.

Status of patients with functioning grafts 6 years after transplantation

Six years after cadaveric renal transplantation, 118 patients have functioning grafts. Medical and social rehabilitation is very good in the vast majority of

Table 3. Causes of death during the period of 6 years after transplantation.

Cause	No.
Bacterial sepsis	7[a]
Myocardial infaction	6
Cerebral hemorrhage	3
Hepatic failure	2
Tuberculosis	2
Pneumonia	3
AIDS	1
Traffic accident	1
Pancreatitis	1
Malignoma (liver/kidney)	2
Total	$n = 28$

[a] 6/7 during 1 year.

these patients (115/118) although some of them are currently confronted with the problem of chronic progressive renal dysfunction.

Current mode of immunosuppression

Ninety-four patients could be maintained on steroid-free immunosuppression (CsA monotherapy); in 17 patients a double-drug therapy consisting of CsA and steroids is applied. Seven patients were converted to conventional immunosuppression; 5 of them were 'early conversions' within the first 3 months after transplantation, the remaining 2 patients had 'late conversion' due to CsA-intolerance (CsA-associated renal damage and intractable arthralgia under CsA-therapy).

Six years after transplantation, best renal allograft function (mean serum creatinine 1.4 mg%) is observed in the small group of patients under conventional immunosuppression. In patients under CsA-monotherapy, mean serum creatinine is 1.8 mg%. Transplant function is poorest in patients who receive a CsA/steroids double drug immunosuppression (Table 4). The reason for this phenomenon will be discussed later.

Table 4. Current mode of immunosuppression in patients started with CsA and steroids 6 years ago.

	Mean dosage CsA	Mean creatinine
CsA alone	4.12 ± 1.8	1.8 ± 0.55
CsA/steroids	4.10 ± 0.8	2.6 ± 1.2
Aza/steroids		1.4 ± 0.5

There is no difference concerning the mean CsA-dose between patients on CsA-monotherapy (mean dose 4.12 mg BW) and patients on combined therapy with CsA and steroids (mean dose 4.10 mg/kg BW).

Factors contributing to long-term graft survival

Number of transplantations

When comparing the late outcome of primary transplants ($n = 206$) to retransplant ($n = 50$), it is interesting to see that while there is a striking difference in one-year graft survival (77% vs 66%), the difference is becoming less throughout the years. Six years after tranplantation, 47% of the first transplants and 40% of the retransplants have preserved allograft function (Figure 2).

Incidence of ATN

Cadaveric renal allotransplants without initial diuresis are known to have a poorer prognosis compared to those with initial function. In our series, one year after transplantation there is a difference of 84% graft function rate in kidneys

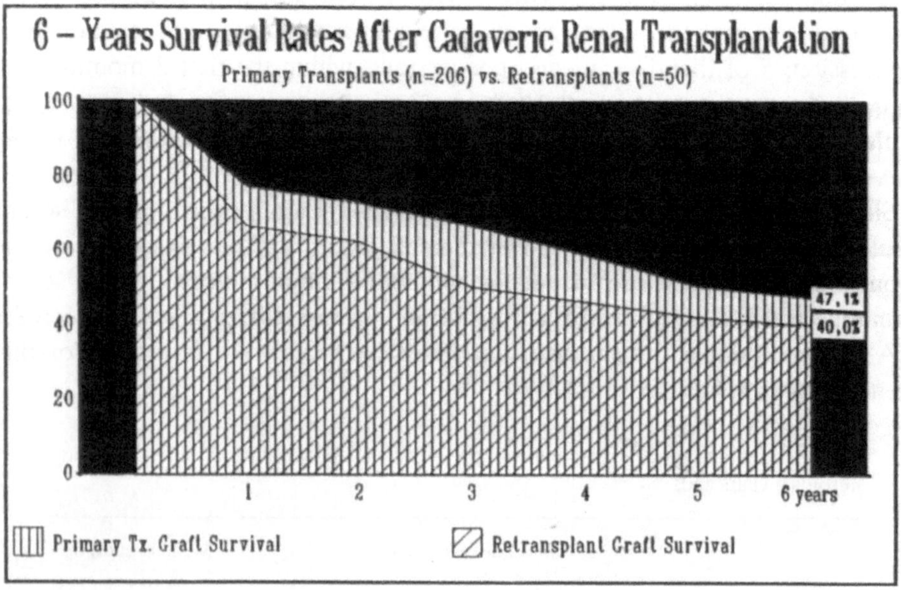

Fig. 2. Six-year graft survival after cadaveric renal transplantation (primary transplants ($n = 206$) vs retransplants ($n = 50$)).

with initial function (n = 118) vs 67% in kidneys with ATN (n = 138). This difference is well preserved up to the sixth year after transplantation where 55% of transplants with initial diuresis have preserved function whereas the 6-year function rate of ATN kidneys is 32.6% (Figure 3).

Early rejection crises

Patients with acute immunologic reaction to their graft have a markedly inferior outcome compared to others. In patients with acute, biopsy-proven, steroid-resistant rejection crises (n = 58), short- and long-term results are poorer compared to patients with no or steroid-sensitive rejection crises (n = 157). One year after transplantation, graft function rates are 70.6% vs 96.1%. Moreover, in the further course after transplantation, the incidence of chronic graft loss is comparatively high in 'early rejectors'. Six years after transplantation, only 26% of the patients with need for serum (ALG/ATG) therapy for acute rejection crisis have functioning grafts while, six years post-transplant, the rate of renal allograft function in patients without acute steroid-resistant rejection crisis is 60.5% (Figure 4).

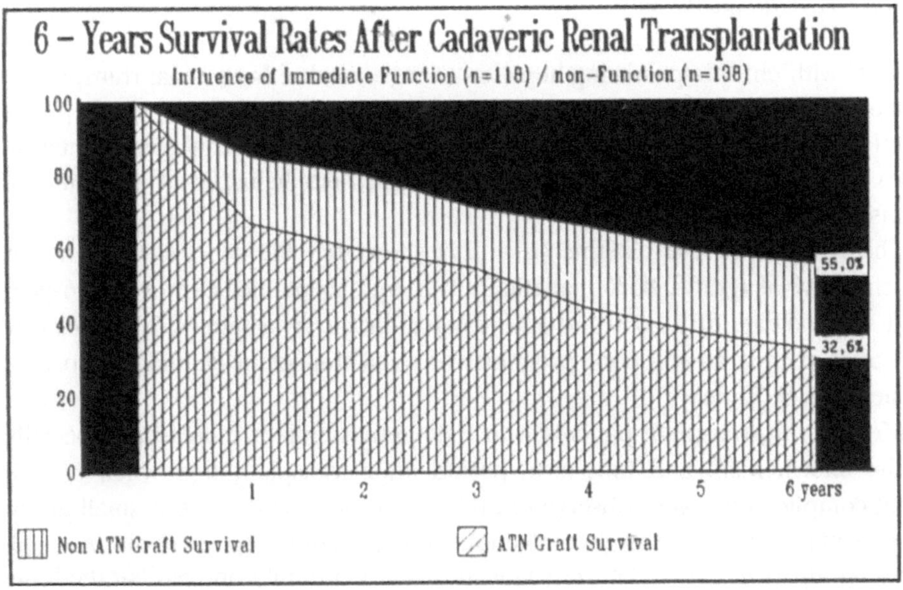

Fig. 3. The influence of immediate function/non-function on the late outcome of cadaveric renal transplantation.

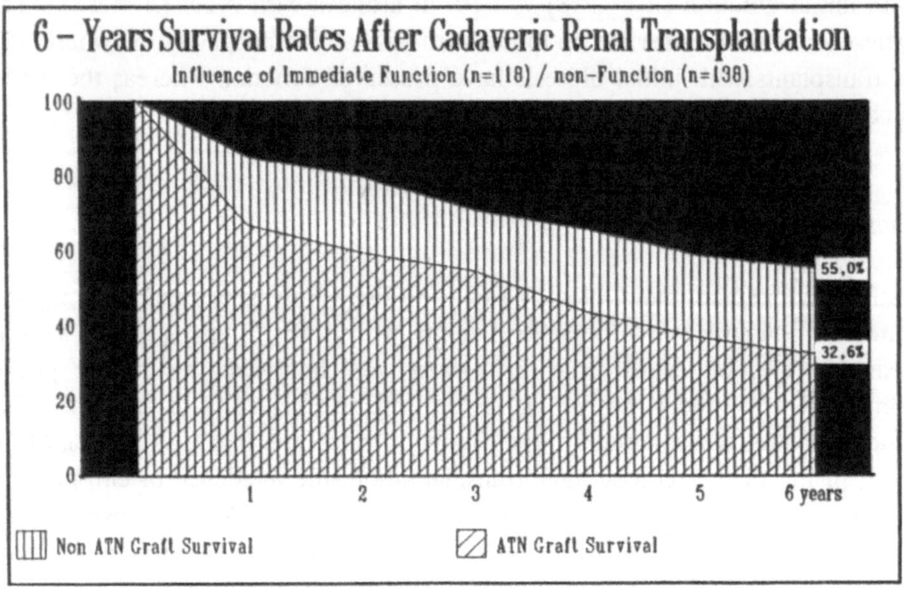

Fig. 4. The influence of early steroid-resistant rejection crises on long-term renal allograft survival (patients with graft loss within the first 3 months are not included).

Chronic HBs-antigenemia

Patients with chronic persisting hepatitis B are excluded from renal transplantation programmes at many centers. At our center, patients with chronic hepatitis B (BHs-antigenemia, HBe-antigenemia) were accepted for renal transplantation when there was no evidence of chronic aggressive hepatitis at the time of admission.

The results in these patients (n = 27) show that the short-term graft and patient survival (grafts, 85%; patients, 93%) are acceptable. However, a 6-year graft survival rate of 29.6% and a 6-year patient survival rate of 70.3% clearly indicate a comparatively poor prognosis of renal transplant candidates positive for hepatitis B (Figure 5).

Mortality in transplant patients with HBs-antigenemia is increased, especially in the intermediate and long-term period after transplantation when 6 of 8 lethal complications were observed in this group of patients. In this small group of patients, death caused by infectious complications (pneumonia n = 3; bacterial sepsis n = 1; AIDS n = 1) is most frequent; only one patient died due to liver failure. However, chronic hepatitis with slow progression towards cirrhosis has also to be observed in 4 more patients with currently functioning renal allograft.

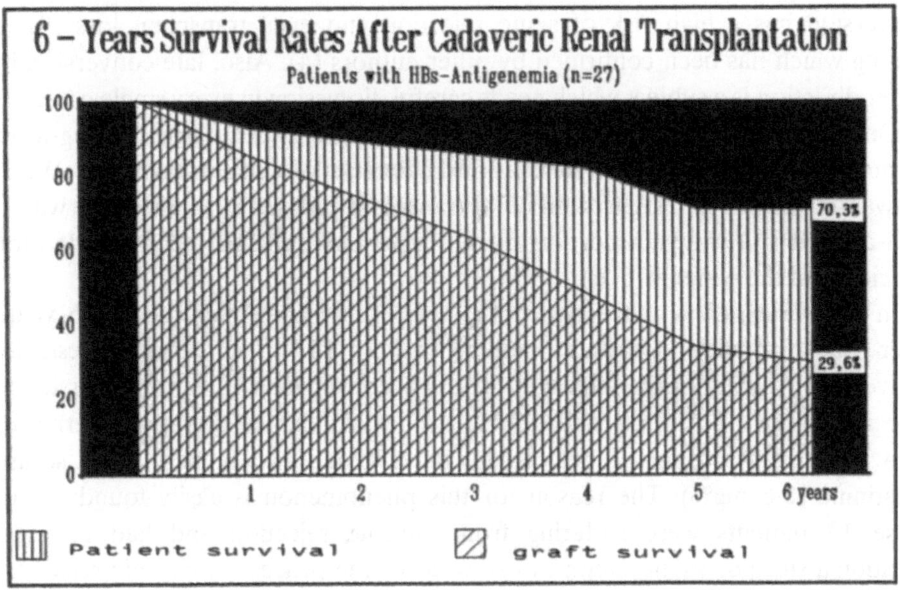

Fig. 5. Six-year graft and patient survival in cadaveric renal transplant patients with HBs-antigenemia ($n = 27$).

Discussion

The results from our 1982/84 series clearly show that CsA contributed much to the solution of early problems — especially rejection — in renal transplantation. It becomes also clear that:

(a) the problems of early rejection and early graft loss are certainly not completely ruled out by the use of CsA;
(b) the problems of chronic toxicity and chronic rejection become more and more important.

Our own results show that in the early series where comparatively high doses of both oral and parenteral CsA were given and where drug monitoring (determination of CsA levels) was at its very beginning, much trouble was caused by CsA overdosage and CsA toxicity. For example, in the 256 patients presented above (years 1982—1984), 45 episodes of acute CsA nephrotoxicity were diagnosed and there is evidence for at least 19 episodes of chronic CsA toxicity in these patients. In contrast, 189 patients transplanted in 1989 and started with oral CsA dosage of 6 mg/kg bodyweight (in combination with azathioprine and steroids), only 5 episodes of acute CsA toxicity were observed. It remains to be evaluated, if chronic nephrotoxicity can be reduced in a similar way.

Conversion to conventional immunosuppression has frequently been discussed in patients with evidence of CsA toxocity. In our own experience, early conversion has a high risk of acute rejection and even transplant loss (3); a finding which has been confirmed by other authors (4). Also, late conversion in either direction is a subject which needs careful discussion in every single case.

One obvious advantage of CsA is the possibility to perform long-term immunosuppression without steroids in recipients of renal transplants. Withdrawal of steroids in CsA-treated renal transplant patients is a procedure with a well-defined risk which, according to our experience, can be recommended for a majority of the patients (5, 6).

In our series, 80% of the patients (94/117) had CsA-monotherapy 6 years after transplantation. Of these patients 5% (6/117) had been successfully converted to azathioprine/steroids (4 early conversions, 2 late conversions). The remaining 17 patients had double drug maintenance therapy in terms of CsA/steroids. As reported before, the latter group had highest mean serum creatinine (2.6 mg%). The reason for this phenomenon is easily found: 10 of these 17 patients were suffering from chronic rejection and had received additional steroids as an attempt to slow down the process of chronic rejection. However, there is no proof that additional steroid treatment has any beneficial effect on the course of chronic progressive renal dysfunction in patients under CsA therapy. Moreover, judging from the results of large multicenter studies, it has to remain unclear if multiple drug maintenance protocols are in any way superior to CsA monotherapy (7).

Considering the factors that have been investigated in order to determine their effect on early and late renal allograft function, it is evident that early rejection and the occurrence of acute renal failure (with oligo/anuria) have the most striking influence on the late outcome.

The inferior results in ATN kidneys need further comment: firstly, it is well known meanwhile that in grafts with acute renal failure post-transplant there is enhanced CsA toxicity (8), especially if the drug is given in high doses, and secondly, never-functioning grafts are usually counted as ATN kidneys. In these kidney grafts, donor factors, circumstances of organ harvesting and perfusion (which, in several cases, are not exactly known) may play a very important role and, therefore it seems advisable to make attempts to separate 'ATN kidneys' from 'never-functioning kidneys' at retrospective investigation.

The quality of HLA matching has often been considered to be also an important factor for early and late results in cadaveric renal transplantation (9). In this report, the results of HLA-typing are not discussed because, especially in 1982, the facilities for DR-typing were not established at every center and therefore a considerable number of cadaveric kidneys were transplanted with unknown DR-type. Future investigations will hopefully contribute to this topic.

Conclusion

The current 6-year results of cadaveric renal transplantation under CsA therapy show the problems and chances of present cadaveric renal transplantation. On the one hand, there are still existing problems of acute and chronic renal allograft rejection with a unsatisfactory graft function rate of below 50% at 6 years as well as the unsolved problems of patient morbidity and mortality under chronic immunosuppression. On the other hand, there is growing experience in handling CsA, reflected by improved results and, for the majority of the patients, the chance of steroid-free long-term immunosuppression.

References

1. Report on the European Multicentre Trial: *Lancet* **2**, 57 (1982).
2. Starzl, T.E., Weil, R., Iwatsuki, S. *et al.*: The use of cyclosporin A and prednisone in cadaver kidney transplantation. *Surg. Gynec. Obstet.* **151**, 17—26 (1980).
3. Land, W., Castro, L.A., Hillebrand, G. *et al.*: Conversion rejection consequences by changing the immunosuppressive therapy from cyclosporine to azathioprine after kidney transplantation. *Transplant. Proc.* **15**(4), Suppl. 1, 356—359 (1983).
4. Wood, R.F.M., Thompson, J.F., Ting, A. *et al.*: A randomized controlled trial of short-term cyclosporine therapy in renal transplantation. *Transplant. Proc.* **17** (1), 1164—1165 (1985).
5. Hillebrand, G., Krumme, D. Schleibner, S. *et al.*: Is withdrawal of steroids hazardous to cadaveric renal transplants under treatment with cyclosporine? *Transplant. Proc.* **20**(3), Suppl. 3, 126—129 (1988).
6. Schleibner, S., Schneeberger, H., Hillebrand, G. *et al.*: Cyclosporine monotherapy — an ideal long-term immunosuppression? *Transplant. Proc.* **22**(4), 1695 (1990).
7. Opelz, G.: *Transplant. Proc.* **20**, 1028 (1988).
8. Klintmalm, G., Gohman, S.O., Sundelin, B. and Wilzcek, H.: Interstitial fibrosis in renal allografts after 12 to 46 months of cyclosporin treatment. Beneficial effects of lower doses early after tranplantation. *Lancet* **ii**, 950 (1984).
9. Opelz, G.: Multicenter Impact of cyclosporin on cadaver kidney graft survival. *Prog. in Allergy* (Karger, Basel) **38**, 329—345 (1986).

24. Transplantation of single and double kidneys from pediatric donors

DAVID E.R. SUTHERLAND, RAINER W.G. GRUESSNER, ARTHUR J. MATAS, GONCAL LLOVERAS, DAVID S. FRYD, DAVID L. DUNN, WILLIAM D. PAYNE and JOHN S. NAJARIAN

The role of pediatric cadaver donors for transplantation of kidneys is controversial; some reports of outcome following pediatric donor transplantation have shown results similar to those with adult donors (1, 2, 3), while others have shown worse results (4, 5). Pediatric donor kidneys can be transplanted singly to two recipients, or both kidneys can be transplanted to a single recipient (16). Single kidney transplants make optimum use of the donor pool; double transplants provide increased renal mass and therefore more functional reserve in the early post-transplant period.

To compare the outcome of double versus single pediatric cadaver kidney transplantation, we reviewed our experience with 131 pediatric cadaver kidneys (donor age $\leqslant$ 10 years) transplanted between 1971 and 1988 (7, 8). Of the group receiving pediatric kidneys, 33 (25%) received double and 98 (75%) received single pediatric kidney transplants.

For recipients of double pediatric cadaver grafts, 1, 5 and 10-year patient survival rates were 88, 81 and 75%, respectively; for recipients of single pediatric grafts, 1, 5 and 10-year patient survival rates were 86, 67 and 53% (p = NS). Graft survival was 78% at one year, 45% at 5 years, and 48% at 10 years in recipients of double pediatric kidney transplants, but only 61% at 1 year, 44% at 5 years, and 34% at 10 years in recipients of single pediatric kidneys ($p = 0.017$). During the same period of time, graft survival in recipients of adult cadaver kidneys ($n = 873$) was 74% at 1 year, 67% at 5 years and 36% at 10 years. When compared to recipients of adult cadaver kidneys, of double pediatric cadaver kidneys had similar short- and long-term outcome ($p = 0.6$), whereas recipients of single pediatric kidneys had significantly decreased graft survival ($p = 0.03$). Causes of graft failures were similar for transplants of double or single pediatric kidneys (7). However, early loss of allograft function (within first 3 months post-transplant) due to rejection was more frequent for single (16%) than in double (3%) pediatric cadaver kidney transplants (NS).

Retransplantation was the only risk factor identified that predisposed to worse results with single than with double pediatric kidneys (8). For primary transplants 1- and 5-year graft survival rates with single pediatric kidneys were 63 and 49%, and with double pediatric kidneys were 76 and 62%. For retransplants, 1- and 5-year graft survival rates with single pediatric kidneys were 35 and 30%, and with double pediatric kidneys were 86 and 29% ($p = 0.037$).

We conclude that double pediatric cadaver kidneys provide an overall higher patient and graft survival than single pediatric kidneys. Except for retransplants, however, the donor pool is optimally used by the transplantation of single pediatric kidneys.

References

1. Wengerter, K., Matas, A.J., Tellis,V.A., Quinn, T. *et al.*: Transplantation of pediatric donor kidneys to adult recipients. *Ann. Surg.* **204**, 172—175 (1986).
2. Brown, M.W., Akyol, A.M., Bradley, J.A., Briggs, J.D. *et al.*: Transplantation of cadaver kidneys from pediatric donors. *Clin. Transplant.* **2**, 87—90 (1988).
3. Hayes, J.M., Novick, A.C., Streem, S.B., Hodge, E.E., Bretan, P.N. *et al.*: The use of single pediatric cadaver kidneys for transplantation. *Transplantation* **45**, 106—110 (1988).
4. Anderson, O.S., Jonasson, O. and Merkel, F.K.: En bloc transplantation of pediatric kidneys into adult patients. *Arch. Surg.* **108**, 35—37 (1974).
5. Hong, J.H., Shirani, K,. Arshad, A., Parsa, I., Matas, A.J. *et al.*: Influence of cadaver donor age on the success of kidney transplants. *Transplantation* **32**, 532—534 (1981).
6. Schneider, J.R., Sutherland, D.E.R., Simmons, R.L., Fryd, D.S. and Najarian, J.S.: Long term success with double pediatric cadaver donor renal transplants. *Ann. Surg.* **197**, 439—442 (1983).
7. Gruessner, R.W.G., Matas, A.J., Lloveras, G., Fryd, D.S., Dunn, D.L. *et al.*: A comparison of single and double pediatric cadaver donor kidneys for transplantation. *Clin. Transplant.* **3**, 209—214 (1989).
8. Gruessner, R.W.G., Matas, A.J., Lloveras, G., Fryd, D.S. *et al.*: Pediatric donors-A risk factor in renal retransplantation. *Clin. Transplant.* **3**, 349—354 (1989).

25. ABO-incompatible living related donor transplantation

M. HABERAL, H. GULAY, S. SERT, G. ARSLAN, M. KOÇ and N. BILGIN

Introduction

In the early years of transplantation, ABO incompatibility was considered as a contra-indication for successful renal transplantation (8). However, some ABO-incompatible cadaver kidneys were transplanted successfully in 1978 without being aware of the incompatibility at the time of surgery. Shortly after, it was realized that blood group A2 kidneys could be transplanted to an O recipient successfully (2, 6, 7). Later G.P.J. Alexandre *et al.* (1) began to use living related ABO-incompatible kidney donors with pretransplant donor platelet transfusions, recipient splenectomy and plasmapheresis with acceptable results.

The requirement for ABO incompatibility for renal transplantation limits the possibilities of organ sources for chronic renal failure patients. Our previous experiences showed that ABO-incompatible relatives could be kidney donors with or without recipient splenectomy but with donor specific skin grafts (3, 4, 5). In the last two years, we designed a donor specific skin graft model for selecting the more convenient ABO-incompatible donors.

Material and method

Among the 729 kidney transplantations which were performed from November 3, 1975 to August 30, 1989 in our centers, 566 (77.64%) were from living donors and 163 (22.36%) were from cadavers. In the last two years we started to use donor specific skin graft to evaluate ABO incompatible donors for kidney transplantation. The donor specific skin graft method which was described previously (4) was used for the selection of suitable donors in 35 chronic kidney failure patients who had a willing but ABO blood group incompatible living donor (Table 1). Sixteen of these patients were rejected due to complete skin graft rejection and another donor was turned down due to cardiac problems (Table 1). Living donor renal transplantation was performed on the remaining 18 patients on the basis of the skin graft reaction. Demographic data on these patients and their donors are given in Table 2.

Table 1. Analysis of 35 ABO-incompatible living related donor candidates.

	No.	%
ABO-incompatible donor candidates (applied)	35	
Rejection of the donor-specific skin graft	16	45.71
Cardiac problem of the donor	1	2.85
Kidney transplantation	18	51.42

Table 2. Analysis of 18 ABO-incompatible living related donors and recipients according to age, sex, ABO incompatibility and HLA mismatch and relation.

	Recipient				Donor			
No.	Age	Sex	ABO	HLA mismatch	Age	Sex	ABO	Relation
1	18	M	O	1	46	F	A_1	Mother
2	36	M	O	0	42	F	A_1	Sibling
3	26	F	A_1	2	65	F	A_1B	Mother
4	24	F	A_1	2	45	F	A_1B	Mother
5	16	M	O	0	38	F	A_1	Mother
6	29	M	B	2	48	F	A_1	Mother
7	29	M	O	2	53	F	B	Mother
8	17	M	A_1	2	40	M	A_1B	Father
9	40	F	O	1	65	M	B	Father
10	18	F	B	0	43	M	AB	Father
11	27	M	O	2	55	F	A	Mother
12	27	M	B	1	33	M	AB	Sibling
13	43	M	B	1	54	F	A	Sibling
14	33	M	A	2	27	M	B	Sibling
15	33	M	B	1	28	F	AB	Sibling
16	38	M	A	2	31	M	AB	Sibling
17	35	F	O	0	32	F	AB	Sibling
18	32	M	A	2	29	F	B	Wife

All ABO-incompatible donor candidates were evaluated with respect to informed consent, HLA typing, and complete medical fitness, the requirements being that the donor was healthy, had at least one haplotype HLA-A, -B, -DR antigens match and a negative crossmatch with the recipient. All donor candidates were subjected to aortagram and bilateral selective renal angiogram. None of the donors was rejected because of multiple arteries.

When the results of these examinations were satisfactory, donor-specific skin grafting was performed. Under local anesthesia, a superficial circular incision with a diameter of 3—4 cm is carried out on the donor thigh and a split thickness skin graft is removed. The skin graft is put in saline with crystalline penicillin and the donor area appropriately dressed. Soon after the recipient is taken to the operating room and under local infiltration anesthesia, a full thickness skin graft with a diameter of 3—4 cm is removed on the front chest wall 3—5 cm below the breast. After hemostasis, the donor specific skin graft is sutured to this bare area with 6/0 atraumatic silk and the graft is appropriately dressed. Following surgery, 0.5 mg/kg prednisone, 2 mg/kg cyclosporine-A and 2 mg/kg azathioprine were started as immunosuppressive agents and continued to the time of rental transplantation. These grafts were closely observed for clinical sign of rejection. Also, iso-aglutinin titers, immunoglobulin levels, white blood cells and platelet counts of the patients were monitored. Starting from the 15th day after skin grafting, lymphocyte crossmatch was performed every week until renal transplantation which was carried out at 3—4 weeks after skin grafting.

In 9 recipients, splenectomy was also performed on the day of skin grafting while, in another 9, no splenectomy was carried out. In addition, prior to transplantation, all recipients received at least two sessions of plasmaphoresis. The above immunosuppression protocol was augmented following transplantation. All rejection episodes were treated with Orthoclone OKT3 and alternate day plasmaphoresis for 10 days.

Results

All the 18 donors were followed regularly and they are all alive and well. The 18 ABO-incompatible kidney transplant recipients were followed for 7—31 months (mean 18 months).

Outcome of skin grafts

The outcome of donor specific skin grafts was one of three categories: In Category I, there was no reaction ($n = 12$); in Category II, there was slight hyperemia over the graft and surrounding tissue ($n = 4$); while in Category III, there was obvious reaction against the skin graft with some necrosis ($n = 2$) (Table 3).

Only 3 patients in Category I experienced any acute rejection episodes and 11 of these are quite well with normal functioning kidney grafts. All the patients in Categories II and III experienced acute rejections; 3 patients lost their kidneys despite antirejective treatment and 1 patient had a second transplant. Two hyperacute rejections were encountered and both grafts were lost. One

Table 3. The outcome of donor-specific skin and kidney grafts in 18 recipients according to the results of skin graft, immediate kidney graft function, rejection episodes of kidney graft and current kidney function.

Cases	Result of skin graft	Immediate kidney graft function	Rejection episode of kidney graft	Current kidney function BUN mg/100	Creatinine mg/100
1	Obvious reaction	+	+	Dialysis	
2	No reaction	+	−	24	1.0
3	No reaction	+	+	26	1.2
4	Slight hyperemia	+	+	Second Graft	
5	No reaction	+	−	28	1.2
6	No reaction	+	−	22	0.9
7	No reaction	+	−	18	1.0
8	Slight hyperemia	+	+	35	1.5
9	Obvious reaction	−	+	Dialysis	
10	No reaction	+	−	18	0.8
11	No reaction	+	−	20	0.9
12	No reaction	+	+	25	1.2
13	No reaction	+	+	35	2.5
14	No reaction	+	−	20	0.9
15	No reaction	+	−	18	0.9
16	Slight hyperemia	+	+	Died of sepsis with functioning graft after 4.5 months.	
17	Hyperemia	−	+	Dialysis	
18	No reaction	+	+	20	1.0

patient in Category I was treated for several rejection episodes and died of CMV infection 5 months after kidney transplantation with functioning grafts.

Immediate function

All of the grafts except 2 functioned immediately and acute rejection episodes were encountered in 4 on the third and seventh days following surgery.

Iso-aglutinin titers

The antibody titers were done using standard commercial anti-A and anti-B sera with dilution method. Patients with rejection episodes had usually higher antibody titers at all times than the patients without rejection episodes. Immunoglobulin G and IgM levels did not change statistically following the transplantation and during the rejection episodes.

Splenectomy vs non-splenectomy

In the splenectomy group more patients developed early irreversible rejections than those in the non-splenectomy group (Tables 4 and 5).

Patient and graft survival

Overall patient survival was 94.5% and graft survival was 72.2% (Table 6). Uncontrolled hypertension was encountered in one of the patients at 7 months which was due to severe stenosis in the proximal part of the renal artery. This patient was treated successfully by ilio-renal Goretex bypass grafting. During the rejection episodes all patients showed leucocytosis as high as 25000/mm^3. The leucocyte counts became normal either after the reversal of the rejection or

Table 4. Outcome of 9 ABO-incompatible living related transplants with splenectomy and donor-specific skin graft.

No.	D: Donor R: Recipient	HLA and DR antigens				ABO	Follow-up (months)	Creatinine (mg/dl)
1	D	A_{26}, A_{32}	—, B_{51}	DR_5 —	DQ_1	A_1	Acute irreversible	
	R	A_{24}, A_{32}	B_{50}, B_{51}	DR_5 DR_3		O	rejection after 1 week	
2	D	A_2, —	B_{44}, —	DR_2 DR_5		A_1	30	1.2
	R	A_2, —	B_{44}, —	DR_3 DR_7		O		
3	D	A_1, A_2	B_{37}, B_{48}			AB	Chronic rejection	
	R	A_3, A_2	B_{52}, B_{48}			A	after 14 months	
4	D	A_{36}, A_{26}	B_{35}, B_{38}	DR_4 DR_6		AB	Acute irreversible	
	R	A_3, A_{26}	—, B_{38}	DR_4 —		A	rejection after 10 days	
5	D	A_1, A_2	—, B_{51}	DR_2 DR_5	DQ_2	A_1	26	1.4
	R	A_1, A_2	B_{35}, B_{51}	DR_9 DR_5	DQ_2	O		
6	D	A_2, A_{29}	B_7, B_{58}	DR_{10} DR_{12}	DQ_1	A_1	22	1.1
	R	A_2, A_{28}	B_7, B_{14}	DR_6 DR_{12}	DQ_1	B		
7	D	A_2, A_{30}	—, B_{44}	DR_5 —	DQ_1	B	22	0.8
	R	—, A_{30}	—, B_{51}	DR_1 DR_7		O		
8	D	A_1, A_2	B_8, B_{44}	DR_1 DR_3	DQ_1	AB	19	1.0
	R	A_1, A_{31}	B_8, B_{27}	DR_8 DR_3	—	A		
9	D	A_{25}, A_{29}	B_{27}, B_{35}	DR_3 —	DQ_1	B	Hyperacute rejection	
	R	A_{30}, A_{29}	B_{27}, B_{35}	DR_3 —	DQ_1	O		

Table 5. Outcome of 9 ABO-incompatible living related transplants with donor-specific skin grafting but without splenectomy.

No.	D: Donor R: Recipient	HLA and DR antigens							ABO	Follow-up (months)	Creatinine (mg/dl)
1	D	–,	A_{24}	B_8,	B_{35}	DR_3	DR_4	DR_7	A_1B	17	0.8
	R	A_1,	A_{24}	B_8,	B_{35}	DR_3	DR_5	DR_9	B		
2	D	A_3,	A_{30}	B_{27},	B_{35}	DR_3	DR_5	DQW_1	A_1	15	0.9
	R	A_{66},	A_{30}	B_{27},	B_{60}	DR_2	DR_5	–	O		
3	D	A_2,	–	B_{44},	B_{51}	DR_3	DR_5		A_1B	13	0.8
	R	A_2,	A_{26}	B_{13},	B_{51}	DR_3	DR_4		B		
4	D	A_2,	A_{11}	B_{35},	B_{52}	DR_2	DR_7		A_1	13	0.9
	R	A_2,	A_1	B_{35},	B_{52}	DR_2	DR_5		B		
5	D	A_2,	A_{24}	–,	B_{35}	DR_4	DR_5		B	12	0.8
	R	A_2,	A_{29}	B_7,	B_{62}	DR_4	DR_1		A		
6	D	A_1,	A_{30}	B_7,	B_{57}	DR_2	DR_3	DQ_1	A_1B	11	0.8
	R	A_1,	A_{30}	B_{35},	B_{57}	–	DR_3	DQ_1	B	11	0.8
7	D	A_3,	A_{29}	B_{18},	B_{51}	DR_3	DR_5		B	Died with functioning kidney 5 months after (CMV infection)	
	R	A_{30},	A_{29}	B_{18},	B_{13}	DR_3	DR_4		A		
8	D	A_2,	A_{11}	B_{35},	B_{51}				A_1	Hyperacute rejection	
	R	A_2,	A_{11}	B_{35},	B_{51}				O		
9	D	A_1,	A_3	B_{35},	B_{44}	DR_1	DR_3		B	6	1.0
	R	A_1,	A_{33}	B_{35},	–	DR_1	DR_4		A		

Table 6. Patient and graft survival in 18 recipients at 3—12 months after transplantation.

	Graft survival		Patient survival	
	No.	%	No.	%
3 months	14/18	77.7	18/18	100
6 months	13/18	72.2	17/18	94.5
12 months	11/16	68.75	17/18	94.5
Overall	13/18	72.2	17/18	94.5

the graft nephrectomy. Platelet counts varied within normal limits and one mortality due to CMV infection, possibly related with over-immunosuppression, was encountered among the recipients.

Discussion

In the early years of transplantation, ABO incompatibility was one of the main problems. While Alexandre and others have reported some success in overcoming this problem, the methods and protocols used are not clinically easy to perform. It was for this reason that we embarked on the donor-specific skin graft model as a clinically practical method for the selection of this group of patients (3, 4, 5). Our present experience with this model showed 94.5% patient survival and 72.2% graft survival in the follow-up period. This result compares well with the results of transplantation from A2 donors to 0 recipient (1, 2, 6, 7).

In this study, the outcome of the skin grafts was parallel to the outcome of kidney grafts. Eleven of the 18 skin grafts did not show any reaction and in the same recipients kidney grafts also did not present any rejection episodes. In contrast, the remaining 7 skin grafts presented slight or obvious reaction and all of these recipients showed acute rejection; unfortunately, 3 patients lost their kidney grafts. These results show that donor-specific skin graft is an easy and practical guide for predicting the outcome of ABO-incompatible kidney transplantation.

There was no difference between splenectomized and non-splenectomized recipients and therefore splenectomy may not be necessary in ABO-incompatible kidney transplantation.

Our iso-aglutinin titers results are similar to some extent to the results of Nelson *et al.* (6) with the recipients of higher levels of iso-aglutinin titers being more prone to rejection. However, we could not find any significant relationship between IgG and IgM levels either after transplantation or during the rejection episodes. The striking discovery was the elevation of total leucocyte counts during or shortly before the clinical and laboratory finding of acute rejection. When leucocytosis occurs in a recipient without any suspicion of infection, rejection should be suspected.

The rejection crises were treated by using OKT3 and alternate day plasmaphoresis. This combined therapy was directed against cellular immunity as well as humoral immunity.

We conclude from this study that donor-specific skin grafting was found to be an easy and applicable method in predicting the outcome of renal transplantation against the ABO blood group barrier. We believe that with this method at least 50% of chronic renal failure patients who have no suitable ABO-compatible living related donor but have a willing ABO-incompatible donor relative can be transplanted with good results.

References

1. Alexandre, G.P.J., Squifflet, J.P. and De Bruyere, M.: Splenectomy as a prerequisite for successful human ABO (incompatible renal transplantation. *Transplant. Proc.* **17**, 138 (1985).
2. Byringer, H., Padberg, L. and Samuelsson, M.: Transplantation of blood group A2 kidney to O recipients. Biochemical and immunological studies of blood group A antigens in human kidneys. *Transplant. Proc.* **17** (6), 2640—2643 (1985).
3. Haberal, M., Gulay, H. and Sert, S.: *Abstract Book, ESSR* (European Society for Surgical Research), Bologna, p. 173 (Presented) (1988).
4. Haberal, M., Gulay, H., Arslan, G. and Bilgin, N.: ABO incompatible kidney transplantation with skin grafting. *Transplant. Proc.* **21** (1), Februrary (1989).
5. Haberal, M.: ABO incompatible kidney transplantation with skin graft. In: M. Haberal (ed.), *Recent Advances in Nephrology and Transplantation*, pp. 163—170, Haberal Educational and Research Foundation (1990).
6. Nelson, P.W., Helling, T.S. and Pierce, G.E.: *Successful Transplantation of Blood* **45** (2), 316—319 February (1988).
7. Slapak, M., Digard, N., Ahmed, K., Shell, T. and Thompson, F.D.: Renal transplantation across the ABO barrier. A five year experience. *Abstract Book of IV Congress of the European Society for Organ Transplantation, Barcelona, Spain*, November 1—4 (1989).
8. Starzl, T.E., Marchioro, T.L. and Holmes, J.H.: Renal homografts in patients with donor recipient blood group incompatibilities. *Surgery* **55**, 195 (1964).

26. The use of single pediatric cadaver kidneys for transplantation into adult recipients

G.M. ABOUNA, P. JOHN, M.S.A. KUMAR, A.G. WHITE, O.S.G. SILVA, E. SHUWAIKH, M. SAMHAN, E.M. PHILIPS and S. AL-DADAH

Introduction

There is a size discrepancy when single small cadaveric pediatric kidneys are transplanted into adult recipients, which may contribute to inadquate function. Additionally, because of the small size of the renal blood vessels and ureter in these kidneys, there is concern that technical complications would ensue, resulting in inferior graft survival.

Here, we describe our experience with transplanting 20 small cadaveric pediatric kidneys as single organs into adult recipients.

Patients and methods

Five hundred and forty renal transplants have been carried out in this Center between March 1979 to May 1990, of which 420 are from living donors and 119 are cadaveric kidneys. Of the 119 cadaveric kidneys, 26 (21%) came from pediatric donors aged 0.25—5 years. Twenty of these were transplanted as single kidneys into adult recipients, 2 sets of kidneys were transplanted en bloc as double grafts into 2 adult recipients and the remaining 2 into two pediatric recipients. In the 20 kidneys transplanted as single kidneys into adult recipients, the mean age of the donors was 1.9 ± 0.84 years (range 0.5—5 years) and the mean body weight was 10.9 ± 3 kg (range 4—15). Most of these kidneys were imported from centers in North America and Europe with a mean preservation period of 48 ± 13 hours (range 20—61 hours). The method of preservation was pulsatile machine perfusion in 2 kidneys and simple ice cooling in 18 (Eurocollins 9, UW solution 9). Many of these kidneys and their donors had additional risk factors such as multiple arteries, maple syrup urine disease, meningitis and renal capsular tears.

The recipients were aged 33 ± 15 (range 20—53 years) with mean body weight of 57 ± 25 kg (42—90 kg). Eighteen of these recipients were maintained on hemodialysis and 2 on peritoneal dialysis prior to transplantation. All the recipients were mismatched for HLA-A, B and DR loci. The transplantation techniques used varied according to number of renal vessels. Basically it involved anastomosis of vascular pedicle to the external iliac vessels, usually through one or more Carrel patches with the ureter tunnelled into the bladder using an antireflux technique (Figure 1).

The post-transplant prophylactic immunosuppression was with azathioprine/prednisone in 4, cyclosporine/prednisone in 5 and sequential triple therapy in 11, consisting of azathioprine/prednisone/ATG until the graft resumed function from acute tubular necrosis with ATG was replaced by cyclosporine. Acute rejections were treated either with intravenous methylprednisolone, ATG or OKT3 (1). The size and function of the kidneys were assessed soon after transplantation and periodically thereafter by serum creatinine, 24 hour creatinine clearance, radionuclide renogram and ultrasound examination.

Early graft function was assessed in terms of primary non-function, requirement of post-transplant dialysis and function at 1 month. The final outcome was expressed as patient survival and graft function at 1 to 5 years using the life table method.

Results

Patient survival was 82% and the graft survival 60 and 50% at 1 and 5 years respectively (Table 1). The causes of patient loss were myocardial infarction in 1, fungal septicemia in 1 and gram negative sepsis in 1, at 10 days, 2 months and 6 years after transplantation respectively.

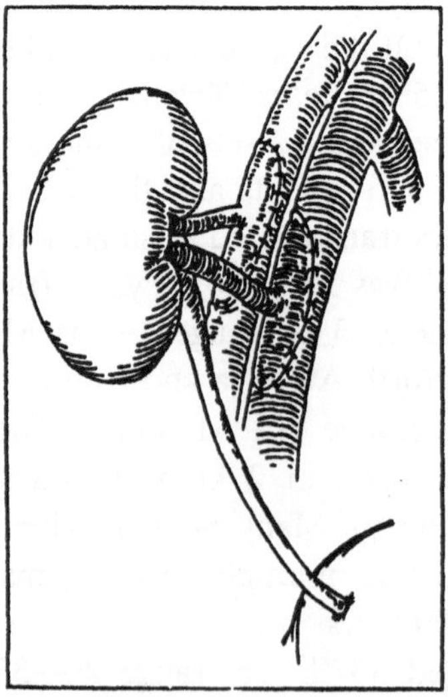

Fig. 1. Technique of transplantation of small pediatric kidneys into adults utilizing Carrel patches of donor aorta and vena cava.

Table 1. Patient and graft survival of pediatric kidneys transplanted into adults ($n = 20$).

Years	Patient survival (%)	Graft function (%)
0.5	90	70
1	82	60
2	82	60
3	82	60
4	82	60
5	82	50

Eight grafts were lost between day 0 and 6 years after transplantation. The causes were primary non-function in 2, acute rejection in 2, patient death in 1, chronic rejection in 1, chronic cyclosporine nephrotoxicity in 1 and renal artery thrombosis in 1.

Primary non-function was seen in 2 (10%), post-transplant dialysis was required in 15 (75%) with function at 1 month in 16 grafts (80%). Serial radioisotope renograms and ultrasound examination of these kidneys showed that the hypertrophy of the transplant kidney was complete by 4—6 weeks after transplantation. The serum creatinine and creatinine clearance improved gradually and stabilized at 6 months after transplantation. Table 2 shows the mean serum creatinine and 24-hour creatinine clearance at 1, 3 and 6 months. Surgical complications were seen in one recipient (5%) who developed renal artery thrombosis at 2 weeks. Fifteen recipients (75%) have controlled hypertension using 1—3 antihypertensive drugs except in 1 recipient with renal artery stenosis in whom hypertension was uncontrolled until the graft was lost at 6 years.

Table 2. Progressive improvement in renal function after transplantation of pediatric kidneys into adults.

		Serum creatinine (mmol/1)		Creatinine clearance (ml/min)	
Time	*n*	Mean	Range	Mean	Range
1 month	16	222 ± 69.1	190—400	14.6 ± 8	5—21
3 months	14	170 ± 40.1	156—270	37.25 ± 16.6	20—45
6 months	11	145 ± 29.9	110—200	50.25 ± 10.7	20—56

Discussion

The first successful transplantation of single pediatric cadaver kidneys into adult recipients was reported by Hume *et al.* in 1966 (2). Elegant experimental evidence by Sibler in 1976 demonstrated that pediatric kidneys show obligatory growth to a natural size which occurs at a standard rate, independent of its environment and a compensatory hypertrophy similar to adult kidneys when there is a need for increased function, which is reversible when the need is removed (3). Thus pediatric kidneys transplanted into adults are capable of twofold growth, obligatory growth and compensatory hypertrophy. There are several reports regarding the satisfactory function of pediatric kidneys transplanted into adult recipients (4, 5, 6). However, the graft loss due to technical and immunological causes may be higher than in adult kidneys resulting in inferior graft survival (7).

In our Center, since June 1983, we have been transplanting pediatric cadaver kidneys as single organs. Our policy is to transplant pediatric kidneys into pediatric recipients. However, because of shortage of organs and in the absence of suitable pediatric recipients, we transplant pediatric kidneys into adults. The adult recipients are selected on the basis of low body weight, HLA matching, a negative crossmatch and preferably without hypertension. In this series, the pediatric kidneys had prolonged cold ischemia time, as many of these were imported from North America and Europe, after the local transplant centers had refused to accept them. The graft survival was comparable to the recipients of adult cadaveric kidneys with prolonged preservation times (1, 8). Technical complication contributed to the loss of only 1 graft (5%) due to renal artery thrombosis. Serial radionuclide renogram and ultrasound examination of these kidneys showed that the compensatory hypertrophy was complete 4—6 weeks after transplantation. However, renal function as assessed by serum creatinine and 24-hour creatinine clearance showed steady improvement up to 6 months after transplantation, indicating that functional hypertrophy precedes the normal obligatory growth with increase in Nephron mass.

Seventy-five percent of the recipients were hypertensive after transplantation compared to 30—40% of the recipients of adult kidneys. Hypertension was more pronounced in recipients of smaller kidneys from very young donors. It is postulated that the cause of hypertension may be due to relative ischemia of the transplant kidney caused by inability of the renal artery to undergo an equally rapid increase in size or be able to accommodate the required blood flow for the rapid compensatory hypertrophy of the kidney. Clearly, there would be better function and possibly less complications by transplanting both kidneys en bloc in an adult recipient, but in this case only one single recipient can have the benefit of transplantation instead of two.

We conclude that with meticulous surgical care it is possible to obtain satisfactory renal function by transplanting single pediatric kidneys into adults and long-term graft survival is comparable to recipients of adult cadaveric kidneys. Furthermore, by giving one kidney to each of two recipients, a greater number of patients can be benefited, especially when there is acute shortage of cadaver grafts.

References

1. Abouna, G.M., John, P., Samhan, M. and Kumar, M.S.A.: Transplantation of single pediatric cadaveric kidneys into adult recipients. *Transplant. Proc.* **22**(2), (April), 407 (1990).
2. Hume, D.M., Lee, H.M., Williams, G.M., White, H.J.O., Ferre, J., Woy, J.S., Prout, G.R. Jr, Slapak, M., O'Brian, J., Kilpatrick, S.J., Kauffman, H.K. Jr and Cleveland, R.J.: Comparative results of cadaver and related donor renal homografts in man and immunologic implications of the outcome of second and paired grafts. *Ann. Surg.* **164**, 352–397 (1966).
3. Silber, S.J.: Growth of baby kidneys transplanted into adults. *Arch. Surg.* **3**, 75–77 (1976).
4. Kootstra, G., West, J.C., Dryburgh, P., Krom, R.A.F., Putnam, C.W. and Weil, R. III: Pediatric cadaver kidneys for transplantation. *Surgery* **83**, 333–337 (1978).
5. Wengerter, K., Tellis, V.A., Soberman, R., Matas, A.J., Quinn, T. and Veith, F.J.: Transplantation of pediatric kidneys to adult recipients. Is there a critical donor age? *Ann. Surg.* **204**, 172–175 (1986).
6. Hong, J.H., Shinani, K., Arshad, A., Parsa, I., Matas, A., Adamsons, R.J. and Butt, K.M.H.: Influence of cadaver donor age on the success of kidney transplants. *Transplantation* **32**, 532–534 (1981).
7. Wetzels, J.F.M., Hoitsma, A.J. and Koene, R.A.P.: Influence of cadaver donor age on renal graft survival. *Clin. Nephrol.* **25**, 256–259 (1986).
8. Kumar, M.S.A., Samhan, M., Philips, E.M. and Abouna, G.M.: Late function in 48 cadaver renal allografts preserved for 48–76 hours. *Transplant. Proc.* **20**(5), 940–941 (1988).

27. Living unrelated donor renal transplantation

S. SERT, H. GULAY, M. KOÇ and M. HABERAL

Introduction

Since kidney transplantation has become a highly accepted and successful therapy for chonic renal failure patients, the demand has increased very rapidly creating a serious shortage in organ supply. It is generally agreed that living related donor kidney transplantation is the first choice for its high success rate, with cadaver donor taking second place and living unrelated donors the third. However, insufficient supply of cadaveric kidney and the good results obtained in patient and graft survivals with the living unrelated donor renal transplantation, it is now widely recognized that living genetically unrelated but emotionally related donors is an acceptable option (1, 2, 3, 4) although some transplant centers refuse kidney transplantation from non-genetically related donors for ethical reasons. Since insufficient cadaveric kidneys continue to be a major problem in our country and other Near Eastern countries, a third organ source (the living unrelated donor) has emerged as an alternative (3, 4). However, some of the so-called unrelated donors are second degree relatives, while spouses are the usual source, since they are the most affected persons for the rehabilitation of chronic renal failure recipients. The other unrelated donor group are emotionally related by friendship. In this study, we present our experience concerning 80 living unrelated kidney transplants with DST and plasmaphoresis.

Material and methods

From October 16, 1985 to October 1, 1989, 415 kidney transplants have been performed in 410 patients at our Center. In 80 recipients, grafts from living unrelated donors were used. Sixty-two of the recipients were males and 18 females with a mean age of 36.7 (range 16—59 years). The donors were 24 spouses (22 wives, 2 husbands); 9 cousins; 12 nephews; 8 maternal uncles; 5 maternal aunts; and 22 were 'friends'. Donors' mean age was 37.6 (between 21 and 61 years). Sixty-nine of living unrelated kidney recipients received DST (3 transfusions of 150 ml each at 10-day intervals) without azathioprine. One patient received an ABO-incompatible graft with donor-specific skin graft. Donor-recipient HLA mismatch were as follows: 3 with 0 mismatch; 20 with 1 mismatch; 23 with 2 mismatches; and 34 with 3 mismatches. Plasmaphoresis was performed in two sessions before transplantation and low-dose triple drug immunosuppressive therapy of prednisone, azathioprine and cyclosporine was administered to all patients after transplantation. Prednisone was started at 1 mg/kg/day; tapered to 20 mg/day when leaving hospital; to 15 mg at 3 months; to 10 mg/day from the fourth month. Azathioprine was given at 2 mg/kg/day while the cyclosporine-A dose was regulated to its blood level using fluorescence polarization immunoassay (FPIA) technique (TDx-Abbot).

Rejection episodes were treated by bolus methylprednisolone 0.5 g intravenously for 3 consecutive days. If necessary, this regimen was repeated once more. When rejection persisted as confirmed by fine needle aspiration biopsy (FNAB), a 10-day course of OKT3, alternating with plasmaphoresis, was used and the standard immunosuppressive drugs being reduced during this period.

Results

All patients were followed for 1—37 months (mean 19 months). Twelve patients rejected their grafts (15%); 4 patients died (5%), 3 due to sepsis and 1 from massive gastrointestinal bleeding with functioning graft. A total of 69 rejection episodes were observed (73.7%). Four patients presented with acute rejection and they lost their grafts in the early post-transplantation period. Thirty-three presented with one rejection episode; 18, two rejection episodes and 4 presented with three rejection episodes. Eight patients developed chronic rejection and all lost their grafts late in the post-transplant period. There were no rejection episodes observed in 21 patients (26.3%). There were 11 steroid-resistant rejections (13.7%). These were treated with combination therapy of OKT3 and plasmaphoresis with rejections being reversed in 9 (81.8%). Overall actuarial patient survival was 95% and graft survival was 80% at 1 and 2 years (Figure 1). HLA-A and B matching did not seem to influence the overall outcome (Table 1).

Discussion

In the early years of kidney transplantation from living unrelated donor, the results were similar to those from cadaveric donor (2). More recently, several studies have shown greatly improved patient and graft survival and lower incidence of rejection episodes in living unrelated transplantation which may be due to better HLA matching, the use of DST or immunosuppression with CyA

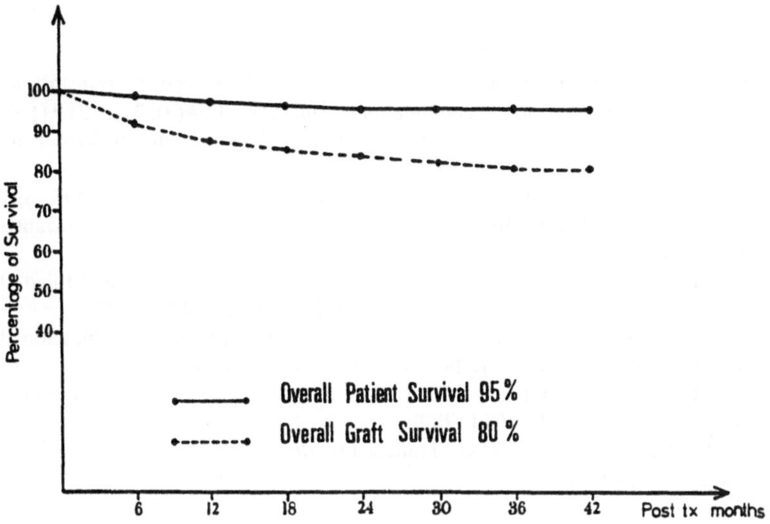

Fig. 1 Overall patient and graft survival in 80 second degree or living unrelated transplantation.

Table 1. HLA compatibility, patient and graft survival in 80 second degree or living unrelated transplant patients.

No. of patients	HLA mismatch	PS (%)	GS (%)
3	0	100	100
20	1	84.7	76.5
23	2	100	85.7
34	3	94.7	78.8

(1, 2, 3, 4, 6, 7). The results from these reported studies are similar: the range of graft survival being 83—92% at 2—4 years. We believe that donor-specific blood transfusions have improved graft survival in these patients (1, 4) either with (1) or without azathioprine (6). In our experience, a combination therapy with OKT3 and plasmaphoresis is highly successful in steroid-resistant rejection (5).

Therefore, we may conclude that living unrelated renal transplantation could be performed since there are not enough cadaveric kidneys available. This should be done with a combination of DST, plasmaphoresis and triple drug immunosuppressive therapy. However, living unrelated kidney transplantation must be performed with strict medical and clinical criteria: lack of living related donor; long and uncertain waiting time for cadaveric kidney; with full understanding and altruistic motivation on the part of the 'emotionally related' donor.

References

1. Sollinger, H.W., Kalayoglu, M. and Belzer, O.F.: Use of donor-specific transfusions protocol in living-unrelated donor recipient combinations. *Ann. Surg.* **3—4**(3), 315—319 (1986).
2. Levey, A.S., Hou, S. and Bush, H.L.: Kidney transplantation from unrelated living donors. *New Engl. J. Med.* **314**(14), 914—916 (1986).
3. Abouna, G.M., Panjavani, D., Kumar, M.S.A., White, A.G., Al-Abdullah, I.H., Silva, O.S.G. and Samhan, M.: The living unrelated donor — a viable alternative for renal transplantation. *Transplant. Proc.* **20**(5), 802 (1988).
4. Haberal, M., Sert, S., Gulay, H., Aybasti, N., Gokce, O., Hamaloglu, E. and Bilgin, N.: Living unrelated donor renal transplantation. *Transplant. Proc.* **20**(5), 805 (1988).
5. Haberal, M., Bulut, O., Sert, S. *et al.*: OKT3 and plasmaphoresis combination therapy of steroid-resistant renal allograft rejection. *Transplant. Proc.* (in press).
6. Haberal, M., Sert, S. and Aybasti, N.: The effect of azathioprine on sensitization due to DST. *Transplant. Proc.* **20**(1), 300-301 (1988).
7. Haberal, M., Bulut, O., Sert, S. *et al.*: Transplantation between husband and wife. *Transplant. Proc.* **22**(2), 342 (1990).

28. Renal transplantation in Tunisia — a three-year experience

H. BEN AYED, A. EL-MATRI, T. BEN ABDALLAH, C. KECHRID, H. BEN MAIZ, A. KHEDER, F. BEN MOUSSA, S. SMERLIE, M. AYED, M. EL-OUAKDI, K. AYED and R. BARDI

Introduction

Until June 1986 renal transplants for Tunisian patients were performed in Europe (2), but since then, a renal transplantation program has started at the Charles Nicolle University Hospital in Tunis. The responsibility for transplantation is shared between nephrologists, urologists and immunologists.

The program was initially restricted to transplants from living related donors (LRD) but later extended to include cadaver donors (CD). Until March 1990, 70 patients were transplanted but we report our experience of 60 transplants performed between June 1986 and June 1989.

Patients and methods

During this 3-year period, 52 living related transplants (86.7%) and 8 cadaveric transplants (13.3%) were performed; 58 were first and 2 were second transplants. Recipients were 39 males and 21 females whose mean age was 28.87 ± 7.8 years. Primary renal disease was chronic glomerulo-nephritis in 26 (43.3%), chronic pyelonephritis in 8 (13.3%), Alport syndrome in 1, cortical necrosis in 1 and unknown in 12 (20%). Initial renal replacement therapy was hemodialysis in 51 cases and CAPD in 9.

For living related transplants, the general health, renal function and urinary tract anatomy of the potential donor is assessed. Only first-degree relatives with informed consent are accepted.

Routine ABO, HLA-A, B and DR typing and lymphocyte crossmatch are performed. All living donors have a pyelogram and a renal arteriogram to assess the anatomy of the kidneys. After removal, the kidney is flushed with Eurocollins solution at 4 °C prior to implantation. In case of cadaver transplants, the kidney is stored in ice then in a refrigerator.

All potential recipients undergo retrograde cystogram, gastroscopy and full medical evaluation. If there is any suspicion of tuberculosis, the patient is treated with antituberculosis therapy for at least 6 months before transplantation.

Three units of random blood transfusions are given in most patients receiving living donor transplants and cytotoxic antibodies screened. The last dialysis is performed 1 day before surgery. Standard surgical technique is carried out with the kidney placed in the right fossa and a uretero-neocystostomy Leadbetter-Politano type performed in all cases.

Initially the patients received conventional maintenance immunosuppression consisting of a combination of prednisone and azathioprine. Triple drug regimen combining cyclosporine with azathioprine and prednisone was used in 18 patients and double drug regimen combining cyclosporine and prednisone in 6 patients. Cyclosporine is administered orally at 6 mg/kg/day then adjusted to clinical state and cyclosporine blood level (radioimmunoassay).

Acute rejection episodes were treated with a combination of methylprednisolone pulses in decreasing doses and antithymocyte immunoglobulin (Thymoglobin* Merieux) at 1.5 mg/kg/day for 7—14 days.

Patient and graft actuarial survival rates are computed using the actuarial method.

Results

Among the 60 transplants, waiting time on dialysis varied. Before 1986, it was 26 ± 25 for LRD and 40 ± 23 days for cadaver, but after that date, it was 10 ± 7 and 10 ± 5 days respectively.

For living transplants, donors were: 23 siblings, 18 parents and 1 child (daughter to mother). HLA matching was: 6 antigen matches in 17 and 3 antigen matches in 35. For cadaveric transplants, HLA matching was 0 to 2 antigens.

After transplantation, acute tubular necrosis occurred in 7/52 (13.5%) LRD and in 3/8 (37.5) cadaveric transplants requiring 1 to 10 sessions of hemodialysis, but all recovered. Acute rejection was encountered in 27/52 (52%) LRD and 5/8 (62%) cadaveric transplants.

Urological complications occurred in 6 cases consisting of 3 urinary leaks (2 required transplant nephrectomy and 1 was repaired surgically) and 3 ureteral stenoses (2 were successfully treated). One urinary stone was effectively treated with shockwave lithotripsy. Vascular complications were seen in 3 cases: 2 were arterial thrombosis and 1 was a perirenal hematoma.

Infectious complications were frequent. Viral infections occurred in 21 cases (35%), mostly CMV and herpes. No HIV infection was seen. Bacterial infection was documented in 12 cases involving urinary tract, skin, mucosa and bone and yeast infection involving skin and gastrointestinal tract in 9. Six patients had scabies; 1 of whom developed an acute glomerulonephritis in the graft.

Twenty patients exhibited hypertension which was related to renal artery stenosis in 3; recurrent glomerulonephritis in 2; chronic rejection in 3, but in 12 patients, hypertension had no organic cause; 7 of these were on cyclosporine. Recurrent glomerulonphritis developed in 4 cases after 1—12 months. Metabolic complications included: diabetes mellitus in 1 case, hyperparathyroidism in 3, hyperlipidemia in 5, cataract in 2, hirsutism in 2 and gingival hyperplasia in 1.

Patient and graft survival

The 3-year actuarial patient and graft survival rates were 95.5 and 90.7% respectively for LRD transplants and 61.3 and 55% for cadaveric transplants.

Mean serum creatinine level ranged between 105 and 120 μmol/l for patients with conventional maintenance immunosuppressive therapy and between 135 and 150 for patients receiving cyclosporine. Three grafts were lost in LRD transplants due to chronic rejection, vascular occlusion and septicemia. Three cadaveric transplants were also lost due to chronic rejection, vascular occlusion and to pyeloureteral necrosis. There were 4 deaths. One patient with cadaveric graft died of massive hemorrhage associated with graft rupture due to hyperacute rejection and another died of septicemia associated with generalized Kaposi's sarcoma. Two patients with LRD grafts died of septicemia.

Discussion

The chronic hemodialysis program in Tunisia, a country of 7.8 million, started in 1968 (1). There are at present time 22 hemodialysis centers and one CAPD unit treating around 800 end-stage renal failure patients at the expense of the community. Until 1986, few cases were sent to Europe for transplantation (2). Since then, the local transplantation program has performed 60 grafts in three years or 20 cases per year, 86.7% of them being living donor transplants.

The patients are treated in conventional internal medicine and urology wards without special rooms or equipment. The program was initially restricted to living related transplants but was extended to cadaveric transplants since Tunisia has had a transplant law, which is similar to the French law where consent is not required (presumed consent). Nevertheless, we insisted on obtaining the family's consent in all cases of cadaveric grafts. Surprisingly, refusal was rare which is encouraging for the future.

Twenty-eight patients received conventional maintenance immunosuppression. Cyclosporine was only used in 8 cadaveric transplants and 24 live transplants, where it was especially needed such as when there was a positive mixed lymphocyte culture or acute rejections which were not controlled with conventional therapy.

Urological and vascular complications were acceptable for a starting program. Infectious complications were as frequent as in European series (4—6), but scabies had a particularly high incidence. One of the patients exhibited an acute glomerulonephritis associated with scabies. Two glomerulonephritis were probably recurrences: one focal glomerulosclerosis and one rheumatoid purpura nephropathy.

Patients and graft survival rate for living donor transplants were as good as those obtained in European Centers (5—7), while that of cadaveric transplants were lower than those reported, but the numbers are too small to be meaningful.

The causes of death and graft loss were in general similar to those encountered in other centers (7). Two patients with severe sepsis were over immunosuppressed. They died with a functional graft.

The local transplantation program could successfully rehabilitate patients with end-stage renal failure at a lower cost and better quality of life than dialysis. Most of those who had a job returned to employment after their transplantation. The cost of the chronic hemodialysis in Tunisia is presently very high compared to the total health expenses in the country. We expect 150—200 new patients coming to dialysis per year. We need to be able to do at least 100 transplants per year to meet the need. We are hopeful that this can be achieved with the establishment of a national cadaveric procurement program, particularly since Tunisia is unique amongst other Middle Eastern countries for having a presumed consent-type law for removal of cadaver organs since 1952.

References

1. El-Matri, A., Ben Abdallah, T., Kechrid, C., Ben Maiz, H., Kheder, A., Ben Moussa, F. and Ben Ayed, H.: Traitement de suppléance de l'insuffisance rénale chronique en Tunisie. *Nephrologie* **7**, 109—113 (1986).
2. El-Matri, A., Ben Abdallah, T., Kechrid, C., Ben Maiz, H. and Ben Ayed, H.: La greffe rénale en Tunisie: de 1977 à 1984. *Tunis Med.* **64**, 39—42 (1986).
3. Eggers, P.W.: Effect of transplantation on the Medicare End-Stage Renal Disease Program. *N.Engl. J. Med.* **318**, 223—229 (1988).
4. Hall, B.M., Tiller, D.J., Hardie, I., Mahoney, M.S.J., Mathew, T., Thatcher, G., Miach, C.B.P., Thomson, N. and Sheil, Ag.R.: Comparison of three immunosuppressive regimens in cadaver renal transplantation. Long term cyclosporine, short term cyclosporine followed by azathioprine and prednisone and azathioprine and prednisone without cyclosporine. *N. Engl. J. Med.* **318**, 1499—1507 (1988).
5. Abouna, G.M., Kumar, M.S.A., White, A.G., Samhan, M., Dadah, S., Silva, S.G. and John, P.B.: Renal transplantation in the Middle East, experience with 250 transplants. *Dialysis and Transplant.* **16**, 81—84 (1987).
6. Hiesse, C. and Benoit, G.: Facteurs de l'amelioration récente des résultats de la transplantation rénale en France. *Sem. Hop. Paris* **64**, 342—345 (1988).
7. Brunner, H.: Survival on renal replacement therapy. Data from the EDTA Registry. *Nephrol. Dial. Transplant.* **2**, 109—122 (1988).

29. Renal transplantation in children

M. SAMHAN, P. JOHN, M.S.A. KUMAR, A.G. WHITE, O.S.G. SILVA,
E. SHUWAIKH, E.M. PHILIPS, S. AL-DADAH and G.M. ABOUNA

Introduction

In the sixties, the outlook for children with end-stage renal disease was grim. As recently as 1970, it was thought that it would be kinder to both the parents and child to let the child die rather than be subjected to prolonged suffering by unproven methods of either dialysis or renal transplantation. Currently, renal transplantation is the preferred method of treatment in children with end-stage renal disease to achieve optimal growth and early rehabilitation.

In Kuwait, since the inception of the renal transplantation programme in 1979, children have been considered for renal transplantation. The first pediatric renal transplant was carried out in 1980, and since that time we have carried out 57 renal transplantations in children. The surgical techniques and the method of immunosuppression have been standardized and here we describe our experience with pediatric renal transplantation for the last 10 years.

Patients and methods

Since the establishment of the transplantation programme in Kuwait in March 1979, over the last 10 years, 57 renal allografts have been carried out in 54 children, of which 54 were primary grafts and 3 secondary grafts. All pediatric patients with end-stage renal disease and free of active infection were considered for transplantation. Twenty-nine of these children were males and 25 females, aged 0.9—16 years (mean 11.6 years). The indications for renal transplantation are shown in Table 1. Of the 57 renal transplants, kidneys were obtained from living donors in 43 (parents, 28; siblings, 10; uncles 2; step mother, 1; friends 2) and from cadaver donors in 14.

In living-donor transplantation, the donors were selected on immunological, medical, ethical and legal criteria according to previously described protocols (1). The immunological selection was based on ABO compatibility, HLA typing at A, B and DR loci and a negative direct lymphocyte crossmatch. Seven recipients received HLA-matched grafts and 36 HLA-mismatched grafts.

Table 1. Indications for renal transplantation.

Original renal disease	No. of recipients
Chronic glomerulonephritis	24
Chronic pyelonephritis	12
Congenital medullary cystic kidney	5
Bladder neck obstruction with chronic pyelonephritis	8
Congenital hypoplastic kidney	3
Oxalosis	1
Neurogenic bladder and bilateral vur	1
Total	54

Of the 14 cadaveric kidneys transplanted in pediatric recipients, 10 were imported from North America with preservation periods of 30—76 hours and the remaining 4 were harvested locally. All the cadaveric kidneys were mismatched with their respective recipients for 2 or more HLA antigens.

Many of these recipients had other associated high-risk factors which included uncontrolled hypertension in 33, bladder neck obstruction in 9, heart failure in 4, pericardial effusion and pulmonary oedema in 2, hepatitis B antigenemia in 5, glucose-6-phosphatase dehydrogenase deficiency in 2, hydrocephalus with ventriculoperitoneal shunt in 1 and neurogenic bladder in 1. Eighteen recipients had dialysis-resistant hypertension prior to transplantation, and in 4 of these bilateral native nephrectomy was carried out and in the remaining 14 simultaneous unilateral nephrectomy was carried out at the time of transplantation, as previously reported (2). In 9 recipients, bilateral or unilateral native nephrectomy was carried out for vesicoureteric reflux. As part of an on-going study and in an attempt to reduce recurrence of focal segmental glomerulosclerosis (FSG) in transplant kidneys, recipients with this disease undergo pre-transplant bilateral nephrectomy following which they are maintained on cylcosporine therapy for 6 weeks before transplantation according to our protocol. Three pediatric recipients with FSG were managed according to this protocol (Table 2). Renal transplantation was a standard procedure similar to that in adults in 48 recipients where the kidney was placed in one of the iliac fossae. In the remaining 9 recipients, with small body build and low body weight, the kidney was placed intra-abdominally and the renal vessels were anastomosed directly to the aorta and inferior vena cava. The ureter was implanted into the bladder using the antireflux technique in 56 recipients. In the remaining recipient with neurogenic bladder, the ureter was brought out as a cutaneous uretrostomy.

Prophylactic immunosuppression therapy in living-donor transplantation was with azathioprine and prednisone in 22 recipients and with triple therapy consisting of azathioprine, prednisone and cyclosporine A in 21 recipients. In

Table 2. Native nephrectomy in pediatric recipients.

	Indication for nephrectomy			
Native nephrectomy	Hypertension	Vesicoureteric reflux	Other	Total
Pre-transplant bilateral nephrectomy	—	2	3[a]	5
Simultaneous unilateral nephrectomy	14	3		17
Simultaneous bilateral nephrectomy	1	3		4
Sequential bilateral nephrectomy	3	1		4
Total	18	9	3	30

[a] Bilateral nephrectomy was carried out for focal segmental glomerulosclerosis in 3 recipients.

cadaver kidney recipients, conventional immunosuppression was used in 3 and triple therapy in 11 recipients. Acute rejection episodes were diagnosed and treated according to our previously described protocols using either intravenous pulse doses of methylprednisolone, or intravenous infusion of antilymphocyte globulin or OKT3 for 10—14 days (3). The height growth patterns of the recipients were recorded regularly in the outpatient clinic. The actuarial survival rates were analyzed using the life table method, and statistical analysis was carried out using the student's '*t*' test and chi-squared analysis.

Results

Living-donor transplantation

The actuarial patient survival in the living donor transplantation is 90% at 1—5 years. Four recipients aged 0.9, 2, 6 and 11 years died due to high output cardiac failure, cardiac arrest, chest infection/septicaemia, reactivation of pulmonary TB and infection on days 3, 3, 60 and 200 after transplantation respectively. A fifth patient died at nearly 7 years from infection.

The overall actuarial graft survival in living donor transplantation is 88 and 70% at 1 and 5 years respectively. In 22 recipients maintained on azathioprine and prednisolone, the graft survival was 86 and 73% at 1 and 3 years, while in the 21 recipients receiving triple therapy with cyclosporine, graft survival was 83% at 1 and 3 years respectively. The difference in the graft survival between the two groups was not significant ($p = 0.95$). The graft loss was due to acute rejection in 3, chronic rejection in 8 and recurrence of original renal disease in 1 and patient death in 3 (Table 3).

In this small series we could not find a correlation between HLA matching and graft survival in living donor transplantation. In the 7 recipients who received matched grafts, the graft survival was 83 and 66% at 1 and 3 years respectively while in the 36 recipients of mismatched grafts, the graft survival was 85 and 77% at 1 and 3 years respectively ($p = 0.45$).

Table 3. Cause and time of graft loss in pediatric recipients of living donor kidneys ($n = 43$)

Cause of graft loss	No.	Time (months)
Chronic graft rejection	8	33, 41, 12, 20 19, 45, 62, 39
Acute graft rejection	3	1, 4, 6
Recipient's death	3	0, 0, 82
Recurrence of PRD	1	48
Total	15	0—82

Cadaver donor transplantation

In cadaveric renal transplantation, the actuarial patient survival is 93% at 1—3 years. One patient died of wound infection at 1 month. The actuarial graft survival of cadaver renal transplantation was 71 and 57% at 1 and 3 years respectively. In cadaver kidney recipients, the statistical analysis with regard to the effect of HLA mismatch, age of recipients and method of immunosuppression on graft survival could not be assessed because of small numbers. The causes of graft loss in this group included chronic cyclosporine nephrotoxicity in 2, chronic rejection in 1, acute rejection in 1, primary non-function of the graft in 2, wound infection in 1 and hyperacute rejection in 1 (Table 4).

Relation between age and survival

Five of the paediatric recipients who died (living donor 4, cadaver 1) were of small build with body weight of less than 15 kg and 4 of these patients were 6 years or younger. In the living donor transplantation group, 30 recipients aged 10 years or more have a graft survival of 93 and 73% at 1 and 5 years

Table 4. Causes and time of graft loss in pediatric recipients of cadaveric kidneys ($n = 14$)

Cause of graft loss	No.	Time (months)
Hyperacute graft rejection	1	0
Acute graft rejection	1	13
Chronic graft rejection	1	44
Chronic CyA nephrotoxicity	2	14, 56
PNF	2	0, 0
Wound infection	1	0.5
Total	8	0–56

compared to 13 recipients aged <10 years with graft survival of 70 and 50% at 1 and 5 years respectively ($p = 0.01$).

Post-transplant complications

There were surgical complications in 7 (wound infection in 1, cerebral bleeding in 1, intestinal obstruction in 3, urethral injury in 1 and transient lower limb paresis in 1). Complications due to steroid therapy were Cushingoid features in 22 and osteoporosis in 2 recipients. Eleven recipients developed post-transplant infections which included bacterial in 4, viral in 6, and protozoal in 1. In 2 recipients, infections were fatal and more caused by pulmonary TB in 1, chest infection and septicaemia in the other.

Rehabilitation and growth

All surviving recipients with functioning grafts are in full-time education or have started employment. Recipients transplanted before chronological age of 11 years and maintained with good graft function have shown considerable improvement in physical growth.

Discussion

Renal transplantation is currently the best mode of therapy for adult patients with end stage renal failure. The same is particularly true for pediatric patients, because of higher patient survival, better quality of life, improved physical growth rates and early and complete rehabilitation as compared to dialysis treatment (4, 5). In Europe, the rate of renal transplantation in children is 4 per million child population (6). There are several reports advocating early transplantation even in those below 1 year of age because of greater likelihood of normal growth in stature and head size (8, 9). The long-term results of renal transplantation in children varies between 40 and 90% at 10 years, depending on the kidney source and HLA matching and are reported to be excellent with regard to rehabilitation, and growth patterns (9, 10). However, the follow-up of these pediatric recipients is not without problem, especially with regard to immunosuppression, infection and surgical complications (10, 11).

In Kuwait, the common indications for renal transplantation in children are chronic glomerulonephritis, chronic pyelonephritis and bladder neck obstruction which is similar to the European series (6). In this series, children form approximately 10% of the transplant population with living donors being the main source of kidneys (75%) because of the shortage of cadaveric organs. In our series, most of the cadaveric kidneys (10/14) were imported from North America and many of these were suboptimal because of prolonged preservation period extending from 30 to 72 hours and/or surgically high-risk kidneys (traumatized or with multiple vessels) and this accounted for poor graft function.

In living-donor transplantation, the patient survival is 90% and graft survival is 88 and 70% at 1 and 5 years respectively. There was no significant difference either in the patient or graft survival when cyclosporine was used as an additional immunosuppressive. Three children (2 females and 1 male) with functioning grafts longer than 5 years have shown normal physical growth patterns. All three recipients were below 11 years of age at the time of transplantation. One of them has taken up employment after completing school and the remaining 2 continue their education at school. Seven children have shown impaired or subnormal physical growth. However, all the children with functioning grafts are fully rehabilitated with regard to physical and educational activities at school and are well adjusted with regard to their social and emotional behavior in the family and society.

Of the 14 cadaveric kidney recipients, 8 have lost the kidneys between 3 weeks to 4 years after transplantation. Three of the 8 recipients who lost their primary cadaver renal grafts have subsequently received secondary grafts from living donors, all of which are functioning. These 3 recipients and the 6 with functioning primary cadaver grafts are fully rehabilitated.

Infection was a major problem and was seen in 11 recipients (19%). These included bacterial, viral and protozoal infections and in 3 recipients it was fatal (2 LD). Surgical complications were minimal and were seen in 7 recipients (12%). Complications due to steroids mainly in the form of Cushingoid features were seen in 22 recipients (38%).

The graft loss due to acute rejection in both living donor and cadaver transplantation was reduced with the introduction of OKT3, ALG/ATG and cyclosporine. In our series, acute rejection was the cause of graft loss in 3 living donor grafts (7%) and in 2 cadaver grafts (14%). However, chronic rejection was the most important cause of graft loss in our series and caused the loss of 19% of living donor grafts.

We conclude that early renal transplantation in children is very worth while and gratifying. We recommend that renal transplantation should be considered as a primary mode of therapy in all children with end-stage renal disease at an early age and even before dialysis becomes necessary since successful renal transplantation results in improved quality of life, near normal physical growth and early rehabilitation, particularly when the source of the graft is a living related donor.

References

1. Abouna, G.M., Kumar, M.S.A., White, A. G. *et al*: Renal transplantation in the Middle East — Experience with 250 transplants. *Dialysis and Transplant* **16**, 81—84 (1987).
2. Abouna, G.M., Samhan, M. and Kumar, M.S.A.: Unilateral native nephrectomy at the time of renal transplantation is effective in the treatment of dialysis-resistant hypertension. *Transplant. Proc.* **21** (1), 2028—2030 (1989).
3. Kumar, M.S.A., White, A.G., John, P. *et al.*: Antilymphocyte infusion in the treatment of acute allograft rejection. in: G.M. Abouna (ed.) *Current Status of Clinical Organ Transplantation*, pp. 49—56. Martinus Nijhoff, The Hague (1984).
4. Fine, R.N., Malekzadeh, M.H., Pennisi, A.H. *et al.*: Long term results of renal transplantation in children. *Pediatrics* **61**, 641 (1978).
5. Doncker, R.A., Broyer, M., Brunner, F. *et al.*: Combined report on regular dialysis and transplantation in Europe 1981. *EDTA Proc.* **19**, 61—68 (1982).
6. Broyer, M., Rizzoni, G., Brunner, H. *et al.*: Combined report on regular dialysis and transplantation of children in Europe XIV 1984. *EDTA Proc.* **23**, 55—79 (1985).
7. So, S.K.S., Nevins, T.E., Chang, P.N. *et al.*: Preliminary results of renal transplantation in children under 1 year of age. *Transplant. Proc.* **17**, 182 (1985).
8. McMahon, Y., MacDonall, R.C. Jr., Richie, R. E. *et al.*: Is kidney transplantation in the very small child (< 10 kg) worth it? *Transplant. Proc.* **21** (1), 2003—2005 (1989).
9. Najarian, J.S., So, S.K., Simmons, R.L. *et al.*: The outcome of 304 primary renal transplants in children (1968—1985). *Ann. Surg.* **204** (3), 246—258, (1986).
10. Lee, H.M., Mendez-Picon, G. and Posmer, M.P.: The status of rehabilitation, morbidity and mortality of long term survivors of pediatric kidney transplants. *Transplant. Proc.* **21** (1), 1989—1991 (1989).
11. Nelson, E.W., Kessler, R. and Holman, P. Jr.: Surgical complications in pediatric renal transplantation: *Transplant. Proc.* **21** (1), 2006—2007 (1989).

30. Kidney donors — long-term follow-up

P. JOHN, M.S.A. KUMAR, H. ABDUL KARIM, M. SAMHAN,
N. AL-SABAWI, S. AL-DADAH, T. ECHE, O.S.G. SILVA,
E. SHUWAIKH, A. KOBRYN, E.M. PHILIPS, and G.M. ABOUNA

Introduction

Improved methods in the management of recipients and the development of new of immunosuppressive protocols has brought wide acceptance of renal transplantation as the method of choice in the treatment of patients with chronic renal failure. In North America and Europe, cadaver donors are the major source of kidneys and other organs for transplantation (1). However, in Kuwait and other developing countries, cadaveric organ procurement is still in its infancy and living donors are the main source of kidneys for transplantation. Even in countries where cadaveric organ procurement is well developed, there is still a shortage of organs because demand exceeds the supply. This is partly met by using kidneys from living donors. In 1984, 32% of kidney transplantations in the U.S.A. were from living donors (2). In our Center, over the last 11 years, living donors form 80% of the source of kidneys for transplantation. Although renal transplantation has gained wide acceptance, kidney transplantation from living donors is being discussed with regard to moral, ethical and medical aspects in view of possible long-term complications such as proteinuria and hypertension (3, 4). In order to examine these adverse but largely theoretical long-term problems, we have followed up and studied in detail the long-term functional, psychological and social effects of nephrectomy on kidney donors who had donated a kidney to a living related recipient 5—10 years previously.

Materials and methods

Between March 1979 and December 1989, some 400 living donor nephrectomies have been carried at our Center without mortality or any serious morbidity. Of these, 176 were carried out 5—10 years previously. The selection of donors was based on strict immunological, medical and ethical criteria according to a previously described protocol (5). However, since our Center is a regional referral centre for transplantation from various countries in the Middle East, many donors who came from abroad had left Kuwait and were not available to be included in this follow-up study. Thirty of these kidneys donors were available locally and agreed to participate in this study. The mean age of these donors at the time of nephrectomy was 36 ± 15 years (range 24—56 years). Sex ratio was 19 : 12 in favour of males. The donor relationship was siblings 15; parents 7; offsprings 4; spouses 3; and nephew 1.

The protocol for the long-term follow-up of these donors included evaluation of medical, functional, psychological and social aspects of kidney donation. These assessments were carried out by transplant surgeons and physicians, nurses and a social worker.

The medical and functional evaluation included complete history and physical examination, measurements of blood pressure in standing and supine positions on at least three different occasions, full hematological and biochemical evaluation comprising, hemoglobin, serum creatinine, blood urea and electrolytes, urine analysis for proteinuria and 24-hour creatinine clearance.

The psychological evaluation comprised a questionnaire regarding their attitude towards life in general and organ donation in particular, their current relationship with their respective recipients and other family members, their views on their own current health and their ability to continue their previous occupation. The questionnaire also included their views on organ donation during life and after death. The data were assessed and compared to the pre-nephrectomy status.

Results

The 30 kidney donors assessed in this study had nephrectomy 6—11 years previously (mean 8 years). The mean age at the time of assessment was 45.4 ± 12.3 (range 31—66). The hematological, biochemical and urinalysis were within normal range and comparable to the pre-nephrectomy data (Table 1). General examination revealed no abnormality. Body weight and blood pressure were within normal range for age and sex. Examination of the nephrectomy scar revealed no residual tenderness with well-healed almost invisible scar in all donors except one who had developed a small keloid at the posterior part of scar.

All the donors were able to go back to their pre-nephrectomy employment without any difficulties. None of the donors regretted kidney donation and all said they would volunteer to donate their organs after death and that they would campaign for cadaveric organ donation. There was marked improvement in the family atmosphere in general and the donor continue to have heightened self-esteem following organ donation.

Discussion

Renal transplantation using either kidneys from living-related or cadaver donors

Table 1. Clinical and renal function parameters in living related donor before and 5+ years after nephrectomy ($n = 30$)

	Pre-nephrectomy mean × s.d. range	Post-nephrectomy (current values) mean × s.d. range
Donor age (years)	36 ± 15 (24—56)	45.4 ± 12.3 (31—66)
Body weight (kg)	73 ± 13 (55—115)	79 ± 14 (58—120)
Blood pressure (mm Hg):		
Systolic	123 ± 11 (96—150)	129 ± 13 (100—168)
Diastolic	75 ± 8 (60—90)	76 ± 8 (58—90)
HB (g/l)	144 ± 13 (117—177)	144 ± 13 (111—185)
Blood sugar	5.2 ± 0.6 (4.0—6.5)	5.4 ± 0.9 (3.5—8.7)
BUN (mmol/l)	4.6 ± 1.2 (2.8—6.2)	5.1 ± 1.2 (3.2—6.6)
Serum creat. (μmol/l)	89 ± 20 (44—141)	93 ± 19 (60—135)
Creat. clearance (ml/min)	104 ± 26 (30—155)	104 ± 24 (80—156)
Urine protein (mg/24 h)	37 ± 31 (13—155)	50 ± 35 (53—165)
Repeated urine cultures	Persistently sterile	Persistently sterile

is now regarded as the primary treatment for most of the chronic renal failure patients. Although, the introduction of cyclosporine in clinical organ transplantation has decreased the gap of 1-year graft survival between living-related (LRD) and cadaver donor transplantation, the long-term results, up to 10 years, remain significantly superior after LRD transplantation. There is also evidence that kidneys from living related donors are less susceptible to cyclosporine nephrotoxicity (6, 7). Additionally, living donor transplantation has been shown to benefit the donor psychologically and emotionally in that it enables him to help a loved one in critical need and raises his own self-esteem (5, 8).

There are however, a few disturbing reports regarding the development of hypertension, proteinuria and even renal failure in kidney donors which have ascribed to the phenomenon of hyperfiltration, although an underlying dormant renal disease many have played a role in their pathogenesis (3, 4, 11). There is no correlation between protein intake and current proteinuria and creatinine clearance, an increased dietary protein intake is reported to result in a significant rise in both serum creatinine and creatinine clearance (12). Following uninephrectomy, there is an initial fall in glomerular filtration rate following which there is hypertrophy and adaptive increase due to hypertrophy and increased glomerular filtration which is complete in 3—4 weeks (9, 10).

In the current study, in 30 kidney donors who underwent uninephrectomy for a mean period of 8 years, there was no deleterious effect detectable with regard to nephrectomy site, blood pressure, proteinuria or renal function. All these donors were happy that they could help their loved ones and none regretted donation. In addition, the process of donation had resulted in a more positive attitude favoring towards organ donation, both in life and after death, in themselves, their immediate family members, friends and relatives. There was a stronger kinship, not only between the donor and recipient, but also within the family as a whole following kidney donation.

Although the number of kidney donors who could be evaluated 5 years or more after nephrectomy is too small to draw any definitive conclusion regarding the long-term effects of uninephrectomy, these findings indicate that at least in the intermediate terms, kidney donation does not have any deleterious effect on the donors or on the function of the remaining kidney. The findings also confirm previous studies that renal hypertrophy compensates adequately for the loss of the opposite kidney.

We recommend that live related kidney donation within the family should be encouraged provided that donor selection protocols are rigorous and complete and that periodic medical evaluation of donors is carried out following nephrectomy.

References

1. Living related kidney donors (editorial). *Lancet* **2**, 696 (1982).
2. Bay, W.H. and Herbert L.A.: The living donor in kidney transplantation. *Ann. Internal Med.* **106**, 719 (1987).
3. Hakim, R.M., Goldszer, R.C. and Brenner, B.M.: Hypertension and Proteinuria: long term sequalae of uninephrectomy in humans. *Kidney Int.* **25** (6), 930 (1984).
4. Zucchelli, P. and Cagnoli, L.: Proteinuria and hypertension after unilateral nephrectomy. *Lancet* **2**, 212 (1985) (letter).
5. John, P.J., Kumar, M.S.A., Samhan, M. and Abouna, G.M.: A series of 100 consecutive renal donors. In: G.M. Abouna (ed.), *Current Status of Clinical Organ Transplantation*, pp. 163—173. Martinus Nijhoff, The Hague (1984).
6. Canadian Transplant Study Group: Examination of parameters influencing the benefit detriment ratio of cyclosporine in renal transplantation. *Amer. J. Kidney Dis.* **5**, 328 (1985).
7. Kumar, M.S.A., Sahman, M., John, P. and Abouna, G.M.: Chronic cyclosporine nephrotoxicity — Is it the effect of preservation? *Transplant. Proc.* **21** (1), 1552—1553 (1989).
8. Kamstra-Hennen, L., Beebe, J., Stenin, S. and Simons, R.G.: Ethical evaluation of related donation: the donor after 5 years. *Transplant. Proc.* **13** (1), 60 (1981).
9. Flanigan, W.J., Burns, R.O., Takacs, F.J. *et al.*: Serial studies of glomerular filtration rate and renal plasma flow in kidney transplant donors, identical twins and allograft recipients. *Amer. J. Surg.* **116**, 788 (1968).
10. Boner, G., Sherp, W.S., Newton, M. *et al.*: Factors influencing the increase in glomerular filtration rate in the remaining kidney of transplant donors. *Amer. J. Med.* **55**, 169 (1973).
11. Tapson, J.S.: End Stage renal failure after donor nephrectomy. *Nephron* **42**, 262 (1986).
12. Cassidy, M.J.D. and Beck, R.M.: Renal function reserve in live related kidney donors. *Amer. J. Kidney Dis.* **9** (6), 468 (1988).

31. Current techniques for permanent vascular access surgery — experience with 930 procedures

S. AL-DADAH, M. KALAWI, M. SAMHAN, P. JOHN,
M.S.A. KUMAR and G.M. ABOUNA

Introduction

Successful construction and maintenance of satisfactory long-term vascular access is the single-most challenging surgical procedure carried out for patients with end-stage renal disease requiring chronic hemodialysis. The Brescia-Cimino fistula between radial artery and cephalic vein at the wrist was described in 1966 and has remained the primary vascular procedure of choice for hemodialysis in most patients (1). When it is not possible to construct this fistula or after a failure of such a fistula, secondary vascular access procedures may have to be carried out which include Brachio cephalic fistula at the elbow, or the use of arterio venous grafts (2—5). The Kuwait Transplant Team has been actively involved in the construction and modification of vascular accesses for the past 10 years.

We describe our experience with the construction of 930 consecutive vascular accesses, procedures, outlining possible complications and their management and indicating the methods of maintaining patency over prolonged periods of 5 to 10 years.

Patients and methods

Between March 1979 to February 1990, 930 chronic vascular access surgical procedures were carried out on patients aged 7—75 years with end-stage renal disease requiring hemodialysis. Arterio venous fistulas were constructed in 730 patients and arterio venous grafts in 200.

Table 1 shows the site and type of the vascular access procedures. All patients were carefully interviewed and examined so as to choose the best type and site for vascular access. The surgical procedure was carried out using local infiltration anaesthesia with 1% Lignocaine. In children and anxious patients, additional intravenous sedation was used. The technique of fistula-construction was carried out using a standard procedure as previously described (6). An Arterio venous fistula was carried out using 6/0 prolene suture after mobilizing

Table 1. Type of vascular access.

Type of access	No.	%
End-to-side Radio-cephalic fistula	593	64
Side-to-side Radio-cephalic fistula	71	7.5
End-to-side Upper arm brachial fistula	66	7.0
Gore-Text Vascular grafts	163	17.5
Bovine heterograft	37	4
Total	930	100

a sufficient length of artery and vein. In an end-to-side fistula, the vein distal of the fistula was ligated to prevent hand edema. The fistula was allowed to mature for 2 to 3 weeks before use for chronic hemodialysis. Arterio venous grafts were constructed using polytetra fluroethylene (PTFE) (Goretex) vascular grafts. Bovine heterografts were used initially in 37 patients but this was discontinued in 1984 with the availability of PTFE synthetic grafts. The arterio venous grafts were placed mostly in the upper arm, between the brachial artery at the elbow and axillary vein at the axilla, and in few cases in the forearm between the radial artery at the wrist and the ante cubital vein at the elbow. In three patients, who had no suitable sites in the upper limb, the graft was placed subcutaneously in the thigh between the femoral artery at mid thigh and the sephenous vein at the groin. All these grafts were straight grafts, with a diameter of 5 to 8 mm depending on the size of the patient and the diameter of the blood vessels.

The patients were assessed periodically with regard to their patency and complications, if any. The follow-up period is 1—10 years. The patency rate is expressed as immediate at 1 month, then 6 months and yearly up to 5 years. The results were analysed statistically using student's '*t*' test, the life table method and chi square.

Results

The immediate patency rate for arteriovenous fistulae was 92 to 97%, depending on the site and type of fistula. The immediate and long-term patency rate of end-to-side and side-to-side RC fistulae are shown in Table 2. End-to-side fistulae have a much better patency rate at 5 years ($P = 0.01$). Table 3 also shows the patency rate for Brachio—Cephalic (BC) end-to-side fistulas.

Table 2. Cumulative patency of fistulae.

Type of access	No.	Patency rate 1 mo	6 mo	1 yr	2 yr	3 yr	4 yr	5 yr
End to side forearm RC	593	96%	92%	88%	85%	83%	81%	80%[a]
Side to side forearm RC	71	92%	82%	78%	75%	72%	70%	60%[a]
End to side upper arm BC	66	97%	94%	91%	84%	78%	75%	73%
Total	730	96%	92%	88%	85%	82%	80%	78%

Patient death counted as failures.
RC = Radio Cephalic. BC = Brachio Cephalic.
[a] $P = 0.01$.

Table 3. Cumulative patency.

Type of access	No.	Patency rate 1 mo	6 mo	1 yr	2 yr	3 yr	4 yr	5 yr
Brescia–Cimino fistula	730	96%	92%	88%	85%	82%	80%	78%
Gore-Tex vascular graft	163	93%	84%	77%	70%	65%	62%	60%[a]
Bovine heterograft	37	92%	81%	73%	67%	59%	54%	48%[a]

Patient death counted as failures.
[a] $P = 0.01$.

The immediate and long-term patency rate for arterio venous grafts is shown in Table 3, where the overall patency rate of arterio venous fistulas is also shown for comparative study.

The early failure rate and complications such as hematoma and infection occurring within one month, were considered to be technical problems, while clotting, varices, aneursysmal formation, steel syndrome occurring after 6 months and late infection were considered as complications due to dialysis procedures. The early and late complications of various types of vascular accesses are shown in Table 4.

Over a follow-up period of five years, 84 fistula and 49 grafts were lost due to patient death and 29 spontaneously occluded after transplantation. In 48 patients (6.5%) the fistulas failed and in 21 (10.5%) the grafts failed, at 1 month to 10 years. Of the 48 patients with failed fistulas, 32 received arterio venous grafts and 16 were converted to peritoneal dialysis. Of the 21 patients with failed grafts, 12 had received secondary grafts on the contralateral side and nine were converted to peritoneal dialysis.

The other complications of vascular access included distal oedema of limbs, varices, aneurysmal dilatation of the veins, steel syndrome, chronic dermatitis/ infection at the fistula site. The incidence of these complications with regard to different vascular accesses is shown in Tables 4, 5 and 6.

Discussion

Today, the Brescia-Cimino fistula remains the primary choice for hemodialysis vascular access (1). However, when this procedure fails or is not possible to construct due to technical reasons, several secondary procedures have been resorted to, such as sephanous vein graft, bovine carotid artery heterograft and, recently, polytetra fluoroetheylene (PTFE) synthetic grafts (2—4). The early success rate for a Brescia-Cimino fistula was reported to be 89—94% and long-term patency at three years 82—89% (5—8). In our study, it is 83% for an end-to-side fistula.

The Brachio cephalic fistula is recommended as a secondary procedure, but it has the advantage over arterio venous grafts in that it is a simple procedure and avoids graft implantation. The reported overall patency rate is 70, 57 and 50% at one, two and three years respectively (9). In this series, it was 78% at three years.

Since its introduction, the PTFE synthetic graft has been widely used as a secondary or tertiary vascular access procedure for hemodialysis (4). The patency rates are reported to be 73—84% at two years (9, 10). However, the incidence of complications such as thrombosis, infection, pseudoaneurysm formation and stenosis of the graft at the venous anastomosis are reported to be much higher (11, 12). In this series, the patency rate was 65% at three years and the late complications rate 39%.

Currently, bovine heterografts and sephenous vein grafts are not commonly used as the incidence of complications are even higher compared to PTFE grafts (13, 14). In this study, it was 51%.

In the current series of 930 vascular access procedures carried out at our Centre, the Brescia-Cimino fistula remains the primary procedure and accounts for 71% of all cases. The procedure is simple, the fistula is well tolerated by the patients with minimal complications and preferred by nursing and medical staff carrying out hemodialysis. The Brachio cephalic fistula was initiated in our Centre in 1984 and forms 7% of all the vascular access surgery. This procedure is usually carried out as a secondary procedure and, in a very small number of patients, as a primary procedure when a Brescia-Cimino fistula cannot be constructed due to technical reasons.

Initially and until 1982, we were using bovine heterografts but since PTFE

Table 4. Complications of Brescia–Cimino fistula.

		Early (surgical)				Late (due to HD)							
Type of Access	No.	Clotting	Haematoma	Infection	Total (%)	Clotting	Oedema	Varices	Aneurysm	Steel syndrome	Infection	Total failure	(%)
End-to-side:													
Radiocephalic	593	22	3	2	4.5	88	—	2	3	1	1	110	18.5
Brachiocephalic	66	2	1	1	6.0	15	1	5	4	1	1	17	10.6
Side-to-side:													
Radiocephalic	71	5	—	—	7.0	16	—	3	1	—	—	21	29.5
Total	730	29	4	3	4.9	119	1	10	8	2	2	148	20.2

NB: Deaths were counted as late clotting.

Table 5. Complications Gore-Tex grafts.

Type of Access	No.	Early (surgical)				Late (due to HD)						Total failure	(%)
		Clotting	Haematoma	Infection	Total (%)	Clotting	Oedema	Varices	Aneurysm	Steel syndrome	Infection		
Upper Arm	144	10	4	1	10.4	41	3	2	5	3	5	51	35
Forearm	17	2	1	—	17.6	10	—	—	—	—	2	12	70
Lower Limb	3	—	1	—	33.3	1	—	—	—	—	1	1	
Total	163	12	6	1	11.6	52	3	2	5	3	8	64	39

NB: Deaths were counted as late clotting.

Table 6. Complications bovine heterografts.

Type of Access	No.	Early (surgical)				Late (due to HD)							
		Clotting	Haematoma	Infection	Total (%)	Clotting	Oedema	Varices	Aneurysm	Steel syndrome	Infection	Total failure	(%)
Upper Arm	33	2	2	1	15.1	15	2	1	7	1	1	17	51.5
Forearm	3	1	—	—	33.3	1	—	—	—	—	1	2	66.6
Lower Limb	1	—	—	—	—	—	—	—	—	—	—	—	—
Total	37	3	2	1	16.2	16	2	1	7	1	2	19	51.3

NB: Deaths were counted as late clotting.

synthetic grafts became available, we have discontinued bovine heterografts as the incidence of complications were high and the long-term patency rates were inferior compared to PFFE grafts. These arteriovenous grafts contribute 22% of the hemodialysis vascular access procedures in our Center.

The patency rate for both fistulas and arterio venous graft in the current series is excellent because of our selection of patients with regard to their suitability to the various types, sites and configurations of the vascular access procedure. The Brescia-Cimino fistula was preferred but was not a mandatory primary procedure. In some patients, an arteriovenous graft was carried out as a primary procedure in the absence of a suitable vein or artery for the construction of a fistula.

Our study indicates that in the majority of patients with end-stage renal disease requiring chronic hemodialysis, the Brescia-Cimino arterio venous fistula is the primary vascular procedure because immediate and long-term patency rates remain excellent with little or few complications. The Brachio cephalic fistula should be considered in the absence of suitable blood vessels in the forearm, as it is simple and effective. Synthetic arterio venous grafts (PTFE) are currently the most suitable and available for hemodialysis vascular access. They are inferior with regard to the long-term patency rates as compared to arterio venous fistulas, and have a higher rate of complications.

For optimal results we recommend proper selection of vascular access to suit the individual needs of the patient, meticulous surgical techniques and hemodialysis procedures.

References

1. Brescia, M.J., Cimino, J.E., Appel, K. and Hurirch, B.J.: Chronic haemodialysis using venepuncture and a surgically created arteriovenous fistula. *N. Engl. J. Med.* **275**, 1089–1092 (1966).
2. May, J., Tiller, D., Johnson, J., Stewart, J. and Shiel, A.G.R.: Saphenous vein arteriovenous fistula in regular dialysis treatment. *N. Engl. J. Med.* **280**, 770 (1969).
3. Chinitz, J.L., Yokoyama, T., Bower, R. and Swartz, C.: Self sealing prosthesis for arteriovenous fistula in man. *Trans. Amer. Soc. Artificial Internal Organs* **1**, 452–455 (1972).
4. Jerkins, A.Mcl.: Gore-tex. A new prosthesis for vascular access. *Br. Med. J.* **2**, 280 (1976).
5. Limet, R.R. and Lejeune, G.N.: Evaluation of 100 subcutaneous arteriovenous fistulae in 100 chronically haemodialysed patient. *J. Cardiovasc. Surg. (Torino)* **15** 573–576 (1974).
6. Dadah, S.K., Samhan, M., Omar, O.F. and Abouna, G.M.: Permanent vascular access for hemodialysis. In: *Current Status of Clinical Organ Transplantation.* G.M. Abouna (ed.), Martinus Nijhoff, The Hague (1984), pp. 147–153.
7. Cohn, H.E. and Solit, R.W.: Arteriovenous fistulas for chronic haemodialysis, *Surg. Clin. North Amer.* **53**, 673–684 (1973).
8. Zerbino, V.R., Tice, D.A., Katz, L.A. and Nidus, B.D.: A 6 year clinical experience with arteriovenous fistulas and bypasses for haemodialysis. *Surgery* **76**(6), 1018–1023 (1974).
9. Dunlop, M.G., Mackinlay, J.Y. and Jenkins, M.: vascular access: Experience with the brachiocephalic fistula. *Ann. Coll. Surg. Engl.* **68**(4), 203–206 (1986).
10. Chatterjee, S.N.: Use of Goretex grafts as vascular access procedure for chronic haemodialy-

sis. Abstract of a paper submitted to the European Society for Artificial Organs Eighth Annual Meeting, Copenhagen, 1981.
11. Anderson, C.B., Sicard, G.A. and Etheredge, E.E.: Bovine carotid artery and expanded polytetrafluorethylene grafts for haemodialysis vascular access. *J. Surg. Res.* **29**, 184—188 (1980).
12. Ziberi, G.B., Rohr, M.S., Landreneau, M.D., Bridges, R.M., DeVault, G.A., Pelty, F.H., Costley, K.J., Brown, S.T. and McDonald, J.C.: Complication from permanent hemodialysis vascular access. *Surgery (United States)* **104**(4), 681—686 (1988).
13. Rizzuti, R.P., Hale, J.C. and Burkart, T.E.: Extended patency of expanded polytetra fluoroethylene grafts for vascular access using optimal configuration and revisions, *Surg. Gynecol. Obstet. (United States)* **166**(1), 23—27 (1988).
14. Butler, H.G., Baker, L.D. and Johnson, J.M.: Vascular access for chronic haemodialysis. Polytetrafluorethylene (PTFE) versus bovine heterograft. *Amer. J. Surg.* **134**(6), 791—793 (1977).
15. Owens, M.L., Stabile, B.E., Gahr, J.A. and Wilson, S.E.: Vascular grafts for haemodialysis: an evaluation of sites and materials. *Dialysis Transplant.* **8** (5), 521—530, (1979).

32. Results of 319 consecutive renal transplants from living related and living unrelated donors in Iran

A.J. GHODS, I. FAZEL, B. NIKBIN, K. RAHBAR, E. ABDI,
H.N. GHASHTI and F. PROOSHANI

Introduction

Chronic hemodialysis started in Iran in 1967. In 1967 an End Stage Renal Disease (ESRD) office was established in the Ministry of Health to cover dialysis expenses for all patients throughout the country (1). The result was that the rate of acceptance of new dialysis patients steadily increased from 179 (5.3 per million) in 1976 to 1060 (21 per million) in 1989. The total number of dialysis patients also rose during this period. At the end of 1980 a total of 700 patients (16 per million) were being dialysed throughout the country, which increased to a total case load of 3100 (62 per million) patients by the end of 1989.

Renal transplantation programs were severely lagging behind in growth, in comparison to hemodialysis activity until 1985. Between 1967 and 1984 only 100 renal transplants had been performed (2). In 1985 the costly hemodialysis program prompted health authorities to encourage renal transplantation. In the last 4 years (1985—1989) 8 renal transplant facilities have been organized and over 850 renal transplants have been performed since. Of these transplants, 319 have been carried out at the Hashemi Nejad Kidney Center between April 1986 and October 1989.

Patients and methods

Of 319 recipients, 213 were male and 106 female. Their age range was 8—68 years. The majority of the grafts, (242) 76% were from LRD (HLA identical, 66; one haplomatch, 168; two haplomismatch, 8) and the remaining (77) 24% from LUD. Selection of recipients and suitable donors was based on a complete clinical, immunological and psychological investigation as well as appropriate laboratory tests and X-rays. All recipients had at least three previous random blood transfusions, 10% having had donor-specific transfusions. Highly sensitized patients who had positive crossmatch test with donor and or high panel cell reactivities were excluded. For all donors true voluntarism of the consent was assessed by a 'Donor Assessment Panel' consisting of transplant surgeon, nephrologist, immunologist and members of nursing staff. Person to person talk was held between panel members and donors at weekly meetings to exclude any possibility of outside pressure being exerted for kidney donation (3).

For immunosuppression cyclosporine was given twice daily at a dose of 4 mg/kg/day. Which was reduced or stopped completely when acute rejection or acute renal failure appeared. Prednisone was started at a dose of 60mg/day, which was tapered gradually to 15 mg/day in 4 weeks and 7.5 mg/day in 6 weeks. Azathioprine was given at a dose of 1.5 mg/kg/day. This was reduced or stopped if the total peripheral white blood count fell below 5000. All patients were also given prophylactic intravenous methylprednisolone at a dose of 1 gm/day for the first 3 postoperative days. Triple therapy with cyclosporine, azathioprine and prednisone was used in 279 patients and conventional therapy in 40 (mostly HLA identical) patients. Antirejection therapy consisted of methylprednisolone 1 gm daily for 3—5 days and plasmaphresis in patients who developed postoperative positive crossmatch tests or high panel cell reactivities.

Results

Patient and graft survival rates in 319 renal transplants are shown in Figure 1. In 18 recipients with a follow-up of more than 3 years, the patient survival rates were 94, 89 and 89% and the graft survival rates 89 and 83% in years 1, 2, 3, respectively. In 95 recipients of more than 2 years follow-up, patient survival rates were 95 and 93% and graft survival rates 92 and 81% at years 1 and 2, respectively. In 209 recipients with more than 1 year follow-up, the patient

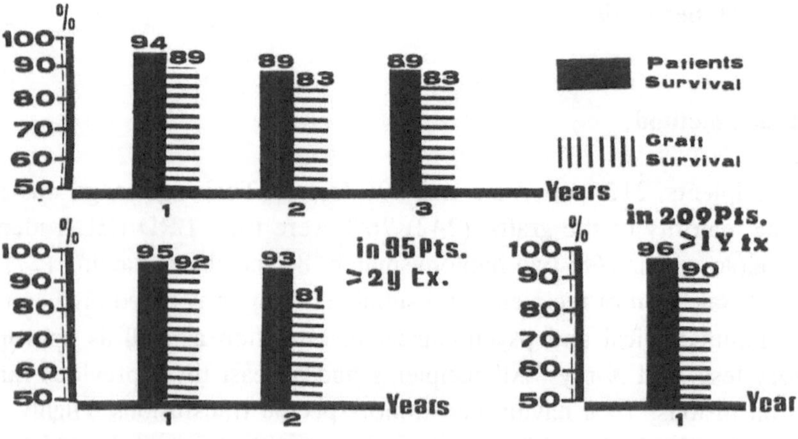

Fig. 1. Patient and graft survival in 319 renal transplantations.

survival was 96% and graft survival 90%. Of a total of 319 recipients (with a follow-up range 1—43 months), 270 (84%) have functioning grafts. Thirty-four patients (11%) have returned to dialysis and 15 (5%) are dead. The causes of death in 15 recipients were: sepsis or pneumonia in 12 cases, gastrointestinal bleeding in 2 cases and C.V.A. in 1 case.

Of 319 renal transplants, 77 have been from LUD, carried out between February 1988 and October 1989. The patient and graft survival rates in these 77 transplants are shown in Figure 2. In 30 recipients who had more than 1 year follow-up, the patient survival was 100% and graft survival 93%. In 52 of these with more than 6 months follow up, patient survival was 98% and graft survival 90%.

In Figure 3, the 1-year patient and graft suvival rates in LRD and LUD transplants, are compared. The 1-year patient survival rate in recipients with LUD, are similar to those with HLA-identical donors, and better than those with one haplomatch LRD. This findings seemed to be due to an increase experience of the transplant team or what is known as the center effect. A comparison of the results of the first 100 and the second 100 consecutive renal transplants are shown in Table 1. In the second 100 consecutive renal transplant cases, however, the number of grafts from LUD increased from 0 to 25%, but one-year patient survival rate improved significantly from 93 to 99%, which is apparently due to the center effect.

Discussion

The first renal transplantation was carried out in Iran 22 years ago. There have been serious problems hindering further development and progression of renal

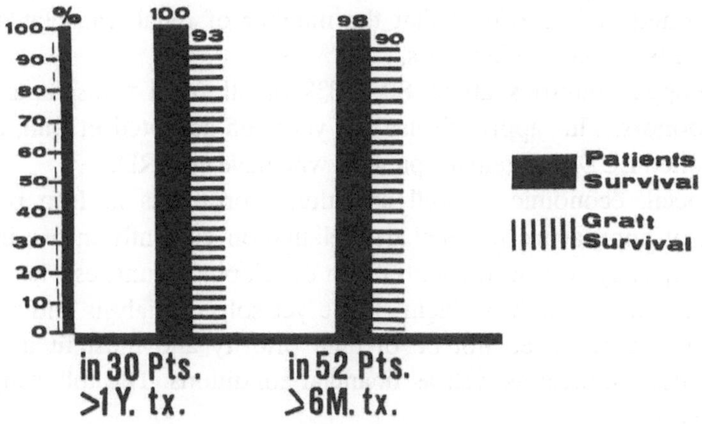

Fig. 2. Patient and graft survival rates in unrelated live donor transplantation.

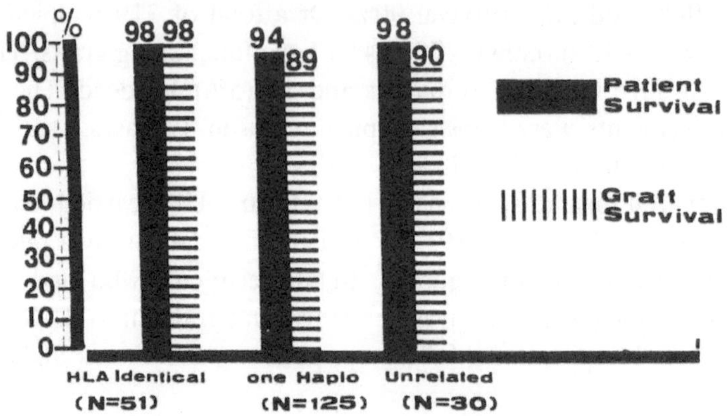

Fig.3. One-year patient and graft survival in live related and unrelated renal transplants.

Table 1. Dialysis and renal transplantation activities in Iran (1979—1989).

	1979—1984	1985—1989
New dialysis patients/year	260—646	649—1016
Total No. of dialysis patients	700—1655	1655—3100
Total No. of transplants	100	850

transplantation until 1985. With the introduction of cyclosporine and improvement of results of organ transplantation the public demand for renal transplantation increased, and health authorities realized that treatment of ESRD by transplantation is much more cost effective. In the last 4 years the renal transplantation programs were fostered and over 850 renal transplants have been performed. It is expected that the number of renal transplantations will steadily increase in the coming years.

In developed countries about 80—90% of all renal transplants are from cadaveric donors. This approach has not yet been accepted in Iran, necessitating a controlled LUD program for patients who have no LRD.

Basic social, economic as well as cultural problems in Iran prevent the adaptation of approaches to renal transplantation currently in use in Western and technologically advanced countries. In developing countries where there are fundamental public health problems to be yet solved, dialysis and renal transplantation programs, need not be of high priority and must fit in with their social, cultural, political as well as financial conditions. The following must be further explored:

1. Factors holding down development of cadaveric transplantation in Iran.

2. Main reasons we use living unrelated donors.
3. Characteristics of our accepted LUD.

The important factors hindering development of cadaveric transplantation in Iran are :

1. Brain death as a human death has not been legally accepted.
2. We have no legislation to allow cadaveric transplantation.
3. There is religious and strong cultural reluctance of the society to accept cadaveric organ donation.

The main reasons for our use of living unrelated donors are:

1. We believe that cadaveric transplantation will not be a reality in Iran in the near future.
2. A large number of our dialysis patients needing transplants have no LRD.
3. In the last 10 years only about 100 Iranian dialysis patients could afford cadaveric transplantation in foreign countries, and few could buy live donor kidneys from India.
4. On the other hand, we have a large number of LUD with true voluntarism.
5. Superior results of these grafts to cadaveric kidneys (4).

The characteristic of our accepted LUD are:

1. True voluntarism of donors has always been explored by our donor assessment panel.
2. The different categories are: spouse to spouse, 2nd degree relatives, friend to friend and person to person. Obviously in the last category there is a role for rewarding gifts.
3. There is no commercialization, no agencies, no middle-man and no coercion among our accepted LUD.
4. Many low-income patients have also been transplanted from LUD.
5. Transplantation from LUD has been on our low priority list (longer waiting list) as compared to transplants from LRD.

The renal transplantation activity will further increase in the coming years. Besides the increasing number of transplants performed, the results obtained are also encouraging.

Another significant finding has been the center effect, which appear in our second 100 consecutive transplant results. The center size has known to have an important effect on the improvement of the results of transplantation. According to EDTA statistics the results of transplantation in centers transplanting over 50 cases a year have been much better than the results of units with a transplant rate of 10—24 grafts per year (5). Having small satellite dialysis units may be a viable concept, but we believe that kidney transplantation should be concentrated in large and experienced centers.

Acknowledgement

The authors acknowledge the help of Miss Agnes Gilana who provided secretarial assistance.

References

1. Ghods, A.J. and Abdi, E.: Dialysis and renal transplantation in Iran. In: M.A. Haberal (ed.), *Chronic Renal Failure and Transplantation*, pp. 103—108. Semith Offset, Turkey (1987)
2. Ghods, A.J., Taghavi, M. and Fazel, I.: Dialysis and renal transplantation in Iran — 1988. In: M.A. Haberal (ed.), *Recent Advances in Nephrology and Transplantation*, pp. 49—55. H.E.V., Turkey (1990).
3. Land, W.: The problem of living organ donation: facts, thoughts, and reflections. *Transplant. Int.* **2**, 168—179 (1989).
4. Abouna, G.M., Kumar, M.S.A. *et al.*: Experience with the first 500 renal transplants in Kuwait (abstract). *The 2nd Int. Congress of the Middle East Society for Organ Transplantation, March 1990 Kuwait* (1990).
5. Jacobs, C., Broyer, M., Brunner, F.P. *et al.*: (1981) Combined report on Regular Dialysis and Transplantation in Europe, XI, 1980, *Proc. Eur. Dial. Transplant. Assoc.* **18**, 4 (1981).

33. Liver transplantation: current status

ROBERT D. GORDON

I have been asked to address the current status of liver transplantation. To understand the current state of the art in this field, one must appreciate what has gone on before, so building on the historical foundation which Dr Lee has provided, I will review with you from a historical perspective where we are today in liver transplantation. I have been greatly assisted by and relied heavily on earlier reviews of the history of developments in liver transplantation provided by my mentor, the man who has paved the path for all working in this field, Thomas Starzl (1).

The first known attempts at experimental orthotopic liver transplantation were reported by Jack Cannon in the *Transplantation Bulletin* in 1956. It was a very brief paper without a title or a description of methods and no animals survived.

In June, 1958 independent programs in experimental orthotopic liver transplantation were begun at the Peter Bent Brigham Hospital in Boston under the leadership of Francis Moore and at Northwestern University in Chicago by Tom Starzl. These early experiences in Boston and Chicago developed the technical approaches to liver replacement, provided the first descriptions of liver graft rejection in the unmodified host, and established the importance of core cooling to preserve donor organ viability. Eventually, using immunosuppression with azathioprine and ALS or ALG chronic survival was achieved by Starzl in mongrel dogs, of which one lived for almost 12 years.

In 1965 Henri Garnier of Paris reported that rejection of liver allografts in the pig was mild compared to dogs and he achieved survival of an animal for more than 35 days without immunosuppression. His observations were soon confirmed by workers in Bristol and Cambridge in England and in Denver. Cable has frequently demonstrated the value of studies of liver transplantation in pigs. Many of his extensive studies of immunology, organ preservation, and hepatic physiology were done using the pig model.

Clinical liver transplantation

Two kinds of transplantation have been attempted clinically — orthotopic transplanation with complete removal of the native host liver and ectopic transplantation of an auxiliary liver. By far, orthotopic transplantation has been the preferred procedure, but much has been learned from experience with the auxiliary method and there has been some renewed interest in auxiliary grafting in the last few years (2).

The first effort to replace the human liver was taken in March 1963 by Starzl at the University of Colorado in Denver. The patient, a 3-year-old boy with biliary atresia, died because of excessive bleeding from venous collaterals and a coagulopathy. Two more transplants were attempted in the next 4 months. The patients lived 22 and 7½ days respectively.

The first 3 Denver cases were reported in 1963. In September 1963 and January 1964 similarly unsuccessful attempts were made in Boston and in Paris. These failures ended clinical trials in liver transplantation for three years. The operation seemed too difficult for practical application, the methods of organ preservation were inadequate, and the immunosuppression available was too primitive.

The sixth and seventh attempts in Denver on October 1966 and May 1967 also failed. Finally, in July 1967, the first extended survival was achieved. A 1½-year-old girl with hepatocellular cancer survived for more than 13 months after transplantation before dying of metastases. In May 1968 Calne and Williams in England treated the first patient in their collaborative program and went on to generate a series of 125 cases.

Thus began the first phase of clinical human liver transplantation which enjoyed limited success through the 1970's: 170 patients were eventually given transplants by Starzl in the Denver series between 1963 and 1980, but 1-year survival remained limited to 33% and 5-year survival was less than 20%. Only 55 patients survived 1 year, but 27 of those patients are still living today. The longest survivor, given a liver transplant at the age of 3 for biliary atresia, is now 20 years since transplantation.

Progress in liver transplantation in the 1980s has been dramatic and can be attributed to developments in several critical areas: immunosuppression, intraoperative management, organ preservation, and improvements in postoperative care.

Immunosuppression

Liver transplantation has followed closely behind the advances in immunosuppression for renal transplantation. Starzl's regimen of double drug therapy with azathioprine and steroids remained the foundation of clinical practice in transplantation for more than 20 years. The introduction of lymphoid depletion by the use of antilymphocyte serum or globulin was a significant advance and such triple drug therapy was used in most liver transplant recipients during 1968–1979. Thoracic duct drainage was also used effectively in Denver but was cumbersome and hazardous. There remained also a significant rate of delayed rejection after discontinuance of ALG or thoracic duct drainage.

The methods used in renal transplantation during this period to circumvent the limitations of available immunosuppression by exploiting developments in tissue typing or by preoperative conditioning of prospective recipients with blood transfusions, were not practical considerations for liver transplantation.

The experimental studies by Borel and the first clinical trials by Calne and associates with cyclosporine A opened up a new era in solid organ transplantation. The most exciting aspect of this groundbreaking work was the observation that almost half of the organ recipients achieved lasting graft function with no agent other than cyclosporine. On the other hand, 10% of their recipients developed lymphomas, none of the recipients has truly normal graft function, and there was a significant patient mortality.

The lymphomas we now know are a complication of overimmunosuppression and Epstein-Barr virus infection and can be appropriately managed in most cases by reduction or temporary withdrawl of immunosuppression. The high mortality in the early series was a price often paid in learning to use a new drug. With increasing experience came a decrease in patient mortality.

The systematic and effective use of combination cyclosporine-steroid therapy in both renal and liver transplantation was begun by Starzl in 1980 in Denver and continued on a much larger scale after transfer of the program to Pittsburgh in 1981. One year patient survival after liver transplantation increased from 33% to 79% and there was an accompanying dramatic increase in caseload and a proliferation of new programs. The development of practical assays for measurements of cyclosporine blood levels has been particularly helpful in liver transplant recipients, since absorption of cyclosporine is unpredictable in the early period after liver transplantation and double route therapy is often required.

Although use of cyclosporine and steroids dramatically improve the graft and patient survival after liver transplantation, overall graft survival at 1 year was about 55% and 22% of the patients required retransplantation, most for uncontrolled rejection. An important advance came in 1981 when Cosimi and his colleagues at the MGH reported their experience with a monoclonal mouse antihuman T-cell antibody preparation, OKT3. Impressed by this report, Starzl began in Pittsburgh in 1984 an extensive trial of OKT3 in liver transplantation (2). In patients treated for steroid resistant acute cellular rejection, retransplantation was necessary in only 6.8% of the patients and 1-year graft survival was better than 75%. This was a significant improvement in both graft survival and the rate of retransplantation when compared to historical controls.

Problems, of course, still remain, including the chronic nephrotoxicity associated with long-term maintenance on cyclosporine, the danger of lymphoproliferative disease, especially in patients requiring heavier levels of therapy to control rejection, the ever present danger of opportunistic infection.

Technical improvements

There have been substantial improvements in the technique of liver transplantation. The biliary reconstruction has sometimes been considered to be the Achilles heel of the operation. In the first human cases, the graft common bile duct was anastomosed to the recipient duct over a T-tube stent. Unfortunately, this approach was abandoned for a time in favor of choledochoduodenostomy, an easier method that had worked well in dogs. However, in clinical use, the incidence of complications including obstruction, fistula, and cholangitis exceeded 30%. During the past decade the method of biliary reconstruction has been standardized and duct-to-duct reconstruction over a T-tube stent or Roux-en-Y choledochoduodenostomy are the procedures of choice. The rate of complications with both methods has been low and the reconstructions have proven to be durable.

When liver transplantation was developed in dogs, operative survival required use of passive veno-venous bypass to transport blood from the inferior vena cava and portal vein to the upper body and thereby to the heart while the venous systems were obstructed after removal of the native liver. Without such a bypass, the capillary beds in the dogs were ruined and the animals died.

Although liver transplantation in humans had for over a decade been performed without a bypass, it was clear that a heavy price was paid in many cases. The persistent venous hypertension during the anhepatic phase resulted in renal venous hypertension and an increased incidence of postoperative renal failure, congestion of the gut, increased bleeding from extensive high pressure venous collaterals in patients with chronic portal hypertension, and cardiodynamic instability. Volume preloading was often required to prior to clamping the portal vein and vena cava with subsequent volume overloading and pulmonary edema after restoration of flow. Deaths in the operating room, including the tragic loss of a teenaged boy in 1982, prompted Starzl to reassess the methodology and initiate an effort to develop a method for venous bypass.

For more than 5 years now, we have routinely used a centripetal force pump driven veno-venous bypass for liver transplantation in adults and larger children. The bypass was developed as a collaborative effort by the liver transplant and cardiac surgical teams in Pittsburgh in 1982 and 1983. It has contributed substantially to reducing operative mortality to under 1% and has permitted us to offer liver transplantation to higher risk patients, including many older patients (Figure 1) patients, who might otherwise have been unable to withstand the rigorous physiological demands of the operation.

Other recent technical advances include the improvements in monitoring a correction of coagulation disorder during surgery, the use of venous jump grafts to reconstruct an occluded recipient portal vein, techniques for reconstruction of multiple hepatic arteries and inadequate recipient hepatic arterial inflow, and the use of reduced and split liver grafts which Professor Broelsch will discuss in Chapter 37.

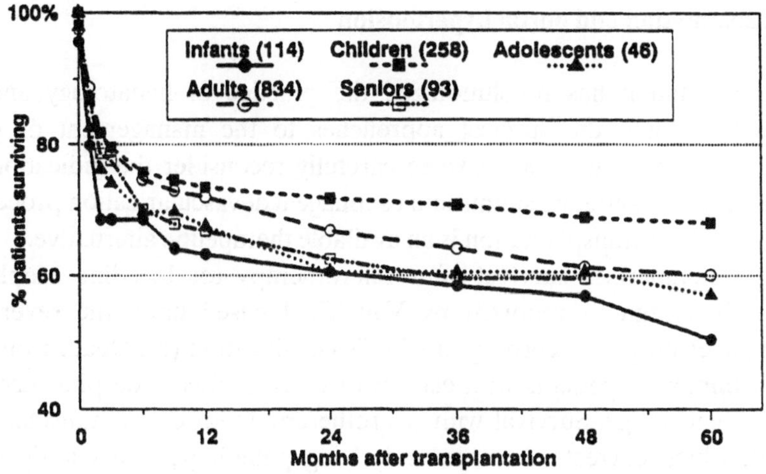

Fig. 1. Actuarial (life table method) patient survival after liver transplantation at the Univeristy of Pittsburgh based upon patient age at the time of transplantation.

Organ removal and preservation

Methods that provided the foundation for techniques of liver preservation used today were developed in Starzl's lab in Denver and Calne's laboratory in England. A major recent advance is development by Belzer and Southard of a new preservation solution which permits the liver to be stored safely well beyond the conventional 8 hour limit (4). I will discuss the development of the techniques for liver preservation and our experience with the 'UW solution' for liver preservation in Pittsburgh later in these proceedings.

Improvements in postoperative care

While there have been significant advances within transplantation itself, improvements in other areas of medical practice have also had an impact on transplantation. The widespread availability of reliable, non-invasive diagnostic tools such as ultrasonography, CT scanning, and magnetic resonance imaging have had great impact on patient management and prompt diagnosis of complications. New drugs such as acyclovir for herpes and Epstein-Barr virus and gancyclovir for cytomegalovirus, have been important additions to our medical armamentarium. Prophylactic Bactrim therapy has dramatically reduced the incidence of Pneumocystis carini pneumonia. Sophisticated critical care units and specialized personnel have advanced the care of our patients during the immediate recovery period after surgery.

Liver transplantation and portal hypertension

Liver transplantation has revolutionized the practice of hepatology and has forced us to rethink the surgical approaches to the management of portal hypertension. In particular, we have to carefully reconsider the indications for conventional porto-systemic shunts and esophageal devascularization procedures in an era when liver transplantation is an available therapeutic alternative.

Figure 2 summarizes survival after sclerotherapy for bleeding esophageal varices in Pittsburgh as reported by Van Thiel based upon the severity of underlying liver disease according to Child's classification (5). Death from liver failure is common in patients with class B or class C disease despite successful control of hemorrhage. Survival with sclerotherapy followed by transplantation (Figure 3), which corrects the true underlying pathology, offers a significant improvement in survival (6).

Shunting operations must be used more sparingly now that an effective alternative exists. Shunts such as the mesocaval shunt or distal splenorenal shunt which avoid the hepatic hilum are preferable.

Summary of current results

Since 1982, we have performed approximately 2000 liver transplantations in Pittsburg. Figure 1 presents patients survival rates (life table method) for infants (age under 2 years), children (age 2—11), adolescents (age 12—17), adults (age 18—59), and seniors (age 60 and above). Figure 4 and 5 present survival rates for the most common indications for liver replacement.

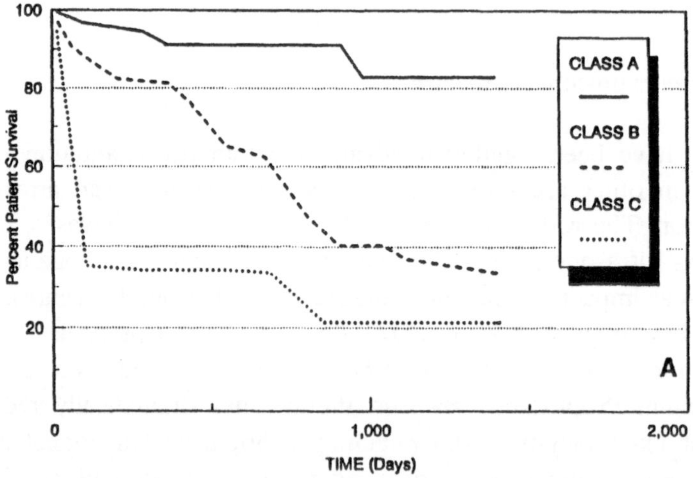

Fig. 2. Survival after esophageal sclerotherapy for variceal hemorrhage based upon the severity of underlying liver disease according to Child's classification (from reference (5)).

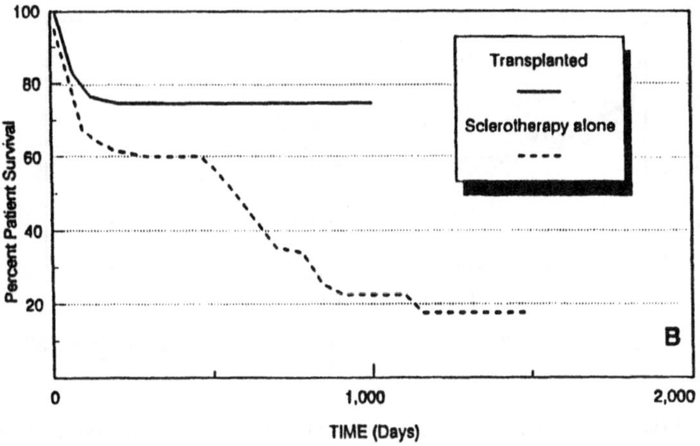

Fig. 3. Survival after esophageal sclerotherapy for variceal hemorrhage with sclerotherapy alone or followed by liver transplantation (from reference (6)).

Two groups of patients clearly stand apart. Patients with surface antigen positive B-virus chronic active hepatitis (HBsAg+) have a significant rate of recurrent infection and risk of recurrent liver disease. Despite this, approximately half of these patients achieve long term survival. Efforts to alter reinfection with passive and active immunization have had some success. A human monoclonal antibody directed against HBsAg has been developed by Sandoz by fusing peripheral blood lymphocytes from an immune adult human to a mouse × human myeloma cell. The resulting human monoclonal HBIgG is 50 000 times more potent than commercially available HBIgG prepared from the pooled serum of immune donors. Whether treatment with this agent can prevent

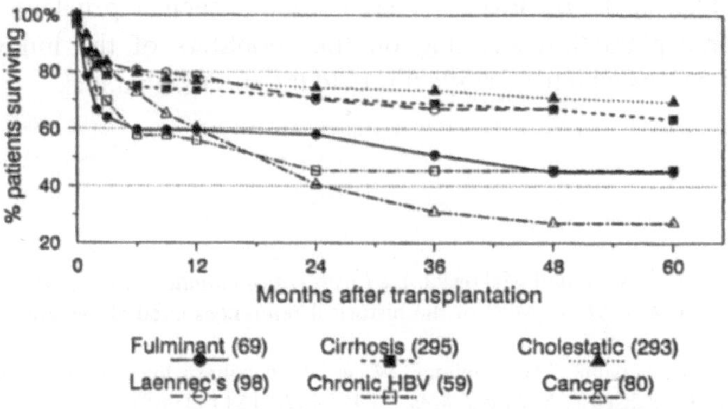

Fig. 4. Actuarial (life table method) patient survival after liver transplantation for fulminant hepatic failure, postnecrotic cirrhosis (excluding hepatitis B virus carriers), cholestatic liver disease (primary biliary cirrhosis, primary sclerosing cholangitis), Laennec's cirrhosis, chronic active B virus hepatitis, and primary hepatobiliary cancer at the University of Pittsburgh.

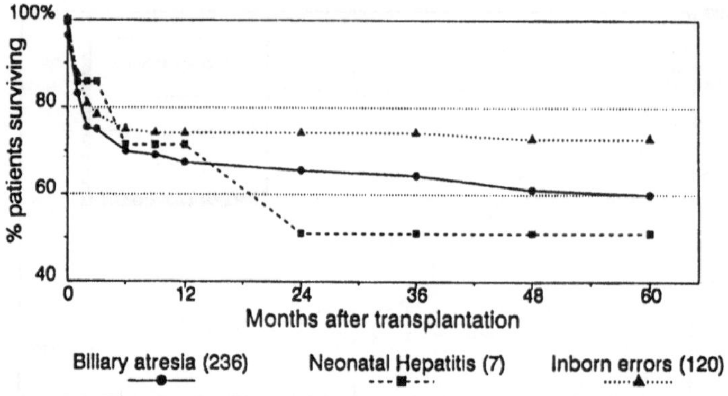

Fig. 5. Actuarial (life table method) patient survival after liver transplantation for biliary atresia, neonatal hepatitis, or inborn errors of metabolism at the Univeristy of Pittsburgh.

or alter the course of clinical reinfection after liver transplantation for HBV is the subject of current clinical trials in Pittsburgh.

Liver transplantation for cancer has been disappointing in every major reported series. Elsewhere in this volume, Dr Wood from Omaha will discuss the results of transplantation for cancer and I will discuss our initial experience in Pittsburgh with a surgical alternative — the cluster resection.

We can expect some significant advances in immunosuppression in the next few years with several new agents likely to be introduced into clinical practice. First among these is FK 506, a macrolide antibiotic that has shown great promise in early clinical trials conducted by Starzl in Pittsburgh (7). I will briefly review the Pittsburgh clinical experience with this agent later in this volume.

It is a very gratifying time to be a liver transplant surgeon. Although there are still many advances to be made, it has certainly been a privilege for me to practice in transplantation standing on the shoulders of the innovative and courageous pioneers who have made this field the success that it is.

References

1. Starzl, T.E., Groth, C.G. and Makowka, L.: *Liver Transplantation. Clio Chirugica.* Silvergirl, Inc., Austin, Texas (1988). (Most of the historical references cited above are reproduced in this volume.)
2. Terpestra, O.T., Schalm, S.W., Weimar, W. *et al.*: Auxiliary liver transplantation for end stage chronic liver disease. *N. Eng. J. Med.* **319**, 1507—1511 (1988).
3. Fung, J.J., Demetris, A.J., Porter, K.A. *et al.*: Use of OKT3 with cyclosporine and steroids for reversal of acute kidney and liver allograft rejection. *Nephron* **46** (Suppl. 1), 494—497 (1987).
4. Belzer, F.O.and Southard, J.H.: Principles of solid organ preservation by cold storage. *Transplantation* **45**, 673 (1988).

5. Garrett, K.O., Reilly, J.J., Schade, R. R. and Van Thiel, D.H.: Sclerotherapy of esophageal varices: long term results and determinants of survival. *Surgery* **104**, 813—818 (1988).
6. Garrett, K.O., Reilly, J.J., Schade, R.R. and Van Thiel, D.H.: Bleeding esophageal varices: treatment by sclerotherapy and liver transplantation. *Surgery* **104**, 819—823 (1988).
7. Second International Workshop on FK506: A potential breakthrough in immunosuppression — clinical implications. *Transplant. Proc.* **22**, 5—113 (1990).

34. An overview of liver transplantation therapy for children

R. PATRICK WOOD, BYERS W. SHAW JR, ROBERT J. STRATTA, ALAN N. LANGNAS and TODD J. PILLEN

Liver transplantation is a proven therapeutic modality for children with a variety of liver disease. At the present time the majority of centers performing pediatric liver transplantation report at least a 65% one-year survival rate. In this brief overview, the authors will review several selected areas in pediatric liver transplantation. These will include the selection and evaluation of patients for transplantation; the short- and long-term survival and follow-up of transplant recipients; and the future of liver transplantation for children. Purposely omitted are discussions of the preoperative preparation of the recipient and timing of the transplant, the transplant procedure, the immediate postoperative care of pediatric recipients, the various immunosuppressive protocols, and the management of the complications following pediatric liver transplantation. Other reviews are available which address these important areas in pediatric liver transplantation (1, 2, 3, 4).

Evaluation and selection of patients

As results have improved, the list of diagnoses for which children receive liver transplants has continued to grow. In most series, biliary atresia represents the most common diagnosis for pediatric recipients. Biliary atresia and the other congenital biliary ductal syndromes (biliary hypoplasia, Alagille's Syndrome) account for over 50% of children transplanted in most series (1—3, 5—10). The next most common indications for transplantation are inborn errors of metabolism followed by posthepatitic cirrhosis (including neonatal hepatitis) and a variety of other disorders including fulminant hepatic failure and primary hepatic malignancies.

Table 1 lists the major indications for the referral of a patient for transplantation. No matter what the underlying diagnosis any pediatric patient who demonstrates a life-threatening complication (hemorrhage from varices or portal hypertensive gastropathy, recurrent episodes of cholangitis) of acute or chronic liver disease despite aggressive management should be referred to consideration of transplantation. In treatment of life-threatening complications requiring

Table 1. Indication for referral for liver transplanation.

I.	*Life-threatening complications*
	A. Variceal hemorrhage
	B. Recurrent cholangitis
	C. Fulminant hepatic failure
II.	*Impaired quality of Life*
	A. Malnutrition
	B. Growth or developmental delay
	C. Encephalopathy
	D. Coagulopathy
	E. Hypersplenism

urgent transplantation, timely referral is the single most important factor to allow sufficient time to both locate a suitable donor liver and to optimize the patient's medical condition before transplantation.

A more difficult decision concerns the best time to refer children who experience complications which are not life-threatening but which impair the quality of the patient's life. Patients with recurrent episodes of encephalopathy, malnutrition, coagulopathy, or growth and developmental retardation should be considered candidates for transplantation. The precise timing of transplantation is difficult and requires close coördination between the referring physicians and the transplant center. With the improved results of transplantation it is unacceptable to allow children to continue to deteriorate until they suffer a life threatening complication prior to offering transplantation. Once the child has failed aggressive medical management and their quality of life is impaired by the underlying liver disease, transplantation is indicated. Put simply, there is nothing to be gained by waiting until a child is sicker before referring them for transplantation.

Pediatric liver diseases requiring transplantation

Biliary atresia

Before the initial reports of Kasai *et al.* (11, 12) on the use of a portoenterostomy procedure in the treatment of patients with biliary atresia, the average survival for patients with untreated biliary atresia was 18 months with survival rates of 4% at a 4 years (13, 14). Since the introduction of the portoenterostomy procedure, the outlook for obiliary atresia patients has brightened but despite a number of encouraging reports (15—25) the majority of patients are not cured following the performance of a portoenterostomy. Detailed studies of large

Table 2. Factors associated with a successful portoenterostomy.

Age:	
	Less than 90 days
Presence of bile flow following portoenterostomy:	
	Bile bilirubin concentration > 8.8mg/dl
	Excretion of > 6 mg bilirubin per day
	Bile clearance ratio (bile/serum bilirubin concentration)
Liver histology:	
	Large bile ducts/ductules in the hilum
	Absence of fibrosis
	Absence of giant cell transformation/parenchymal degeneration
Experience of the surgeon	
Technically adequate portoenterostomy procedure	

Source: Reference (30).

numbers of children undergoing portoenterostomies have identified certain factors (Table 2) which are associated with greater chance of success following the portoenterostomy (15—17, 21, 24—28). When these favorable characteristics are present, biliary drainage will be achieved in over 90% of patients. However, even in the most favorable group of patients, the majority of patients will eventually develop chronic liver disease despite good initial biliary drainage. Only 20—30% of patients with biliary atresia are cured by their portoenterostomy (15—19, 29).

In a recent report by Wood *et al.* (30) patients undergoing transplantation for biliary atresia were compared with patients receiving liver transplants for other liver diseases. Despite the fact that the patients with biliary atresia were younger, of a smaller size and had all undergone portoenterostomy procedures prior to transplantation, there were no significant differences between the two groups of patients in any of five intraoperative parameters compared (Table 3). A trend was noted in all of the intraoperative parameters for the transplant procedure to be somewhat more difficult in the biliary atresia patients. Statisti-

Table 3. Intraoperative parameters comparing biliary atresia vs non-biliary atresia patients.

Preparation time
Operation time
Total anesthesia time
Blood volume transfused
Ischemic time of donor liver

Source: Reference (30).

cally significant differences in all five operative parameters were identified when the biliary atresia patients who had undergone a portoenterostomy involving the creation of a stoma were compared with non-biliary atresia patients or other biliary atresia patients. The authors felt that while a single portoenterostomy procedure did not increase the risk of a subsequent liver transplant, those patients with biliary atresia who undergo multiple prior operative procedures, especially those which include the creation of a stoma, are more difficult to transplant from a technical standpoint.

In view of the results of their study and the excellent results achieved with liver transplantation, Wood *et al.* (30) developed the algorithm presented in Figure 1 for the management of the jaundiced infant with suspected biliary atresia. At the present time a portoenterostomy procedure is the primary therapy of choice for these patients with biliary atresia who have the favorable characteristics as shown in Table 2. However, patients referred beyond 3 months of age having no obvious manifestations of chronic liver disease may require laparotomy to fully assess the chances for a successful portoenterostomy. Patients found to have obvious cirrhosis, marked portal hypertension, or unfavorable histology are best served by aborting the portoenterostomy in view of the extremely low chance of achieving sustained biliary decompression (18, 19). They should be immediately referred for transplantation. Only patients who have experienced a period of adequate biliary drainage and suffer a sudden decrease or cessation of bile flow will benefit from a revision of their portoen-

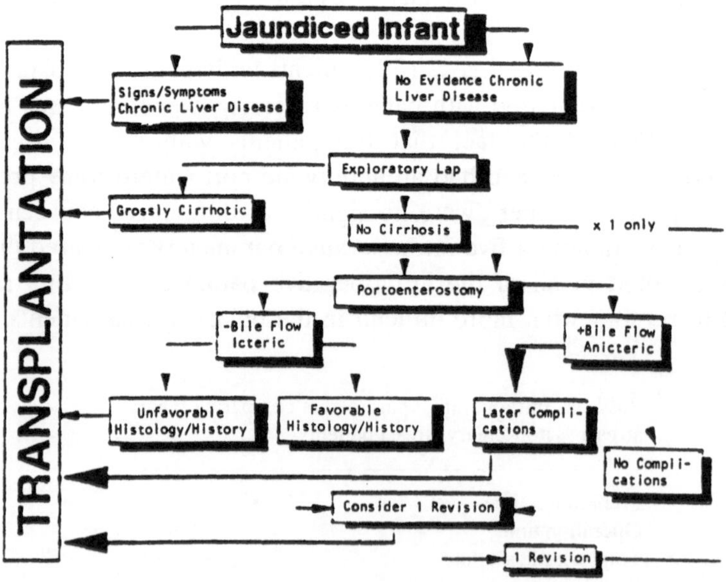

Fig. 1. Algorithm for the treatment of the jaundical infant with biliary atresia. (*Source*: Reference (30).)

terostomy (16—22, 28, 31—37, 39). Patients in whom adequate biliary drainage is not achieved are unlikely to be improved by revision of the failed portoenterostomy and should be referred for transplantation before they develop manifestations of chronic liver disease.

In the final analysis, portoenterostomy and liver transplantation are both appropriate procedures in the treatment of properly selected patients with biliary atresia.

Metabolic disorders

Lists of disorders of metabolism for which liver transplantation has been carried out includes alpha$_1$-antitrypsin deficiency, Wilson's disease, hereditary tyrosinemia, glycogen storage diseases, galactosemia, Crigler—Najjar syndrome type I, hyperlipoproteinemia types I and IV, protoporphyria, sea-blue histiocyte syndrome, Gaucher's disease, hemophilia A, cystic fibrosis, and primary hyperoxaluria. Liver replacement either eliminates or substantially ameliorates the metabolic defect in a number of these disorders.

Alpha$_1$-antitrypsin. Alpha$_1$-antitrypsin deficiency occurs in 1 in 2000 live births (1, 40). This disorder rsults in a variable clinical presentation in infancy with almost 50% of children with the homozygous deficiency having elevated serum aminotransferase levels as evidence of chronic liver dysfunction during the first 4 years of life. Of those patients who develop liver disease, 75% will manifest signs of cholestasis during infancy. While the majority of cholestatic infants will eventually become anicteric, fewer than 25% will recover without some evidence of liver disease and over 50% of these will die by early adulthood of complications of chronic liver disease.

The recipient proteinase inhibitor (P_i) type becomes that of the donor and serum alpha$_1$-antitrypsin levels are restored to normal following successful transplantation (41, 42). In the only report of long-term survival, 4 patients transplanted before 1981 for alpha$_1$-antitrypsin deficiency are alive without evidence of progressive disease in any other organ system (1). The effect of liver transplant on pre-existing extrahepatic lesions remains unknown and studies on larger number of patients with long-term follow-up will be necessary to truly define the long-term results in patients with this disease. In the future it is possible that liver transplantation will be carried out in patients with alpha$_1$-antitrypsin deficiency without evidence of liver disease in order to protect other organ systems from developing progressive disease.

Wilson's disease. The medical management of patients with Wilson's disease has improved to the point that liver transplantation is required only in those patients who develop fulminant hepatic failure or fail medical therapy. Fulminant hepatic failure secondary to Wilson's disease is almost always fatal if transplantation is not carried out. Following transplantation copper metabolism is returned to normal. In addition, the neurologic sequelae which occurs as part of the spectrum of Wilson's disease appear to be reversed following transplantation (43).

Hereditary tyrosinemia. Hereditary tyrosinemia occurs in one of every 100 000 live births and is inherited as an autosomal recessive trait. The two clinical presentations of this disorder are acute fulminant hepatic failure within the first few weeks of life or a more gradual presentation usually after 6 months of age with nodular cirrhosis, kidney dysfunction, rickets and failure to thrive (1, 4, 44). The disease is slowly progressive in the latter group of patients and is frequently complicated by the development of hepatomas. The diagnosis is made by positive succinylacetone in the urine but the diagnosis can be suspected when markedly elevated tyrosine and methionine levels are found in the serum (1, 45). One report (46) has claimed that transplantation restores serum tyrosine levels to normal and eliminates further risk of hepatoma. There is, at the present time, insufficient data to determine if transplantation reverses pre-existing changes in other organ systems, or whether progression of dysfunction is prevented in the other organ systems which are effected in this disorder.

Other metabolic disorders. The variety of other metabolic disorders treated occasionally with transplantation were previously mentioned. In the majority of these disorders transplantation has been confined to limited numbers of patients described in isolated case reports (1, 47—52). A detailed review of all of these disorders is beyond the scope of this paper. It is anticipated in the future, however, that many more disorders will be identified that may be amendable to therapy with either complete replacement of the liver or the use of partial liver transplants in an auxiliary position as described later in this review.

Post-hepatic cirrhosis

This group of disorders basically presents in one of two general patterns (1, 4). Patients with neonatal hepatitis (the precise etiology of which is often unknown) may present in infancy with rapidly progressing liver dysfunction. These children often require urgent transplantation and referral of these patients for transplant should be made as soon as the diagnosis is confirmed. Patients who contract non-A, non-B, or type B hepatitis, or who develop autoimmune hepatitis are often in their teens before they develop significant liver dysfunction. The indications for referral and transplantation of these patients are the same as for adults with these disorders, namely, the development of life-threatening complications of their liver disease or significant impairment in their quality of life as a direct consequence of the liver disease.

Acute fulminant hepatic failure

Two of the major etiologies for acute fulminant hepatic failure have been discussed previously in the sections on tyrosinemia and Wilson's disease. The majority of other patients who present with fulminant hepatic failure have either acute viral hepatitis or toxin-induced liver failure. In general the most significant difficulty in dealing with patients with fulminant hepatic failure is the fact that these patients are often referred for transplantation only after their condition has become critical (53—56). No matter what their age, any patient with suspected fulminant hepatic failure should be referred to a transplant center. Unless early referral is made, in view of the severe shortage of pediatric donor livers, there may be insufficient time to locate a suitable donor liver before the patient's condition becomes critical. Once evaluated at a transplant center, the patient can be placed on the transplant list as a high priority and reassessed at the time that a donor organ becomes available. If the patient is showing signs of improvement, the donor liver can be passed on to another recipient. If no improvement is evident, transplantation may be carried out. As is the case in all patients requiring transplantation, but especially in patients with acute fulminant hepatic failure, the results with transplantation will only be further improved by more timely referral of these patients.

Hepatic malignancies

As compared to the variety of tumors transplanted in adult patients, the majority of patients requiring transplantation for malignant disease in the pediatric age group have hepatoblastomas (57—60). Koneru (61) has collected data on 12 children who had been transplanted for hepatoblastoma in North America. Six remained alive with a mean follow-up of 44 months. Only 3 of the deaths were from tumor recurrence. Vascular invasion and predominance of embryonal and/or anaplastic epithelium was associated with a poor prognosis while focal lesions and intrahepatic tumors had a much better prognosis. At the University of Nebraska, 2 patients have been transplanted with hepatoblastomas, one of whom is alive over 3 years after transplantation and the second is alive without evidence of a tumor recurrence less than 1 year following his transplant. In addition, 2 children have been transplanted whose native livers were found at the time of pathologic sectioning to contain unsuspected hepatomas. Both of these patients are alive without evidence of tumor recurrence.

Congenital hepatic fibrosis

Congenital hepatic fibrosis rarely requires transplantation during childhood.

The majority of patients who develop significant portal hypertension can be managed by non-transplant measures including endoscopic sclerotherapy or portosystemic shunts. A large number of these patients, however, will require transplantation during adulthood due to progression of their liver disease (62).

Survival and rehabilitation

The first major symposium on pediatric liver transplantation was held in Brussels in October, 1986 (3). At this time a number of centers from around the world presented data on their survival rates and Figure 2 (1) shows data extracted from the symposium on the two-year survival rates from the presenting centers. In general, the reported survival rates for pediatric patients receiving liver transplantations exceed 65% at most centers (63) with selected reports of survival rates up to 90% at one year. In adult patients, it has been well demonstrated that the mortality of patients following transplantation is related to the patient's preoperative status. This has not been demonstrated in pediatric patients. In fact, in a report by Malatack *et al.* (64) there appeared to be no correlation between the survival of pediatric patients and the severity of disease prior to transplantation. In contrast, however, in the report by Wood *et al.* (30) it was noted that the survival rate in the non-biliary atresia patients was

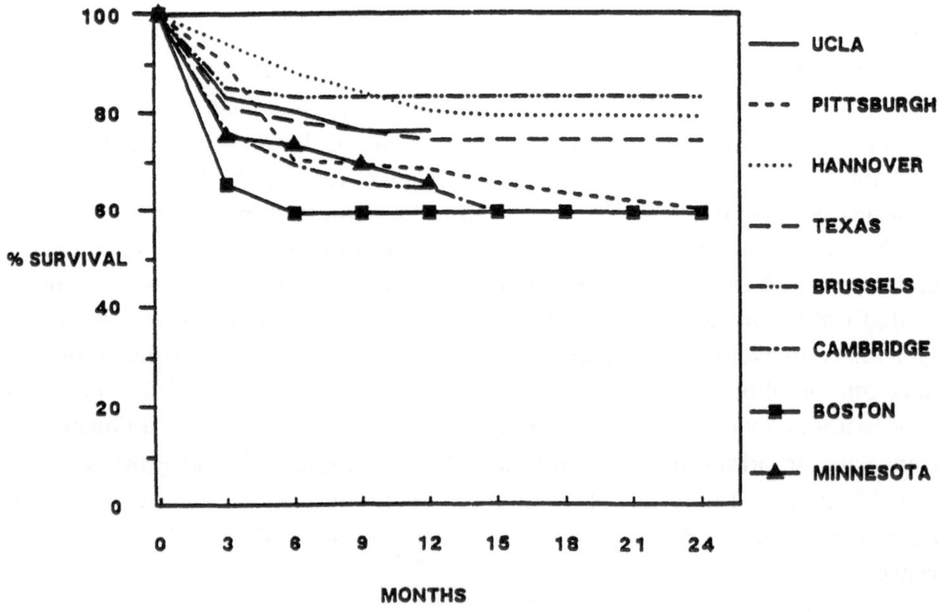

Fig. 2. Actuarial 2-year survival of pediatric liver recipients at various centers as extrapolated from data presented in Brussels at the first European Symposium on Liver Transplantation in Children in October 1986. (*Source*: Reference (1).)

lower than the survival rate of patients transplanted for biliary atresia. This was attributed to the fact that 9 of the 11 patients who died in the non-biliary atresia group were in the intensive care unit at the time of their transplant indicating the severe nature of their clinical condition. In addition, a report from Otte *et al.* (65) on the use of reduced-size liver transplants clearly demonstrates the much reduced success rate of this procedure in patients requiring urgent transplantation when compared to patients electively transplanted. It remains, therefore, our clinical impression that patients who are sufficiently debilitated by their liver disease to require the intensive care unit are high-risk candidates for transplantation.

Long-term follow-up

The long-term results of pediatric liver transplantation have been the subject of a limited number of reports (66—68). Urbach *et al.* (68) found that 29 children followed for at least 1 year after transplantation fell into one of three categories when compared for growth and development. Eighteen children (62%) either maintained normal growth along established percentile lines or experiences 'catch-up growth' with their growth curves crossing percentile lines. The second group of patients (14%) were growing at a normal rate at the time of transplantation and maintained normal growth after the procedure. Of the 7 remaining patients, all 7 fell off their normal growth curves and 4 of these patients had been growing normally before surgery. The reasons for failure in growth in this latter group of patients were often related to the requirement for additional immunosuppression to treat episodes of rejection. In addition, a number of these patients had experienced complications during the postoperative period. It would appear, therefore, that for all pediatric patients the potential appears to be real for eventual normal or near normal growth and development. In the majority of pediatric liver recipients the use of cyclosporine has allowed the maintenance dose of steroids to be tapered rapidly and kept at an extremely low level so that previous concerns over premature closure of bone epiphyses (primarily stemming from observations in pediatric kidney recipients before the cyclosporine era) may not be relevant in this group of patients. In addition, new immunosuppressive agents such as FK 506, rapamycin, etc., may allow even lower baseline steroid doses or even no steroids in some patients.

A report by Stewart *et al.* (70) from Dallas on the 1-year follow-up on 29 pediatric patients noted that steroid dosage had a significant negative impact on growth. In addition, at 1 year following transplantation, older subjects had a significantly improved social competence and there were significant increments of growth in weight, head circumference and arm anthropomorphic measurements but no change in linear growth rate. It should be noted that a follow-up of 1-year may be too short to demonstrate significant changes in growth due to the greater requirement for immunosuppression during the first postoperative year.

In addition to excellent growth and development, 90% of the 57 children reported by Zitelli *et al.* (71) have returned to normal quality of life following transplantation. Forty-four of the 57 children (77.2%) were in age-appropriate and standard school classes or only 1 year behind. Ninety percent of the children (18 of 20 tested) had normal or above-normal intelligence quotients (72) and all were performing at an acceptable level in their school work. Behavior adjustments were assessed by parent completed questionnaires that examined changes in three areas: gross motor control; parent-sibling behavior; and attendance and behavior at school. Statistically significant improvements in all areas were noted by the patients after transplantation. In all patients using the Vineland Social Maturity Scale, the majority of children were well below age-appropriate norms before transplantation but reached or exceeded these normal values beyond one year following transplantation (72).

Despite these results, parents of liver transplant recipients remain concerned about a number of issues. While these concerns vary depending on the parent, the recipient and the postoperative course of the patient, the most common concerns include rejection of the transplanted liver, side effects of medications, costs of medications and follow-up medical care, impact of the transpant on the family and especially siblings, and the unknown regarding long-term results of pediatric orthotopic liver transplantation.

Many parents also worry that they are being overprotective of their transplanted child, especially in those situations where the child was quite ill for a long period of time before the transplant (73). Thus, while the quality of life following transplant is excellent in the majority of surviving patients it is never 'normal'. The prior liver disease is replaced by a new 'disease', a transplanted liver, which requires lifelong medication, at least at the present state-of-the-art of pediatric liver transplantation.

The future of pediatric liver transplantation

The list of indications for pediatric liver transplantation continues to grow. As the procedure has become safer, with a better survival rate, patients should be transplanted before they suffer the ravages of chronic liver dysfunction. There is little justification for allowing the patients to get sicker to justify the use of transplant. Rather, patients should be referred for liver transplant as soon as it is obvious that their disease is unresponsive to medical management. New surgical techniques such as reduced-size or split livers may allow the use of heterotopic transplantation of partial liver grafts to cure metabolic disorders that do not directly effect the function of the native liver.

As stated by Shaw in a recent review, 'The disturbing irony that has surfaced in the new era of pediatric liver transplantation involves the crisis in the availability of donor organs. At the same time that the probability of surviving transplantation has reached levels that make it the treatment of choice for a growing variety of hepatic disorders, the increase in demand for donor organs has made transplantation less available' (1). It is widely quoted that between 25 and 30% of children on active transplant waiting lists in this country will die before they can be treated solely because of the lack of donor organs (1).

In an attempt to increase the number of available donors, legislative measures have been instituted which require hospitals to have in place a mechanism to identify and refer potential donors. Despite these laws there is as yet little evidence that the number of pediatric livers available for transplantation has increased. In view of this shortage, a number of centers have resorted to the use of partial liver grafting to attempt to reduce the number of children dying while awaiting transplantation (74—78). These new surgical techniques may have a positive impact in the future by providing transplantation to children who might otherwise have died while awaiting a whole organ. Enthusiasm for this new technology must, however, be tempered by several factors. The first is the fact that all of these reports have shown a lower success rate in the use of these partial liver grafts in the urgent situation, including re-transplantation, which is precisely the time when locating a donor liver is most critical. The second is the fact that the follow-up on recipients of reduced-size and split livers is very short. The third is the potential depletion of the donor pool of larger children or small adults for reduced-size transplants and theoretically, at least, depriving older children or small adults of these organs. Finally, the development of this technology has opened the potential for living related transplants as described by the group in Chicago (79) as another potential source of livers for infants and small children. However, in view of the factors noted above and the diverse ethical and scientific questions about the procedure, this remains an experimental procedure.

While the enthusiasm for pediatric liver transplantation remains high, it must be tempered by the large number of questions which remain unanswered. Some of these as yet unanswered questions include the fact that despite the increased activity over the last several years there remains no truly long-term follow-up on large numbers of pediatric liver recipients. Data on growth and development as well as quality of life in the long-term remain sketchy and isolated to small numbers of patients. Whether long-term immunosuppressive medications have adverse effects on the rapidly growing child and the potential for the late development of complications such as de-novo malignancies remain areas of concern. Finally, the precise role that new technologies such as reduced-size transplants and living related transplants will assume in the future remains to be evaluated.

Summary

End stage liver disease affects approximately 300 children each year the United States. Liver transplantation now offers children a 65% chance of surviving at least two years postoperatively and returning to a near 'normal' quality of life. A variety of factors have contributed to the improved results in pediatric liver transplantation recipients the most important of which is improved immunosuppression. However, much remains to be learned regarding the optimal preoperative and postoperative management of pediatric patients transplanted for a vareity of liver disease. The development of new immunosuppressive agents such as FK 506 will also require extensive evaluation to decide on the optimal use of these agents in the pediatric population. At the present time, it is most likely that further improvements in pediatric liver transplantation will only be recognized through the application of state-of-the-art pediatric hepatology to maintain patients in optimal condition prior to liver transplantation and the early referral of patients for liver transplantation before they develop complications and require urgent liver transplantation. The addition use of reduced-size and split livers for pediatric transplantation may also reduce the number of pediatric patients dying on the liver transplant waiting lists.

References

1. Shaw, B.W. Jr, Wood, R.P., Kaufman, S.S. *et al.*: Liver transplantation in children: In: E. Lebenthal (ed.), *Textbook of Gastroenterology and Nutrition in Infancy*, pp. 1045—1066, Raven Press, New York (1989).
2. Shaw, B.W. Jr, Wood, R.P., Kaufman, S.S. *et al.*: Liver transplantation therapy for children: Part I, *J. Pediat. Gastroent. Nutr.* **7**, 157—166 (1988).
3. Shaw, B.W. Jr, Wood, R.P., Kaufman, S.S. *et al.*: Liver transplantation therapy for children: Part II. *J. Pediat. Gastroent. Nutr.* **7**, 797—815 (1988).
4. Kaufman, S.S., Scrivner, D.J. and Gest, J.E.: Preoperative evaluation, preparation, and timing of orthotopic liver in the child. *Semin. Liver Dis.* **9**, 176—183 (1989).
5. Iwatsuki, S., Shaw, B.W. Jr and Starzl T.E.: Liver transplantation for biliary atresia. *World J Surg* **8**, 51—56 (1984).
6. Malatack J.J., Zitelli, B.J., Gartner, J.C. Jr and Shaw, B.W. Jr: Pediatric liver transplantation under therapy with cyclosporine A and steroids. *Transplant. Proc.* **15**, 1292—1296 (1983).
7. Iwatsuki, S., Starzel, T.E., Shaw, B.W. Jr *et al.*: Pediatric liver transplantation. In: C.H. Gips and R.A.F. Krom (eds.), *Orthotopic Liver Transplantation*, pp. 196—207, Martinus Nijhoff, The Hague (1985).
8. Krom, R.A.F., Gips, C.H., Houthoff, H.J. *et al.*: Orthotopic liver transplantation in Groningen, The Netherlands (1979—1983). *Hepatology* **4** (Suppl. 1), 61—66S (1984).
9. Busuttil, R.W., Memsic, L.D.F., Quinones-Baldrich, W., Hiatt J.R. and Ramming K.P.: Liver transplantation at UCLA. *Amer. J. Surg.* **152**, 75—80 (1986).
10. Jenkins, R.L.: The Boston Center for Liver Transplantation (BCLT). *Arch. Surg.* **121**, 424—430 (1986).
11. Kasai, M. and Suzuki, S.: A new operation for 'non-correctable' biliary atresia: Hepatic portoenterostomy. *Shujutsu (Jpn)* **13**, 733—739 (1959).
12. Kasai, M., Kimura, S., Asakura, Y. *et al.*: Surgical treatment of biliary atresia. *J. Pediatr. Surg.* **3**, 665-675 (1968).

13. Hays, D.M. and Synder, W.H. Jr: Life-span in untreated biliary atresia. *Surgery* **54**, 373–375, (1963).
14. Adelman, S.: Prognosis of uncorrected biliary atresia: an update. *J. Pediatr. Surg.* **13**, 389–391 (1978).
15. Lilly, J.R. and Altman, R.P.: Liver transplantation and Kasai operation in the first year of life: Therapeutic dilemma in biliary atresia. *J. Pediatr. Surg.* **110**, 561–562 (1987).
16. Lilly, J.R., Karrer, F.M., Hall, R.J. *et al.*: The surgery of biliary atresia: A personal experience. Presented at the American Surgical Association Annual Meeting, Colorado Springs, April 10–12, 1989.
17. Altman, R.P.: Biliary atresia — Update. *Proc. ACS Ann. Clin. Cong.* **71**, 13–15 (1985).
18. Stewart, B.A., Hall, R.J. and Lilly, J.R.: Liver transplantation and the Kasai operation in biliary atresia. *J. Pediatr. Surg.* **23**, 623–626 (1988).
19. Grosfeld, J.L., Fitzgerald, J.F., Predaina, R. *et al.*: The efficacy of hepatoportoenterostomy in biliary atresia. *Surgery* **106**, 692–701 (1989).
20. Lilly, J.R. and Altman, R.P.: Hepatic portoenterostomy (the Kasai operation) for biliary atresia. *Surgery* **78**, 76–85 (1975).
21. Hitch, D.C., Shikes, R.H. and Lilly, J.R.: Determinants of survival after Kasai's operation for biliary atresia using actuarial data. *J. Pediatr. Surg.* **14**, 310–314 (1979).
22. Suruga, K., Miyano, T., Arai, T.*et al.*: A study on hepatic portoenterostomy for the treatment of atresia of the biliary tract. *Surg. Gynecol. Obstet.* **159**, 53–58 (1984).
23. Lilly, J.R. and Carr, F.M.: Contemporary surgery of biliary atresia. *Pediatr. Clin. North Amer.* **32**, 1233–1245 (1985).
24. Andrews, H.G., Zwiren, G.T., Caplan, D.B. *et al.*: Biliary atresia: An evolving perspective. *South. Med. J.* **79**, 581–584 (1986).
25. Vazquex-Estevex, J., Stewart, B., Shikes, R.H. *et al.*: Biliary atresia: Early determinants of prognosis. *J. Pediatr. Surg.* **24**, 48–51 (1989).
26. Ohi, R., Hanamatsu, M., Mochizuki, I. *et. al*: Progress in the treatment of biliary atresia. *World J. Surg.* **9**, 285–293 (1985).
27. Weber, T.R., Grosfeld, J.L. and Fitzgerald, J.F.: Prognostic determinants after hepatoportoenterostomy for biliary atresia. *Amer. J. Surg.* **141**, 57–60 (1981).
28. Lawrence, D., Howard, E.R., Tzannatos, C. *et al.*: Hepatic portoenterostomy for biliary atresia. *Arch. Dis. Child.* **56**, 460–463 (1981).
29. Alagille, D.: Liver transplantation in children — Indications in cholestatic states. *Transplant. Proc.* **19**, 3242–3248 (1987).
30. Wood, R.P., Langnas, A.N., Stratta, R.J. *et al.*: Optimal therapy for patients with biliary atresia: Portoenterostomy ('Kasai' procedure) versus primary transplant. *J. Pediatr. Surg.* **25**, 153–161 (1990).
31. Pettit, B.J., Zitelli, B.J. and Rowe, M.I.: Analysis of patients with biliary atresia coming to liver transplantation. *J. Pediatr. Surg.* **19**, 779–785 (1984).
32. Zitelli, B.J., Gartner, J.C. Jr, Malatack, J.J. *et al.*: Pediatric liver transplantation: Patient evaluation and selection, infectious complications, and life-style after transplantation. *Transplant. Proc.* **17**, 3309–3316 (1987).
33. Bismuth, H. and Houssin, D.: Reduced-sized orthotopic liver graft in hepatic transplantation in children. *Surgery* **95**, 367–370 (1984).
34. Broelsch, C.E., Emond, J.C., Thistlethwait, J.R. *et al.*: Liver transplantation, including the concept of reduced-size liver transplants in children. *Ann. Surg.* **208**, 410–420 (1988).
35. Kasai, M., Kimura, S., Asakura, Y. *et al.*: Surgical treatment of biliary atresia. *J. Pediatr. Surg.* **3**, 665–675 (1968).
36. Hays, D.M. and Synder, W.H. Jr: Life-span in untreated biliary atresia. *Surgery* **54**, 373–375 (1963).
37. Adelam, S.: Prognosis of uncorrected biliary atresia: An update. *J. Pediatr. Surg.* **13**, 389–391 (1978).
38. Ohi, R., Hanamatsu, M., Mochizuki, I. *et al.*: Reoperation in patients with biliary atresia. *J. Pediatr. Surg.* **20**, 256–259 (1985).
39. Freitas, L., Gauthier, F. and Valayer, J.: Second operation for repair of biliary atresia. *J. Pediatr. Surg.* **22**, 857–860 (1987).

40. Balistreri, W.F. and Schubert, W.K.: Liver disease in infancy and childhood. In: L. Schiff and E.R. Schiff (eds.), *Diseases of the Liver*, pp. 1297—1299, J.B. Lippincott, Philadelphia (1982).
41. Putnam, C.W., Porter, K.A., Peters, R.L., Ashcavai, M., Redeker, A.G. and Starzl, T.E.: Liver replacement for alpha$_1$-antitrypsin deficiency. *Surgery* **81**, 258—261 (1977).
42. Van Furth, R., Kramps, J.A., van der Putten, A.B., Korm, R.A. and Gips, C.H.: Change in alpha$_1$-antitrypsin phenotype after orthotopic liver transplant. *Clin. Exp. Immunol.* **66**, 669—672 (1986).
43. Zitelli, B.J., Malatack, J.J., Gartner, J.C. Jr, Shaw, B.W. Jr, Iwatsuki, S. and Starzl, T.E.: Orthotopic liver transplantation in children with hepatic-based metabolic disease. *Transplant. Proc.* **15**, 1284—1287 (1983).
44. Lloyd-Still, J.D.: Mortality from liver disease in children; implications for hepatic transplantation programs. *Amer. J. Dis. Child.* **139**, 381—384 (1985).
45. Balistreri, W.F. and Schubert, W.K.: Liver disease in infancy and childhood. In: L. Schiff and E.R. Schiff (eds.), *Diseases of the Liver*, pp. 1292—1293, Lippincott, Philadelphia (1982).
46. Starzl, T.E., Zitelli, B.J., Shaw, B.W. Jr *et al.*: Liver replacement for hereditary tyrosinemia and hepatoma under cyclosporine and steroids. *J. Pediatr.* **106**, 604—606 (1985).
47. Starzl, T.E., Bilheimer, D.W., Bahnson, H.T. *et al.*: Heart-liver transplantation in a patient with familial hypercholesterolemia. *Lancet* **1**, 1382—1383 (1984).
48. Shaw, B.W. Jr, Bahnson, H.T., Hardesty, R.L., Griffith, B.P. and Starzl, T.E.: Combined transplantation of the heart and liver. *Ann. Surg.* **202**, 667—672 (1985).
49. Kaufman, S.S., Wood, R.P., Shaw, B.R. Jr *et al.*: Orthotopic liver transplantation for type I Crigler-Najjar syndrome. *Hepatology* **6**, 1259—1262 (1986).
50. Wolff, H., Otto, G. and Giest, H.: Liver transplantation in Crigler-Najjar syndrome. A case report. *Transplantation* **42**, 84 (1986).
51. Mowat, A.: Liver disorders in children: The indications for liver replacement in parenchymal and metabolic diseases. *Transplant. Proc.* **19**, 3236—3241 (1987).
52. Gartner, J.C. Jr, Bergman, I., Malatack, J.J. *et al.*: Progression of neurovisceral storage disease with supranuclear ophthalmoplegia following orthotopic liver transplantation. *Pediatrics* **77**, 104—107 (1986).
53. Iwatsuki, S., Esquivel, C.O., Gordon, R.D. *et al.*: Liver transplantation for fulminant hepatic failure. *Semin. Liver Dis.* **5**, 325—328 (1985).
54. Rueff B. and Benhamou J.P.: Acute hepatic necrosis and fulminant hepatic failure. *Gut* **14**, 805 (1973).
55. Saunders, S.J., Hickman, R., MacDonald, R. *et al.*: The treatment of acute liver failure. *Prog. Liver Dis.* **4**, 333 (1972).
56. Sherlock, S. and Panboo, S.P.: The management of acute hepatic failure. *Postgrad. Med. J.* **47**, 493 (1971).
57. Bismuth, H., Ericzon, B.G., Rolles, K. *et al.*: Hepatic transplantation in Europe: First report of the European Liver Transplant Registry. *Lancet* **2**, 674—676 (1987).
58. Iwatsuki, S., Gordon, R.D., Shaw, B.W. *et al.*: Role of liver transplantation in cancer therapy. *Ann. Surg.* **202**, 401—407 (1985).
59. O'Grady, J.J., Polson, R.J., Rolles, K. *et al.*: Liver transplantation for malignant disease: Results in 93 consecutive patients. *Ann. Surg.* **207**, 373—379 (1988).
60. Starzl, T.E., Toto, S., Tzakis, A. *et al.*: Abdominal organ cluster transplantation for the treatment of hepatic malignancies. *Ann. Surg.* **210**, 374—385 (1989).
61. Koneru, B. (personal communication).
62. Balistreri, W.F. and Schubert, W.K.: Liver disease in infancy and childhood. In: L. Schiff and E.R. Schiff (eds.), *Diseases of the Liver*, p. 1318, J.B. Lippincott, Philadelphia (1982).
63. *Transplant. Proc.* **19**, 3227—3380 (1987).
64. Malatack, J.J., Schaid, D.J., Urbach, A.H. *et al.*: Choosing a pediatric recipient for orthotopic liver transplantation. *J. Pediatr.* **111**, 479—489 (1987).
65. Otte, J.B., DeVille de Goyet, J., Sokal, E. *et al.*: Size reduction of the donor liver is a safe way to alleviate the shortage of size-matched organs in pediatric liver transplantation. *Ann. Surg.* **211**, 146—157 (1990).
66. Gartner, J.C. Jr, Zitelli, B.J., Malatack, J.J., Shaw, B.W. Jr, Iwatsuki, S. and Starzl, T.E.:

Orthotopic liver transplantation in children: 2-year experience with 47 patients. *Pediatrics* **74**, 140–145 (1984).
67. Zitelli, B.J., Malatack, J.J., Urbach, A.H. *et al.*: Pediatric hepatology: A three-year experience with pediatric liver transplantation with cyclosporine and steroids. In: P.M. Winter and Y.G Kang (eds.), *Hepatic Transplantation*, pp. 61–73, Praeger, New York (1986).
68. Urbach, A.H., Gartner, J.C. Jr, Malatack J.J. *et al.*: Linear growth following pediatric liver transplantation. *Amer. J. Dis.Child.* **141**, 547–549 (1987).
69. Riley, C.M.: Thoughts about kidney homotransplantation in children. *J. Pediatr.* **65**, 797 (1964).
70. Stewart, S.M., Uauy, R., Waller, D.A. *et al.*: Mental and motor development, social competence, and growth one year after successful pediatric liver transplantation. *J. Pediatr.* **114**, 579–581 (1989).
71. Zitelli, B.J., Gartner, J.C. Jr, Malatack, J.J. *et al.*: Pediatric liver transplantation: Patient evaluation and selection, infectious complications, and life-style after transplantation. *Transplant. Proc.* **19**, 2399–2402 (1987).
72. Miller, J.W.: Parents' perceptions of behavior of children with congenital liver disease one-year after liver transplantation [Dissertation]. Pittsburgh, Pennsylvania: University of Pittsburgh (1985).
73. Smith, E.I., Miyano, T., Kimura, K., Arai, T. and Kojima, Y.: Improved results with hepatic portoenterostomy. A reassessment of its value in the treatment of biliary atresia. *Ann. Surg.* **195**, 746–755 (1982).

35. Current anesthetic management in clinical liver transplantation

YOOGOO KANG

Intraoperative management of orthotopic liver transplantation is quite complex because of the presence of multiple organ dysfunction in potential recipients combined with the difficulty of this surgical procedure. In addition to impaired hepatic function, candidates for liver transplantation frequently suffer from hepatic encephalopathy, a hyperdynamic circulatory state, hepatopulmonary and hepatorenal syndromes, coagulopathy, and imbalances in electrolytes and in the acid-base state. Patients undergoing liver transplantation are prone to hemodynamic instability as a result of massive bleeding and manipulation of major vessels. The anhepatic state and the postreperfusion syndrome impose severe stress on liver recipients. And finally, the perioperative course of such recipients depends on the function of the newly grafted liver. Therefore, a clear understanding of the pathophysiologic changes that occur in liver recipients and tight control of homeostasis are essential for a successful outcome.

Altered physiology of liver recipients

Hepatic encephalopathy of various degrees is common, ranging from subtle confusion (stage 1), to gross mental confusion (stage 2), to somnolence and stupor (stage 3), and to deep coma with response only to pain (stage 4). Cortical atrophy and EEG abnormalities may be seen in patients suffering from chronic liver disease; while brain edema and elevated intracranial pressure are evident in approximately half of the patients with acute fulminant hepatic failure (1).

The hyperdynamic circulatory state is characterized by high cardiac output and low vascular resistance (2). Low vascular resistance is caused by circulating vasodilators and arteriovenous shunting (3) and is less responsive to catecholamines (4). Blood volume is increased 10–20% above the normal value (5), but it can be depleted by diuretic therapy or overloaded by fluid administration. Ventricular function is frequently normal (6, 7), but it may be impaired in patients with Laennec's cirrhosis, Wilson's disease, or hemochromatosis (8–10). Ischemic heart disease is relatively uncommon but pulmonary hypertension may occasionally be seen (11).

Hypoxemia results from decreased ventilation, increased ventilation-perfusion mismatch, and intrapulmonary right-to-left shunting. Tidal volume, vital capacity, and functional residual capacity are reduced. The adult respiratory distress syndrome resulting from hepatic failure improves after liver transplantation (12).

The hepatorenal syndrome results in sodium retention and in impaired renal water clearance and concentration capacity. *Hyponatremia* results from the increased activity of antidiuretic hormone and from decreased water excretion. *Hypokalemia* is caused by a depletion of total body potassium and by diuretic therapy, and *hyperkalemia* is caused by renal dysfunction. Other abnormalities associated with hepatorenal syndrome are *ionized hypocalcemia, hypophosphatemia*, and *hypomagnesemia. Metabolic alkalosis* results from vomiting and hyperaldosteronism, and *metabolic acidosis* occurs with rapidly deteriorating hepatic function.

Hypochromic microcytic or *macrocytic anemia* is commonly found in cirrhotic patients (13), and most have *coagulopathies* (14). The levels of all coagulation factors except for fibrinogen and Factor VIII are decreased. Platelet count is low in more than two-thirds of the patients, and platelet function is frequently impaired (15). Fibrinolytic activity is increased (16), and low-grade intravascular coagulation may occur.

Chronic liver disease is associated with *glucose intolerance* and insulin resistance (17) and fulminant hepatic failure is associated with severe *hypoglycemia*. The *biotransformation* of drugs is impaired, but drug dispositions are inconsistent. In general, patients are sensitive to sodium thiopental and resistant to pancuronium bromide and to d-tubocurarine. The half-lives of pancuronium, thiopental, morphine sulfate, meperidine hydrochloride, fentanyl citrate, and diazepam are prolonged (18—19).

Preparation and maintenance of anesthesia

Premedication is usually not given to liver patients because of their hepatic encephalopathy and poor physical state. Blood type and the presence of antibodies should be determined, and serologic tests for hepatitis and AIDS should be performed. Adequate quantities of blood products (20 units of red blood cells and 20 units of fresh frozen plasma) should be available at all times. Monitoring devices and equipment necessary during surgery are listed in Table 1.

The operating table is prepared with a warming blanket and padding. Both of the patient's arms are abducted without undue tension, and ECG electrodes and apulse oximeter probe are secured. Two 8.5 French catheters are inserted for fluid administration; one in the right antecubital vein and another in the left internal or external jugular vein. Blood pressure is monitored by a femoral

Table 1. Equipment for liver transplantation.

1.	Anesthesia machine and ventilator with compressed air supply
2.	Inspired gas humidifier
3.	Mass spectrometer or CO_2 analyzer
4.	Pulse oximeter
5.	Multiple-channel vital sign monitor
6.	Cardiac output computer with on-line mixed-venous oxymetry
7.	Thrombelastograph
8.	Rapid infusion system
9.	Autotransfusion system
10.	Blood pump and blood warmer
11.	Warming blanket
12.	Cardiac defibrillator
13.	Telephone

arterial catheter (18 gauge). In addition, a radical arterial catheter (20 gauge) is used for back-up pressure monitoring, and a pulmonary artery catheter with oximetry is placed via the right internal jugular vein. An indwelling urinary catheter, a rectal thermistor, an esophageal stethoscope, and a nasogastric tube are inserted. Heat loss is minimized by wrapping the head and extremities with vinyl covers.

A rapid-sequence technique is used for the induction of anesthesia because of a delayed gastric emptying time and the urgency of the surgery. Thiopental (4 mg/kg), etomidate (300—500 μg/kg), or ketamine hydrochloride (2 mg/kg) is used depending on the hemodynamic stability of the individual patient. Endotracheal intubation is facilitated by succinylcholine chloride (1—2 mg/kg), and anesthesia is maintained with an inhalation agent and/or narcotics. Isoflurane is used most commonly, because hepatotoxicity, cardiovascular depression, and biotransformation are minimal. In addition, short-acting narcotics (fentanyl), muscle relaxants (pencuronium), and amnesics (lorazepam) are administered as needed. Nitrous oxide is not used because it can cause myocardial depression and distension of bowel loops (20). Ventilation (50% oxygen in air and PEEP, 5 cm H_2O) is adjusted to maintain P_aCO_2 between 35 and 40 mmHg.

Intraoperative management

Orthotopic liver transplantation is divided into three stages. The *preanhepatic stage* extends from skin incision to the skeletonization of the hepatic vasculature. The *anhepatic stage* begins with hepatectomy and ends when cascular anastomosis of the inferior vena cava (IVC) and portal vein is complete. The *neohepatic stage* begins with reperfusion of the grafted liver via the portal vein and it is followed by reconstruction of the hepatic artery and bilary drainage system.

The cardiovascular system

High cardiac output, low vascular resistance, and relative tachycardia continue during the preanhepatic stage. Blood pressure and filling pressures are generally within the normal range. However, high central venous pressure (CVP) and pulmonary capillary wedge pressure (PCWP) may occur as a result of fluid overloading, and pleural and pericardial effusion; and these conditions should be treated. Pulmonary vasodilators may be used for severe pulmonary hypertension, although the result is not promising. A vasopressor (dopamine, 2—5 μg/kg per minute) may be given to improve cardiac performance, but alpha-vasopressors are avoided because they may increase the shunt fraction and interfere with tissue perfusion. The major hemodynamic instability seen during the preanhepatic stage is caused by acute changes in preload due to surgical bleeding and compression of major vessels. Lost blood should be replaced, and hypotension associated with compression should be reported to the surgeons.

A reduction in venous return of up to 50% is unavoidable when the IVC, portal vein, and hepatic artery are clamped during the anhepatic stage (21). The resulting decrease in preload and visceral congestion leads to hypotension, acidosis, hematuria, and surgical bleeding. Although these can be partially ameliorated by volume expansion and vasopressors (22), *veno-venous bypass* is the most physiologic technique (23). The bypass consists of cannulae in the protal and femoral veins for drainage of venous blood, a cannula in the axillary vein for venous return, and a centrifugal pump (Biopump^R, Biomedicus, Minn.) (24). The system carries up to 40% of the cardiac output, minimizing the hemodynamic changes associated with vascular cross-clamping except for some degree of reduction in cardiac output and an increase in vascular resistance. However, an inadvertent decrease in bypass flow caused by obstructed cannulae, kinked tubing, excessive centrifugal pump force, or low preload, should be corrected by repositioning of the catheter or increasing the intravascular volume. When the portal cannula is removed during anastomosis of the portal vein (*partial bypass*, femoral-axillary bypass only), cardiac output and blood pressure usually decrease. Unless negative hemodynamic changes are very severe, this transient hypovolemia is tolerated to avoid inadvertent overloading when the grafted liver is reperfused. Although a veno-venous bypass maintains hemodynamic stability, there are potential complications, including air emboli from the cannulation site and pulmonary thromboembolism. During anastomosis of the infrahepatic IVC, the donor liver is flushed with lactated Ringer's solution (300—500 ml) via the hepatic artery to remove the preservation solution, air, and metabolites.

Acute physiologic changes that occur on reperfusion of the grafted liver are challenge to anesthesiologists. These changes include cardiovascular collapse, severe coagulopathy by fibrinolysis and a heparin effect, hyperkalemia, hyperglycemia, acidosis, lactatemia, and acute hypothermia. Changes in the cardiovascular system (*postreperfusion syndrome*) consist of precipitous hypotension, bradycardia, dysrhythmia, a decrease in vascular resistance, and variable cardiac output. The postreperfusion syndrome occurs in about 30% of liver recipients (25), occasionally requiring cardiopulmonary resuscitation. The postreperfusion syndrome may be caused by an acute influx of hyperkalemic, acidotic, cold preservation solution from the grafted liver, or by right ventricular dysfunction associated with air emboli (26). However, dialyzable vasoactive substances released from the grafted liver appear to be responsible for the hemodynamic changes, since the hypotensive episode is not related to the degree of hyperkalemia, and it persists even when blood temperature is greater than 34 °C. Furthermore, clinically significant air embolism occurs very rarely.

Several measures can be taken to minimize the hemodynamic effects of the postreperfusion syndrome. Before reperfusion of the grafted liver, all laboratory values, especially potassium and ionized calcium levels, are normalized and the intravascular volume is corrected. The prophylactic administration of calcium chloride may increase cardiac output, but it does not prevent hypotension and bradycardia (27). Once the postreperfusion syndrome develops, calcium chloride (1 g) and sodium bicarbonate (50 mEq) are given to treat symptomatic hyperkalemia and acidosis. Hypotension is treated with small doses of epinephrine (in 5—10 μg increments) to increase cardiac contractility and to restore heart rate. Atropine sulfate (0.4—1 mg) may be given to increase the heart rate. A severely low output state requires immediate cardiopulmonary resuscitation including closed- and open-chested cardiac massage. When dysrhythmia is the cause of a low output state, it can be treated by antiarrhythmic drugs and, occasionally, by a transvenous pacemaker. An epinephrine drip infusion may be required for persistent hypotension. Treatment of hyperkalemia is not necessary because the potassium level returns to its baseline value by redistribution in the next 5—10 minutes. Recipients generally recover from the postreperfusion syndrome within 5—30 minutes, but the filling pressure may remain high and vascular resistance low. From this point on, intraoperative course can be relatively smooth, but high filling pressures and alpha-vasopressors should be avoided to minimize hepatic congestion and ischemia. Hypertension may be seen at the end of surgery from fluid overload or from the side effects of cyclosporine. A small dose of hydralazine (2.5—10 mg) is effective in treating hypertension, although a nitroprusside infusion may be required in extreme cases. Closure of the abdominal cavity may decrease blood pressure by increasing intrathoracic pressure.

The pulmonary system

Generally, gas exchange is not a clinical problem, and drainage of pleural effusion and ascites improves oxygenation within 1—2 hours. Ventilation should be adjusted according to end-tidal carbon dioxide tension. Pulmonary edema is avoided by careful titration of fluid administration and by normalization of the ionized calcium level to preserve myocardial contractility. Pulmonary thromboembolism, an infrequent complication, may be caused by migration of preexisting thrombi in the venous system.

Renal function and electrolyte balance

Relatively normal urine output is maintained by proper titration of intravascular blood volume, unless renal insufficiency or the hepatorenal syndrome is severe. Dopamine (2—3 μg/kg per minute) and mannitol have been reported to increase urine output (28), but maintaining adequate intravascular volume and perfusion pressure appears to be more important. Hematuria and oliguria, complications of a simple cross-clamping technique, very rarely occur when the veno-venous bypass technique is used during the anhepatic stage.

Hyponatremia and hypokalemia are gradually corrected by the administration of fresh frozen plasma and a balanced electrolyte solution. Rapid correction of hyponatremia should be avoided, since it may precipitate central pontine myelitis. Progressive hyperkalemia may occur in patients with renal dysfunction or in patients requiring a massive blood transfusion. In order to avoid lethal hyperkalemia on reperfusion, hyperkalemia should be treated aggressively by infusion of glucose and insulin or by transfusion of washed red blood cells using an autotransfusion system (29). The reuptake of potassium at the end of surgery may lead to hypokalemia (30), and a small dose of potassium (10—40 mEq) can be supplemented. Citrate intoxication caused by the inadequate metabolism of citrate in the banked blood (31), invariably occurs during liver transplantation. The ionized calcium level should be determined frequently, and abnormal levels should be treated to avoid myocardial depression and pulmonary edema.

Metabolism and hepatic function

Body temperature gradually decreases to as low as 31 °C, particularly during the anhepatic stage and on reperfusion of the grafted liver. It gradually returns to 34—35 °C at the completion of surgery. Progressive metabolic acidosis develops during surgery and is treated with sodium bicarbonate to avoid myocardial depression. Metabolic alkalosis, which may occur at the end of surgery, appears to be associated with a hormonal imbalance rather than with the volume of blood transfused or the dosage of sodium bicarbonate (32). The blood glucose level is maintained between 100—200 mg% by transfusions of glucose-containing blood, although hypoglycemia may occur during the anhepatic stage. Sudden hyperglycemia occurs on reperfusion, because of the massive release of glucose from the donor liver, and it does not appear to respond to insulin. The blood glucose level returns towards normal values in 24 hours (33).

The function of the grafted liver is detectable about 2 hours after reperfusion: citrate, lactate, and blood glucose levels decrease gradually, coagulopathy improves, and bile is produced. Persistent citrate intoxication, lactic acidosis, hyperglycemia, and coagulopathy are considered poor prognostic signs.

Fluid administration and coagulation

Fluid volume is administered by a rapid infusion system as indicated by hemodynamic profiles and urine output. Fluids adminstered consist of electrolyte solution to replace interstitial space loss, colloids to maintain oncotic pressure, fresh frozen plasma to supplement coagulation factors, and red blood cells to maintain oxygen-carrying capacity. Blood transfusion procedures and management of coagulation are described in Chapter 39 [The diagnosis and management of massive blood loss during liver transplantation].

At the end of surgery, liver recipients are monitored by ECG and blood pressure while they are transported to the intensive care unit (ICU). Ventilation and hemodynamic monitoring are continued in the ICU while the patient recovers from anesthetics and muscle relaxants. Subsequent postoperative care is a challenge to intensivists, who must manage potential complications such as immunosuppression, rejection, infection, and multiple organ failure (34).

References

1. Gazzard, B.G., Portmann, B., Murray-Lyon, I.M. *et al.*: Causes of death in fulminant hepatic failure and relationship to quantitative histological assessment of parenchymal damage. *J. Med. Qtly.* **44**, 615 (1975).
2. Bradley, S.E., Ingelfinger F.J. and Bradley, G.P.: Hepatic circulation in cirrhosis of the liver. *Circ.* **5**, 419 (1952).
3. Calabresi, P. and Abelmann, W.H.: Porto-caval and porto-pulmonary anastomoses in Laennec's cirrhosis and in heart failure. *J. Clin. Invest.* **36**, 1257 (1957).
4. Lunzer, M.R., Manghani, K.K., Newman, S.P. *et al.*: Impaired cardiovascular responsiveness in liver disease. *Lancet* **2**, 382 (1975).
5. Eisenberg, S.: Blood volume in patients with Laennec's cirrhosis of the liver as determined by radioactive chromium-tagged red cells. *Amer. J. Med.* **20**, 189 (1956).
6. Baley, T.J., Segel, N. and Bishop, J.M.: The circulatory changes in patients with cirrhosis of the liver at rest and during exercise. *Clin Sci.* **26**, 227 (1964).

7. Mathews, E.C. Jr, Cardin, J.M., Hentry, W.L. *et al.*: Echocardiographic abnormalities in chronic alcoholics with and without overt congestive heart failure. *Amer. J. Cardiol.* **47**, 570 (1981).
8. Limas, C.J., Guiha, N.H., Lekagul, O. *et al.*: Impaired left ventricular function in alcoholic cirrhosis with ascites. *Circulation* **49**, 755 (1974).
9. Kuan, P.: Fatal cardiac complications of Wilson's disease. *Amer. Heart J.* **104**, 314 (1982).
10. Buja L.M. and Roberts, W.C.: Iron in the heart: Etiology and clinical significance. *Amer. J. Med.* **51**, 209 (1971).
11. Lebrec D., Capron, J.P., Dhumeaux, D. *et al.*: Pulmonary hypertension complicating portal hypertension. *Amer. Rev. Respir. Dis.* **120**, 849 (1979).
12. Matuschak, G.M., Rinaldo, J.E., Pinsky, M.R. *et al.*: Effect of end-stage liver failure on incidence and resolution of the adult respiratory distress syndrome. *J. Crit. Care Med.* **2**(3), 162 (1987).
13. Sheehy, J.W. and Berman, A.: The anemia of cirrhosis. *J. Lab. Clin. Med.* **56**, 72 (1960).
14. Ragni, M.V., Lewis, J.H., Spero, J.A. *et al.*: Bleeding and coagulation abnormalities in alcoholic cirrhotic liver disease. *Clin. Exp. Res.* **6**, 267 (1982).
15. Ballard, H.S. and Marcus, A.J.: Platelet aggregation in portal cirrhosis. *Arch. Int. Med.* **136**, 316 (1976).
16. Fletcher, A.P., Biederman, O., Moore D. *et al.*: Abnormal plasminogen-plasmin system activity (fibrinolysis) in patients with hepatic cirrhosis: its cause and consequences. *J. Clin. Invest.* **43**, 681 (1964).
17. Flier, J.S., Kahn, C.R. and Roth, J.: Receptors, antireceptor antibodies and mechanisms of insulin resistance. *New Engl. J. Med.* **300**, 413 (1979).
18. Shideman, F.E., Kelly, A.R., Lee, L.E. *et al.*: The role of the liver in the detoxification of thiopental (penthotal) by man. *Anesthesiol* **10**, 421 (1949).
19. Hug, C.C. Jr, Aldrete, J.A., Sampson, J.F. *et al.*: Morphine anesthesia in patients with liver failure. *Anesthesiol* (Abstr) **51**, S30 (1979).
20. Eisele, J.H., Smith, N.T.Y.: Cardiovascular effects of 40 percent nitrous oxide in man. *Anesth. Analg.* **51**, 956 (1972).
21. Papas, G., Palmer, W.M., Martineau, G.L. *et al.*: Hemodynamic alterations caused during orthotopic liver transplantation in humans. *Surgery* **70**, 872 (1971).
22. Walls, W.J., Grant, D.R., Duff, J.H. *et al.*: Blood transfusion requirements and renal function in patients undergoing liver transplantation without venous bypass. *Transplant. Proc.* **19** (Suppl. 3), 17 (1987).
23. Shaw, B.W. Jr, Martin, D.J., Marquez, J.M. *et al.*: Advantages of venous bypass during orthotopic transplantation of the liver. *Semin. Liver Dis.* **5**, 344 (1985).
24. Griffith, B.P., Shaw, B.W. Jr, Hardesty, R.L. *et al.*: Veno-venous bypass without systemic anticoagulation for transplantation of the human liver. *Surg. Gynecol. Obstet.* **160**, 270 (1985).
25. Aggarwal, S., Kang, Y., Freeman, J.A. *et. al.*: Postreperfusion syndrome: Cardiovascular collapse following hepatic reperfusion during liver transplantation. *Transplant. Proc.* **19** (Suppl. 3), 54 (1987).
26. Lichtor, J.L., Ellis, J.E., Uitvlugt, A. *et al.*: Transesophageal echocardiography during liver transplantation. *Anesth. Analg.* (Abstr) **66**, S104 (1987).
27. Martin D.J., Marquez, J.M., Kang, Y.G. *et al.*: Liver transplantation: hemodynamic and electrolyte changes seen immediately followinig revascularization. *Anesth. Analg.* (Abstr) **63**, 246 (1984).
28. Polson, R.J., Parks, G.R., Lindop, M.J. *et al.*: The prevention of renal impairment in patients undergoing orthotopic liver transplantation by infusion of low dose of dopamine. *Anaesthesia* **42**, 15 (1987).
29. Belani, K.G. and Estrin, J.A.: Biochemical and hematologic effects of intraoperative processing of CPDA-1 and AS-1 packed red cells. *Anesthesiology* (Abstr) **67**, A156 (1987).
30. Abouna, G.M., Aldrete, J.A. and Starzl, T.E.: Changes in serum potassium and pH during clinical and experimental liver transplantation. *Surgery* **69**, 419 (1971).

31. Marquex, J., Martin, D., Kang, Y.G. *et al.*: Cardiovascular depression secondary to citrate intoxication during hepatic transplantation in man. *Anesthesiology* **65**, 457 (1986).
32. Fortunato, F.L. Jr, Kang, Y., Aggarwal, S. *et al.*: Acid-base status during and after orthotopic liver transplantation. *Transplant. Proc.* **19** (Suppl. 3), 59, (1987).
33. Mallett, S.V., Kang, Y., Freeman, J.A. *et al.*: Prognostic significance of blood glucose levels during liver transplantation. *Anesthesiology* (Abstr) **67**, A313 (1987).
34. Wood, R.P., Shaw, B.W. Jr and Starzl, T.E.: Extrahepatic complications of liver transplantation. *Semin. Liver Dis.* **5**, 377 (1985).

36. Risk factors in adult liver transplant recipients

R. PATRICK WOOD, BYERS W. SHAW JR., ROBERT J. STRATTA, ALAN N. LANGNAS, and TODD J. PILLEN

The earliest attempt to identify risk factors which might be important in the success of liver transplantation was by the Pittsburgh group in 1983. In preparation for the National Institutes of Health Census Development Conference on Liver Transplantation the survival of patients following liver transplantation was analyzed in terms of the severity of the patient's underlying liver disease (1). The measure of the severity of liver disease used by the Pittsburgh Group then was the location of the patient at the time of transplantation. Significant differences in survival rates were found between the patients who were in the intensive care unit (ICU) when compared to patients who were on the regular hospital ward or at home just piror to transplantation. The 6 month survival rates for the latter two groups were 84 and 68% respectively compared to only 42% for those who were in the ICU at the time of transplantation.

In 1984, in a paper describing the improved results with transplantation following the introduction of the venous bypass system, the Pittsburgh Group again demonstrated that the premorbid status of the patient had a significant impact on the success of subsequent transplantation (2). In this report it was noted that the 30 day survival for the patients in the bypass group was significantly higher than the survival rate for historical controls that had received transplants without the use of the venous bypass. However, by 90 days the improved survival rate was no longer present and survival rates between the groups were statistically equivalent. When the groups were closely analyzed it became clear that the mortality which occurred between 30 and 90 days was confined primarily to those patients who had been in the ICU prior to transplantation and were thus considered high-risk. These findings suggested that the use of the venous bypass system allowed more patients to survive the operative procedure and the early postoperative period but that high-risk patients went on to die of complications over the subsequent 2 months. Not surprisingly these complications appeared to be directly related to the patient's preoperative morbidity.

In 1985, Shaw *et al.* (3), reported the results of a multi-variant analysis of 23 different patients characteristics reviewed in an effort to determine which of these were associated with mortality in the initial 6 months following transplantation. This study was limited to adult patients. In all, 23 different variables were examined and statistical correlations between these variables and whether the patients were alive or dead at 6 months were examined. This allowed the development of a scoring system that took into account each of the most important correlates with mortality weighing each one by different amounts until the greatest difference between scores for living and dead patients were obtained. Results of this study and the exact scoring system have been previously published (3). The variables included in the scoring system are age, coma, ascites, total bilirubin, malnutrition, prothrombin time, and intraoperative blood loss. By using the so-called 'Shaw' scoring system, the authors were able to define a group of patients with low scores and high survival rates and a group of high scores and low survival rates. They likewise identified a group that was intermediate between the low- and high-risk groups with more variability even for small changes in score. The explanation for this becomes clear when one looks at a curve describing their relationship between risk score and mean survival rate (Figure 1). Medium-risk scores fall on the steep portion of the sigmoid curve and small changes in the score result in greater changes in survival rates. Based on the application of this scoring system to 119 adult patients receiving liver transplants, the survival rates for the high, medium, and low scores at 6 months were 22, 73, and 74%, respectively.

Since the beginning of our transplant program at the University of Nebraska Medical Center all adult patients have been prospectively scored and we recently reported a second analysis of these patients (4). This included 101 adult patients transplanted from July 1985 through July 1988. The present

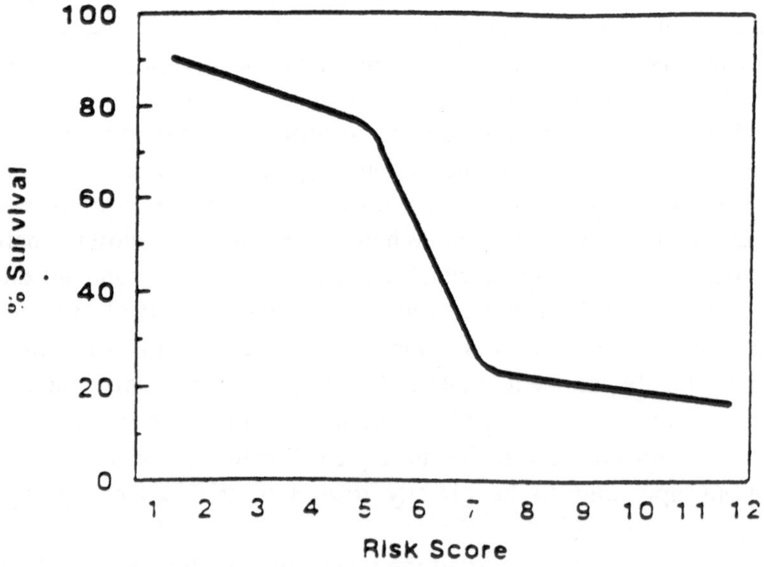

Fig. 1. Proposed relationship between the risk score or any of its component variables and survive probability (see text). (Adapted from reference (7).)

report expands the analyses to include 168 adult liver transplant recipients. The survival rates by group of the 168 adults at 6 months are 87.3% for low-risk patients, 68.7% for medium-risk patients, and 50% for high-risk patients, remarkably similar to the survival rates reported in the initial 101 patients.

In order to further test the validity of this scoring system it was compared to the Child's-Pugh classification (5, 6) for patients with liver disease. Of the 168 patients, 118 were classified as low-risk patients by the Shaw scoring method. Twenty-two (18.6) of these patients were Child's A, 69 (58.5%) were Child's B and 27 (22.9%) were Child's C. As noted above, the overall survival rate for these low-risk patients was 87.3%. Of the 168 patients only 22 were classified as Child's A patients. Within this group of 22 patients, all 22 were low-risk by the Shaw scoring system and the survival rate for Child's A patients in our series is 86.4%. Of the 168 patients, 22 were classified as moderate-risk patients. None of these patients were Child's A, 4 (18.2%) were Child's B and 18 (81.6%) were Child's C. The overall survival in this group is 68%. Based on the Child's-Pugh classification, 74 patients were Child's B. Of these 74 patients, 69 (93.2%) were low-risk by the Shaw scoring system, 4 (5.4%) were moderate-risk and 1 (1.4%) was high-risk. The overall survival for Child's B patients is 86.5%.

Of the 168 patients, 28 patients were classified as high-risk. All but one of these patients (96.4%) were Child's C. The survival rate for high-risk patients was 50%. Seventy-two of the 168 patients were classified as Child's C. Of these, 27 (37.5%) were low-risk by the Shaw scoring system, 18 (25%) were moderate-risk, and 27 (37.5%) were high-risk. The survival rate in Child's C patients is 68.1%.

This analysis illustrates the greater sensitivity of the Shaw scoring system in identifying those patients who are at significant risk of dying within the first 6 months following transplantation. By noting the survival rate of 50% in the patients classified as high-risk as compared to the 70% survival of the Child's C patients it becomes clear that the Shaw system identifies a group of patients who are higher risk.

The utility of this scoring system was further confirmed by examining the causes of death of patients dying following transplantation. In a paper on the stratification of the causes of death, Shaw *et al.* (4) categorized deaths following transplantation into one of four categories. The first category included those deaths related to preoperative morbidity, the second those deaths related to technical complications or management errors, third those deaths related to complications of immunosuppression and the fourth those deaths from unusual or unpredicted complications. In this report it was noted that 5 of the 8 deaths that occurred in adults with high-risk scores were from causes directly related to preoperative morbidity (category 1). In contrast, 4 of the 5 deaths in adults with low-risk scores were related to unusual or unpredicted (category 4) causes and the fifth to a technical error (7).

If one examines the cause of death in 3 of the major diagnostic groups undergoing transplantation, the utility of this scoring system is again confirmed. Of 35 patients transplanted for primary biliary cirrhosis, 33 were classified as low-risk and 2 as high-risk. One of the two high-risk patients died of complications directly related to preoperative morbidity. Two othe deaths occurred, both in the low-risk patients, but neither of these was from complications related to preoperative morbidity. Survival rate in patients with primary biliary cirrhosis is 93.1% as would be expected by the fact that the vast majority of these patients were low-risk.

Twenty-five patients with sclerosing cholangitis underwent transplantation during this period. Twenty patients were low-risk, 1 was moderate-risk and 3 were high-risk. The 2 deaths in the high-risk patients were directly related to preoperative morbidity and the 1 death in the moderate-risk patient was likewise due to unresolved preoperative morbidity. The overall survival rate of 84% in patients with sclerosing cholangitis again is indicative of the large percentage of good-risk patients in this group.

Seventeen patients were transplanted for acute fulminant hepatic failure. Of these 3 were low-risk, 4 were moderate-risk, and 10 were high-risk patients. Four of the 5 deaths in the high-risk patients and the 1 death in a moderate-risk patient were the result of unresolved preoperative morbidity.

Finally, in addition to providing a prediction of the risk of mortality following transplantation, the Shaw risk score provides an interesting means to analyze the costs of transplantation. The mean cost for patients who survive a transplant is approximately $80 000 in low-risk patients approaches $190 000 (Figure 2). This illustrates the fact that these high-risk patients, in addition to being at an increased risk of dying, are severely debilitated and require prolonged hospitalizations even when the transplant is successful.

Implications of the risk-score analysis extend to the present system of distributing the limited resource of donor livers in the United States. At the present time the greatest number of points in the United Network of Organ Sharing system used to distribute donor livers to potential recipients is given for the severity of the patients' liver failure. Those patients who are in the intensive care unit or experience fulminant hepatic failure receive a disproportionately higher point total and are more likely to be transplanted than good-risk patients who are awaiting transplantation at home. It is inevitable that as the competition for donor livers becomes more intense because of the expanding numbers of centers and the broadening of indications for transplantation, including new populations of patients such as acute and chronic alcoholics, the present system which provides livers for the sickest paitent may require re-evaluation in light of data as presented in this report. In view of the better success rates with transplantation before patients become end-stage, good-risk patients should be afforded an equal opportunity to receive a transplant.

In the final analysis, however, it would appear that this data demonstrates the

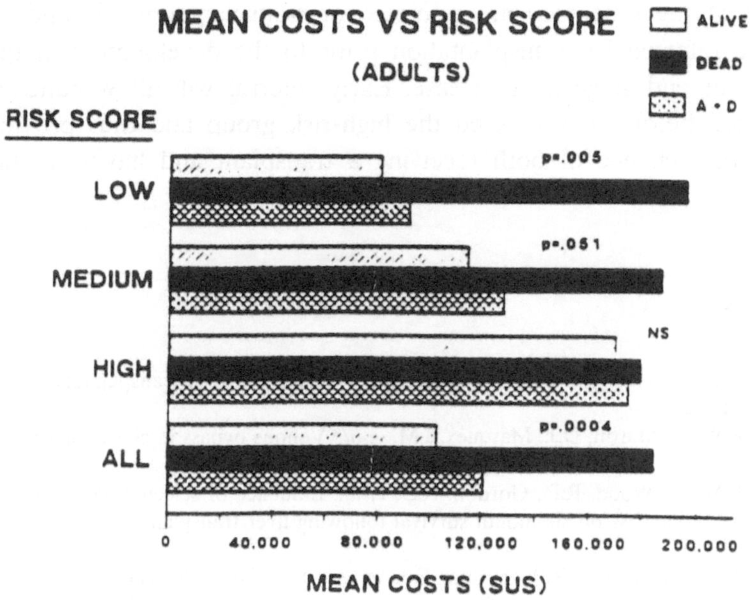

Fig. 2. Mean costs of transplantation as a function of risk score and clinical status (alive vs dead). (Adapted from reference (4).)

need for and advantage of early referral of patients for liver transplantation. The data supports the concept of aggressive use of transplantation while patients are in the best shape to survive and recover from the procedure. There is no reason at the present time to allow patients to become profoundly debilitated by their liver disease, reserving transplantation only as a last ditch effort to salvage patients. As aptly put by one of our hepatologists, 'transplantation can no longer be looked on as the "diving catch" of hepatology'. Rather this therapy must be aggressively utilized by hepatologists at anytime that the patient becomes refractory to medical or other form of surgical intervention.

Summary

The Shaw risk factors scoring system accurately identifies patients at high-risk of dying within 6 months of transplantation. This risk scoring system is more sensitive than the Child's-Pugh classification system which is presently widely employed to assess preoperative risk.

The key to further improving survival rates in patients undergoing hepatic transplantation is two fold. First is the aggressive application of state-of-the-art hepatology to the care of patients with liver disease. These patients should be aggressively supported and maintained so that they remain in the best possible condition at the time they are referred for transplantation. Second, patients should be referred for transplantation prior to the development of the complications of end stage liver disease. Early referral will allow patients to be transplanted before they entered the high-risk group and thus provide them with the best chance of both receiving a transplant and having a successful outcome.

References

1. Starzl, T.E., Iwatsuki, S., van Thiel, D.H. *et al.*: Evolution of liver transplantation. *Hepatology* **2**, 614 (1982).
2. Shaw, B.W. Jr, Martin, D.J., Marquex, J.M. *et al.*: Venous bypass in clinical liver transplantation. *Ann. Surg.* **200**, 524 (1984).
3. Shaw, B.W. Jr, Wood, R.P., Gordon, R.D. *et al.*: Influence of selected patient variables and operative blood loss on six-month survival following liver transplantation. *Semin. Liver Dis.* **5**, 385 (1985).
4. Shaw, B.W. Jr, Wood, R.P., Stratta, R.J. *et. al.*: Stratifying the causes of death in liver transplant recipients: An approach to improving survival. *Arch. Surg.* **124**, 895 (1989).
5. Conn, H.O.: A peek at the Child-Turcotte classification. *Hepatology* **1**, 673–676 (1981).
6. Pugh, R.W.H., Murray-Lyon, I.M., Dawson, J.L. *et al.*: Transection of the oesophagus for bleeding oesophageal varices. *Brit. J. Surg.* **60**, 646–649 (1983).
7. Shaw, B.W. Jr: Exclusion criteria for liver transplant recipients. *Transplant. Proc.* **21**, 3484 (1989).

37. The concept of reduced-size liver transplantation, including split-liver and living related liver transplantation

X.M. ROGIERS, J.C. EMOND, P.F. WHITINGTON, T.G. HEFFRON, K.L. KING, M.D. YANG and C.E. BROELSCH

Liver transplantation is the accepted treatment for end-stage liver disease and the number of liver transplants performed each year has increased steadily. The increasing demand for cadaveric livers can scarcely be met at present and further evolution is dependent on donor availability.

Donor scarcity is a life-threatening problem in pediatric liver transplantation. The reason for this is the discrepancy between the age distribution of children with end-stage liver disease and of potential cadaveric liver donors (Figure 1) (1, 2). Thus the mortality on the transplant waiting list for children in various major liver transplant centers in the U.S.A. as well as in Europe amounted to 20—30% (3, 4).

Strategies to increase the number of suitable donors include legislative and administrative measures as well as public information (e.g. the creation of organ procurement agencies, presumed consent law in some European countries, required request law in the U.S., etc.). Early recognition and optimal management of potential donors will also contribute to the number of cadaver donors available for transplantation.

Another way to improve donor liver availability is the application of new surgical techniques including reduced liver transplantation, split-liver transplantation and living related liver transplantation. All these techniques are based on the segmental anatomy of the liver (Figure 2 (a)) and on experience obtained from hepatic resections (5, 6). The techniques for graft reduction and splitting were described in previous publications (7—12).

Reduced-size liver transplantation

Reduction of the liver allows for a substantial mismatch between donor and recipient liver size which previously was the limitation to transplant children with more readily available livers from adult or juvenile donors. The different types of reduced grafts are illustrated in Figure 2(b). Right lobe transplantation can conveniently be performed from a donor who is twice the weight of the recipient, a left lobe can come from a donor who has 4 times the weight of the

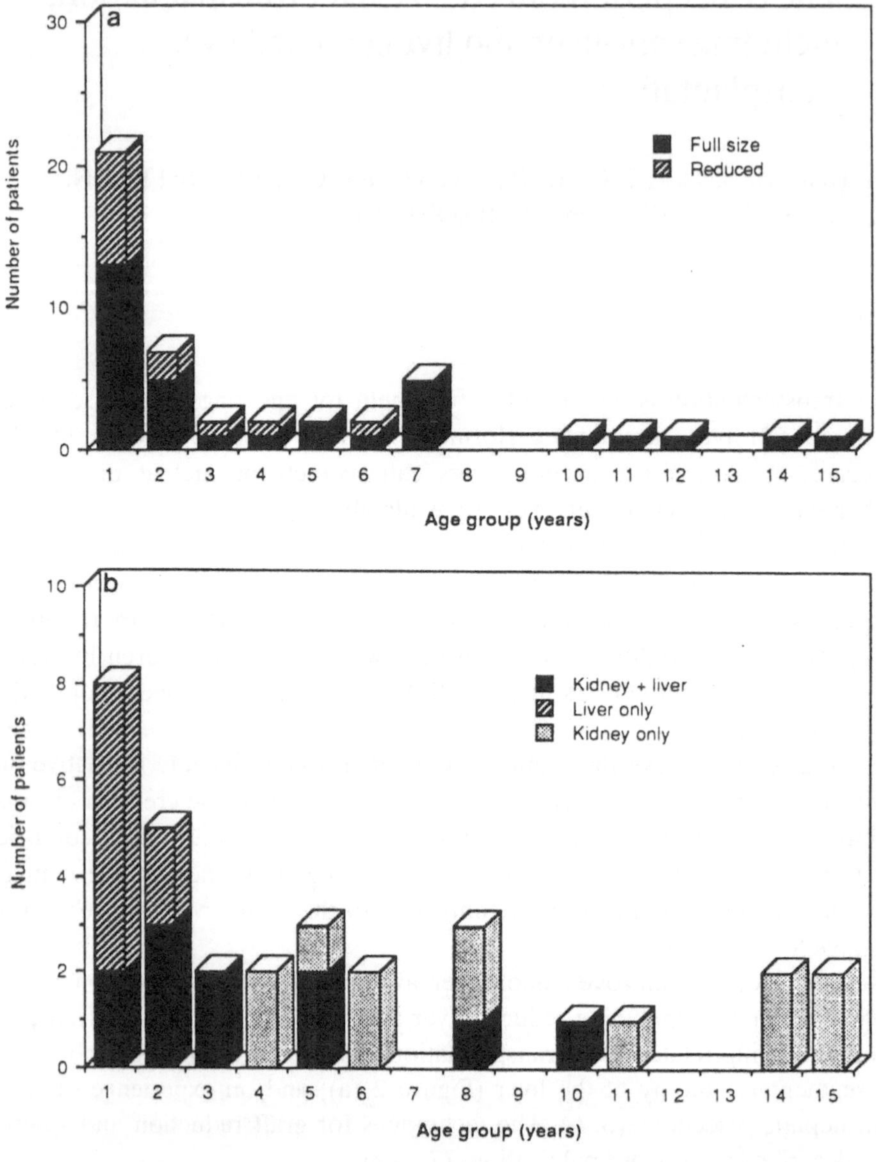

Fig. 1. (a) Distribution of ages of recipients of full-size and reduced-size OLT. (b) Age distribution of cadaveric visceral donor available in 1 year through the Regional Organ Bank of Illinois. (After reference (3).)

recipient and a left lateral segment transplantation allows for a size discrepancy of up to 10 times the recipient weight.

At the University of Chicago 2 right, 11 left and 10 left lateral lobes were transplanted between November 1986 and February 1990. The results are shown in Table 1.

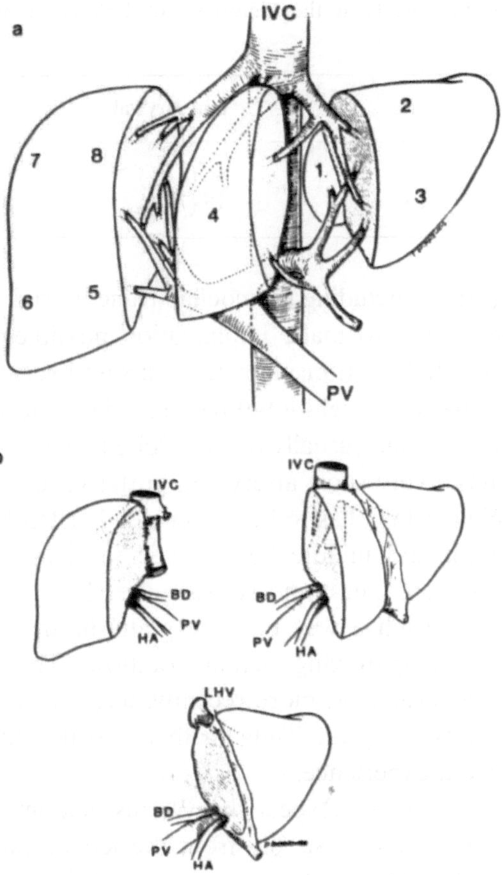

Fig. 2. (a) Segmental anatomy of the human liver. Functional allografts can be constructed from segments that have discrete vascular supply and bile drainage. (b) In practice, the right lobe graft consists in segments 5 to 8, the left lobe graft of segments 1 to 4 and the left-lateral segment graft of segments 1 to 3. IVC = inferior vena cava; PV = portal vein; HA = hepatic artery; LHV = left hepatic vein; BD = bile duct. (After reference (3).)

Split-liver transplantation

While reduced-size grafting had proven to be as successful as whole liver grafting, it became conceivable that using the remaining portion of the liver as a second transplant could be achieved successfully (10, 13). 'Split-liver' transplantation allows one donor organ to be used for two smaller recipients thus being even more efficient in achieving the goal of reducing the pediatric donor liver shortage.

However the 'split-liver' concept faces the surgeon with a number of technical problems. In reduced-size transplantation the graft received the necessary

Table 1. Pediatric liver transplants at the University of Chicago from November 1986 to February 1990.

	No.	6 m survival	Retransplanation
Whole liver	57	46 (81%)	24%
Reduced liver	23	18 (78%)	17%

vascular structures (artery including the coeliac trunc, portal vein, inferior vena cava) in appropriate length to make implantation possible with the standard techniques used for whole liver transplantation. In split-liver transplantation one of the grafts (preferentially the right lobe) has essentially the same anatomy as a reduced size graft. The second (usually the left) lobe however lacks the presence of a vena cava and has a very short artery and portal vein. During the recipient hepatectomy the recipient IVC has to be preserved. The left hepatic vein orifice is closed and the right and middle hepatic vein orifices are connected and extended to allow a wide anastomosis with the donor hepatic vein. This anastomosis is made in such a way that the graft sits in a stable position in the abdomen without jeopardizing venous outflow. The hepatic artery is anastomosed using iliac artery or, more recently, inferior mesenteric vein from the donor as an interposition graft. Thus far this does not influence the rate of arterial thrombosis in our experience.

Attention has to be paid to respect the venous anatomy of the liver. The quadrate lobe receives its blood supply from the left portal vein and hepatic artery. It should not be transplanted in continuity with the right lobe since portal blood supply, venous drainage and biliary drainage are compromised when the liver is transected in the plane of the round ligament.

Biliary drainage is achieved in the usual fashion using a Roux en Y bilioenteric anastomosis. Biliary complications (27%) occurred more frequently than in whole liver or segmental grafting. These were due to two factors: (a) devascularization of the bile duct during graft preparation or ligation of a segmental bile duct during preparation of a left lateral lobe graft; (b) in the event of arterial thrombosis ($n = 3$) bile lduct breakdown is unavoidable. Increased experience with the anatomy and awareness of abnormalities, particularly in venous and biliary drainage, should reduce the incidence of these complications. At the University of Chicago 21 split-liver transplant procedures were performed on children. Ten of these were right lobes, 5 left lobes and 6 left lateral lobes. The 6-month patient survival was 67% and the retransplantation rate was 35%.

Split-liver transplantation is the answer of modern liver transplant surgery to the shortage of livers for small children with end-stage liver disease. Increasing experience with the technical pitfalls of the procedure will make this a standard operation in pediatric liver transplant centers capable of handling the logistics of two simultaneous transplant procedures.

Living related liver transplantation

The concept of living related liver transplantation is derived from the experience with split-liver transplantation, proving that a suitable segment of the liver can be procured without traumatizing the rest of the liver, and of the experience with liver resections, allowing for liver dissection with maximum of safety and minimal blood loss (14, 15).

An ethical analysis concerning the issue of informed consent, to be obtained from the donor, has been presented on an institutional and national level (16). It was concluded that within an investigative protocol this procedure should be carried out in children with the greatest need for liver transplantation and the highest likelihood of deterioration without a transplant or while waiting for a transplant. Consequently, children with less than 3 years of age and biliary atresia are being selected.

In the first 3 cases, a left hepatic lobectomy was performed on the donor, followed by further cut down of the graft to a left lateral segment. In the following 8 cases a suitable graft could be obtained by carrying out only a left lateral segment (segments 2 and 3) resection in the donor. However, vascular reconstruction had to be used in these cases.

Eleven living related liver transplants have been performed at the University of Chicago since November 1989. All the donors are alive and well. One recipient had to be regrafted with a cadaver liver because of hepatic artery thrombosis. The survival of the recipients is 100%.

Organs from living related donation have been shown to have superior early function and a greater resistance to further stresses than cadaveric livers. A study to evaluate 20 consecutive cases is under way.

Conclusion

Reduced-size liver transplantation as well as split-liver transplantation have been proven to be valuable solutions to the shortage of organs for small children with end-stage liver disease. Cadaveric transplantation using split livers becomes our first line treatment for pediatric patients. Early experience with living related liver transplantation is even more promising and could become more applicable, particularly in countries where donor availability is very restricted.

References

1. Singer, P.A., Lantos, J.D., Whitington, P.F., Broelsch, C.E. and Siegler, M.: Equipose and the ethics of segmental liver transplantation. *Clin. Res.* **36**, 539—545 (1988).

2. *Vital Statistics of the U.S. 1982 Mortality*, Parts A, B Hyattsville, MD, Vol. 2, p. 186 (1986).
3. Emond, J.C., Whitington, P.F., Thistlethwaite, J.R., Alonso, E.M. and Broelsch, C.E.: Reduced-size orthotopic liver transplantation: use in the management of children with chronic liver disease. *Hepatology* **10**, 867—872 (1989).
4. Otte, J.B., de Ville de Goyet, J., Sokal, E. *et al.*: Size reduction of the donor liver is a safe way to alleviate the shortage of size-matched organs in pediatric liver transplantation. *Ann. Surg.* **211**(2), 146—157 (1990).
5. Bismuth, H., Castaing, D. and Garden, O.J.: Segmental surgery of the liver. In: L. Nyhus (ed.), *Surg. Ann.* (20), pp. 291—310. Norwalk, Appleton & Lange (1988).
6. Couinaud, C.: Le foie: études anatomiques et chirurgicales. Masson, Paris (1957).
7. Broelsch, C.E., Emond, J.C., Thistlethwaite, J.R., Whitington, P.F., Zucker, A., Baker, A.L., Aran, P.F., Rouch D.A. and Lichtor, J.L.: Liver transplantation, including the concept of reduced size liver transplants in children. *Ann. Surg.* **208**, 410—420 (1988).
8. Broelsch, C.E., Emond, J.C., Thistlethwaite, J.R., Rouch, D.A., Whitington, P.F. and Lichtor, J.L.: Liver transplantation with reduced-sized donor organs. *Transplantation* **45**, 519—523 (1988).
9 Broelsch, C.E. and Emond, J.C.: Transplantationof hepatic segments. In: S. Bengmark (ed.), *Progress in Surgery of the Liver, Pancreas and Biliary System*, pp. 379—393. Martinus Nijhoff, The Hague (1987).
10. Emond, J.C., Whitington, P.F., Thistlethwaite, J.R., Cherqui, D., Alonso, E.A., Woodle, E.S., Vogelbach, P., Busse-Henry, S.M., Zucker, A.R. and Broelsch, C.E.: Transplantation of two patients with one liver: Analysis of a preliminary experience with 'Split Liver' grafting. *Ann. Surg.* (1990; in press).
11. Pichlmayr, R., Ringe, B., Gubernatis, G., Hanos, T. and Burdelski, H.: Transplantation einer Spenderleber auf zwei Empfanger (Split liver transplantation). Eine neue Methode in der Weitzentwicklung der Lebersegment Transplantation. *Langenbecks Archiv. Chir.* **373**, 127—130 (1989).
12. Ringe, B., Bunzendahl, H., Gubernatis, G., Burdelski, M. and Pichlmayr, R.: Partielle Lebertransplantation: Indication, Technik und Ergebnisse. *Langenbecks Arch. Chir.* (1990; in press).
13. Otte, J.B., Yandza, T., de Ville de Goyet, J., Tan, K.C. and Salizzoni, M. de Hemptinne: Pediatric liver transplantation: Report on 52 patients with a 2-year survival of 86%. *J. Pediatr. Surg.* **23**, 250—253 (1988).
14. Cherqui, D., Emond, J.C., Pietrabissa, A. *et al.*: Segmental liver transplantation from living donors in the dog. *World. J. HPB Surg.* (in press).
15. Raia, S., Nery, J.R. and Mies, S.: Liver transplantation from live donors. *Lancet* **2**, 497 (1989).
16. Singer, P.A., Siegler, M., Whitington, P.F. *et al.*: Ethics of liver transplantation with living donors. *New Engl. J. Med.* **321**, 620—622 (1989).
17. Bismuth, H. and Houssin, D.: Reduced-size orthotopic liver graft in hepatic transplantation in children. *Surgery* **95**, 367—372 (1984).
18. Broelsch, C.E., Emond, J.C., Whitington, P.F., Thistlethwaite, J.R., Baker, A.L. and Lichtor, J.L.: Application of reduced-size transplants as split grafts, auxiliary orthotopic grafts, and living related segmental transplants. *Ann. Surg.* (in press).
19. Esquivel, C.O., Koneru, B., Karrer, F. *et al.*: Liver transplantation before 1 year of age. *J. Pediatr.* **110**, 545—548 (1987).
20. Kalayoglu, M., Sollinger, F.W., Stratta, R.J., D'Alessandro, A.M., Hoffman, R.M., Pirsch, J.D. and Belser F.O.: Extended preservation of the liver for clinical transplantation. *Lancet* **1**, 617—619 (1988).
21. Lilly, J.R. and Hall, R.J.: Liver transplantation and Kasai operation in the first year of life: therapeutic dilemma in biliary atresia. *J. Pediatr.* **110**, 561 (1987).
22. Lynch, S.V., Balderson, G., Armstrong, G. *et al.*: Mortality in patients on liver transplant waiting lists; an avoidable tragedy. *Transplant. Proc.* **21**, 1—3 (1989).
23. Starzl, T.E., Iwatsuki, S., Van Thiel, D. *et al.*: Evolution of liver transplantation. *Hepatology* **2**, 614—636 (1982).

38. Immunological factors contributing to outcome in liver transplantation

ROBERT D. GORDON

For many years it was thought that transplantation of the liver was not subject of the common prohibitive barriers that must routinely be observed in renal transplantation. For example, incompatibility for ABO blood group antigens and the presence of preformed anti-lymphocytotoxic antibody directed against HLA specificies are prohibitive for kidney transplants but were not considered to be so for liver transplantation. However, as the expanded case experience of the last decade became available for analysis, we have come to learn that some of the factors not previously considered important in liver transplantation are indeed relevant.

Preformed antibody

It is now well established from both clinical studies and in several experimental animal models that antibody-mediated hyperacute rejection of the liver can and does occur. However, it cannot be predicted with the same degree of reliability in the clinical setting as it can for renal transplantation and the clinical presentation differs significantly.

Presenisitization of rats, pigs and subhuman primates has been shown to produce hyperacute rejection of liver allografts characterized by antibody deposition and hemorrhagic necrosis. A similar pathological picture has been described for liver transplantation performed in humans across and ABO blood group incompatibility. Furthermore, analysis of a large series of liver transplantation has shown graft survival to be significantly less when such transplantation is performed across ABO incompatibility (1).

Demetris *et al.* analyzed 51 ABO incompatible grafts in 49 recipients and found a 46% failure rate within 30 days after transplantation compared to an 11% failure rate for a comparison series of ABO compatible grafts matched for age, sex, and clinical priority (2). Rejection was characterized clinically by persistent rise in serum aminotransferases, coagulopathy, and hemorrhagic necrosis of the liver with arterial deposition of antibody and complement demonstrable by immunoflourescent. Tissue bound donor-specific isoagglutinins were shown by elution studies.

Liver transplantation across an ABO compatible mismatch (O to A, O to B, O to AB) also has been shown to have a potential penalty, since passenger lymphocytes from the graft may produce antibodies against recipient ABO isoantigens resulting in hemolytic anemia usually within 12 to 21 days after transplantation (3). Although this often responds to conservative treatment or an increase in immunosuppression, in some cases splenectomy or even retransplantation may be required. Rapid rise in serum bilirubin with a corresponding fall in hematocrit and free haptoglobin in a patient who has received an ABO mismatched graft is characteristic of this graft versus host reaction.

The significant of pre-formed anti-HLA antibody in liver transplantation is less clear (4). In our own experience with over 2000 liver transplantations, we have been unable to make a correlation between graft outcome and historical or current panel reactive antibody or the donor-specific antibody crossmatch. We have been unable to correlate early irreversible rejection of ABO compatible grafts with conventional crossmatch results, although we believe that vigorous early cellular rejection may be more common in patients with a positive donor-specific crossmatch. It may well be that donor lymphocytes, the target cells used in conventional assays, do not adequately reflect the relevant antigenic composition of the liver. The distribution and expression of relevant antigens in the liver may differ significantly from the kidney. In addition, the functional anatomy of the liver including its capacity as a sinusoidal and reticulo-endothelial organ, many enable it to tolerate antibody better than a capillary structured organ such as the kidney.

The Mayo Clinic liver transplant group has reported a correlation between the vanishing bile duct syndrome (VBDS) and a positive lymphocytotoxic crossmatch and a class II histocompatibility mismatch (5). Also, Demetris has reported that following transplantation, but not before, the preferential targets of rejection such a bile duct epithelium, portal and central vein, and hepatic artery, express DR/Ia antigens (class II) (6). On the other hand, the Cambridge group has reported a higher incident of VBDS in patients with a class I mismatch and partial or complete matching for class II (7). They also reported a higher incident of anti-class I antibody in patients who developed VBDS when compared to patients without VBDS. Further study is necessary to better define how the expression of histocompatibility antigens on bile duct epithelium influences the course of rejection.

Marino *et al.* analyzed the transfusion requirements in patients receiving liver transplants in Pittsburgh (8). They found that operative requirements for platelets, packed red cells, fresh frozen plasma, and cyroprecipiate were all significantly higher in patients with a high (70%) panel reactive antibody (PRA) at the time of transplantation. Postoperative platelet counts were also significantly lower in patients with a high PRA. The presence of high titers of performed anti-HLA antibody may adversely affect transfused platelets and result in coagulation abnormalities and higher transfusion requirements in presensitized patients undergoing liver transplantation.

Major histocompatibility antigens

It is difficult to analyze the influence of HLA matching on graft outcome in liver transplantation, since prospective matching is not routinely practiced and, even in large clinical series, there are relatively few high grade matches. In our own experience, we have found some survival advantage for HLA *mismatched* grafts (9, 10). It has been suggested that HLA matching might facilitate viral or other immune mediated diseases since antigen presentation is known to occur in association with MHC gene products. For example, the Cambridge group has reported that a 1—2 HLA-DR match with cytomegalovirus (CMV) infection carried a high risk of development of VBDS whereas either CMV infection or HLA-DR match alone had a low association with VBDS (11). This suggests a relationship between the development of chronic rejection and CMV-induced HLA-expression.

Although the immunobiology of liver allograft rejection remains incompletely understood, there is ample evidence that the T-lymphocyte plays an important role. In the cellular infiltrates seen in rejecting allografts, T cells bearing IL-2 receptors can be demonstrated and these cells can be retrieved in biopsy specimens and propagated in vitro in medium containing exogenous IL-2 (12, 13). These cells show reactivity patterns are for a limited number of donor HLA antigens and their reactivity can be blocked by specific antisera. Furthermore, a pattern of sequential infiltration, first by class I reactive cells seen in early biopsy specimens followed by predominantly class II or a mixture of class I and class II reactive cells in later biopsies has been observed.

Patterns of antigens expression can also be studied by testing tissue recovered from allograft biopsy specimens with monoclonal antibody typing reagents (14). After transplantation, an increased expression of class I antigen is seen on hepatocytes and HLA-DR expression on bile duct epithelium which is intensified during acute rejection.

The characterization of T-cell reactivity and antigen expression on hepatic tissue can be summarized in the working hypothesis proposed in Figure 1. Adherence of class I reactive recipient T cells to donor vascular endothelium results in the release of various cytokines and promotion of class II antigen expression on vascular endothelium. This results in the adherence and migration class II reactive cells which reorganize class II antigen expressed on biliary epithelium. The subsequent immunological attack on the bile ducts results in the increase in cannalicular enzymes and the historical picture of bile duct injury that is a hallmark of liver rejection.

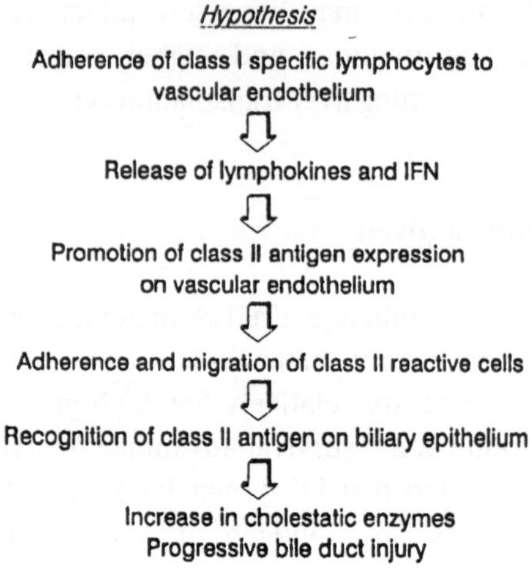

Fig 1. Hypothetical mechanism of T-cell mediated liver allograft rejection.

As has always been the case in immunology, this hypothesis is undoubtedly an oversimplification of the immune mechanisms of liver rejection and will be modified by outgoing investigation in the years ahead.

Acknowledgement

This work was supported by research grants from the Veterans Administration and Project Grant No. DK29961 from the National Institutes of Health, Bethesda, MD.

References

1. Gordon, R.D., Iwatsuki, S., Esquivel, C.O., Tzakis, A., Todo, S., and Starzl, T.E.: Liver transplantation across ABO blood groups. *Surgery* **100**, 342—348 (1986).
2. Demetris, A.J., Jaffe, R., Tzakis, A. *et al.*: Antibody-mediated rejection of human orthotopic liver allografts: A study of liver transplantation across ABO blood group barriers. *Amer. J. Pathol* **132**, 489—502.
3. Ramsey, G., Nusbacher, J., Strazl, T.E. and Linsday, G.D.: Isohemmaglutinins of graft origin after ABO unmatched liver transplantation. *New Eng. J. Med.* **311**, 1167—1170 (1984).
4. Gordon, R.D., Fung, J.J., Markus, B., *et al.*: The antibody crossmatch in liver transplantation. *Surgery* **100**, 705—715 (1986).
5. Demetris, A.J., Lasky, Van Thiel, D.H. *et al.*: Induction of DR/IA antigens in human liver allografts. An immunocytochemcial and clinicopathological analysis of twenty failed grafts. *Transplantation* **40**, 504—509 (1985).
6. Demetris, A.J., Lasky S., Van Thiel, D.H. *et al.*: Induction of DR/IA antigens in human liver allografts. An immunocytochemical and clinicopathological analysis of twenty failed grafts. *Transplantation* **40**, 504—509 (1985).

7. Donaldson, P.T., Alexander, G.J., O'Grady, J. *et al.*: Evidence for an immune response to HLA class I antigens in the vanishing-bile duct syndrome after liver transplantation. *Lancet* **1**, 945–951 (1987).
8. Marino, I.G., Weber, T., Kang, Y.G. *et al.*: HLA alloimmunization and blood requirements in orthotopic liver transplantation. *Transplant. Proc.* **21**, 789–791 (1989).
9. Markus, B.H., Fung, J.J., Gordon, R.D. *et al.* HLA histocompatibility and liver transplant survival. *Transplant. Proc.* **19** (4, Suppl. 3), 63–65 (1987).
10. Markus, B.H., Duquesnoy, R.J., Gordon, R.D. *et al.*: Histocompatibility and graft outcome: Does HLA exert a dualistic effect? *Transplantation* **46**, 372–327 (1988).
11. O'Grady, J.G., Alexander, G.J., Sutherland, S. *et al.*: Cytomegalovirus infection and donor/recipient HLA antigens: interdependent co-factors in pathogenesis of vanishing bile duct syndrome. *Lancet* **2**, 302–305 (1988).
12. Markus, B.H., Demetris, A.J., Fung, J.J. *et al.*: Allsospecificity of liver allograft-derived lymphocytes and correlation with clinicopathological findings. *Transplant. Proc.* **20**, 219–222 (1988).
13. Markus, B.H., Fung, J.J., Zeevi, A. *et al.*: Analysis of T-lymphcytes infiltrating human hepatic allografts. *Transplant. Proc.* **19** (1, Pt. 3), 2470–2473 (1987).
14. Steinhoff, G., Wonigeit, K., Pichlmayr, R.: Analysis of sequential changes in major histocompatibility complex expression in human liver grafts after transplantation. *Transplantation* **45**, 394–401 (1988).

39. Transplantation for hepatobiliary malignancies

R. PATRICK WOOD, BYERS W. SHAW JR., ROBERT J. STRATTA, ALAN N. LANGNAS and TODD J. PILLEN,

The use of liver transplantation in the treatment of hepatobiliary malignancies remains controversial. In the early experience with liver transplantation, patients with hepatobiliary maligancies were considered the ideal candidates for transplantation because, in most cases, they had not experienced the sequelae of chronic end stage liver disease. The operative procedure was straightforward and the early success rates were better than for any other group of patients. However, with longer follow-up an extremely high recurrences rate for these tumors (> 80% at 2 years) led a number of transplant centers to abandon the use of transplantation for the treatment of patients with hepatobiliary malignancies. This review will briefly discuss the results of liver transplantation for hepatobiliary malignancies and outline the potential future applications of this therapy. The experience from several centers will be reviewed. The overall actuarial survival for all types of malignancies ranges from 20 to 40% at 3 years in these series (1—5).

Hepatocellular carcinoma (HCC)

At the present time the only potential for cure of patients with HCC is surgical resection. There is no effective chemotherapy or radiation therapy for these patients. Unfortunately, only 20—30% of patients presenting with HCC can be considered for curative resection. Although longer survival is occasionally observed, the median survival from the time of diagnosis for patients with unresectable tumors is 2—4 months. The operative mortality for patients undergoing elective hepatic resection for HCC ranges from 5 to 8% and the 5-year survival rates following curative resection range from 20 to 40%.

To be considered a candidate for liver transplantation the patient with HCC must have a tumor which is not amendable to resection. This may be because the tumor is bilobar, centrally located or because coexisting liver disease compromises resectability. In addition, there should be no evidence of extrahepatic spread of the primary hepatic tumor.

Koneru *et al.* (1) in 1989 reported on the Pittsburgh experience with transplantation for HCC. Of their 35 patients transplanted in the cyclosporine era with non-fibrolamellar HCC, 14 had tumors which were known prior to total hepatectomy (incidental tumors). Thirteen of these patients were alive with follow-up from 3 to 73 months. The only death in a patient with an incidental tumor was from recurrent tumor at 23 months after transplantation. In the remaining 21 patients whose primary indication for transplantation was the presence of the tumor, the recurrence rate was 56%. Only 6 of these patients were alive with follow-ups ranging from 6 to 54 months. The 3-year survival rate for patients transplanted for hepatocellular carcinoma in this series was 20%.

Nine patients in the Pittsburgh series were transplanted for the fibrolamellar variant of HCC. Three of these died of causes unrelated to the tumor. Two of the 6 remaining patients died as a direct consequence of recurrent tumor and 1 of the 4 surviving patients was alive but with a recurrent tumor. The mean survival rate for the group with fibrolamellar HCC was 30.3 months.

In 1989, Iwatsuki *et al.* (6) at the Fourth Congress of the European Society for Organ Transplantation reported on the prognostic factors which influence the success of transplantation in patients with HCC. Iwatsuki identified four factors that independently affected survival. These were the presence of vascular invasion, the number of tumor nodules (single vs multiple), tumor shape (circumscribed vs non-circumscribed), and the presence of lymph node metastasis. In addition, four factors were identified which were associated with a higher incidence of tumor recurrence. These included tumor size greater than 5 cm, multiple nodules (2 or more), vascular invasion, and tumor shape (non-circumscribed).

Ringe *et al.* (5) in 1989 reported on the Hannover group's experience with transplantation of hepatobiliary malignancies. Fifty-two patients were transplanted for HCC, 4 with the fibrolamellar variant. Fifty-two percent of these patients developed recurrent tumor and only 15 remained alive at the time of the report. The 3-year survival rate for this group of patients was 20% with a median survival of 8.94 months. This group reviewed their experience based on determination of the TNM classification of the hepatocellular carcinomas. Their results clearly showed that patients with Stage 4 disease had a much worse prognosis than those with Stage 2 disease. In addition, as has been the experience at most other centers, no patient with lymph node metastasis at the time of transplantation survived beyond 1 year.

O'Grady *et al.* (3) reported the experience from Cambridge in 1988. They reported 50 patients transplanted with HCC, 7 of whom had the fibrolamellar variant. In the patients surviving beyond 3 months the recurrence rate of HCC was 64.9%. Tumor recurrence accounted for almost 60% of the deaths that occurred in the patients surviving beyond 3 months. The 2-year survival rate in this series was 38%. There were, however, 2 long-term survivors at 4.8 and 11.8 years.

In a report from 32 centers in the European Transplant Registry in 1987, Bismuth *et al.* (7) reviewed the results in 217 patients transplanted with HCC. The 2-year survival rate for these patients was 30%.

Cholangiocarcinoma

Bile duct cancers may arise either from the major extrahepatic bile ducts outside of the liver substance or from the biliary ductual epithelium within the liver parenchyman. Technically, only those cancers arising in the intrahepatic bile ducts should be classified as cholangiocarcinomas. Cholangiocarcinoma accounts for 5—20% of primary carcinomas of the liver and is the second most common primary hepatic malignancy. It may arise in a normal liver or be associated with sclerosing cholangitis. It is a relatively slow-growing tumor and metastasizes relatively late in its course. Because of its location, obstructive jaudice may appear while the tumor is still relatively small. The hilar type of cholangiocarcinoma is often referred to as a Klatskin tumor (8).

In reviewing the results of transplantation for cholangiocarcinoma, it is difficult, at times, to distinguish between patients who have Klatskin type tumors and those with proximal bile duct carcinomas. It would appear, in general, that the proximal bile duct tumors have a better prognosis than the Klatskin tumors. Koneru *et al.* (1) in 1989 reported the Pittsburgh experience in 11 patients transplanted for cholangiocarcinoma. Seven of these 11 patients developed recurrence and only 3 remained alive at the time of the report, 2 at 15 months and on at 13 months following transplantation. Stieber *et al.* (9) in 1989 reported the Pittsburgh experience with cholangiocarcinoma in patients with sclerosing cholangitis. In this series of 10 patients, 7 of whom were included in the previously mentioned report, only 3 patients remained alive at follow-ups of 24 months (2 patients) and 6 months (1 patient) following transplantation. Of interest, in only 3 of these 10 patients was the presence of the cholangiocarcinoma known prior to transplantation. There was, however, little data on the precise location of these tumors in either of the Pittsburgh reports.

In the report by O'Grady *et al.* (3) there were 14 patients with cholangiocarcinomas. The 1-year survival rates were similar for 'central' and 'peripheral' cholangiocarcinomas (30.7 and 38.4% respectively). Of the 7 patients with central cholangiocarcinomas who survived 3 months, 6 had documented recurrence leading to death at a median of 34 weeks following transplantation. Six of the 7 patients with peripheral cholangiocarcinomas likewise experienced recurrent tumor. The median survival for this subgroup was 1.4 years longer than for the central cholangiocarcinoma patients. In the report by Ringe *et al.* (5), 4 of their 10 patients with cholangiocarcinomas had extrahepatic involvement at the time of transplantation. All of the patients died within 1 year of transplantation with the exception of 1 patient who survived 25 months following transplantation. Of their 20 patients with proximal bile duct carcinoma, 8 patients remained alive and free of disease at a maximum follow-up of 35 months. Of interest was the fact that within the group of patients with proximal bile duct carcinomas, those patients who were free of lymph node metastasis at the time of transplantation has a survival rate at 2 years of 64.1%.

Other primary hepatic tumors

Hemangioendotheliomas

Much less is known about the treatment of primary hepatic malignancies other than hepatoma and cholangiocarcinoma by transplantation has not been well studied. In a collection of small numbers of patients the results with transplantation of patients with hemangioendotheliomas appear to be promising with 1-year survival rates in excess of 80% (1, 5, 10—13).

Hepatoblastomas

Hepatoblastoma represents the most common tumor requiring transplantation in the children. There appears to be a relationship between the histologic type of the tumor and the long-term survival with the pure fetal-cell type having the best prognosis. In most series resectability may be increased with preoperative chemotherapy, usually a combination of adriamycin and cisplatin. Koneru (14) has gathered data on the American experience with the transplantation of children with hepatoblastomas. This was a combined series of 12 children from 10 different centers. Six of the 12 children were alive with mean follow-up of 14 months. Only 3 of the 6 deaths were the result of tumor recurrence. Vascular invasion and the predominance of embryonal or anaplastic epithelium were associated with a poor prognosis while unifocal and intrahepatic tumors had a much better prognosis.

Metastatic tumors to the liver

In their review Flye *et al.* (15) identified 30 patients in the literature who had been transplanted for metastatic disease. There were no 5-year survivors reported in any of these series although the follow-up in several series was short. Makowka and collegues (16) reported a series of 5 patients transplanted for metastatic endocrine tumors. This included 2 patients with carcinoid tumors, 2 patients with glucagonomas and 2 patients with gastrinomas. With a limited follow-up of 7—34 months, 2 patients had died while 3 patients were alive without evidence of recurrent tumor.

In 1989 Starzl *et al.* (17) reported the Pittsburgh experience with the abdominal cluster operation. The premise for this operative procedure was that radical excision of most of the embryonic foregut would extirpate all malignancy and local spread arising within the derivatives of the original duodenal outpouchings. The operative procedure involves removing the liver, spleen, stomach, pancreas, duodenum, proximal jejunum, terminal iluem, and ascending and transverse colons. The cluster graft consists of the liver, pancreas, duodenum and variable amounts of proximal jejunum. In this initial report the results were somewhat promising. However, at the Second International Congress Middle East Society for Organ Transplantation, Dr Robert Gordon (18) presented data which demonstrated that with longer follow-up the incidence of recurrent tumor was greater than 50% in patients surviving the cluster operation. This operation remains an experimental procedure.

Conclusions

In view of the poor long-term success rates with the transplantation of most hepatic malignancies, certain recommendations can be made. Patients with unresectable hepatocellular or cholangiocarcinomas should be transplanted only at centers with well designed protocols which include adjuvant therapy in addition to transplantation. In spite of some isolated long-term successes and the opinion of some transplant surgeons that transplantation provides satisfactory palliation, we believe that, in view of the shortage of donor organs, transplantation of the liver in patients with hepatocellular carcinoma or cholangiocarcinoma is not justified except as part of carefully considered protocols. Exceptions to this may include patients with the fibrolamellar variant of hepatocellular carcinoma, patients with hemangioendotheliomas and selected patients with metastatic endocrine tumors. We believe that there is essentially no role for the use of transplantation in other patients with metastatic tumors to the liver. Transplantation will not be an important part of the therapy for the majority of patients with primary or secondary hepatocellular malignancies.

In general the best results with transplantation for malignancies have been in patients who are found after total hepatectomy to have an unsuspected hepatocellular carcinoma. In the vast majority of these patients the tumors are small and asymptomatic. Selected patients with chronic liver disease who are found on routine screening to have small asymptomatic tumors may be transplanted without the need for adjuvant therapy.

In summary, we do not believe that the use of transplantation for the treatment of hepatic malignancies should be abandoned. However, the use of this therapy can only be fully evaluated in carefully controlled trials with appropriately selected patients. Until more potent adjuvant therapies are developed, hepatic transplantation will remain of limited utility in the treatment of the majority of patients with primary or secondary hepatobiliary malignancies.

References

1. Koneru, B., Casavilla, A., Bowman, J. *et al.*: Liver Transplantation for malignant tumors. *Gastroenterology Clinic N.A.* **17**, 177–193 (1988).
2. Iwatsuki, S., Gordon, R.D., Shaw, B.W. *et al.*: Role of liver transplantation in cancer therapy. *Ann. Surg.* **202**, 401 (1985).
3. O'Grady, J.J., Polson, R.J., Rolles, K. *et al.*: Liver transplantation for malignant disease: Results in 93 consecutive patients. *Ann. Surg.* **207**, 373 (1988).
4. Pichlmayr R: Is there a place for liver grafting for malignancy? *Transplant. Proc.* **20**, 478 (1988).
5. Ringe, B., Wittenkind, C., Bechstein, W.O. *et al.*: The role of liver transplantation in hepatobiliary malignancy: A retrospective analysis of 95 patients with particular regard to tumor stage and recurrence. *Ann. Surg.* **209**, 88 (1989).
6. Iwatsuki, S.: Presented at the Fourth Congress of the European Society for Organ Transplantation in Barcelona, Spain, November 1989.
7. Bismuth, H., Ericzon, B.G., Rolles, K. *et al.*: Hepatic transplantation in Europe: First report of the European liver transplant registry. *Lancet* 674 (1987).
8. Klatskin, G.: Adenocarcinoma of the hepatic duct at its bifurcation within the porta hepatis. *Amer. J. Med.* **38**, 241 (1965).
9. Stieber, A.C., Marino, I.R., Iwatuski, S., and Stanzl T.: Cholangiocarcinoma in sclerosing cholangitis. The role of liver transplantation. *Int. Surg.* **79**, 1–3 (1989).
10. Scoazec J.Y., Lamy, P., DeGott, C. *et al.*: Epitheloid hemangioendothelioma of the liver: Diagnostic features and the role of liver transplantation. *Gastroenterology* **94**, 1447 (1988).
11. Clements D., Hubscher, S., West, R. *et al.*: Epitheloid haemangioendothelioma: A case report. *J. Hepatol.* **2**, 441 (1986).
12. Forbes, A., Portmann, B., Johnson, P. *et al.*: Hepatic sarcomas in adults: A review of 25 cases. *Gut.* **28**, 668 (1987).
13. Mesmic LDF: Survival after liver transplantation. In: R.W., Busuttil (Moderator) *Liver Transplantation Today. Ann. Int. Med.* **104**, 377 (1986).
14. Koneru, B. (personal communication).
15. Flye, M.W., and McCullough, C.S.: Liver transplantation for malignant disease: *Prin. Pract. Oncology* **3**, 1–12 (1989).
16. Makowka, L., Tzakis, A., Mazzafeno, V. *et al.*: Transplantation of the liver for metastatic endocrine tumors of the intestine and pancreas. *Surg. Gynecol. Obstet.* **168**, 107–111 (1989).
17. Starzl, T.E., Todo, S., Tzakis, A., *et al.*: Abdominal organ cluster transplantation for the treatment of upper abdominal malignancies. *Ann. Surg.* **270**, 374–385 (1989).
18. Gordon, R.D.: Presented at the Second International Congress Middle East Society for Organ Transplantation. March 11–15, 1990, Kuwait City, Kuwait.

40. The diagnosis and management of massive blood loss during liver transplantation

YOOGOO KANG

Massive bleeding of up to 300 units in 12 hours is unavoidable during liver transplantation (1). Therefore, a thorough understanding of the coagulation system and of the management of massive blood transfusion is critically important for intraoperative-care of liver transplant recipients. The goal of blood transfusion is to maintain normovolemia, oxygen-carrying capacity, and medical hemostasis. But transfusion is frequently complicated by decreases in coagulation factors, in body temperature, and in 2,3 DPG, and by the introduction of citrates, potassium acids, aggregates, antibodies, and viruses (2).

Mode of transfusion

Traditionally, blood products are transfused according to estimated blood loss using pressurized transfusion devices. However, this technique is not adequate during liver transplantation: blood loss can be greatly underestimated, and conventional transfusion devices have several drawbacks (3). The maximum flow rate of a conventional transfusion device is approximately 130 ml/min; therefore several devices are necessary during massive transfusion. The blood-warming capacity of these devices is very limited ($<25°$) and hypothermia is a frequently experienced complication. The blood transfusion volume is difficult to control, and cycles of hypovolemia and hypervolemia may occur. The composition of blood products given to the patient may be inconsistent, resulting in variable hematocrit and coagulation factor levels. Most of all, the management of transfusion using this technique requires a great deal of staff effort.

To overcome these difficulties, blood transfusion is guided by measurement of the hemodynamic profile and of urine output, rather than by estimates of blood loss. The continuous monitoring of mixed-venous hemoglobin oxygen saturation is helpful in assessing preload levels. In addition, a blood transfusion device that can minimize the potential complications of conventional transfusion technique is necessary. The ideal transfusion device should deliver up to 1.5 l/min blood volume, it should have an efficient heat exchanger, and it should be easily controllable. These goals have been met by a rapid-infusion system developed by Sassano at the University of Pittsburgh, and manufactured by Haemonetics, Inc. (Braintree, Mass.) (Figure 1) (4).

This system consists of a cardiotomy reservoir that holds up to 2.5 L of premixed blood, an efficient heat exchanger, a variable-speed roller pump, a micropore filter, and various safety features. The cardiotomy reservoir has four large spikes to facilitate rapid transfer of blood from blood bags. Generally, one unit (300 ml) of packed red blood cells is mixed with one unit (200 ml) of fresh frozen plasma and 250 ml of calcium- and glucose-free isotonic solution (PlasmaLyte A, Travenol, Deerfield, Ill). This mixture yields a solution of consistent hematocrit (26—28%) and coagulation factor levels (30—50% of normal) (5). The heat exchanger in this system is very efficient: cold blood (<10 °C) can be warmed to greater than 33 °C in one cycle, and warmer blood (20 °C) can be warmed to greater than 36 °C (6). The roller pump delivers up to 1.5 l/min of blood, with a range from 1 ml/h to 1.5 l/min. Two fluid-challenge modes deliver 100 ml or 500 ml at a flow rate of 400 ml/min. The recirculation mode returns warmed blood to the reservoir where it is mixed and kept warm. A macropore filter (170 μm) lining the cardiotomy reservoir and an online micropore filter (40 μm) remove most of the aggregates. Two large-caliber tubings are attached to two 8.5 French intravenous catheters for rapid delivery of the blood. Safety features include two air detectors, a temperature sensor, and a pressure sensor. The detection of air, of extreme temperatures in the blood, or the excessive pressure in the system prevents the system from transfusing blood. This system has been shown to resolve most problems

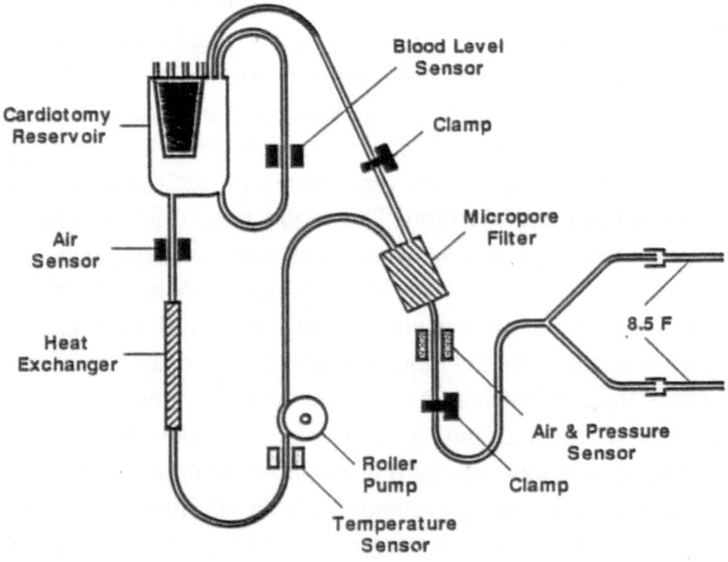

Fig. 1. A schematic diagram of the Rapid Infusion System (Haemonetics, Inc., Braintree, Mass.).

associated with massive blood transfusion, and it has become an essential piece of equipment for liver transplantation. The transfusion of premixed blood from the reservoir prevents hypothermia, hypovolemia, and fluctuation of composition of the transfused blood with minimal staff effort.

This method of transfusion has several potential complications, although they are unlikely to occur. Over transfusion may occur when the continuous infusion mode is used at a high flow-rate. Therefore, an intermittent fluid-challenge mode is preferred to a continuous-infusion mode. Air emboli may occur when the reservoir is empty, although the air detector should stop transfusion in this case. Blood in the system may clot when the blood is mixed with a calcium-containing solution, such as lactated Ringer's solution.

Autotransfusion

The use of red blood cells, and complications of banked blood transfusion, such as transmission of blood-borne disease, isoimmunization, and hemolytic reaction, can be reduced by using an autotransfusion system (7). However, potential complications of autotransfusion such as the occurrence of hemolysis, the effects of residual anticoagulants, the contamination by tissue thromboplastin, the dissemination of infection or malignancy, and the creation of air and fat emboli can be very serious in liver transplant recipients (8). Recent studies reported that autotransfusion can salvage up to 30 or 40% of the lost red blood cells (9). Furthermore, when the salvaged blood is anticoagulated with a citrate solution (6 ml/min) and washed with 1 l of PlasmaLyte-A, the effects of autotransfusion on coagulation, electrolyte balance, and plasma-free hemoglobin levels were clinically satisfactory (10). Although bacterial contamination was seen in the processed blood, the quantity of bacteria was clinically negligible, and bacteria cultures were negative after autotransfusion suggesting that occasional contamination by a few bacteria is not clinically significant in patients who receive prophylaytic antibiotic therapy (11). Therefore, autotransfusion during liver transplantation appears to be clinically acceptable, although it is not recommended in patients with intra-abdominal infection, neoplasms, or the positive hepatitis antigens.

Management of coagulation

Coagulopathy is a common feature of liver transplantation candidates. It is characterized by generalized decreases in coagulation factors, quantitative and qualitative defects in platelets, and some degree of intravascular coagulation and fibrinolysis (5, 12). The major intraoperative changes in coagulation are listed in Table 1.

Table 1. Coagulopathy during liver transplantation.

Preanhepatic stage	Dilution Fibrinolysis (mild)
Anhepatic stage	Dilution Heparin effect (with veno-venous bypass) Fibrinolysis (moderate) Intravascular coagulation (?)
Neohepatic stage (early)	Fibrinolysis (explosive) Heparin effect Effects of inhibitors (?) Hypothermia
Neohepatic stage (late)	Gradual recovery

Dilutional coagulopathy associated with surgical bleeding is the most common coagulation problem during the preanhepatic stage, although some degree of fibrinolysis may be detected. The absence of the liver during the anhepatic stage results in the depletion of coagulation factors and the lack of hepatic clearance of activated coagulation factors and inhibitors. Therefore, very low levels of coagulation factors and a gradual increase in fibrinolytic activity are frequently seen and some degree of intravascular coagulation may occur. Dilutional coagulopathy may persist, although surgical bleeding is less severe than that at the preanhepatic stage. When a venovenous bypass is used, a heparin effect is seen at the onset of the anhepatic stage, and is caused by the small dose of heparin (1000—2000 units) used in the bypass priming solution. This heparin effect dissipates without treatment at the end of the anhepatic stage. During this stage, the administration of platelets and epsilon-aminocaproic acid is reserved for severe cases of thrombocytopenia or fibrinolysis to avoid a potential thromboembolism in the unheparinized veno-venous bypass system (13).

Reperfusion of the grafted liver is associated with severe coagulopathy: explosive fibrinolysis caused by the release of tissue plasminogen activator from the donor liver, a heparin effect caused by the release of heparin or heparin-like substances from the donor liver, dilutional coagulopathy caused by an influx of preservation solution, the inhibition of coagulation caused by unknown substances, and acute hypothermia (13, 14). Thereafter, coagulopathy improves gradually when the function of the grafted liver is adequate.

These severe changes in coagulation require proper monitoring and treatment. A conventional coagulation profile (prothrombin time [PT], activated partial thromboplastin time [aPTT], platelet count, fibrinogen level, euglobulin lysis time, and fibrin degradation products) has several drawbacks. PT is considered to be a hepatic function test and the clinical significance of PT and aPTT is questionable, since they are prolonged in most patients. Platelet function is difficult to assess in the presence of thrombocytopenia. Euglobulin lysis time measures plasminogen activity, but ignored the balance between fibrinolysis and its inhibition. The presence of fibrin degradation products does not necessarily mean intravascular coagulation. Furthermore, a coagulation profile requires a laboratory facility, results may not be available for several hours, and the interpretation of the test results is difficult.

Thrombelastography (TEG) is found to be an extremely valuable monitoring tool during liver transplantation (15). It measures the coagulability of whole blood, not the quantity of coagulation factors. TEG also monitors the entire coagulation process including coagulation and fibrinolysis, and it provides clinically useful information within 30 minutes. Generally, the following TEG variables are measured: reaction time (r) is the initial latency period, which reflects the function of the coagulation cascade; clot formation rate (alpha) is a measure of the function of fibrinogen; maximum amplitude (MA) quantifies platelet function; and fibrinolysis time (F) reflects the balance between fibrinolysis and its inhibitors. In general, deficiency in coagulation factors is corrected by the administration of fresh frozen plasma that has been premixed in a rapid-infusion system. Fresh frozen plasma contains a small quantity of factor V, but it is sufficient to maintain blood coagulability. However, additional two units of fresh frozen plasma are administered when the reaction time is longer than 15 min. A decrease in platelet function indicated by a decrease in the maximum amplitude in thrombelastographic monitoring ($MA < 40$ mm) is corrected by the transfusion of 10 units of platelets. The transfusion of 10 units of platelets increases the platelet count to 40 000—50 000/mm^3 (15). Six units of cryoprecipitate when the clot formation rate is persistently less than 40°, since it contains fibrinogen, factor VIII, and factor XIII.

This TEG-guided replacement therapy successfully treats dilutional coagulopathy, but it is not effective against generalized oozing caused by pathologic coagulation, such as fibrinolysis or a heparin effect. These types of pathologic coagulation require differential diagnosis and selective treatment, as illustrated in Figure 2. The TEG pattern of blood drawn 5 minutes before reperfusion was within the normal range. However, a blood sample taken 5 minutes after reperfusion showed severe coagulopathy, including prolonged reaction time, poor clot-formation rate, poor platelet function, and fibrinolysis. In comparison, blood treated with epsilon-aminocaproic acid (EACA, 0.09%) exhibited an improvement in reaction time, clot formation rate, and platelet function, and an inhibition of fibrinolysis. In addition, blood treated with protamine sulfate displayed an improved reaction time and clot formation rate, but this treatment did not influence fibrinolysis. These *in vitro* findings suggest the presence of fibrinolysis and heparin activity, and the consequent effectiveness of EACA and

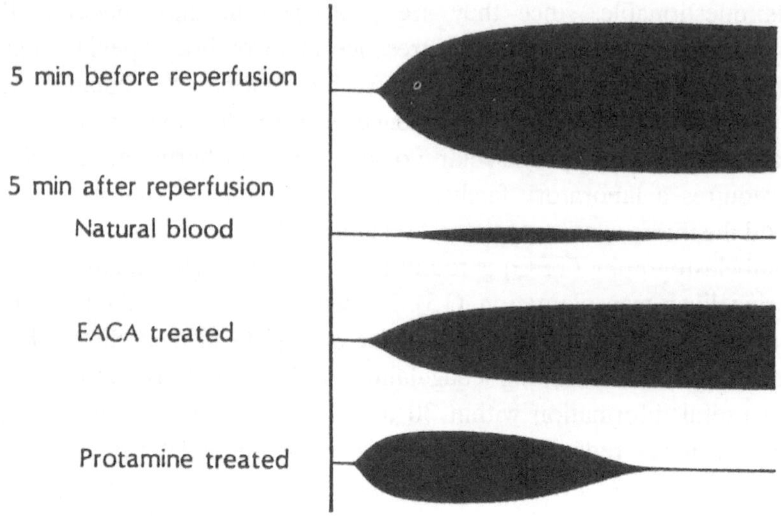

Fig. 2. Effects of pharmacologic agents in blood of a patient undergoing liver transplantation. (From Kang (15), by permission of the publisher.)

protamine sulfate in preventing severe coagulopathy. These observations led to the clinical introduction of pharmacologic coagulation therapy (13). A single dose of EACA (0.5—1 g) is administered to the patient when fibrinolysis occurs (F < 120 min) and fibrinolysis is absent in EACA-treated blood *in vitro*. However, only severe fibrinolysis (F < 60 min) is treated during the anhepatic stage with veno-venous bypass. This antifibrinolytic therapy has been successful in treating fibrinolysis without thrombotic complications in all patients. It is unclear whether fibrinolysis seen during liver transplantation is primary or secondary to intravascular coagulation (16). However, it is believed to be caused by primary fibrinolysis because of the association of fibrinolysis with disproportional decreases in factor VIII : C and factor V (17), a low level of fibrin monomers (13), a high level of tissue plasminogen activator (18), and a steady level of antithrombin III (19). Therefore, antifibrinolytic therapy is justified, since a small single dose (1 g) can stop severe transient fibrinolysis without thrombotic complications. This antifibrinolytic therapy can be very effective when TEG is used to identify any imbalance between fibrinolytic activity and the activity of inhibitors.

A heparin effect can be reversed in a similar fashion, although most heparin activity is reversed within one hour without treatment. Protamine sulfate (25—50 mg) is administered to the patient when a heparin effect is severe and the reaction time is shortened *in vitro* in blood treated with protamine sulfate (20).

Electrolyte balance and the acid-base state

Although electrolyte imbalance and metabolic acidosis have been recognized as major contributing factor for intraoperative mortality, and correction of these abnormalities has been emphasized, severe hypocalcemia, hyperkalemia, and acidosis still occur during massive blood transfusion (21).

Hypocalcemia

Generally, in apatient weighing 70 kg who has normal hepatic function, transient ionic hypocalcemia occurs when the transfusion rate is greater than 50 ml/min. Significant hypocalcemia (Ca^{++} < 0.55 mM) is seen when the transfusion rate exceeds 150 ml/min following citrate loading from banked blood (22). During liver transplantation, ionic hypocalcemia invariably occurs, particularly during the anhepatic stage: the serum citrate level nearly equals the level in banked blood (23). However, the serum citrate level decreases gradually after reperfusion and once the grafted liver begins to function. Ionized hypocalcemia (Ca^{++} < 0.56 mM) is associated with myocardial dysfunction (decreased blood pressure, cardiac index, and stroke-work index), but these negative hemodynamic changes can be reversed by the administration of calcium chloride. Therefore, the ionized calcium level should be monitored hourly, or more frequently, and it should be normalized to prevent serious hemodynamic complications.

Hyperkalemia

Progressive hyperkalemia (up to 7—8 mEq/l) inevitably occurs when a large volume of banked blood with a high potassium content is transfused rapidly (24). This is particularly so in patients with poor renal function. Untreated hyperkalemia is a serious complication, since a frequently occurring combination of hyperkalemia and tissue acidosis may precipitate severe cardiovascular instability. A relatively mild form of hyperkalemia can be treated with the infusion of glucose (12.5 g) and insulin (5—10 units). However, the transfusion of potassium-free blood should be considered when hyperkalemia is more pronounced (> 5.5 mEq/l) or when a massive blood transfusion is anticipated. Potassium-free blood is available in the blood bank by washing red blood cells, but it can also be obtained by washing red blood cells using an autotransfusion system (25). When an autotransfusion system is used to wash banked blood, a saline solution is used instead of with PlasmaLyte-A during a wash cycle to reduce the potassium load. Symptomatic hyperkalemia is treated using calcium chloride and sodium bicarbonate, as described in Chapter 34 [Current anesthetic management in clinical liver transplantation].

Acidosis

Progressive metabolic acidosis is a common complication of massive blood transfusion, particularly when the hepatic metabolism of acidic substances is impaired. Because of myocardial dysfunction and inadequate tissue respiration during the acidotic state, metabolic acidosis is treated with sodium bicarbonate to maintain a base deficit less than 5, particularly immediately before and after reperfusion. Lactic acidosis may occur simultaneously, owing to inadequate tissue perfusion. This should be treated by optimizing the circulatory physiology. Postoperative metabolic alkalosis was considered to be a result of the hepatic metabolism of the citrate and sodium bicarbonate loads. However, recent information suggests that postoperative metabolic alkalosis is not related to the volume of blood transfused, or to the dose of sodium bicarbonate (26).

In conclusion, massive blood transfusion can be performed safely with minimal complications. Hypovolemia, hypothermia, and the introduction of aggregates are prevented by using a rapid-infusion system. Proper blood component replacement and pharmacologic coagulation therapy are not difficult with the use of TEG. Complications related to electrolyte imbalance and acidosis can be prevented by frequent monitoring and anticipation. Autotransfusion, can reduce the banked blood usage, the incidence of viral transmission, and excessive antibody formation. Other complications appear to be irrelevant in the acute care of patients: for example, low levels of 2,3, DPG are restored to normal spontaneously after transfusion.

References

1. Bontempo, F.A., Lewis, J.H., Van Thiel, D.H., Spero, J.A., Ragni, M.V., Butler, P., Israel, L. and Starzl, T.E.: The relation of preoperative coagulation findings to diagnosis, blood usage, and survival in adult liver transplantation. *Transplantation* **39**, 532 (1985).
2. Collins, J.A.: Problems associated with the massive transfusion of stored blood. *Surgery* **75**, 274 (1974).
3. Dula D: Flow rate variance of commonly used IV infusion techniques. *J. Trauma* **21**, 480 (1981).
4. Sassano, J.J.: The rapid infusion system. In: P.M. Winter and Y.G. Kang (eds), *Hepatic Transplantation: Anesthetic and Perioperative Management*, p. 120 Praeger, New York (1986).
5. Kang, Y.G., Martin, D.J., Marquez, J.M. *et al.*: Intraoperative changes in blood coagulation and thrombelastographic monitoring in liver transplantation. *Anesth. Analg.* **64**, 888 (1985).
6. Kang, Y: Anesthesia for liver transplantation. *Anesth. Clin. North Amer.* **7**, 551 (1989).
7. Ellison, N. and Wurzel, H.A.: The blood shortage: is autotransfusion an answer? *Anesthesiol.* **43**, 288—290 (1975).

8. Hauer, J.M. and Thurer, R.L.: Controversies in autotransfusion. *Vox Sang.* **46**, 8—12 (1984).
9. Van Voorst, S.J., Peters, T.G., Williams, J.W., Vera, S.R. and Britt, L.G.: Autotransfusion in hepatic transplantation. *Amer. Surg.* **51**, 623—626 (1985).
10. Kang, Y., Virji, M.A., Lewis, J.H., *et al.*: Autotransfusion during liver transplantation. *Anesthesiol* **67**, A83 (1987).
11. Kang, Y., Aggarwal, S., Pasculle, A.W., *et al.*: Bacteriologic study of autotransfusion during liver transplantation. *Transplant. Proc.* **21**, 3538 (1989).
12. Ragni, M.V., Lewis, J.H., Spero, J.A. *et al.*: Bleeding and coagulation abnormalities in alcoholic cirrhotic liver disease. *Clin. Exp. Res.* **6**, 267 (1982).
13. Kang, Y., Lewis, J.H., Navalgund, A. *et al.*: Epsilonaminocaproic acid for treatment of fibrinolysis during liver transplantation. *Anesthesiol.* **66**, 766 (1987).
14. Groth, C.G., Pechet, L. and Starzl, T.E.: Coagulation during and after orthotopic transplantation of the human liver. *Arch. Surg.* **98**, (1969).
15. Kang, Y.G.: Monitoring and treatment of coagulation. In: P.M. Winter and Y.G. Kang (eds), *Hepatic Transplantation: Anesthetic and Perioperative Management*, p. 151. Praeger, New York (1986).
16. Bloom, A.L.: Intravascular coagulation and the liver. *Brit. J. Haematol.* **30**, 1—7 (1975).
17 Lewis, J.H., Bontempo, F.A., Kang, Y.G. *et al.*: Intraoperative coagulation changes in liver transplantation. In: P.M. Winter and Y.G. Kang (eds), *Hepatic Transplantation: Anesthetic and Perioperative Management*, p. 142. Praeger, New York (1986).
18. Porte, R.J., Bontempo, F.A., Knot, E.A.R. *et al.*: Tissue-type plasminogen activator associated with fibrinolysis in orthopic liver transplantation. *Transplant. Proc.* **21**, 3542 (1989).
19. Lewis, J.H., Bontempo, F.A., Ragni, M.V. and Starzl, T.E.: Antithrombin III during liver transplantation. *Transplant. Proc.* **21**, 3543 (1989).
20. Kang, Y., Borland, L.M., Picone, J. *et al.*: Intraoperative changes in coagulation during liver transplantation in children. *Anesthesiol.* (Abstr) **67**, A525 (1987).
21. Kang, Y., Aggarwal, S. and Freeman, J.A.: Intraoperative mortality during liver transplantation. *Transplant. Proc.* **20**, (Suppl. 1) 600 (1988).
22. Denlinger, J.K., Nahrwold, M.L. and Gibbs, P.S.: Hypocalcemia during rapid blood transfusion in an anaesthetized man. *Brit. J. Anaesth.* **48**, (1976).
23. Marquez, J., Martin, D., Kang, Y.G. *et al.*: Cardiovascular depression secondary to citrate intoxication during hepatic transplantation in man. *Anesthesiol.* **65**, 457 (1986).
24. Young, L.E.: Complications of blood transfusion. *Ann Int. Med.* **61**, 136 (1964).
25. Brown, M.R. and Ramay, M.A.: Exchange autotransfusion using the cell saver during liver transplantation. *Anesthesiol.* **70**, 168 (1989).
26. Fortunato, F.L., Jr., Kang, Y., Aggarwal, S. *et al.*: Acid-base status during and after orthotopic liver transplantation. *Transplant. Proc.* **19**, (Suppl. 3), 59 (1987).

41. Early clinical experience with cluster resection and transplantation for right upper quadrant abdominal malignancy

ROBERT D. GORDON, SATORU TODO, ANDREAS G. TZAKIS and THOMAS E. STARZL

Liver transplantation for primary tumors originating in the liver or biliary tree, not suitable because of location of extent for subtotal hepatic resection, has been disappointing. So has liver transplantation for tumors metastatic to the liver. Although many patients receiving a liver transplant for malignant disease are technically easier to operate on than patients with cirrhosis and such patients often make a swift postoperative recovery, disease recurrences within 6 to 18 months is common despite the additional field of resection a transplant hepatectomy can provide. Patients with disease extending beyond the liver capsule, into regional lymph nodes, or into major vascular structures such as the portal vein or vena cava, have a particularly poor prognosis and are probably not suitable candidates for liver transplantation alone.

New approaches are needed if patients with right upper quadrant abdominal malignancies are to be helped. Either additional surgical resection or additional modes of chemotherapy or biological modification may be needed. Actually, a combination of innovative surgical and medical techniques may be needed.

The liver and pancreas develop as outpouchings of the foregut region which ultimately becomes the duodenum. Tumors arising in one of these organs tend to spread into one of the other organs or to the transverse mesocolon or colon. This prompted our transplant surgeons to consider whether a more radical en-bloc excision of the right upper quadrant viscera, including the liver, duodenum, pancreas, right colon, and all or part of the stomach, and the associated regional lymphatic drainage, followed by liver or liver-pancreas replacement, might be of benefit in the management of right upper quandrant abdominal cancer.

Starzl long ago realized the surgical feasibility of the solid organ abdominal cluster transplant (1). In 1962 he published a description of transplantation in the dog of an abdominal organ cluster, including the liver, stomach, spleen, pancreas, small bowel and colon based on an aortic stalk (Figure 1). Venous return was provided by reanastomosis of the infrahepatic and suprahepatic vena cava. This early experience was finally applied to clinical practice 27 years later when in 1987 a child with short gut syndrome and hepatic failure was successfully transplanted in Pittsburgh and survived for 6 months (2). The current

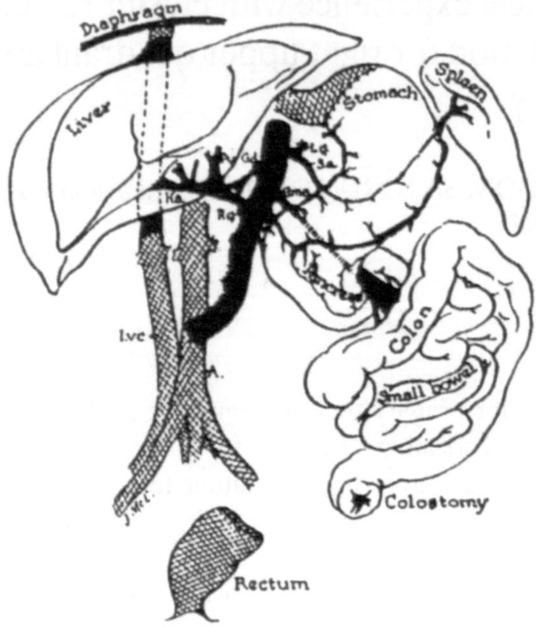

Fig 1. Starzl's original experimental approach to the abdominal cluster organ transplant in the dog. The abdominal viscera are based on an aortic stalk reimplanted end-to-side to the recipient aorta. The only venous reconstruction required is the supra- and infra-hepatic vena cava. (From reference (1).)

surgical methods used for organ cluster resection and transplantation (Figure 2) and our earliest results were recently reported by Starzl *et al.* (3). A modification of the procedure in which liver transplantation alone (Figure 3) is used to replace the resected organs was recently described by Tzakis *et al.* (4). Subsequent experience with the first 34 patients to undergo such a procedure is summarized in Table 1. Seventeen patients were given a liver transplant after upper abdominal organ cluster resection and 17 received a composite liver-pancreas graft (organ cluster graft).

Sixteen of the original 34 patients are surviving 4—9 months after operation. Four survivors are known to have recurrent disease. Thus, there are 12 (35.3%) survivors presently believed to be disease free. Serious technical complications have most often been related to complications of the pancreatic portion of the graft and have included pancreatitis, abscess, sepsis, and mycotic aneurysm. For this reason, we have used simple liver replacement and pancreatic enzyme and insulin replacement therapy in later parts of our experience. Malnutrition associated with total pancreatectomy or the extensive upper GI tact resection, has been the most significant cause of morbidity in surviving patients.

A few of the patients with early recurrence of cancer were probably inaccurately staged and may have already had microscopically disseminated tumor

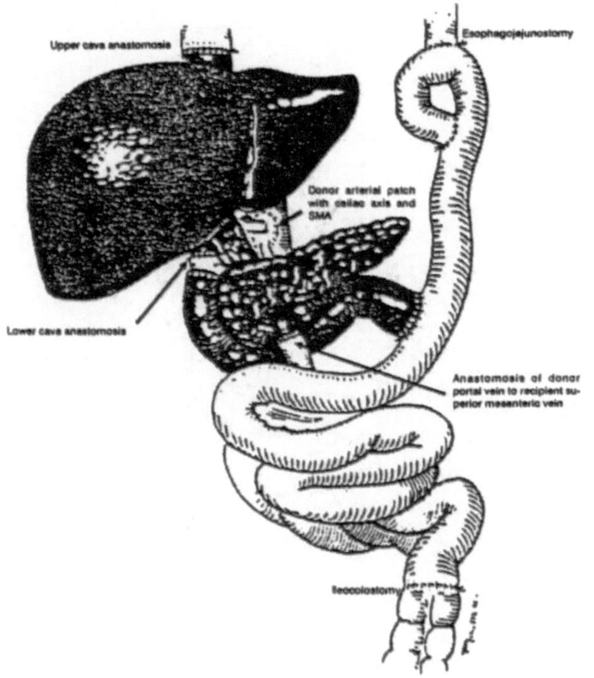

Fig 2. The organ cluster transplant for replacement of vital abdominal organs after right upper quadrant exenteration (organ cluster resection). In the operation shown, the arterial reconstruction is a Carrel patch of donor aorta containing both the celiac axis and the superior mesenteric artery to preserve blood supply to both the liver and pancreas. The venous reconstruction requires anastomosis of the donor portal vein to the recipient superior mesenteric vein and the supra- and infrahepatic vena cava anastomoses. Biliary reconstruction is not needed. (Adapted from reference (3).)

beyond the bounds of resection prior to operation. Clearly accurate staging of disease is important before undertaking such surgery and new technology may need to be applied to accomplish this. Nevertheless, although our experience is limited and follow-up for most of the patients is relatively short, we have a small but encouraging set of patients surviving beyond 6 months after surgery who are out of the hospital and so far appear free of cancer.

At the present time, this unique approach to the management of conventionally unresectable cancer must still be considered experimental. We are still learning how to best stage these patients for surgery, which tumors are best suited for this type of management, what adjunctive therapy is indicated, and how to minimize the technical complications and reduce the morbidity of the procedure. The use of cluster resection with liver replacement only has eliminated the complications associated with intraabdominal pancreas transplantation, but has added diabetes and nutritional complications. Increased surgical experience has already reduced the incidence and severity of technical com-

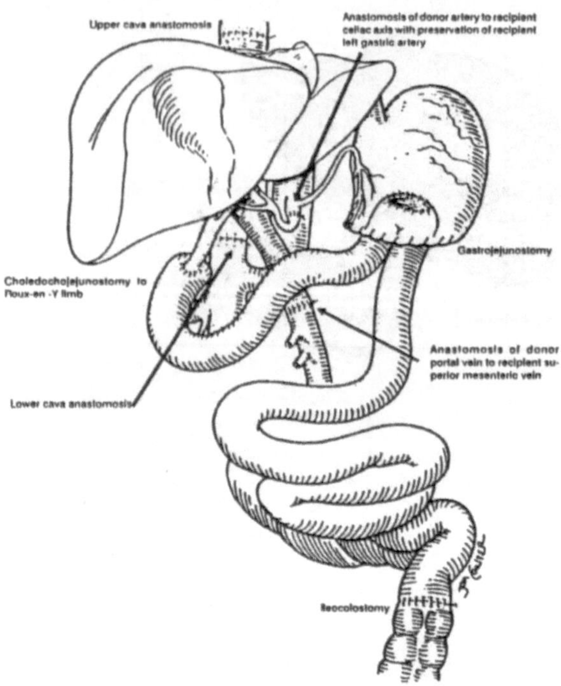

Fig 3. Liver transplantation (without cluster) for reconstruction after right upper quadrant exenteration (organ cluster resection). In the procedure shown, the proximal celiac axis and left gastric artery of the recipient have been retained which permits preservation of the proximal stomach. (Adapted from reference (4).)

Table 1. Outcome after cluster resection and transplantation for right upper quadrant malignancy (4 to 9 months follow-up).

Indication for resection	Alive	Dead
Cholangiocarcinoma	9 (3)	10
Hepatocellular carcinoma	2 (1)	4
Carcinoid tumor	2 (0)	1
Spindle cell sarcoma	1 (0)	1
Neuro-endocrine tumor	2 (0)	0
Islet cell tumor	0	1
Pancreatic cancer		1
Total	16 (4)	18

plications in subsequently treated patients. The use of home hyperalimentation for a prescribed period is being tried and may help with management of the early nutritional problems.

Acknowledgement

This work was supported by research grants from the Veterans Administration and Project Grant No. DK29961 from the National Institutes of Health, Bethesda, MD.

References

1. Starzl, T.E., Kaupp, H.A., Brock, D.R. *et al.*: Homotransplantation of multiple abdominal viscera. *Amer. J. Surg.* **103**, 219—229 (1962).
2. Starzl, T.E., Rowe, M.I., Todo, S. *et al.*: Transplantation of multiple abdominal viscera. *J. Amer. Med. Assoc.* **261**, 1449—1457 (1989).
3. Starzl, T.E., Todo, S., Tzakis, A.G. *et al.*: Abdominal organ cluster transplantation for the treatment of upper abdominal malignancies. *Ann. Surg.* **210**, 118—130 (1989).
4. Tzakis, A.G., Todo, S., and Starzl, T.E.: Upper abdominal exenteration with liver replacement: a modification of the cluster procedure. *Transplant. Proc.* **22** 273—274 (1990).

42. Lung transplantation: current techniques and outcomes

R. MORTON BOLMAN III

Introduction

With the pioneering work of Cooper and the Toronto Lung Transplant group, transplantation of the lung has joined the ranks of other vital organs which can be successfully transplanted. This work stands as a landmark achievement and is a tribute to the combination of careful laboratory investigation coupled with meticulous clinical application of laboratory principles (1). Lung transplantation has also been made possible by the advent of cyclosporine-based immunosuppressive regimens.

Patient Selection

Patients to be considered for lung transplantation must have end-stage pulmonary parenchymal or vascular disease and should be disabled and requiring supplemental oxygen support. Most individuals are deemed to be experiencing the last 12—24 months of their natural life if transplantation is not performed. Accordingly individuals to be considered for transplantation must have end-stage lung disease not amendable to any conventional medical or surgical therapeutic intervention. Individuals should be 60 years of age or younger to be suitable candidates for lung transplantation and should have adequate psychosocial support mechanisms in place.

Contraindications to lung transplantation include necessity for mechanical ventilation prior to transplantation, any steroid administration within 30 days, non-reversible extrathoratic organ system dysfunction, and severe irreversible right ventricular decompensation with or without severe tricuspid regurgitation. Table 1 outlines the recipient selection criteria and contraindications to the procedure of single lung transplantation.

Although the initial patients undergoing transplantation have had primarily forms of pulmonary fibrosis, other diagnoses are now being successfully treated by this modality. Table 2 demonstrates the recipient diagnosis in patients transplanted at the University of Minnesota since the beginning of 1989. Two

Table 1. Recipient selection criteria for single lung transplantation.

End-stage pulmonary parenchymal or vascular disease:	
last 12—24 months of natural life	
disabled, requiring supplemental O_2.	
Age 60 years or younger	
Adequate psychosocial support	
Contraindications:	Mechanical ventilation prior to transplant
	Steroid administration within 30 days
	Non-reversible extrathoracic organ dysfunction
	Severe right ventricular failure

Table 2. Recipient diagnosis, University of Minnesota.

$Alpha_1$-antitrypsin deficiency	2
Lymphocytic interstitial pneumonitis	1 (retransplant at 1 month)
Idiopathic pulmonary fibrosis	1
Bronchiolitis obliterans	1
Lymphangio leiomyomatosis	1
	7 transplants in 6 patients

patients had successful transplantation with a diagnosis of emphysema due to $alpha_1$-antitrypsin deficiency. It was formerly thought that obstructive physiology precluded successful single lung transplantation due to potential air trapping in the remaining native lung. This has not however been a problem and our center and others are successfully performing single lung transplants in patients with obstructive pulmonary diseases. Both our patients with $alpha_1$-antitrypsin deficiency are doing well 10 and 8 months postoperatively respectively. One patient had lymphocytic interstitial pneumonitis and required retransplantation at 1 month for failure of the initial donor lung. She is now doing well 7 months following her second transplant. One patient had idiopathic pulmonary fibrosis and is doing well 5 months postoperatively. One 10 year-old girl who had undergone previous heart-lung transplantation had single lung transplantation for bronchiolitis obliterans and expired preoperatively from hypoxic brain injury. One patient with lymphangioleiomyomatosis received a lung transplant and is doing well 1 year following transplantation. This patient has had an airway complication as she developed a stricture at the site of her anastamosis which has required repeat bronchoscopic dilatations and laser therapy with successful resolution.

Donor Selection

Fewer than 20% of potential heart donors are suitable for lung donation because of problems of pulmonary contusion, nosocomial pneumonia and neurogenic pulmonary edema accompanying brain death and prolonged intubation. Size match is important between donor and recipient for lung transplantation. The donor and recipient heights should correspond as an index of lung volume. The chest radiograph in the donor should be clear and gas exchange should be normal (PaO_2 of greater than 100 mmHg on FiO_2 of 0.4). Lung compliance should be normal and there should be an absence of purulent pulmonary secretions. Presence of fungus or gram-negative rods in the pulmonary secretions should contraindicate transplantation. Both lungs from a single donor can be used successfully for two separate recipients and this has been performed on two occasions in our experience.

The operation

The donor operation proceeds as part of a multiple organ retrieval. Heart and lungs should be visualized at the initiation of the procedure to ascertain if they are indeed suitable for transplantation and that no unsuspected findings such as an occult pulmonary contusion is present. Retrieval of the abdominal visceral organs then proceeds and when nearing completion, cannulas are placed in the ascending aorta and main pulmonary artery. When cardiopulmonary harvesting can proceed, the aorta is cross-clamped and the heart is arrested with a cold potassium cardioplegia solution while the lungs are being preserved with a solution of modified Euro-Collins solution. The lungs are gently ventilated with room air during this infusion and 30—50 ml/kg is infused over a 5—8 min period, with attention directed to maintaining the infusion pressure low. Both heart and lungs are bathed continuously during this infusion period with ice-cold lactated Ringer's solution. The ventilation of the lungs is felt to improve the uniformity of cooling of the lung parenchyma. The tip of the left atrial appendage is amputated to provide egress for the pulmonary cooling solution as it passes throughout the left atrium. Heart and lungs can be separated either *in situ* in the donor or following removal from the donor. It is generally more expeditious to separate the heart from the lung bloc in the donor. An incision is made in the left atrium halfway between the left inferior pulmonary vein and the coronary sinus and from the inside of the left atrium this incision is carried around leaving generous cuffs of left atrium surrounding pulmonary veins on both the right and the left. It is essential to adequately develop the interatrial plane between right and left atrium on the right aspect of the heart to allow for an adequate cuff of left atrium to be preserved surrounding the right pulmonary veins. This will uniformly leave adequate left atrial tissue for the heart implant. There is plenty of left atrium for suitable heart and bilateral individual lung donation. The pulmonary artery is then transected just proximal to the bifurcation into right and left main pulmonary arteries. Superior and inferior vena cave and aorta are divided in routine fashion and the heart is removed. The lung bloc is then removed from the donor by electrocautery dissection of the posterior mediastinal attachments of the lungs and inferior pulmonary ligaments. The trachea is encircled with a TA-30 mechanical stapling device with the lungs partially inflated with room air. The lungs are then removed. For single lung transplantation, the lungs can be separated into two separate lungs for transplantation into two separate recipients. Generous amounts of donor pericardium accompany the lungs and can be used to reinforce the bronchial anastamosis. The donor lungs are then packaged in sterile containers packed in ice and returned to the transplant hospital.

The procedure in the recipient has evolved with experience. Recipients are now positioned such that the abdominal and thoracic portions of the procedure can be performed with the patient in one position on the operating table. The patient is positioned in the lateral decubitious position with the shoulders and hips rolled back to allow access to the midline of the abdomen and to the ipsilateral groin for the institution of cardiopulmonary bypass should it be necessary. Either right or left lung can be transplanted with equal facility. For purposes of discussion I will discuss left single lung transplant. The patient is intubated with a double lumen endotracheal tube. The patient is positioned in the right lateral decubitious position with the shoulders and hips posteriorly displaced for access to the midline of the abdomen and the left groin for institution for cardiopulmonary bypass should it be necessary. A posterolateral thoracotomy is fashioned, the left lung ventilation is ceased and the pleural covering of the hilum and inferior pulmonary ligament is divided. The pulmonary artery is encircled and clamped to prevent shunting through this lung. The artery is ligated distally and divided. The pulmonary veins are individually doubly ligated and divided and the bronchus is transected just above its bifurcation into the upper and lower lobe bronchi. The lung is removed and hemostatis is secured in the mediastinum. With the lung removed the pericardium is entered around the pulmonary veins and a generous cuff of left atrium is created. If time allows, the abdomen is opened in the midline at this point and the omentum is mobilized from the transverse colon. It is passed through a subcostal incision in the diaphragm into the left chest and tacked loosely to the diaphragmatic hiatus to prevent herniation of abdominal contents. This procedure can be delayed if the lung ischemia time is becoming prolonged. The donor lung is then brought to the field. The bronchus is opened and cultures are taken of the donor airway for assistance in postoperative management of infection. The donor bronchus is transected two cartilaginous rings above bifurcation into upper and lower lobe and implantation of the lung begins with anastomosis of donor and recipient bronchus. This is a very important anastamosis and should be performed carefully with interrupted suture technique. The membranous portion of the bronchus is first anastamosed with interrupted 4-0 PDS suture with knots on the outside of the bronchus. Next the cartilaginous portion of the bronchus is approximated again with interrupted 4-0 PDS suture and if possible the donor bronchus is telescoped into the recipient bronchus for 1—2 mm. At this point the omentum is wrapped around the anastamosis and then sutured loosely to itself with 4-0 suture. The donor and recipient pulmonary arteries are joined end to end using 5-0 Prolene and finally a partial occlusion clamp is placed across the base of the left atrium at the cuff encompassing both pulmonary veins. The cuff of atrium is then created by connecting incisions in the pulmonary veins and donor and recipient left atria are joined using running 4-0 Prolene. Retrograde and antegrade flushing of the lung is carried out and the clamps are removed restoring perfusion to the lung as ventilation is also restored to the lung. Homostatis needs to be meticulous in the hilum and in the chest.

If the patient does not tolerate single lung anesthesia, cardiopulmonary bypass can be instituted through the ipsilateral femoral artery and vein using a venous cannula that passes to the right atrium and conventional arterial cannulation. Should this prove inadequate, the thoracotomy incision can be readily extended across the sternum and access to the heart thereby obtained for institution of bypass via the aorta and right atrium.

Once meticulous hemostasis has been assured, the midline abdominal incision is closed in routine fashion. Large-bore chest drainage catheters are placed one posteriorly to the apex and a right angle tube in the costophrenic sulcus and the chest is closed in routine fashion.

Immunosuppression

Recipients of lung allografts receive standard triple drug immunosuppression with minor modifications (2). Patients receive preoperative low doses of cyclosporine (3—5 mg/kg) and high dose azathioprine (3 mg/kg/PO). Perioperatively patients receive menthylprednisolone. Steriods are then withheld for the subsequent 2 weeks to enhance airway healing. Postoperatively patients are maintained on low dose cyclosporine both orally and supplemented with a low dose intravenous infusion (1—2 mg/h as a continuous infusion). Little attention is directed to achieving adequate cyclosporine levels for the first several days in the interest of preserving renal function adequate to allow diuresis and expedite extubation. Azathioprine doses remain 2.5—3 mg/kg/day. At 2 weeks patients are begun on 30 mg/day of predisone as well as cyclosporine and imuran and are maintained on triple drug therapy indefinitely. Cyclosporine levels are targeted to a 12-h trough level of 200—250 ng/ml (HPLC). Azathioprine is targeted to a white blood cell of 4000—5000 per cubic millimeter and prednisone is tapered to a maintenance dose of 5—10 mg per day by 3 months. All patients receive trimethoprim sulfamethoxazole as prophylaxis against pneumocystis and nocardia infection. High dose acyclovir and mycostatin are administered for 3 months as prophylaxis against viral and fungal infections respectively.

Postoperative surveillance

Lung allograft recipients are followed carefully for evidence of infection and rejection. Bronchoscopy with bronchoalveolar lavage and transbronchial biopsy are performed liberally for the diagnosis of these entities. Histology of lung rejection consists of perivascular or intraendothelial infiltrates of mononuclear cells. Rejection can manifest as low grade temperature elevation coupled with subtle perihilar changes in the chest radiograph. Patients may experience shortness of breath. It is important to rule out infection prior to initiating therapy for rejection. Rejection is treated with pulse methylprednisolone therapy. Infection is diagnosed and treated aggressively as it can be devasting in the immunocompromised host. Most patients experience one episode of rejection during the first 1—2 weeks following transplantation.

Quantitative perfusion scans are performed to demonstrate laterization of blood flow to the transplanted lung. With successful transplantation most pulmonary blood flow should be directed to the transplanted lung. Pulmonary function studies are also performed shortly after transplantation and frequently in the postoperative course to monitor progressive improvement and to herald possible rejection or infection episodes. A representative chest radiograph and quantitative perfusion scan in shown in Figure 1. This patient with alpha^1-antitrypsin deficiency underwent single lung transplantation. His chest radiograph and quantitative perfusion scan at 3 months following transplantation are shown. Figure 2 demonstrates the pulmonary function tests in this same patient both before surgery and through 6 weeks following his transplant demonstrating a progressive and dramatic rise in FEV_1 and DLCO.

Conclusions

Lung transplantation has been shown to be an effective modality for treatment of parenchymal or vascular disease of the lung with preservation of adequate cardiac function. With further development and experience, this procedure will become the mainstay of the armamentarium of treatment of end-stage lung disease not amenable to conventional medical and surgical therapies. The ability to benefit three individual recipients from a single donor makes single lung transplantation more attractive than heart-lung transplantation on a logistic basis. Both procedures are plagued with bronchiolitis obliterans and much work remains to optimize long-term results.

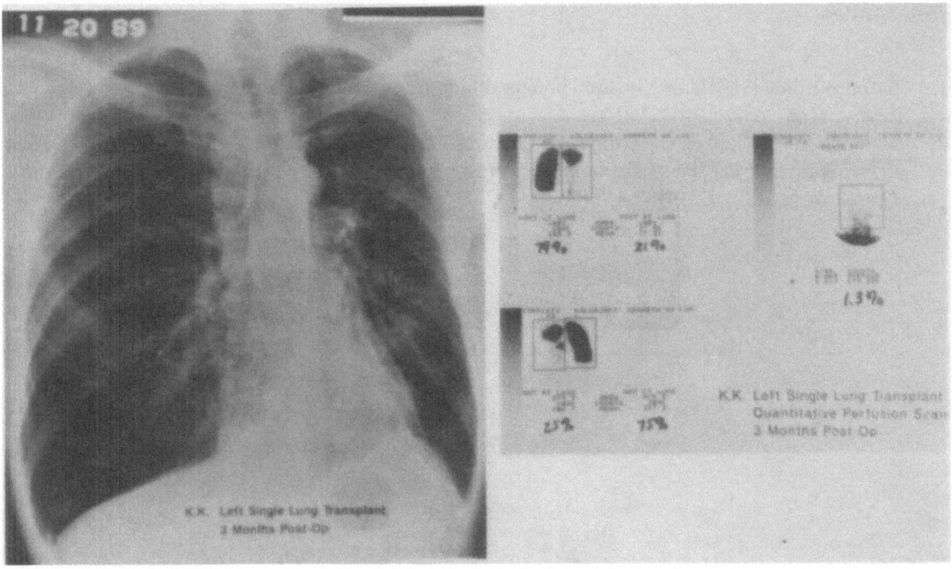

Fig. 1. Chest radiograph of patient with alpha$_1$-antitrypsin deficiency 3 months following left single lung transplant. On the right is a quantitative perfusion scan demonstrating that most of the blood flow enters the transplanted lung.

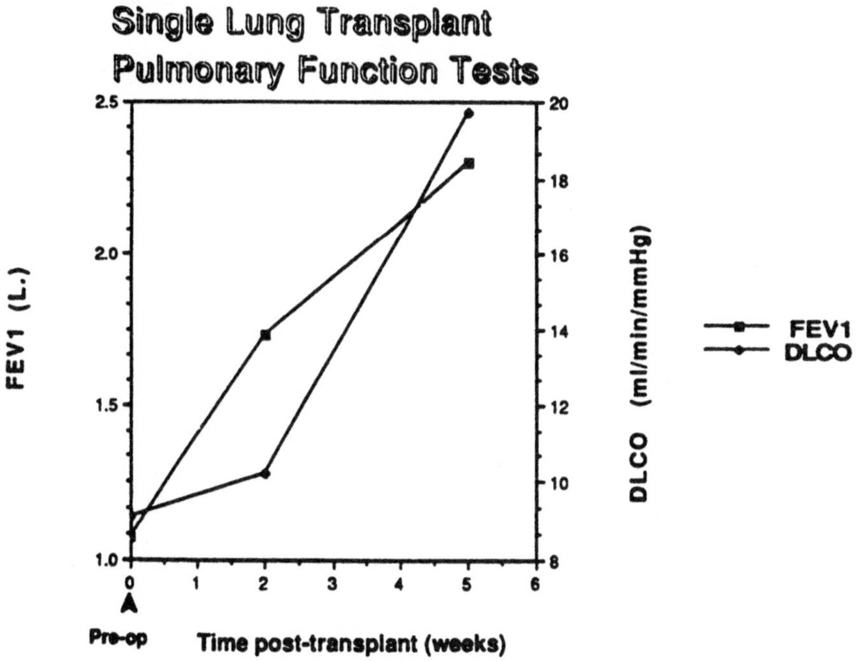

Fig. 2. Pulmonary function tests over time in patient from Figure 1. FEV$_1$ and DLCO, both severely depressed pretransplant, demonstrate marked improvement during the first 6 weeks post-transplant.

References

1. Toronto Lung Transplant Group: Unilateral lung transplantation for pulmonary fibrosis. *New Engl. J. Med.* **314**, 1140 (1986).
2. Bolman, R.M., Cance, C., Spray, T., Genton, R., Weiss, C., Saffitz, J. and Eisen, H.: The changing face of cardiac transplantation: Washington University program 1985—1987. *Ann. Thorac. Surg.* **45**, 192—197 (1988).

43. Heart-lung transplantation at the University of Minnesota

R. MORTON BOLMAN III

Heart-lung transplantation was pioneered by Reitz and his collegues at Stanfrod University following a long period of preparation in primate laboratory investigation (1). This major step forward in thoracic transplantation was made possible both by the dedicated efforts by these individuals as well as the availability of cyclosporine-based immunosuppressive regimens. The ability to transplant the heart-lung bloc successfully and to achieve healing of the airway anastamosis lent great impetus to the development of lung transplantation as a therapeutic modality. Indeed the field of lung transplantation had been plagued by almost uniform failure of healing of the airway anastamosis. The demonstration by Reitz that tracheal healing following heart-lung transplantation could be achieved was of critical importance. The restoration to health of these desperately ill individuals for whom no previous treatment had been available ranks among the most noteworthy achievements in the field of thoracic surgery.

Recipient selection

Patients with end-stage pulmonary vascular disease have proven the most suitable candidates for heart-lung transplantation. Individuals with primary pulmonary hypertension and secondary pulmonary hypertension with congenital heart defects (Eisenmenger's syndrome) have formed the bulk of patients transplanted to date (2). Patients must have end-stage parenchymal or vascular disease of the lung associated with the severe heart failure. They must have an absence of extra-thoracic organ dysfunction that is non-reversible. As with all transplantation candidates an adequate psycho-social support structure is necessary. Table 1 demonstrates the recipient diagnosis in patients transplanted at the University of Minnesota. Eight of 17 patients had primary pulmonary hypertension, 5 had Eisenmenger's syndrome, these two diagnoses together forming the majority of patients transplanted.

Contraindications to transplantation include necessity for mechanical ventilation, any steriod administration within 30 days and a major prior thoracotomy due to risk of excessive hemorrhage at time of transplantation from adhensions.

Table 1. Recipient diagnosis in heart-lung recipients at the University of Minnesota.

Primary pulmonary hypertension	8
Eisenmenger's syndrome	5
Cystic fibrosis	1
Lymphocytic interstitial pneumonitis	1
$Alpha_1$-antitrypsin deficiency	2
Total	17

Donor selection

Fewer than 20% of potential heart donors are suitable for heart-lung donation. Reasons for pulmonary unsuitability are neurogenic pulmonary edema, thoracic trauma and constusion to the lung and pneumonia from long-term ventilatory support. Critical features for donor selection are shown in Table 2. The donor should have a clear chest radiograph. There should be no purulent pulmonary secretions and Gram stains should reveal no fungus or gram-negative organisms. Gas exchange should be normal with a PaO_2 100 mmHg or greater on FiO_2 of 0.4. Lung compliance should be normal. Size match between donor and recipient is important and the donor heart lung bloc should be smaller than that being replaced in the recipient to avoid overcrowding of the lungs in the recipient and resultant atelectasis.

Operation

Donor harvest of the heart-lung bloc occurs in concert with multiple organ retrieval, often at a hospital distant from the transplant center. Careful coordination between the retrieving teams is essential and the heart-lung bloc should be implanted in the recipient within 4—5 hours of removal from the donor. Heart and lungs are examined early in the harvest procedure to assure suitability for transplantation. At that time the recipient operation can begin. When the vital organs are ready to be removed, heart and lungs are preserved.

Table 2. Donor selection criteria for heart-lung transplantation.

Clear chest radiograph
Absent purulent secretions
Normal gas exchange: PaO_2 100 mgHg or greater on FiO_2 of 0.4
Normal lung compliance: peak airway pressure of 30 mmHg on normal TV
Size match: donor organs same size or smaller than recipient

The aorta is cross-clamped and the heart arrested with cardioplegia infusion into the aortic root in combination with topical cooling. Simultaneously an infusion of a cold Euro-Collins solution is infused into the pulmonary artery in the amount of 30—50 ml/kg body weight (3). The lungs are gently ventilated and topical cooling solution is liberally bathed over the heart and lungs (3). The tip of the atrial appendage is amputated to allow egress of the pulmonary preservation solution. The heart-lung bloc is then removed by division of the posterior mediastinal attachments with electrocautery. The aorta is divided just proximal to the innominate artery. The trachea is clamped well above the carina with a TA-30 stapler with the lungs partially inflated and the heart-lung bloc is removed. The bloc is placed in a sterile container, packed in ice and returned to the transplant hospital.

The recipient operation should begin 2—3 hours before the anticipated arrival of the donor heart-lung bloc. The chest is opened through a midline sternotomy. The pleural cavities are explored for adhesions. If any are found they are divided. The pericardium is then opened and the patient placed on bypass. The heart is removed leaving a long cuff of aorta and a generous cuff of right atrium. The lungs are then individually removed. The phrenic nerves bilaterally are isolated on a generous pedicle of pericardium from the pulmonary artery to the diaphragm. It is important to leave a segment of left pulmonary artery in place to avoid damage to the recurrent laryngeal nerve. The inferior pulmonary ligaments are then divided using electrocautery and the lungs individually are removed following application of the TA-55 surgical stapler. Hemostatis is secured along the staple pulmonary hila. The trachea is then isolated between the aorta and the superior vena cava. The individual left and right main stem bronchi are removed and the trachea divided just above the carina. Hemostatis is secured in the posterior mediastinum. It is imperative to remove most of the left atrium from the recipient heart to allow easy passage of the heart-lung bloc behind the right atrium. The heart-lung bloc is then brought to the field and the lungs passed into their respective pleural cavities. Anastamosis of donor and recipient tracheas is carried out with running 3-0 monofilament suture. This anastamosis is then reinforced with circumferential wrapping with donor pericardium. Aortic anastamosis follows between donor and recipient aortas and when completed reperfusion of the organs can be accomplished and gentle ventilation initiated in the lungs. As rewarming in being completed, the donor and recipient right atrial remnants are joined completing the procedure.

The heart-lung transplant operation removes all surgical planes in the chest cavity. This allows large amounts of bleeding to occur and to be relatively inapparent to the surgeon if not carefully searched for. A common site of bleeding is the posterior right atrium. If there is a patent foramen ovale or other communication between right and left atrium in the recipient heart, this can cause bleeding which is very difficult to control with the new organs in place.

Once hemostatis is secured, chest catheters are placed. One straight catheter is passed to the apex of each chest and one right angled catheter just over the diaphragm of each chest. It is not necessary to drain the mediastinum *per se* since all areas of the chest communicate freely. The chest catheters on the right and left are attached to separate drainage systems to allow laterialization of postoperative bleeding in case re-exploration is necessary.

Immunosuppression

As a result of our large experience in heart transplantation and the application of triple drug immunosuppression, we have adapted this regimen for heart-lung recipients as well (4). All patients receive low dose cyclosporine in the perioperative period in the interest of preserving renal function to allow aggressive diuresis and early extubation. Azathioprine is also administered and patients receive perioperative corticosteroid therapy for the first 24 hours and then no further corticosteriods for the first 2 weeks. Patients may receive a short 3-day course of antilymphocyte globulin for additional immunosuppression during the time when cyclosporine levels are being maintained low. Maintenance therapy consists of cyclosporine, azathioprine and prednisone. Prednisone is begun at 30 mg/day at 2 weeks and tapered to 5 mg/day at 3 months.

Surveillance for infection and rejection

Aggressive surveillance for postoperative infection and rejection is of paramount importance to successful heart and lung transplantation. In conjunction with our pulmonology collegues, we have developed an aggressive program of bronchoscopy with frequent bronchoalveolar lavage (BAL) and transbronchial biopsy (TBB). BAL is very useful for the diagnosis of infection and TBB for the diagnosis of rejection as well as some invasion infections (fungus, CMV, etc.). Bronchoscopy with BAL and TBB has yielded a sensitivity of 79% and a specificity of 100% in the diagnosis of perioperative pulmonary dysfunction in these patients. In fully 32% of the case, an unsuspected finding has been observed at bronchoscopy, demonstrating the great utility of this procedure in the postoperative management of these patients. Frequent chest radiographs are also of great utility in the screening for perioperative pulmonary dysfunction. Figure 1 is a chest radiograph demonstrating pleural effusion and infiltrates in a young woman 2 weeks following heart-lung transplantation*. Figure 2 is the

* Bronchoscopy was performed, BAL was negative for infection and this patient received therapy for rejection.

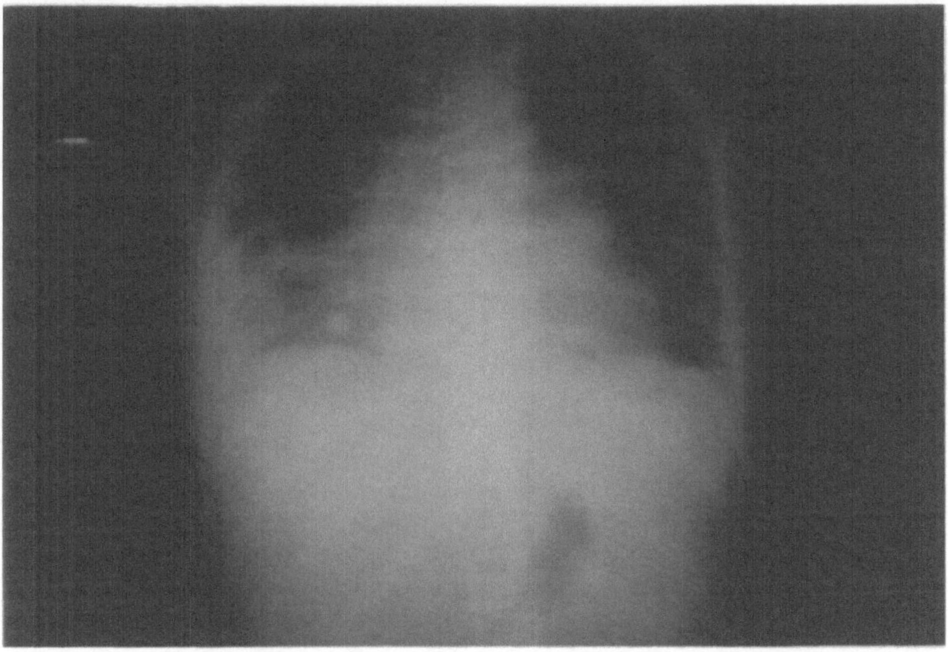

Fig. 1. Chest radiograph two weeks after heart-lung transplantation demonstrating pulmonary infiltrates and right pleural effusion. Bronchoscopic cultures were negative and a diagnosis of rejection was made.

chest radiograph of this lady following treatment for rejection. The diagnosis of rejection rests on clinical grounds supported by TBB and the absence of demonstrable infection. Treatment consists of 3 days of intravenous pulse therapy with methylprednisolone.

Results

There have been 17 heart-lung transplants performed at the University of Minnesota. All patients have survived to hospital discharge. There has been no perioperative mortality. There have been 3 late deaths from bronchiolitis obliterans and a fourth patient has recently been diagnosed with this disorder. All patients have experience rejection during the transplant hospitalization which has successfully been treated with steriod therapy. Late out of hospital rejection has been rare in this experience. Bronchiolitis obliterans, felt to be a manifestation of chronic lung rejection, has accounted for 17% late mortality in this series. This disease is heralded by diminished exercise tolerance, recurrent dyspnea and a decrease in the small airways flow measurements in pulmonary function testing. This entity when it occurs can sometimes be stabilized with

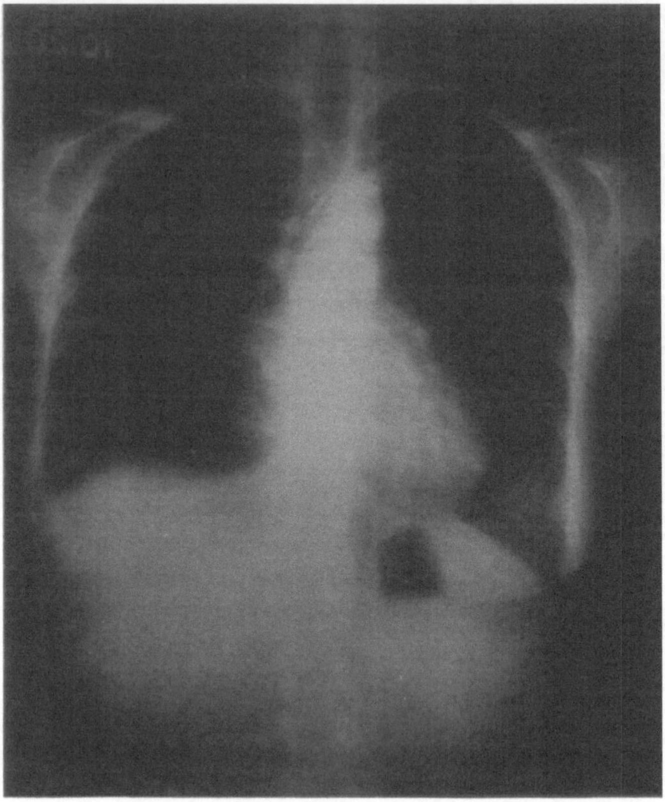

Fig. 2. Chest radiograph in same patient as Figure 1. Findings of infiltrates and effusion have resolved following three days of intravenous methylprednisolone therapy for rejection.

additional immunosuppression but tends to run an inexorable downhill course eventuating in the patient's death.

Conclusions

Heart-lung transplantation, though a relatively infrequently performed procedure, has had an impact on the field of thoracic organ transplantation far beyond its numbers. The successful application of this procedure has ushered in the era of lung transplantation which will undoubtedly benefit many more patients in the future. Reitz and his collegues deserve great credit for their pioneering work in this field. As single lung transplantation evolves, this procedure will become the mainstay of our treatment armamentarium against end-stage diseases of the lung. Limited donor organs will dictate that more recipients can benefit from single lung transplantation than heart-lung transplantation and single lung transplantation will be applied to an increasing variety of disorders formerly thought amendable only to heart-lung transplantation. Nonetheless, heart-lung transplantation will reserve a place in the treatment of end-stage heart and lung disease when the heart function is severly compromised or the congential defect is too complex to repair in conjuction with simultaneous single lung transplantation. Heart-lung transplantation has paved the way for successful transplantation of the lungs and deserves its rightful place in the annals of thoracic organ transplantation.

References

1. Reitz, B.A., Wallwork, J.L., Hunt, S.A. *et al.*: Heart-lung transplantation: Successful therapy for patients with pulmonary vascular disease. *New Engl. J. Med.* **306**, 557 (1982).
2. Fragomeni, L.S. and Kaye, M.P.: The Registry of the International Society for Heart Transplantation: 5th Official Report, 1988, *J. Heart Transplant.* **7**, 249 (1988).
3. Baldwin, J.C., Frist, W.H., Starkey, T.D. *et al.*: Distant graft procurement for combined heart and lung transplantation using pulmonary artery flush and simple topical hypothermia for graft preservation. *Ann. Thorac. Surg.* **43**, 670 (1987).
4. Bolman, R.M., Olivari, M.T., Sibley, R., Saffitz, J., Spadaro, J., Cance, C. and Elick, B.: Current results with triple therapy for heart transplantation. *Transplant. Proc.* **19**, 2490–2491 (1987).

44. Specificity and sensitivity of the cytoimmunological monitoring (CIM): differentiation between cardiac rejection, viral, bacterial, or fungal infection

C. HAMMER, D. KLANKE, P. DIRSCHEDL, B.M. KEMKES, B. REICHART M. GOKEL AND F. KROMBACH

Introduction

Postoperative survival of human heart recipients depends mainly on the early diagnosis and prevention of inflammatory events. Different therapeutic regimens, e.g. immunosuppressive drugs or antibiotics, enable transplant surgeons to treat such complications successfully. Non-invasive and reliable methods for the early detection of inflammation in graft recipients are desired in order to avoid major organ damage.

Following heart transplantation (HTP) the postoperative course of the recipients and their grafts is usually monitored by daily physical examinations, using different electrodiograms (ECGs), analysis of enzyme and neopterin levels in the peripheral blood or the urine, two-dimensional echocardiography, endomyocardial biopsies (EMB)(1), and microbiological and serological test for infections. The methods are either invasive biopsies or not useful to discriminate between acute graft rejections and infections. Therefore, a cytoimmunological monitoring (CIM) has been established in order to supply further information on inflammatory processes threatening patients' lives.

The non-invasive and atraumatic cytoimmunological monitoring was developed for early diagnosis of inflammatory events in the postoperative period of HTP. CIM consists of phenotyping mononuclear cells for HTP according to their degree of activation. Normal lymphocytes (Ly) are distinguished from activated lymphocytes (ALy), lymphoblasts (Lb), or monocytes (2). The degree of activation of these lymphoid cells, mainly the percentage of Lbs, allows a staging of the immunological condition of the recipient, including rejection episodes, and bacterial, fungal, or viral infections. Monoclonal antibodies (MoAbs) analyzing lymphocyte subsets help to distinguish rejection from various types of infection. The reduction of traumatic and EMBs invasive under CIM stimulated a retrospective statistical analysis of the sensitivity and specificity of CIM, in correlation with EMB, and its gradation.

Material and methods

The study included 108 HTPs (64 males and 44 females). Their ages ranged from 19 to 54 years. For statistical evaluation 72 patients could be taken into consideration. Selection criteria and indication for transplantation as well as immunosuppression has been published.

Cytoimmunological monitoring

The technique of CIM has been described extensively (3); in short:

Fast test. Only 10 μl of PB are needed for a smear for differentiation of leukocytes; 40 μl for total leukocyte counting. The mononuclear cells (MNC) separated from 500 μl of heparinized peripheral blood (hpB) over a Ficoll micro-gradient (d = 1.077) are spread on a slide using a cytocentrifuge. All smears are stained according to Pappenheim. All leukocyte subsets and their activated forms are taken into consideration. As long as no signs of activation or other exceptional observations are found, an additional procedure is not necessary.

Extended test. If any of the subpopulations is activated, the second test must be applied: MNC out of hpB are counted using a cytofluorometer. The interesting subpopulations are distinguished by means of MoAbs. The most important lymphocytes are those labelled by CD4 and CD8 MoAb.

The following parameters were investigated: (a) leukocyte number (Coulter-counter), (b) differential blood count (Pappenheim staining), (c) mononuclear concentrate (Pappenheim staining), (d) mononuclear concentrate (flow-cytometry/MoAb).

Statistical analysis

Statistical analyses used, were: Estimation of reliability of lymphoblasts (Lb), counts of two raters; a multiple logistic regression (i.e. discriminant analysis to select the best discriminating variables); the construction of a ROC-curve (receiver operating characteristic curve) to find an optimal operation point; a life table analysis (i.e. the Kaplan-Meier estimator), and a non-parametric discriminant method for further investigation. The method called CART (classified and regression trees) has shown to be asymptotically efficient with respect to the error rates (4).

Results

Acute cellular rejection

The most alarming cells, indicating acute inflammatory events in the grafts, are lymphoblasts and activated lymphocytes and cells of the monocytemacrophage series described elsewhere (5, 6, 7). During acute rejections inflammatory cells accumulate in the graft. The intensity of inflammation associated with rejection can be quantified from the pB and HTP and expressed as an activation index.

In a case of severe rejection, an activated MNC including more than 7% blast cells or 20% activated lymphocytes, is found. The ratio of cells expressing the phenotypes CD4/CD8 is approximately 1.5. B-cell numbers are lower than 15%. EMBs are used to estimate the severity of rejection as defined by the extent of edema and by nature and number of infiltrating cells. (Fig. 1).

Infection

Viral infection. During viral infection, the activated MNC is characterized by a CD4/CD8 ratio lower than 1.0. At the climax of infection, the ratio is often as low as 0.1. The percentage of B-cells remains unchanged or is slightly increased. So-called 'large granular lymphocytes' (LGL), supposed to be natural killer cells, exceed 5% of leukocytes; these LGLs sometimes comprise 40%—50% of the lymphocyte population. Mainly cytomegalovirus, hepesvirus, and Epstein — Barr virus induce such phenomena. Serological methods and virus isolation are still the method of choice for diagnosis of viral infection (Fig. 2).

Bacterial infection. The diagnosis of bacterial or fungal infections by CIM is possible. There infections induce activation but no change in the CD4/CD8 ratio. A significant increase of B-cells and juvenile polimorphonuclear cells is found. Often this increase of promyelocytes makes the reading and distinction of cells of the lymphocyte line difficult. The isolation and cultivation of bacteria or fungi and measurements of chemiluminescence activity of phagocytes in pB or aspirates of grafts supports the CIM of microbial infections (8) (Fig. 3).

- **Activated Mononuclear Concentrate**
- **T4 / T8 ≥ 1.0**
- **Ly 2 pos. B-cells < 20 %**

Fig. 1. Acute rejection.

- **Activated Mononuclear Concentrate**
- **T4 / T8 < 1.0**
- **Ly 2 pos. B-cells < 20 %**
- **Large Granular Lymphocytes > 5 %**

Fig. 2. Viral infection.

- **Activated Mononuclear Concentrate**
- **T4 / T8 = 1.0 - 1.5**
- **B-cells > 20 %**
- **Juvenile Granulocytes**

Fig. 3. Bacterial, i.e., fungal, infections.

Clinical diagnosis

Beside CIM, other non-invasive methods such as Fast-Fourier-transformed ECG (9) and Echocardiography are applied. As soon as CIM together with another test is positive, CIM remaining the leading parameter, the patient is treated for rejection, and the process is then controlled by endomyocardial biopsies.

A typical follow-up of a patient shows the behavior of activated lymphocytes and blasts. An increase of ALYs and LBs at day 5 heralds a rejection sensitive to methylprednisolone. The peak at day 25, due to a bacterial infection, was negative in EMB (Fig. 4).

Statistical evaluation

The estimation of reliability, reflecting in this application an equivalent to the IRC (interrater correlation) for measurements, shows a nearly perfect concordance of LB-counts of two raters. The correlation coefficient of 0.99 supports this finding. The results of CIM were compared with those of EMB.

Histograms of LB and ALY correlated to the histological finding, which were graded according to Billingham. To show the heterogeneity of LB classes in EMB groups, a cutpoint is set at LB <6 and LB >7. This comparison leads to a contingency table (Fig. 5).

In 72 heart transplant patients, 33 CIMs and EMBs simultaneously diagnosed AR (Fig. 6). In 5 cases CIM was positive without clinical correlate. In 39

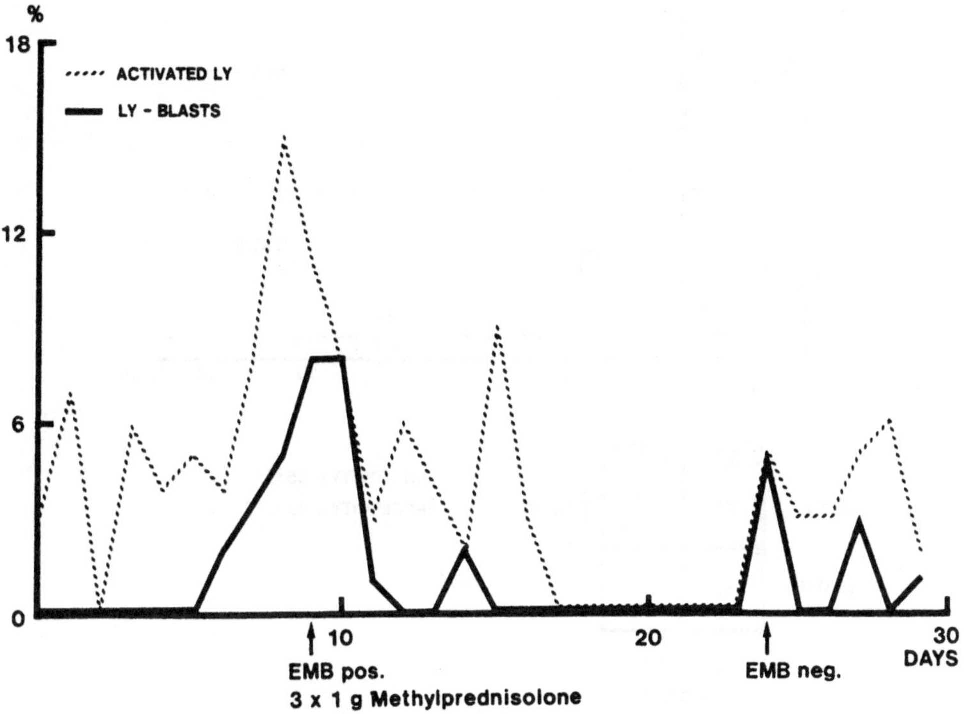

Fig. 4. Follow up of LBs and aLys of a heart transplant patient suffering from acute rejection (day 7 to day 10) and bacterial infection (day 25).

cases, EMBs and CIMs were both negative, and in 5 patients, positive EMB was not accompanied by signs of activation in CIM.

According to this analysis the sensitivity of CIM is 85% and its specificity 90% ($p < 0.0000001$) (4).

Discussion

The simple and atraumatic CIM method, with a sensitivity of 85% and a specificity of 90%, is a valid and reliable method for diagnosis of acute rejection. EMB should, therefore, be used only to monitor the effects of medication during acute rejection.

CIM allows reduction in the frequency of EMB in the postoperative phase of HTP. The construction of an ROC curve provides a preliminary definition of an optimal operational point a > 7% of lymphoblasts, in order to decide whether further or more potent therapy is necessary to control acute rejection. Correlation with EMB indicated that this index coincides with the intramural inflammation episodes in the graft. Concerning the prognostic value of CIM, it is also useful to take the slope of acceleration of lymphoblasts into considerations. The

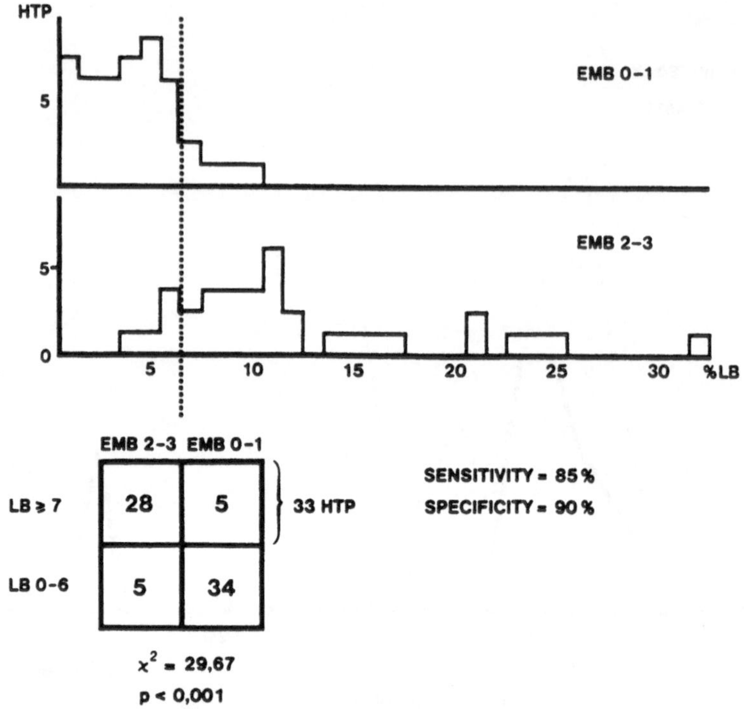

Fig. 5. Histogram and contingency table for %LBs during the first inflammatory event after cardiac transplantation.

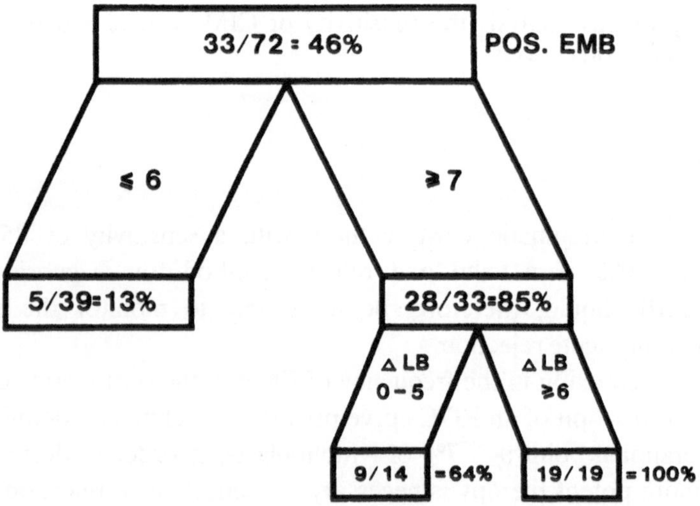

Fig. 6. Decision tree for acute rejection after cardiac transplantation (CART).

life table analysis supports the hypothesis that recipients undergoing a moderate or severe rejection as their first inflammatory event are at highest risk.

The construction of an ROC-curve provided a preliminary definition of an optimal operational point at 6% Lb, to decide whether further or more potent therapy is necessary to control AR. The correlation with EMB indicates that this index coincides with the intramural inflammation events in the graft. Concerning the prognostic value of CIM, it is also useful to take the slope of acceleration of Lbs into consideration. The life table analysis supports the hypothesis that recipients undergoing a moderate/severe rejection as their first inflammatory event have the highest risk.

As these three different statistical analyses lead to the same result, it can be concluded that CIM, with its high sensitivity and specificity, provides good information about the extent of inflammation in the graft, thus providing an opportunity for early treatment and control of acute rejection.

As these three different statistical analyses lead to the same result, it can be concluded that CIM, with it high sensitivity, provides good information about the extent of inflammation in the graft, thus giving a chance for early treatment and control of acute rejection.

References

1. Caves, P.K., Stinson, G.B., Billingham, E. and Shumway, N.E.: Percutaneous transvenous endomyocardial biopsy in human heart recipients. *Ann. Thorac. Surg.* **16**, 325—329 (1973).
2. Hammer, C.: *Cytology in Transplantation.* Schulz-Verlag (1989).
3. Hammer, C., Reichenspurner, H., Ertel, W., Lersch, C., Plahl, M., Brendel, W., Reichart, B., Überfuhr, P., Welz, A., Kemkes, B.M., Reble, B., Functius, W. and Gokel, M.: Cytological and immunologic monitoring of Cyclosporine-treated human heart recipients. *Heart Transplant* **3**, 228—232 (1984).
4. Klanke, D., Dirschedl, P., Kemkes, B.M., Reichart, B., Gokel, M. and Krombach, F.: Sensitivity and specificity of cytoimmunological monitoring in correlation with endomyocardial biopsies in heart transplant patients. *Transplant. Proc.* **21**, 3781—3783 (1987).
5. Häyry, P. and Willebrand, E.: Practical guidelines for needle aspiration biopsy of human renal allografts. *Ann. Clin. Res.* **13**, 288—306 (1981).
6. Hammer, C., Land, W., Stadler, J., Koller, C. and Brendel, W.: Lymphocyte subclasses in rejecting kidney grafts detected by monoclonal antibodies. *Transplant. Proc.* **11**, 356—360 (1983).
7. Hammer, C. and Lersch, C.: Hematological cytology in organ transplantation. In: Baethmann and Messmer (eds), *Surgical Research: Recent Concepts and Results*, pp. 173—180, Springer (1989).
8. Schödel, F., Krombach, F., Lersch, C., Hammer, C. and Brendel, W.: Chemoluminescence of polymorphonuclear leukocytes during allograft rejection. *Transplant. Proc.* **17**, 2534—2535 (1985).
9. Haberl, R., Weber, M., Reichenspurner, H., Kemkes, B.M., Osterholzer, G., Anthuber, M. and Steinbeck, G.: Frequency analysis of the surface electrocardiogram for recognition of acute rejection after orthotopic *Circulation* **76**, 101—108 (1987).

45. International Pancreas Transplantation Registry report

DAVID E.R. SUTHERLAND, KRISTIN GILLINGHAM and
KAY C. MOUDRY-MUNNS

The International Pancreas Transplant Registry (IPTR) has collected information prospectively on all pancreas transplant cases in the world since 1980 (1), and has retrospective information on all cases before 1980 dating back to the first case performed in 1966 (2). Several previous reports of the Registry have been made (3—13). Some of the results of an analysis performed on August 22, 1989, of cases submitted to the Registry as of June 30, 1989, and reported in greater detail elsewhere (14, 15), are summarized here.

Methods

Information on location of the transplants, methods of duct management; duration of graft preservation; HLA type of donor and recipient; the presence or absence of a kidney transplant in the pancreas recipients and their fate; and complications of the transplant were analyzed. Patient and graft survival rates were calculated by actuarial techniques on the University of Minnesota Health Science CDC Cyber Computer using SPSS software. Pancreas grafts were considered functioning for a long as the recipients were insulin-independent. p-values comparing survival rates between groups over the entire survival experience were calculated by the Lee-Desu variant of the Gehan test (16), and were considered statistically significant when $p \leqslant 0.05$.

Registry results

Overall analysis of outcome by era

Between December 17, 1966 and December 31, 1989, 2292 pancreas transplants were reported to the Registry, including over 400 in both 1988 and 1989. Only the 2004 pancreas transplants in 1876 diabetic patients that were reported to the Registry as of June 30, 1989 were analyzed. Outcome was compared for four eras, 1966—77 (n = 64), 1978—83 (n = 336), 1984—85

($n = 364$), and 1986—89 ($n = 1220$). The one-year pancreas graft functional survival rates were 6, 36, 55, and 70%, and the corresponding patient survival rates were 39, 71, 80, and 87% in the respective ears.

Analysis of 1986—89 Cases

The 1986—89 cases were analyzed separately to multiple factors. In this era there were 241 (20%) technical failures. Of 979 technically successful (TS) cases, the one-year functional survival rate was 70%.

The one-year actuarial pancreas graft functional survival rates for 1986—89 cases within multiple subgroups are shown in Table 1, and the comparisons for which p values are $\leqslant 0.05$ are given. The number of pancreas transplants performed during this time were nearly equal to North America and Europe, and these continents account for nearly all of the cases. Pancreas graft survival rates were slightly higher ($p = 0.05$) in North America than Europe.

In regard to management of the pancreatic duct and exocrine secretions, the functional survival rate was significantly higher for bladder- than for either intestinal-drained or duct-injected grafts ($p < 0.05$). The functional survival rate with duct-injection was also significantly higher than with enteric drainage, but the difference was not statistically significant.

In regard to preservation time, more than half of the grafts were stored for <6 h, but longer preservation times are being reported and more than one-seventh were stored for over 12 h, including 27 for more than 24 h (2%). The highest graft functional survival rate was in the >24 h group, but there were no significant differences in functional survival rates between grafts stored <6, 6—12, 12—24, and >24 h.

Recipients of grafts mismatched for 0 DR antigens had significantly higher ($p \leqslant 0.02$) graft survival rates than those mismatched for 1 or 2 DR antigens. The same relative differences were seen in the analysis of TS cases, and the comparison of 0 vs 2 DR mismatches was significant ($p = 0.05$).

In regard to recipient category, pancreas graft survival rates differed according to whether a kidney was or was not transplanted and according to the kidney transplant. Most pancreas transplants continue to be performed in recipients of kidney transplants and the majority of these were performed simultaneous with the kidney. Less than 15% of the transplants performed during the 1986—89 period were in non-kidney transplant recipients. The pancreas graft survival rates were significantly higher ($p < 0.05$) in recipients of simultaneous kidney transplants than in recipients of a pancreas after a kidney or in a non-uremic, non-kidney transplant recipients of pancreas transplants alone.

Although pancreas graft survival rates were higher in recipients of simul-

Table 1. Graft actuarial functional (insulin-independent) survival rates at one year for pancreas transplants reported to the Registry between January 1, 1986 and June 30, 1989, and analyzed August 22, 1989.

	Category (*N*)	Percent functioning at one year	*p* values ⩽ 0.05
A.	All cases (1604)	56%	1 vs 2
	1. North America (798)	59%	
	2. Europe (783)	53%	
	3. Other (23)	55%	
B.	Duct management		
	1. Bladder drainage (785)	59%	1 vs 2
	2. Polymer injection (274)	54%	1 vs 3
	3. Intestinal drainage (785)	47%	
C.	Preservation time		
	1. <6 hours (626)	56%	
	2. 6—12 hours (314)	52%	
	3. 12—24 hours (164)	57%	
	4. >24 hours (27)	66%	
D.	HLA-DR mismatches (all cases)		
	1. 0 (89)	68%	
	2. 1 (436)	56%	1 vs 3
	3. 2 (390)	51%	
E.	HLA-DR mismatches (TS cases)		
	1. 0 (74)	84%	1 vs 3
	2. 1 (337)	72%	1 vs 2
	3. 2 (321)	62%	2 vs 3
F.	Association with and timing of kidney Tx		
	1. Px Simul with Kid Tx (865)[a]	63%	1 vs 2
	2. Px after Kid Tx (186)	45%	1 vs 3
	3. Px Alone (165)	37%	

[a] 1 year kidney function rate = 79%.

taneous kidney pancreas transplants, patient survival rates were lowest in this category (86% at one year), and were significantly higher in the recipients of a pancreas transplant alone (89% at one year) or recipients of a pancreas after a kidney (94% at one year) ($p \leqslant 0.05$).

In recipients of simultaneous pancreas/kidney transplant during the 1986—89 period, the overall one-year kidney graft survival rate was 79%, similar to that reported for cyclosporine-treated uremic diabetic recipients of kidney transplants alone by the UCLA Kidney Transplant Registry of Terasaki (17).

Discussion

As in previous analyses of Registry data, pancreas transplant results continue to improve. The improvement occurred in all recipient categories, but the same relative differences were seen as in the previous analyses. For 1986—89 cases, pancreas graft survival rates were highest in the recipients of simultaneous kidney transplants and lowest in non-uremic, non-kidney transplant recipient of pancreas transplant alone. Pancreas graft survival rates were also higher with bladder drainage than with other duct management techniques. Preservation times are being extended, and the functional survival rates for pancreas grafts stored for more than 24 was not significantly different than for grafts stored for shorter periods of time. Almost all grafts stored for >24 h were in UW or plasma-based solutions (15). HLA-DR matching influences the results, and the highest pancreas graft survival rates were with 0 DR mismatches.

Acknowledgements

A portion of the data on U.S. cases included in the analysis were collected under a subcontract with the United Network for Organ Sharing. The Registry is also supported by a NIH grant from the National Institute of Diabetes, Digestive and Kidney Disease. Computer services of the Clinical Research Center at the University of Minnesota, supported by NIH Grant RR-400, were also used.

References

1. Sutherland, D.E.R.: *Transplant. Proc.* **12** (4, Suppl. 2), 229—236 (1980).
2. Gerrish, E.W.: Final Newsletter. American College of Surgeons/National Institutes of Health Organ Transplant Registry, Chicago, Illinois, pp. 1—4, June 30, 1977.
3. Sutherland, D.E.R.: *Diabetes* **31** (Suppl. 4), 112—116 (1982).
4. Sutherland, D.E.R.: *Transplant. Proc.* **15**, 1303—1307 (1983).
5. Sutherland, D.E.R.: *World J. Surg.* **8**, 270—271 (1984).
6. Sutherland, D.E.R. and Kendall, D.: *Transplant. Proc.* **17**, 307—311 (1985).
7. Sutherland, D.E.R. and Moudry, K.C.: Report of the Pancreas Transplant Registry. In: P.I. Terasaki (ed.), *Clinical Transplants*, pp. 7—15. UCLA Press, Los Angeles (1986).
8. Sutherland, D.E.R. and Moudry, K.C.: *Clin. Transplant.* **1**, 3—17 (1987).
9. Sutherland, D.E.R. and Moudry, K.C.: *Pancreas* **2**, 473—488 (1987).
10. Sutherland, D.E.R. and Moudry, K.C.: Report of the International Pancreas Transplant Registry. In: P.I. Terasaki (ed.), *Clinical Transplants 1987*, pp. 63—101. UCLA Press, Los Angeles (1987).
11. Sutherland, D.E.R. and Moudry, K.C.: *Diabetes* **38** (Suppl. 1), 46—54 (1989).
12. Sutherland, D.E.R. and Moudry, K.C.: *Transplant. Proc.* **21**, 2759—2761 (1989).
13. Sutherland, D.E.R., Chow, S. and Moudry-Munns, K.C.: *Clin. Transplant.* **3**, 129—149 (1989).
14. Sutherland, D.E.R. and Moudry-Munns, K.C.: *Transplant. Proc.* **22**(4) 1605 (1990).

15. Sutherland, D.E.R., Moudry-Munns, K.C. and Gillingham, K.: Pancreas Transplantation: Report from International Registry and Preliminary Analysis of U.S. Results from New United Network for Organ Sharing (UNOS) Registry. In: P.I. Terasaki (ed.), *Clinical Transplants 1989*, pp. 19—44, UCLA Press, Los Angeles (1990).
16. Gehan, E: *Biometrika* **52**, 203—221 (1965).
17. Terashita, G.Y. and Crook, J.D.: Original disease of the recipient. In: P.I. Terasaki (ed.), *Clinical Transplant 1987*, pp. 373—379. UCLA Press, Los Angeles (1987).

46. Techniques and experience of pancreatic transplantation with bladder drainage

ROBERT J. CORRY AND JOHN L. SMITH

Introduction

Our group at Iowa was the first to show that combined liver-pancreas retrievals could be accomplished with successful implantation of both organs into different individuals (1). We and others have subsequently performed this procedure routinely, and it has been shown that results of liver transplantation are not compromised (2).

In the early years of our program, exocrine drainage was accomplished by means of duodenal enterostomy. The inability to diagnose rejection and the higher rate of wound infections led us to adopt the bladder drainage technique advocated by Sollinger. However, we altered the technique slightly by maintaining the short duodenal segment and joining this directly to the dome of the bladder in a side-to-side fashion (3). This procedure has been adopted nationally and is now the procedure of choice in the United States.

This chapter will briefly outline the technique of combined liver-pancreas retrieval and whole-organ pancreatic transplantation with bladder drainage. In addition, overall results will be presented and the bladder drainage technique will be compared with the intestinal drainage.

Donor Operation

The details of the donor operation are outlined elsewhere (4). A standard midline incision is made dividing the sternum and extending to the symphysis pubis. The pericardium is opened and the heart is dissected appropriately for subsequent removal. The spleen and the tail of the pancreas are freed from retroperitoneum. An extensive Kocher maneuver is accomplished and the structures in the porta hepatis are totally dissected free. Attention is then turned to the origin of the celiac artery. The diaphragm is divided at the level of the aorta to obtain exposure above the celiac artery. Dissection is carried along either side of the aorta, dividing the lymphatic and neural tissue. The origin of the superior mesenteric artery is dissected free and the origins of both renal arteries are exposed. Frequently, the right renal artery emerges close to the origin of the superior mesenteric artery. Encircling tapes are placed above the celiac artery and below the superior mesenteric artery. Dissection is then carried out on the inferior surface of the pancreas, particularly in the area of the uncinate process. The superior mesenteric artery and vein are identified. The inferior mesentric vein is divided. After the pancreas has been freed from the retroperitoneum and the celiac artery has been totally dissected so that its branches can be identified, the left gastric artery is ligated, and the origins of the gastroduodenal and splenic artery are dissected free. Following this, it is then determined whether or not there is an aberrant right hepatic artery arising from the superior mesentric artery. If not, dissection of that vessel can cease at this point. If there is an aberrant right hepatic artery, dissection of the vessel is carried out so that the superior mesenteric artery can go along with the liver.

The kidneys are then dissected free from the retroperitoneum and the ureters are divided as they traverse over the pelvic brim. At this point, a cannula is placed in the distal aorta for washout with University of Wisconsin solution. A drainage catheter is placed in the inferior vena cava.

When the heart is stopped for immediate removal, a vascular clamp is placed above the celiac artery occluding the aorta and the *in situ* washout is begun. At this point the portal vein is divided as it emerges from the pancreas. The common bile duct had been ligated earlier. It's important to divide the portal vein earlier after the initiation of *in situ* washout so that pressure does not build within the pancreatic parencyma. The aorta is divided above the celiac artery and below the superior mesenteric artery. The splenic artery is divided a few millimeters distal to its origin on the hepatic artery, and the gastroduodenal artery is ligated and divided. If there is a single hepatic artery, the liver is then removed, having been dissected free earlier. If there is a right hepatic emerging from the superior mesenteric, then the aortic tube containing both the superior mesenteric and the celiac arteries are removed and kept with the liver. The superior mesenteric artery is divided distal to the origin of the aberrant right hepatic artery. The liver is then removed and taken to the back table for additional flush through the portal vein. The pancreas is removed after dividing the duodenum with a stapling device just distal to the pylorus and 7—8 cm distal to that, preserving the ampulla of Vater. The pancreas is then taken to the back table, where it is flushed gently with 50—60 cc of UW solution through both the superior mesenteric and splenic arteries. The kidneys are then removed in the usual fashion.

Reconstruction of the pancreas with implantation

On a few occasions, it has been necessary to divide the superior mesenteric high, just adjacent to the origin of the inferior pancreatic duodenal artery. If there is not an aberrant right hepatic artery, the superior artery can be taken with the pancreas. The Y graft technique joins the donor external iliac artery to the splenic artery in an end-to-end fashion and the superior mesenteric artery or inferior pancreatic duodenal artery is joined to the internal iliac artery (5). The common iliac is used for the recipient anastomosis. The short portal vein is similarly lengthened by utilizing an external iliac vein extension graft obtained from the donor. The duodenum is opened and washed out with chilled neomycin solution. Lembert sutures are used to turn in both ends of the stapled duodenum.

The recipient operation has been described elsewhere (6). We still prefer an oblique incision similar to a renal transplant incision. We believe this gives better exposure to the iliac vessels. The iliac vessels are freed and either the common iliac Y graft or a patch of aorta with the superior mesenteric and celiac arteries is joined in an end-to-side fashion to either the common or external iliac artery. The extended portal vein is then joined to the external iliac vein 2—3 inches below the arterial anastomosis. It is important to avoid kinking of this vessel, and we have found that anastomosis to the distal external iliac vein accomplished this by relaxing the splenic vein-portal vein angle. Clamps are released and great care is taken to achieve hemostasis. The duodenotomy is widened to about 1.5 inches and a standard side-to-side two-layer anastomosis is accomplished to the dome of the bladder. It's important to have this anastomosis fairly wide which provides is free drainage of duodenal mucus and pancreatic contents into the bladder.

The kidney transplant is then accomplished through another incision or through the same midline incision if that has been chosen.

Results

We have preferred the technique utilizing bladder drainage by means of duodenoystostomy, rather than intestinal drainage for two reasons. First, we have felt that there has been a lower incidence of infection since entry into the jejunum has been avoided. Second, bladder drainage allows one to monitor urinary amylase levels on a sequential basis. In fact, a sustained drop in urinary amylase has usually coincided with a rejection episode (7).

Graft survival rates in the patients with bladder drainage are compared with those with intestinal drainage (Figure 1). This superiority of the bladder-drained patients may in part be due to the fact that most of our early experience was with intestinal drainage, whereas our later experience was largely with bladder drainage. Our overall results are shown in Figure 2 and our more recent results with the simultaneous pancreas and kidney procedure are in Figure 3.

A review of our patients who were one or more years post-successful

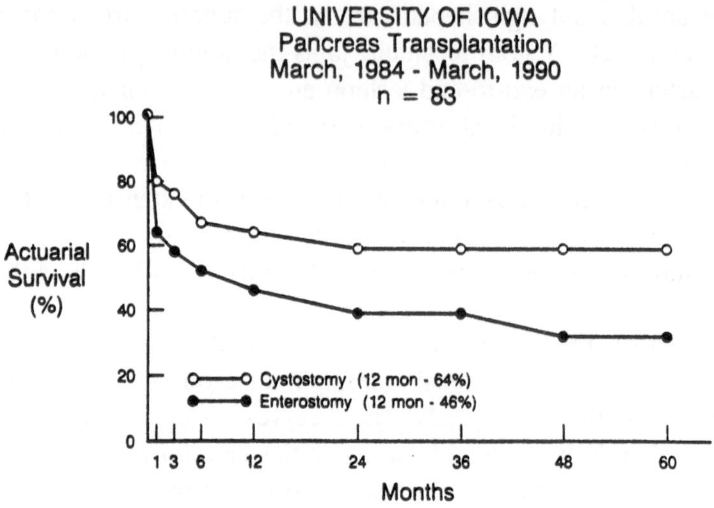

Fig. 1. Graft survival for all patients comparing bladder drainage (open circles) with intestinal drainage (closed circles).

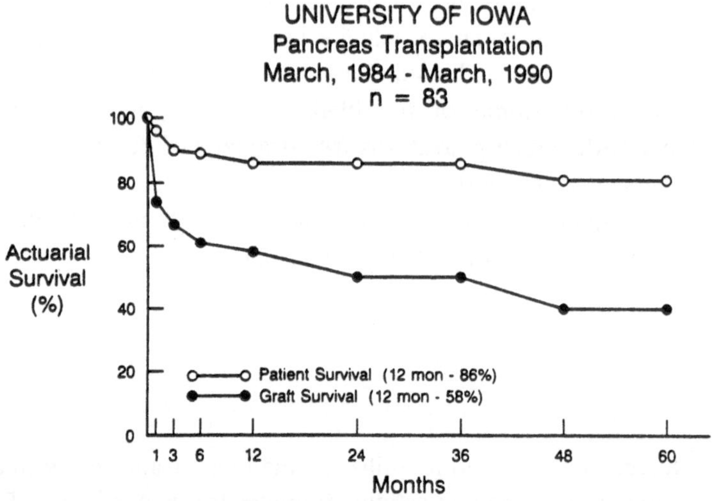

Fig. 2. Overall patient and graft survival of all patients since 1984.

pancreas transplantation has shown marked improvement in subjective symptoms of enteropathy, gastropathy, neuropathy, and general well-being (8,9).

Discussion

At the present time, we believe that the technique described herein offers the best opportunity for successful pancreatic transplantation. The bladder drainage

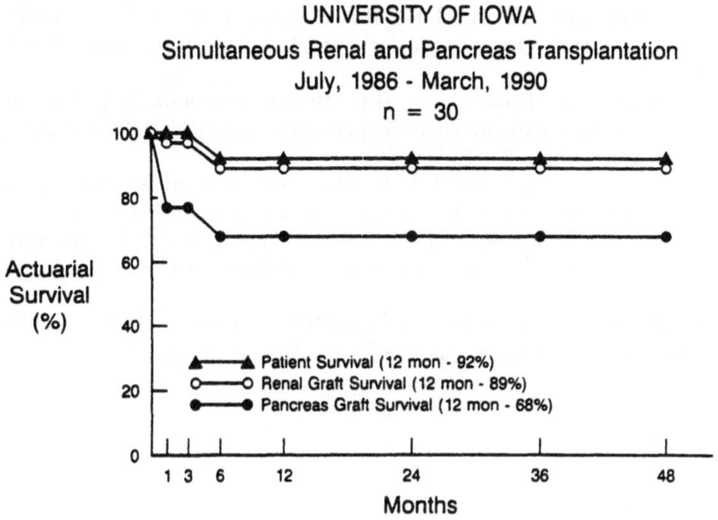

Fig. 3. Results of simultaneous kidney-pancreas transplantation since July 1986. Pancreas survival at 4 years approaches 70%.

technique has a lower incidence of wound infection, as well as permitting continuous monitoring of urinary amylase values, as well as IL2 levels.

Although not the subject of this report, complications of bladder drainage include metabolic acidosis secondary to the fixed bicarbonate losses, erosive cystitis in a few patients, which are probably secondary to incomplete bladder emptying, and a higher incidence of urinary tract infection, which will be reported elsewhere. Nevertheless, bladder drainage appears to be somewhat better than intestial drainage with its attendant risks of wound infection.

We are exploring the concept of portal venous rather than systemic drainage. Our group has been concerned about the problem of persistent hyperinsulinemia in these patients and whether or not a more physiologic arrangment should be the preferred procedure. In addition, we are exploring the technique of fine needle aspiration as a more precise method of diagnosing rejection.

References

1. Corry, R.J.: Pancreatic-duodenal transplantation with urinary tract drainage. In: Carl Groth (ed.), *Pancreatic Transplantation*, pp. 147—153. Grune & Stratton, London (1988).
2. Schulak, J.A.: Survey of American Society of Transplant Surgeons Scientific Advisory Committee, presented at ASTS Annual Meeting (1989).
3. Nghiem, D.D. and Corry, R.J.: Technique of simultaneous renal pancreaticoduodenal transplantation with urinary drainage of pancreatic secretion. *Amer. J. Surg.* **153**, 405—406 (1987).
4. Nghiem, D.D., Schulak, J.A. and Corry, R.J.: Duodenopancreatectomy for transplantation. *Arch. Surg.* **122**, 1201—1206 (1987).

5. Marsh, C.L., Perkins, J.D., Sutherland, D.E.R., Corry, R.J. and Sterioff, S.: Combined hepatic and pancreaticoduodenal procurement for transplantation, *Surg. Gynecol. Obstet.* **168**, 254—258 (1989).
6. Corry, R.J., Nghiem, D.D., Schulak, J.D., W.D., Beutel and Gonwa, T.A.: Surgical treatment of diabetic nephropathy with simultaneous pancreatic duodenal and renal transplantation. *Surg. Gynecol. Obstet.* **162**, 547—555 (1986).
7. Nghiem, D.D., Gonwa, T.A., Corry, R.J.: Metabolic effects of urinary diversion of exocrine secretions in pancreas transplantation. *Transplantation* **43**(1), 70—73 (1987).
8. Wright, F.H., Zehr, P., Schanbacher, B.A., Smith, J.L. and Corry, R.J.: Improved functional status of patients after successful pancreas transplantation. *Diabetes* **38** (Suppl. 1), 264 (1989).
9. Corry, R.J. and Zehr, P.: The quality of life in diabetic recipients of kidney transplantation is better with the addition of the pancreas. *Clin. Transplant.* (in press).

47. Pancreas transplantation in non-uremic diabetic recipients

DAVID E.R. SUTHERLAND, DAVID L. DUNN,
KAY C. MOUDRY-MUNNS, KRISTIN GILLINGHAM, and
JOHN S. NAJARIAN

Most pancreas transplants have been performed in diabetic patients with end-stage nephropathy who also received kidney transplants, either simultaneous with or before the pancreas graft (1). Such patients have been selected for the procedure because they were already obligated to immunosuppression in lieu of the kidney transplant, and the only risk incurred in order to achieve an insulin-independent, normoglycemic state, was that of the surgery itself, a risk that is currently very low (2—8). In addition, in such patients a kidney graft can be used to monitor for rejection episodes that in most instances effect both grafts simultaneously, with a rise in serum creatinine as a manifestation of renal allograft rejection preceding pancreas allograft dysfunction, allowing treatment to be initiated in time to preserve endocrine function. For this reason, pancreas graft survival rates are higher in recipients of simultaneous kidney transplants than in recipients of solitary pancreas transplants (8).

Application of pancreas transplants to non-uremic, non-kidney transplant (NUNK) diabetic patients has been much less common, primarily because such patients are subjected to the side effects of immunosuppression and antirejection drugs, side effects that must be weighed against the problems to which the potential recipients are, or will be subjected, if they choose to remain diabetic. Until recently (9, 10), there also was uncertainty as to whether a completely normoglycemic state could stabilize or reverse established secondary lesions of diabetes.

For more than a decade our institution has accepted non-uremic patients with early lesions of diabetic nephropathy (albuminuria creatinine clearance >50 ml/min) and other secondary complications, or diabetic patients with or without secondary complications whose blood glucose control on insulin is so liable (unpredictable extremes of hypo- or hyperglycemia) that their day-to-day quality of life is extremely poor, for pancreas transplantation (11). The results of this experience is briefly updated in abstract form here.

Between July 1978, and December 1989, 147 of 327 pancreas transplants at the University of Minnesota were in NUNK recipients in whom the problems and complications associated with their diabetes were judged more serious than the potential side effects of antirejection therapy. In all NUNK recipients of

PTA (3 open duct, 13 duct occlusion, 68 enteric drained and 63 bladder drained; 115 primary, 32 retransplants), the 1- and 3-year patient survival rates (PSRs) were 92 and 89%, and the 1- and 3- year graft survival (insulin-independent) rates (GSRs) were 43 and 28%; for TS cases (n = 112), the 1- and 3 year GSRs were 56 and 36%.

Since November 1984, we have used the bladder drainage (BD) technique in 63 NUNK recipients of pancreas transplants alone (PTA) and a quadruple immunosuppressive therapy regimen (6), consisting of antilymphocyte globulin for induction during the first 1—2 weeks, and cyclosporine, azathioprine and prednisone for maintenance. In NUNK recipients of non-bladder drained grafts, rejection episodes were diagnosed and treated based on a rise of blood glucose, and were rarely reversed (12). In NUNK recipients of BD grafts, rejection episodes were diagnosed and treated when urine amylase activity declined by 25 to 50%, based on experimental (13, 14) and clinical (12, 14, 15) evidence that a decrease in urine amylase preceded a rise in plasma glucose as a manifestation of rejection.

In NUNK recipients of BD PTA, the 1- and 3-year PSRs were 96 and 90%, and the 1- and 3-year GSRs were 58 and 34%; for TS BD PTA cases (n = 55) the 1- and 3-year GSRs were 66 and 40%.

The results in the NUNK recipients of BD PTA can be compared to those in the two other recipient categories. For recipients of BD pancreas transplants after a kidney (PAK), the 1- and 3-year PSRs were 95 and 90% and the 1- and 3-year GSRs were 52 and 42%; for TS BD PAK cases (n = 29), the 1- and 3-year pancreas GSRs were 68 and 61%. As in other series, the best results were in recipients of simultaneous pancreas and kidney transplants (SPK). For all SPK recipients of BD pancreas transplants (n = 75), the 1- and 3-year patient survival rates were 86 and 86% and the 1- and 3-year pancreas graft survival rates were 63 and 60%; for TS BD SPK cases (n = 61), the 1- and 3-year pancreas GSRs were 78 and 75%.

The above analyses included both primary and retransplant cases. In a separate analysis, of all primary BD transplants, the 1- year and 3-year GSRs were 54 and 26% for the NUNK recipients of PTA (n = 41), 53 and 46% for the PAK recipients (n = 21), and 68 and 65% for SPK recipients (n = 63). For TS primary BD pancreas transplants, the 1- and 3-year GSRs were 64 and 31% for PTA (n = 36), 75 and 75% for PAK (n = 18), and 83 and 80% for SPK (n = 52).

In the analysis of BD cases, pancreas graft survival rates were higher in SPK than in the PAK and PTA groups. More recently, however, the results have been similar in all three groups. For all 1988—89 BD cases, the 1-year actuarial pancreas GSRs were 69% in the PTA (n = 33), 57% in the PAK (n = 27), and 62% in the SPK (n = 56) categories. For the corresponding 1988—89 TS BD cases, GSRs were 75% in the PTA (n = 30), 67% in the PA (n = 23) and 77% in the SPK (n = 46) categories.

HLA matching at the HLA-DR loci was also found to be associated with significantly better patient survival rates. For all 1984—89 BD PTA cases, 1- and 3-year functional survivial rates for recipients of grafts with a 2 DR match (n = 8) were 70 and 70%, with a 1 DR match (n = 22 were 71% and 36%, and with a 0 DR match (n = 29) were 48 and 23%. For the corresponding TS 1984—89 BD PTA cases, the 1- and 3-year graft functional survival rates with a 2 DR match (n = 8) were 70 and 70% (no TF in this subgroup), with a 1 DR match (n = 19) were 83 and 41%, and with a 0 DR match (n = 25) were 56 and 27%.

The results were similar in an analysis carried out according to number of DR mismatches. For the 1984—88 BD PTA, 1- and 3-year cadaver donor graft survival rates with a 0 DR mismatch (n = 11) were 78 and 78%, with a 1 DR mismatch (n = 28) were 63 and 29%, and with a 2 DR mismatch (n = 20) were 45 and 25%. For the corresponding TS 1984—89 BD PTA cases, the 1- and 3-year graft functional survival rates with a 0 DR mismatch (n = 11) were 78 and 78% (no TF in this subgroup), with a 1 DR mismatch (n = 23) were 77 and 35%, and with a 2 DR mismatch (n = 18) were 50 and 28%.

Thus, it is apparent that with BD and HLA-DR matching, a high GSR can be achieved in PTA recipients. Further improvement should be possible with prospective application of deliberate HLA-DR matching.

Currently, we have over 50 NUNK patients with pancreas tranplants alone functioning for >1 year. Studies of the course of secondary applications of diabetes in this cohort have been reported elsewhere (9—11, 16). In regard to nephropathy, serial biopsies beginning at baseline and carried out 2 and more years after the transplant, have shown that the native kidneys of patients with functioning grafts exhibit a decrease in glomerular mesangial volume (9), the latter being a hallmark lesion of diabetic nephropathy (17). In cyclosporine-treated recipients, serum creatinine usually increased and creatinine clearance usually decreased by a magnitude of 40% during the first 6 months (18). However, thereafter serum creatinine and creatinine clearance values remained stable in most patients (11).

In regard to retinopathy, in NUNK patients with functioning pancreas grafts, progression to a higher grade occurred in approximately 30—40% over the next 1—3 years, while the lesions remained stable in the remaining 60—70% (11, 6). Deterioration has not been seen after 3 years, in patients with failed grafts retinopathy has continued to worsen after 3 years (16).

In regard to neuropathy, motor nerve conduction velocities were significantly increased and muscle action potentials remain stable in most patients with functioning grafts studied between 1 and 4 years, while in patients in whom the pancreas transplants failed there has been a significant decrease in evoked muscle action potentials and deterioration of other parameters (10, 11). Autonomic nerve function also stabilized in patients with functioning grafts while continuing to deteriorate in the control patients with failed grafts (10).

Quality of life studies have also been performed in pancreas transplant recipients, and have shown improvement on several of the standard scales used to measure this parameter in patients with chronic illness (19). Insulin independence itself has a positive effect independent of the state of secondary complications for diabetic patients in whom blood sugar management is a disabling problem.

Pancreas transplants alone have also been given to a few patients in our series in whom the diabetes was secondary to total pancreatectomy for benign disease. In some patients exocrine deficiency was corrected by enteric drainage, while in others bladder drainage was used because the primary problem related to lack of an endocrine pancreas (20).

In summary, a sustained euglycemic, insulin-independent state can be established in most non-uremic, non-kidney diabetic recipients of pancreas transplants alone, with a beneficial effect on neuropathy, lack of an immediate benefit on advanced nephropathy, an effect on nephropathy compounded by the influence of CsA on renal function, and an improvement in day-to-day quality of life. However, widespread application to the general population awaits development of antirejection strategies with fewer side effects than those currently employed. This still leaves a substantial number of diabetic patients who can benefit from a solitary pancreas transplant (1).

References

1. Sutherland, D.E.R.: Who should get a pancreas transplant? *Diabetes Care* **11**, 681—685 (1988).
2. LaRocca, E., Dubernard, J.M., Sangeverno, R. *et al.*: Results of simultaneous pancreatico-renal transplanation. *Transplant. Proc.* **19** (Suppl. 4), 44—47 (1987).
3. Tyden, G., Brattstrom, C., Lundgren, G. *et al.*: Improved results in pancreatic transplantation by avoidance nonimmunological graft failures. *Transplantation* **43**, 674—676 (1987).
4. Wright, F.H., Smith, J.L., Ames, S.A. *et al.*: Function of pancreas allografts more than 1 year following transplantation. *Arch. Surg.* **124**, 796—800 (1989).
5. Cosimi, A.B., Auchiniloss, H., Delmonico, F. *et al.*: Combined kidney and pancreas transplantation in diabetics. *Arch. Surg.* **123** 621—628 (1988).
6. Sutherland, D.E.R., Dunn, D.L., Goetz, F.C. *et al.*: A ten year experience with 290 pancreas transplants at a single institution. *Ann. Surg.* **210**, 274—288 (1989).
7. Illner, W.D., Schleibner, S., Abendroth, R. *et al.*: Recent Improvement in Clinical Pancreas Transplantation. *Transplant. Proc.* **19**, 3870—3871 (1987).
8. Sollinger, H.: Experience with simultaneous pancreas kidney transplantation. *Ann. Surg.* **208**, 475—483 (1988).
9. Bilous, R.W., Mauer, S.M., Sutherland, D.E.R. and Steffes, M.V.: Glomerular structure and function following successful pancreas transplantation for insulin-dependent diabetes mellitus. *Diabetes* **36**, 43A (1987).
10. Kennedy, W.R., Navarro, X., Goetz, F.C., Sutherland, D.E.R. and Najarian, J.S.: The effects of pancreas transplantation of diabetic neuropathy. *New Engl. J. Med.* **322**, 1031—1037 (1990).
11. Sutherland, D.E.R., Kendall, D.M., Moudry, K.C., Navarro, X., Kennedy, W.R., Ramsay, R.C., Steffes, M.W., Mauer, S.M., Goetz, F.C., Dunn D.L. and Najarian, J.S.: Pancreas transplantation in non-uremic, type I diabetic recipients. *Surgery* **104**, 453—464 (1988).

12. Prieto, M., Sutherland, D.E.R., Goetz, F.C., Rosenberg, M. and Najarian, J.S.: Pancreas transplant results according to technique of duct management: bladder versus enteric drainage. *Surgery* **102**, 680–691 (1987).
13. Prieto, M., Sutherland, D.E.R., Fernandez-Cruz, L., Heil, J. and Najarian, J.S.: Urinary amylase monitoring for early diagnosis of pancreas allograft rejection in dogs. *J. Surg. Res.* **40**, 597–604 (1987).
14. Prieto, M., Sutherland, D.E.R., Fernandez-Cruz, L., Heil, J., Najarian, J.S.: Experimental and clinical experience with urine amylase monitoring for early diagnosis of rejection in pancreas transplantation. *Transplantation* **43** 71–79 (1987).
15. Sollinger, H.W., Stratta, R.J., Kalayoglu, M. *et al.*: Pancreas transplantation with pancreaticocystostomy and quadruple immunosuppression. *Surgery* **102**, 674–679 (1987).
16. Ramsay, R.C., Goetz, F.C., Sutherland, D.E.R., Mauer, S.M., Robinson, L.L., Cantrill, H.L., Knobloch, W.H. and Najarian, J.S.: Progression of diabetic retinopathy after pancreas transplantation for insulin-dependent diabetes mellitus. *New Engl. J. Med.* **318**, 208–214 (1988).
17. Mauer, S.M., Steffes, M.W., Ellis, E.N., Sutherland, D.E.R., Brown, D.M. and Goetz, F.C.: Structural-functional relationship in diabetic nephropathy. *J. Clin. Invest.* **74**, 1143–1155 (1984).
18. DeFrancisco, A.M., Mauer, S.M., Steffes, M.V., Goetz, F.C., Najarian, J.S. and Sutherland, D.E.R.: The effect of cyclosporine on native renal function in non-uremic diabetic recipients of pancreas transplants. *J. Diab. Compl.* **1**, 128–131 (1988).
19. Zehrer, C. and Gross, C.: Quality of life in pancreas transplantation. *Diab. Care* **13** 539–541 (1990).
20. Sutherland, D.E.R., Dunn, D.L., Gruessner, R. and Najarian, J.S.: Pancreas and islet transplantation for treatment of type I diabetes and as a surgical adjuvant for treatment of pancreatic disease. In: J.S. Najarian and J.P. Delaney (eds), *Progress in Gastrointestinal Surgery 1990*, pp. 357–369. Yearbook Medical Publishers, Chicago (1990).

48. Early observation in pancreas transplantation using the bladder drainage procedure

W.D. ILLNER, D. ABENDROTH, H. SCHNEEBERGER,
S. SCHLEIBNER, M. STANGL, J. THEODORAKIS, R. LANDGRAF
and W. LAND

Improved results in pancreas transplantation using the whole organ and a duodenal segment for diversion of exocrine secretion (1, 2) led to the introduction of this technique at the Munich Transplant Centre, too. This technique permits monitoring of the pancreatic exocrine secretion in the urine. There is accumulating suggestion that reduction in urine amylase activity might be an early marker of pancreatic allograft rejection. As an extension to our experience with the duct-occlusion technique we started a controlled study comparing both surgical techniques.

Patients and methods

So far 91 combined pancreas and kidney transplantation and 7 isolated pancreas transplantations have been performed using prolamine for duct occlusion. The bladder drainage technique was used in 16 diabetics, 11 simultaneously and 5 pancreas alone. Clinical results of our experience with the duct-occlusion technique have been published elsewhere (3).

Donor and recipient operation

The whole pancreas with spleen and a short duodenal segment is removed from the donor after complete *in situ* flushing using UW solution. In 4/16 organ procurements we harvested the whole pancreas together with the liver for grafting. Priority of vascular supply was given to the liver, consisting of the celiac axis plus an aortic patch and the portal vein. The whole pancreas graft includes the splenic artery, divided just distal to its origin on the celiac axis, superior mesenteric artery with an aortic patch and the remaining portal vein plus the superior mesenteric vein. After the Kocher maneuver a short duodenal segment is provided using a GIA stapler. The combined removal of liver and whole pancreas requires an arterial and venous reconstruction for the pancreatico- duodenal graft with the donor iliac vessels (4). The pancreaticoduodenal graft is placed intraperitoneally along the ascending colon with a transrectal incision. Arterial and venous anastomoses were carried out between the reconstruction pancreatic vessels and the recipient's external iliac vessels. For the bladder-duodenal anastomosis we use the two layer side-to-side technique (inner layer: running: 3/0 Vicryl and outer layer: interrupted 3/0 Vicryl).

Immunosuppressive protocol

Since 1984 a quadruple drug induction therapy is routinely used in pancreatic transplantation. It consists of CsA, Aza 'high' dose of steriods and ATG/ALG for a short period of time. Maintenance treatment consists of steriods, CsA and Aza for a period of 6 months, followed by double drug maintenance treatment with CsA and Aza.

More recently we have used a quadruple drug induction therapy with CsA, Aza, 'high' dose of steriods and ATG or OKT3 in a controlled study. The preliminary results were presented in Barcelona (5).

Problems and complications according to different surgical techniques

Using the duct-occlusion technique we are confronted with two major problems. Firstly, the occurrence of a primary irreversible venous thrombosis. Secondly, the development of a pancreatic fistula with the high risk of a secondary infection. The rate of this complication is shown in Table 1. The need of an anticoagulation therapy is required.

Despite of duct-occlusion with prolamine the residual exocrine secretion remains unsolved at the present time.

According to the new technique our clinical results show a hight incidence of intraparanchymal graft abscesses with subsequent loss of the pancreatic graft

Table 1. Early complications after stimultaneous pancreas and kidney transplantation.

Surgical technique	Venous thrombosis	Local infection		Pancreatic fistula
		Intragraft	Perigraft	
Dust occlusion ($n = 59$)	15% ($n = 9$)	0	20% ($n = 12$)	20% ($n = 12$)
Bladder drainage ($n = 11$)	0	36% ($n = 4$)	18% ($n = 2$)	0

(Table 1). This complication is very common in association with an urinary tract infection.

Results

Patients and graft survival probability rates for 1 year are comparable in both groups (Figures 1 and 2). Long-term results are demonstrable for the duct occlusion technique only (Figure 3).

Summary

Mortality and morbidity rates after pancreas transplantation are low and comparable in both groups talking into account that the number of patients transplanted using the bladder technique is still low and the observation period limited. The 1-year pancreas graft function rate is 60% in both groups. The early phase post-transplant using the duct obliteration in a segmental allograft bears the risk of an irreversible venous thrombosis and the development of a pancreatic fistula with subsequent graft loss. As a consequence of prolamine,

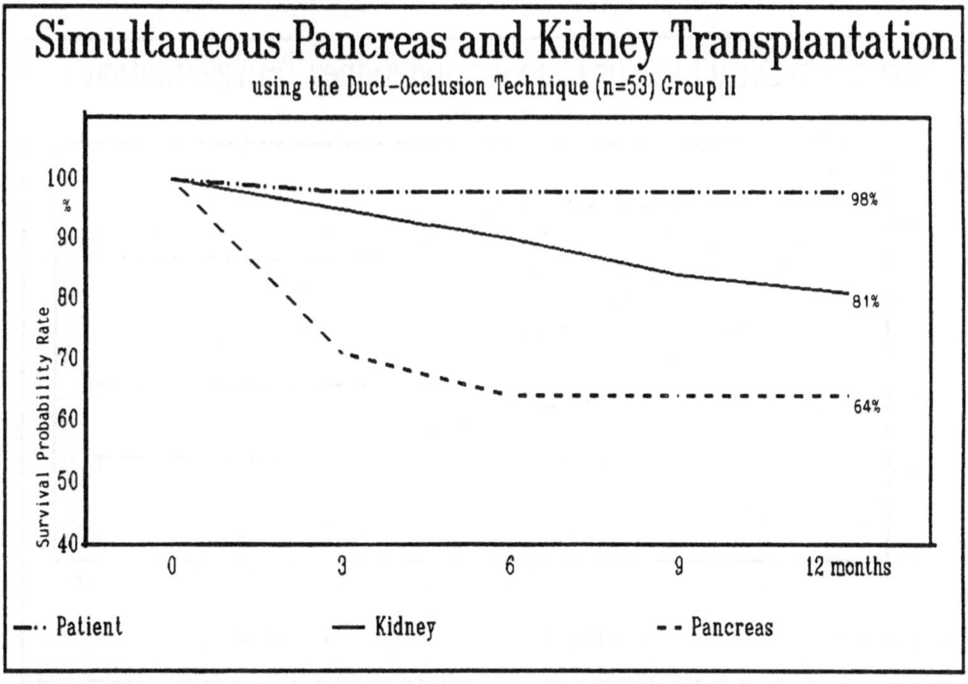

Fig. 1. Patients and graft survival probability in stimultaneous pancreas and kidney transplantation using the duct-occlusion techniques ($n = 53$) (Cutler/Ederer formula).

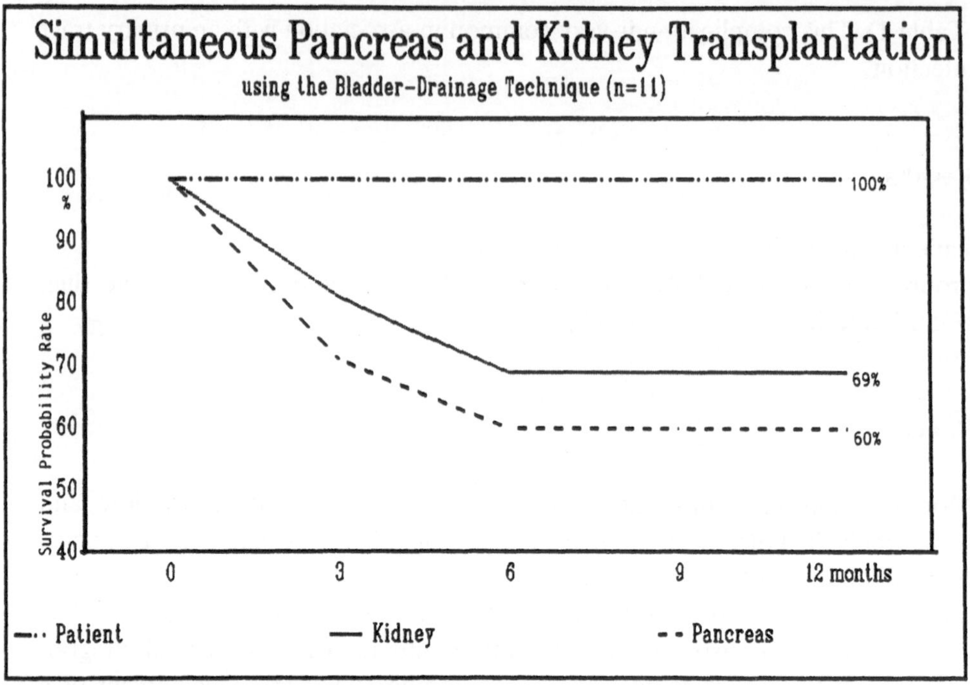

Fig. 2. Patient and graft survival probability in combined pancreas and renal transplantation using the bladder-drainage technique ($n = 11$) (Cutler/Ederer formula).

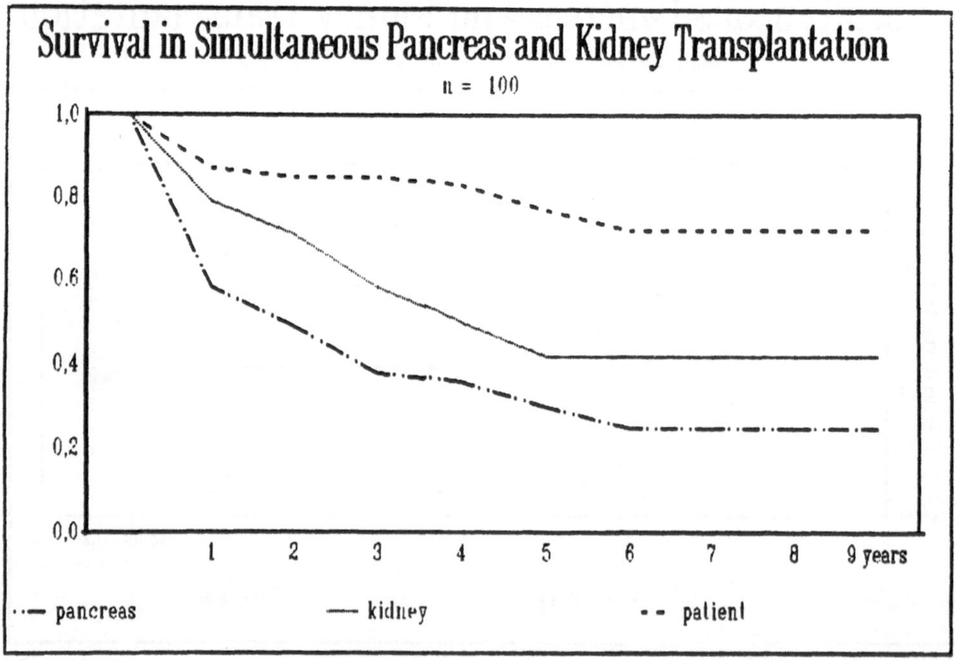

Fig. 3. Long-term results in simultaneous pancreas and kidney transplantation in duct-occluded segmental allografts ($n = 100$) (Cutler/Ederer formula).

the result in the long-run is a vascularized islet cell graft without any exocrine activity and with no risk for the recipient. The induced destruction of exocrine tissue by prolamine is not associated with a deterioration of the endocrine function. Our early clinical observations with the bladder drainage show a remarkably high rate of local infection-complication following urinary tract infection also with subsequent graft loss. Patients with a history of bladder dysfunction as a side effect of long-term diabetic disease might therefore be better candidates for the duct-occlusion technique.

The surgical complication rate is acceptable. Still unsolved is the problem of a transplanted gland with an aggressive enzymatic secretion at the bladder mucosa, as well as for the recipient himself. With this technique postoperative complications may not only develop on the side of the pancreas but also from the duodenal segment. Further experience and long-term results must be gained to find out the best surgical technique.

References

1. Sollinger, H.W. and Belzer, F.O.: Pancreas transplantation with urinary tract drainage. In: C.G. Groth (ed.), *Pancreatic Transplantation*, pp. 131—146. W.B. Saunders (1988).
2. Corry, R.J.: Pancreatico-duodena transplantation with urinary tract drainage. In: C.G. Groth (ed.), *Pancreatic Transplantation*, pp. 147—168. W.B. Saunders (1988).
3. Land, W., Landgraf, W.-D., Illner *et al.*: Clinical pancreatic transplantation using the prolamine duct occlusion technique. The Munich experience. *Transplant. Proc.* **19** (4, Suppl. 4), 75—83 (1987).
4. Gubernatis, G., Abendroth, D., Haverich, A. *et al.*: Technik der Mehrorganentnahme. In: *Der Chirung*, 59. Jg., Heft 7, 461—468 (1988).
5. Illner, W.-D., Theodorakis, J., Abendroth, D. *et al.*: Quadruple drug induction therapy in combined renal and pancreas transplantation — OKT3 versus ATG. *Transplant. Proc.* (in press).

49. Results of pancreas transplantation with irradiated spleen and segment of duodenum

G. KOOTSTRA, J.P. VAN HOOFF, H. PELTENBURG, C.J. VAN DER LINDEN, R. WIJNEN, P. VAN DEN BERG-LOONEN, J.A.M. DE JONG, T. VERSCHUEREN and G. HEIDENDAL

Introduction

At the introduction of our Pancreas Transplant Program in 1985, we decided to try to prevent graft thrombosis by including the spleen in the graft (1). In those days the incidence of graft thrombosis was as high as 25% (2). We based our policy on the work of Starzl (3), who introduced the inclusion of the spleen in pancreatic transplantation. The assumption is, that preservation of the normal vascular architecture of the pancreas will maintain the normal flow pattern. We presume that the pancreas receive about 1% of the heart minute volume and the spleen about 5%, and therefore, inclusion of the spleen might increase several times the amount of flow through the graft. But the pathophysiology of the thrombotic episode is not totally clear and other factors as edema due to ischemia and preservation or pancreatic enzyme damage to vascular endothelium (4), and eventually the pancreas being a low-flow state organ (5), all may play a role.

In April 1986 Deierhoi *et al.* published a case report of lethal graft versus host disease (GVHD) in a recipient of a pancreas spleen transplant (6), and in most centers the inclusion of the spleen was abolished based on the serious risk of GVHD. We decided from our second patient on to irradiate the spleen *ex-vivo*, with a dose of 6 Gy. This dose is supposed to reduce the replication of the stem cells, although for kill of the stem cells a higher dose f.i. 25 Gy might be indicated due to anoxia and low temperature in the *ex-vivo* situation. The technique of *ex-vivo* irradiation has been described elsewhere (1, 7). We report the results of 11 patients, with the exception of one (patient 1), who had an irradiated spleen in their pancreas graft, with special emphasis on the long-term outcome of the spleen. Our immunosuppressive protocols and surgical procedure have been published previously (1, 7).

Results

Patient and graft survival

The patient and graft survival is presented in Table 1. Nine of the 11 patients

Table 1. Patient and graft survival of the segment of duodenum-pancreatic-spleen grafts.

No.	Patient Initial	Age	Sex	Donor sex	Kidney simultaneously	Outcome
1	A[a]	24	M	F	Yes	Chronic rejection after 2 years; some pancreas function
2	M	24	F	M	Yes	Suicide 9 months; chronic rejection; moderate pancreas function
3	M	41	M	F	No	Chronic rejection after 3 years; some pancreas function
4	B	47	M	F	Yes	Chronic rejection after 3 years; some pancreas function (chimerism 20%)
5	N	37	M	F	No	Rejection after 6 months; no function left (chimerism 1/7 cells ♀)
6	de JvE	35	F	M	No	Thrombosis day 1; splenectomy; graft loss
7	SB	33	F	M	Yes	Graft loss 5 weeks mycotic aneurysm; rejection
8	SvB	51	F	F	No	Rupture of spleen, day 3; acute rejection; graft loss
9	F	36	M	M	No	Lethal CMV 6 weeks; good graft function; rejection
10	Z	29	F	M	No	Chronic rejection; no function
11	vdK	23	F	M	No	Acute rejection; lethal pneumonia

[a] The spleen in this patient was not *ex-vivo* irradiated.

rejected their graft, either acute or chronic. Transplantectomy for thrombosis early in the postoperative course, and for mycotic aneurysm in another patient, had to be performed. The case history of this patient is described elsewhere (8). This patient was treated for rejection as well and it is evident that all our 10 patients who had their graft long enough for presentation of rejection, indeed went through one or several courses of rejection.

GVHD and chimerism

All patients were carefully examined on multiple occasions for clinical signs of GVHD. No such physical signs were observed. Several but not all patients were investigated for chimerism. Basically three methods have been applied: (a) cytotoxic tests with recipient lymphocytes and for donor cells specific antisera; (b) labeling of donor origin lymphocytes of the recipient lymphocytes with HLA antisera against donor antigens; and (c) karyotyping of lymphocytes when donor and recipient have different sex. We were able to determine in 2 patients that they went through a temporary chimerism, being 20% of the lymphocytes in one and ± 14% in another patient. Again, no clinical side effects were observed.

The incidence of thrombosis

We observed one case of thrombosis of the SPS graft (Table 1) in a patient who received only a pancreas graft. In this patient (Pat. 6) the SPS graft was placed extraperitoneally in the groin, as is the kidney in renal transplantation. At exploration within 24 hours the splenic vessels were twisted through malpositioning of the spleen. This might have served as the start of the factual thrombosis. In none of the grafts simultaneously transplanted with a kidney was thrombosis observed.

Histology of removed spleens

Seven spleens were removed either separately (pat. 6 and 8), with the graft (pat. 7 and 10), or at autopsy (pat. 2, 9 and 11). There are three clusters: within 2 days, between 36 and 49 days, and at 7 and 9 months. The spleens removed after several weeks showed no signs of irradiation with marked fibrosis, areas with necrosis, and proliferation of the vessel wall.

Discussion

It is evident from the data presented in Table 1 that our patient and graft survival is rather poor. With the exception of patient 9, who died at 6 weeks, with excellent graft function, from pulmonary CMV infection, all grafts lost function. Comparatively, the grafts transplanted simultaneously with kidneys did better than pancreas alone. This is in accordance with data from the World Pancreas Registry, that pancreas alone has a high failure rate, and 2 our of 3 will fail in the first year. Our patients with a simultaneous transplant had at least 1 month, 9 months, 2 and 3 years' function of their pancreatic graft. Although our results are somewhat overshadowed by the relative large representation of pancreas alone cases, we have the impression that inclusion of the irradiated spleen in the pancreatic graft coincides with a high number of rejections, which are particularly difficult to treat. In small animal studies the transplantation of the spleen has been associated with an improvement of pancreas graft survival (9).

Dafoe *et al.* (10) studied the inclusion of the spleen in the porcine pancreaticoduodenal allograft. They demonstrated that the inclusion of the spleen was detrimental to graft survival. The increased graft loss was due to rejection (11). Evidently we need stronger or other combinations of immunosuppressive drugs. Although we have not observed GVHD, several cases have been reported (12, 13, 14), including one lethal case. This is the reason that all programs have abandoned the use of this technique.

Irradiation has been used in the clinical setting (13) to reverse signs of possible GVHD. Schulak and Sharp (15) observed in rats with a not-irradiated pancreatic spleen graft severe GVHD, which could be prevented with whole body donor irradiation (5 and 2.5 Gy) or with *ex-vivo* graft irradiation (10 Gy or 5Gy). Delay of graft irradiation until 3 days after transplantation failed to prevent GVHD. Cells derived from the irradiated grafts failed to stimulate lymph node enlargement in a popliteal lymph node assay for GVHD. The effect of irradiation of the donor spleen before transplantation was studied in the pig by Dafoe *et al.* (10). They concluded that the detrimental effect of inclusion of the spleen on graft survival in their porcine model could be abrogated by irradiation (10 Gy) of the spleen. Ten Gy was chosen based on studies that this dose is lethal to splenocytes (16) and they presume that a lower dose might have selectively depleted radiosensitive suppressor cells, perhaps fostering a rejection episode. We have used a dose of 6 Gy, and it is just guesswork whether this might have played a role in our poor results. Nevertheless, there is experimental (10, 15) and clinical evidence (our data) that pretransplant irradiation of the spleen can abrogate the risk of GVHD in the pancreas spleen transplants.

In our series only one graft was lost due to thrombosis. There is only one other documented case of graft loss due to thrombosis in a pancreas-spleen graft (17). In the world literature a total 34 transplants of the pancreas with the spleen can be traced. They are compiled in Table 2. The overall incidence of failure through thrombosis is about 6%. This is rather a low figure and suggests that inclusion of the spleen might have the expected positive effect on the hemodynamics of the graft.

Table 2. Literature search for pancreatic grafts that included the spleen. Incidence of thrombosis.

Authors	No. of transplants	Thrombosis
Starzl *et al.* (3)	3	0
Sollinger *et al.* (18)	9	0
Munda *et al.* (19)	4	0
Dafoe *et al.* (14)	1	0
Corry *et al.* (17)	5	1
Grassi *et al.* (20)	1	0
Kootstra *et al.* (00)	11	1
Total experience	34	2 (±6%)

Starzl (3) mentions that his patients had suffered increased morbidity due to inclusion of the spleen in the graft. This is not the case in our patients, although 1 patient sustained a rupture of the spleen. In the literature the spleen has been removed on several occasions early in the postoperative course for thrombocytopenia. We have observed this phenomeno as well (1), but a splenectomy was never indicated or performed for this reason.

In conclusion it can be stated that inclusion of an irradiated spleen in a pancreatic graft might reduce the chance for thrombosis. Irradiation abrogates the risk for GVHD, but at a dose of 6 Gy it does not reduce the rate of rejection.

References

1. Kootstra, G., Van Hooff, J.P., Jörning, P.J.G., Leunissen, K.M.L., van der Linden, C.J., Beukers, E. and Buurman, W.A.: A new variant for whole pancreas grafting. *Transplant. Proc.* **19**, 2314—2318 (1987).
2. Sutherland, D.E.R. and Moudry, K.C.: Pancreas Transplant Registry: history and analysis of cases, 1966 to October 1988. *Pancreas* **2**, 473—488 (1987).
3. Starzl, T.E., Iwatsuki, S., Shaw, B.K., Green, D.A., Van Thiel, D.H., Nalesnik, M.A., Nusbacher, J., Dilix-Perc, H. and Hakala, Th.R.: Pancreaticoduodenal transplantation in humans. *Surg. Gynec. Obstet.* **159**, 265—272 (1984).
4. Sibley, R.K.: Pathology of pancreas grafts. In: J.M. Dubernard and D.E.R. Sutherlands (eds.), *International Handbook of Pancreas Transplantation*, pp. 203—223. Kluwer Academic Publishers, Dordrecht, Boston, London (1989).
5. Calne, R.Y., McMaster, P.E., Rolles, K. and Duffy, T.J.: Technical observations in segmental pancreas allografting. Observations on pancreatic bloodflow. *Transplant. Proc.* **12**, 51—57 (1980).
6. Deierhoi, M.H., Sollinger, H.W., Bozdeck, M.J. and Belzer, F.O.: Lethal graft versus hosts disease in a recipient of a pancreas-spleen transplant. *Transplantation* **41**, 544—545 (1986).
7. Kootstra, G., Van Hooff, J.P., Jörning, P.J.G., Leunissen, K.M.L., van der Linden, C.J., Beukers, E. and Buurman, W.A.: Pancreatic transplantation in patients with type-2 diabetes: the experience in Maastricht with a new model. *Neth. J. Surg.* **39**, 32—36 (1987).
8. Walstra, B.R.J., Jörning, P.J.G., Kootstra, G., Van Hooff, J.P. and Janevski, B.K.: Pancreas transplantation complicated by a mycotic false aneurysm: diagnostic features. *J. Med. Imaging* **2**, 133—136 (1988).
9. Bitter-Suermann, H. and Shevach, E.M.: Induction of transplantation tolerance in guinea pigs by spleen allografts. I. Operative techniques and clinical results. *Transplantation* **33**, 45—51 (1982).
10. Dafoe, D.C., Campbell, D.A., Marks, W.H., Borgstrom, A., Lichter, A.S. and Turcotte, J.G.: The effect of irradiation of the donor spleen on rejection of porcine pancreataico-duodenosplenic allografts. *Transplantation* **42**, 686—687 (1986).
11. Dafoe, D.C., Campbell, D.A., Marks, W.H., Borgstrom, A., Lloyd, E.V. and Turcotte, J.G.: Inclusion of the donor spleen in pancreaticoduodenal transplantation is associated with rejection. *Transplantation* **40**, 579—584 (1985).
12. Sollinger, H.W., Kalayoglu, M., Hoffmann, R.M., Deierhoi, M.H. and Belzer, F.O.: Experience with pancreaticocystostomy in 24 consecutive pancreas transplants. *Transplant. Proc.* **17**, 141—143 (1987).
13. Gonwa, T.A., Goeken, N.E., Schulak, J.A., Nghiem, D.D. and Corry, R.J.: Failure of cyclosporine to prevent in vivo T cell priming in man: studies in allogenic spleen transplantation. *Transplant. Proc.* **40**, 299—304 (1985).

14. Dafoe, D.D., Campbell, D.A., Marks, W.H., Wilson, G.N. and Turcotte, J.G.: Karyotypic chimerism and rejection in a pancreaticoduodenosplenic transplant. *Transplantation* **40**, 572–574 (1985).
15. Schulak, J.A. And Sharp, W.J.: Graft irradiation abrogates graft-versus-host disease in combined pancreas-spleen transplantation. *J. Surg. Res.* **40**, 326–331 (1986).
16. Thomas, E.D., Storb, R. and Buckner, C.D.: Total-body irradiation in preparation for marrow engraftment. *Transplant. Proc.* **8**, 591–593 (1976).
17. Corry, R.J., Nghiem, D.D. and Schulak, J.A.: Surgical treatment of diabetic nephropathy with simultaaneous pancreatic duodenal and renal transplantation. *Surg. Gynecol. Obsted.* **162**, 547–555 (1986).
18. Sollinger, H.W., Kalayoglu, M. and Hoffmann, R.M.: Results of segmental and pancreatosplenic transplantation with pancreaticocystostomy. *Transplant. Proc.* **17**, 360–362 (1985).
19. Munda, R., First, M.R. and Jaffe, S.N.: Experience with pancreatic allografts in renal transplant recipients. *Transplant. Proc.* **17**, 353–357 (1985).
20. Grassi, C.J., Lee, R.G., Hill, Th.C. and Clouse, M.E.: Technetium-99m sulfur colloid imaging of vascular thrombosis in pancreaticosplenic transplant. *J. Radiology* **18**, 558–559 (1986).

50. Experience with pancreas transplants from living related donors

DAVID E.R. SUTHERLAND, FREDERICK C. GOETZ, DAVID M. KENDALL, R. PAUL ROBERTSON, KRISTIN GILLINGHAM, KAY C. MOUDRY-MUNNS, and JOHN S. NAJARIAN

The rationale to perform transplants of any organ from related donors rather than cadaver donors is twofold: there is a shortage of cadaver (CAD) donors for the number in need of a transplant, and the rejection rate will be less with grafts from living related donor (LRDs). Either of these two alone will justify the use of LRDs, and for kidney transplants both rationales pertain.

In most parts of the world, there is not a shortage of CAD donors for the number of diabetics who are currently considered for pancreas transplantation. Thus, the main benefit of an LRD pancreas transplant, is the need for less immunosuppression and less rejection long term. For kidney transplants, the technical failure rate is equally low for LRD and CAD donor transplants (or lower for LRD kidneys). For pancreas transplants, the technical failure is actually higher for LRD than for CAD donor transplants because only a segment of the organ can be used, and only short lengths of vessels are available (1). The higher technical failure rate with pancreas grafts from LRDs than from CAD donors partically offsets the immunological gain in the overall results. However, in an individual recipient, if the pancreas transplant is technically successful, the probability of long-term success is better with an LRD.

The University of Minnesota began to use LRDs for pancreas transplants in 1979 (2). Of 327 pancreas transplants performed at this institution from July 1978 through December 1989, 72 were segmental grafts from LRDs (30 HLA-identical siblings, 9 identical twins, 33 HLA-mismatched relatives). All recipients had been diabetic for at least 10 years and all donors were at least 10 years older than the age of onset of diabetes in the recipient; in the case of sibling donors, no other siblings or family members other than the recipients were diabetic. When these demographic features pertain, the risk of future diabetes developing is no greater than for the general population (3).

Changes in blood glucose and insulin levels have occurred in most donors postoperatively, but oral glucose tolerance tests have remained normal in two-thirds of those tested and all but 3 donors have been completely normoglycemic during the follow-up (fasting and post-prandial blood sugars within the range of the non-diabetic, non-pancreatectomized referenced population). The donors that had abnormal glucose tolerance tests postoperatively were those whose insulin levels during preoperative stimulatory tests were below the thirtieth percentile or so of a normal reference population (4). Approximately one-half of the donors whose preoperative insulin secretory response to stimulation was below the thirtieth percentile of normal had abnormal glucose tolerance test results postoperatively. Since this correlation was made, only individuals with a post-stimulatory insulin level above the thirtieth percentile of normal have been accepted as donors (5).

Surgical complications of segmental pancreatectomy have occurred in 10 (13.8%) of the 72 related donors: need for splenectomy in 3 (4.2%), one at 2 days because of a total infarct, one at 1 month for rupture occurring during minor trauma, and one at 4 years for bleeding from esophageal varices formed in the splenic venous collaterals; sterile fluid collections treated by percutaneous aspiration without recurrence in 4 (5.5%); an abcess drained percutaneously in 1 (1.4%); and need for reoperation in 2 (2.8%), 1 to religate the pancreatic duct at the site of transection, and 1 to retrieve a sponge.

All the LRD pancreas transplants were solitary (without a concomitant kidney transplant), either a pancreas transplant alone (PTA, $n = 45$), or a pancreas after a kidney (PAK, $n = 27$). For comparison, there were 180 solitary CAD donor pancreas transplants (PTA, $n = 102$; PAK, $n = 78$). (In addition, we did 75 simultaneous pancreas/kidney (SPK) transplants, all the pancreas grafts being from CAD donors; there were no LRD pancreas transplants performed simultaneous with a kidney transplant. All SPK transplants were done with the bladder drainage technique.) For the solitary pancreas transplants (Sox Px Tx), a variety of duct management techniques were used, including open duct intraperitoneal drainage (OD) in 15 (5 LRD, 10 CAD), duct occlusion (DO) in 44 (6 LRD, 38 CAD), enteric drainage (ED) in 80 (53 LRD, 37 CAD), and bladder drainage (BD) in 103 (8 LRD, 95 CAD). The overall results and results in technically successful pancreas transplants are summarized in Table 1.

In the overall series of Sol Px Tx, the 1- and 3-year functional survival rates for grafts from LRDs ($n = 72$) were 42% and 36% and for grafts from CAD donors ($n = 180$) were 39% and 26% (p = ns). (For the SPK cases, $n = 75$, 1- and 3-year pancreas (Px) graft functional (Fxn) survival rates were 63 and 60%.) In the two Sol Px Tx subgroups, there also were no significant differences. For PTA, 1- and 3-year Px Fxn survival rates for LRD grafts ($n = 45$) were 42 and 34% and for CAD grafts ($n = 102$) were 44 and 24% ($p = 0.2$). For PAK transplants 1- and 3-year Px Fxn survival rates for LRD grafts ($n = 27$) were 44 and 40% and for CAD grafts ($n = 78$) were 34 and 28%. Even though the differences between the LRD and CAD donor Px Fxn graft survival curves overall were not statistically significant, long-term ($\geqslant 3$ years) Px graft Fxn rates were significantly higher for LRD transplants. Patient survival rates showed the same trends, and for all Sol Px Tx cases at 1 and 3 years were 94 and 93% for recipients of LRD and 90 and 85% for recipients of CAD donor grafts.

Table 1. Comparison of living related versus cadaver pancreas transplants at the University of Minnesota 1978–89.

	No. LRD	Txs CAD	One yr LRD (%)	Fxn CAD (%)	Three yr LRD (%)	Fxn CAD (%)	*p* value
All cases							
Sol Px Txs	72	180	42	39	36	26	NS
PxTx alone	45	102	42	44	34	24	NS
Px after kid.	27	78	44	34	40	28	NS
Simult. Px/kid.	–	75	–	63	–	60	N/A
Tech. suc. cases							
Sol Px Txs	46	143	64	48	54	32	0.01
PxTx alone	30	82	59	55	47	30	0.22
Px after kid.	16	61	74	40	67	35	0.02
Simult. Px/kid.	–	61	–	78	–	75	N/A

The immunological advantage of LRD over CAD pancreas transplant was seen in the analysis of technically successful cases (TS). The reason this difference did not show up in the analysis of all cases was because of the high technical failure rate, leading to early graft losses, but by 3 years this handicap had been overcome. The technical failure rate for all solitary pancreas transplant was 36% for LRD and 21% for CAD donor grafts (compared to 18% for SPK CAD pancreas transplants). In an analysis of all TS solitary transplants (7 OD, 36 DO, 58 ED, 88 BD), 1- and 3-year Px Fxn survival rates for grafts from LRDs (n = 46) were 64 and 54% and for those from CAD donors (n = 143) were 48 and 32% (p = 0.01). (For TS SPK transplants, n = 61, the 1- and 3-year Px graft Fxn rates were 78 and 75%.) In the two subgroups of the Sol Px Tx cases, similar differences were seen in one. In the PTA group, the 1- and 3-year Px graft Fxn survival rates for LRD transplants (n = 30) were 59 and 47% and for CAD donor transplants (n = 82) were 55 and 30% (p = 0.22). For TS PAK transplants, 1- and 3-year Px graft Fxn survival rates for grafts from LRDs (n = 16) were 74 and 67% and for grafts from CAD donors (n = 61) were 40 and 35% (p = 0.02).

The advantage of LRD pancreas transplant is largely reflected in the long-term graft functional survival rates. We have 30 LRD grafts functioning between 1 and 9 years, 19 in the PTA and 11 in the PAK categories.

There is one aspect of the LRD experience that deserves special comment: the course of 6 TS identical twin transplants and the serendipitous observation that in the absence of immunosuppression the graft is susceptible to isletitis and recurrence of disease (6, 7). The first 3 twins were not prophylactically immunosuppressed; all 3 became hyperglycemic between 6 and 12 weeks, and biopsies showed isletitis (appreciated in retrospect in the first case). The second and third twin recipients received antilymphocyte globulin (ALG) and azathiopprine (AZA) after the diagnosis of recurrence of disease was made. In one AZA was stopped because of the lack of a clinical response, while in the other, the need for a permanent return to exogenous insulin was obviated for 1 year and this recipient remains on AZA with a partially functioning graft at 6 years (8). The fourth identical twin transplant recipient received AZA prophylactically; she was normoglycemic for 3 years, at which time hyperglycemia occurred and a biopsy showed isletitis; she received a course of ALG and cyclosporine was added to her regimen, and had an initial clinical response, but at 5 years post-transplant resumed insulin permanently. The fifth recipient of an identical twin transplant received AZA and cyclosporine (CsA) prophylactically; a biopsy of the pancreas graft at 1 year showed normal islets and she remains normoglycemic at 2½ years. The sixth also received AZA and CsA prophylactically; she had slight elevations of blood sugar levels at 6 months; a graft biopsy showed mild isletitis for which she received ALG, and she remains normoglycemic at 1½ years.

Type I diabetes mellitus is known to be an autoimmune disease in which the beta cells are selectively destroyed (9). The natural history of pancreatic pathology in diabetes was recapitulated in the first few twin transplants, and this observation provided one of the strongest bits of evidence that type I diabetes has an autoimmune etiology. Isletitis has also been seen in grafts transplanted from non-twin HLA-identical siblings to recipients who were only minimally immunosuppressed with low-dose cyclosporine alone or low-dose azathioprine and prednisone (9, 10), but the clinical manifestation of recurrence of disease was at a slower rate and the process was reversed in some by an increase in immunosuppression (8). It is apparent that recurrence of disease can be prevented by adequate immunosuppression, and this may be why such a process has not yet been recognized in any cadaver donor pancreas transplants where immunosuppressive doses have been higher because of the known greater propensity to rejection. The amount of immunosuppression needed to prevent isletitis may exceed that needed to prevent rejection of cadaveric pancreas allografts. Recurrence of disease appears to be prevented by adequate immunosuppression in twins as well as in non-twin cases, and steroids have not been used in any of the twin cases, including the last two that so far remain successful.

In summary, in 72 related donor pancreas transplants, metabolic changes were seen in one-third of the donors. The insulin secretory response to intravenous glucose can be used as a screening test, and individuals with first phase insulin response above the thirtieth percentile can be chosen as donors with the assurance that they will remain normal after segmental pancreatectomy. In recipients of solitary TS pancreas transplants, long-term functional survival rates are higher with grafts from LRD than CAD donors. Scientifically, the detection of recurrence of isletitis in absence of immunosuppression and the prevention of recurrence of disease by adequate immunosuppression has been the most interesting aspect of the LRD pancreas program. If the technical failure rate can be lowered, LRD pancreas transplants could be applied more liberally since the long-term graft functional survival rates are superior to CAD transplants for TS cases. If immunosuppression is improved to the point where pancreas transplants could be considered in all diabetic patients, the number of CAD donors would be the limiting factor, and the rationale for LRD pancreas donation would be completely analogous to that of the kidney. However, at this time, we limit LRD pancreas transplants to situations in which both the donor and recipient and entire family understands the trade-off of accepting a higher probability of an immediate technical failure for a higher probability of long-term function, if the graft is technically successful. Only in a diabetic individual who is so highly sensitized that a CAD donor transplant is extremely unlikely to occur, and in whom a negative crossmatch can be obtained only with an HLA-identical sibling, is an LRD pancreas seen as the only practical option if transplantation is deemed the best treatment for the patient.

At this time, pancreas transplantation is an appropriate treatment for diabetic patients already obligated to immunosuppression by lieu of a kidney transplant, or to a non-kidney transplant recipient whose problems with diabetes are more serious than the potential side effects of the antirejection drugs or of immunosuppression in general (12). Since the need for immunosuppression is less with LRD transplants, this option expands the diabetic subpopulation than can benefit from this procedure.

References

1. Sutherland, D.E.R., Goetz, F.C. and Najarian, J.S.: Pancreas transplants from living related donors. *Transplantation* **38**, 674—679 (1984).
2. Sutherland, D.E.R., Goetz, F.C., Rynasiewicz, J.J. *et al.*: Segmental pancreas transplantation from living related and cadaver donors: A clinical experience. *Surgery* **90**, 159—169 (1981).
3. Barbosa, J., King, R. Goetz, F.C. *et al.*: Histocompatibility antigens (HLA) in families with juvenile insulin dependent diabetes mellitus. *J. Clin. Invest.* **60**, 989—999 (1977).
4. Kendall, D.M., Sutherland, D.E.R., Goetz, F.C. and Najarian, J.S.: Metabolic effect on hemipancreatectomy in donors: preoperative prediction of postoperative oral glucose tolerance. *Diabetes* **38** (Suppl. 1), 101—103 (1989).
5. Kendall, D.M., Sutherland, D.E.R., Najarian, J.S., Goetz, F.D. and Robertson, R.P.: Effects of hemi-pancreatectomy on insulin secretion and glucose tolerance in healthy human donors. *New Engl. J. Med.* (in press).
6. Sutherland, D.E.R., Sibley, R., Zhu, X-Z., Michael, A., Srikanta, S., Taub, F., Najarian, J.S. and Goetz, F.C.: Twin-to-twin pancreas transplantation: reversal and reenactment of the pathogenesis of type I diabetes. *Trans. Assoc. Amer. Phys.* **XCVII**, 80—87 (1984).
7. Sibley, R.K., Sutherland, D.E.R., Goetz, F. and Michael, A.F.: Recurrent diabetes mellitus in the pancreas iso- and allograft. A light and electron microscopic and immunohistochemical analysis of four cases. *Laboratory Investigation* **53**, 132—144 (1985).
8. Sutherland, D.E.R., Goetz, F.C. and Sibley, F.K.: Recurrence of disease in pancreas transplants. *Diabetes* **38** (Suppl. 1), 85—87 (1989).
9. Eisenbarth, G.S.: Type I diabetes mellitus: a chronic autoimmune disease. *New Engl. J. Med.* **314**, 1360—1368 (1986).

10. Sutherland, D.E.R., Goetz, F.C., Elick, B.A. and Najarian, J.S.: Experience with 49 segmental pancreas transplants in 45 diabetic patients. *Transplantation* **34**, 330—338 (1982).
11. Sibley R.K. and Sutherland D.E.R.: Pancreas Transplantation: an immunohistologic and histopathologic examination of 100 grafts. *Amer. J. Pathol.* **128**, 151—170 (1987).
12. Sutherland, D.E.R., Dunn, D.L., Goetz, F.C. *et al.*: A ten year experience with 290 pancreas transplants at a single institution. *Ann. Surg.* **210** 274—288 (1989).

51. Islet transplantation – the World Transplant Registry

R.G. BRETZEL, B.J. HERING and K.F. FEDERLIN

Introduction

The realization that conventional insulin treatment of type I diabetes mellitus is apparently insufficient to prevent and even stabilize the secondary complications of diabetes, generated interest in endocrine pancreas replacement therapy with the hope that normoglycemia achieved by the replacement of normally functioning islets may prevent, stop or even reverse late diabetic complications (Table 1). Besides this, pancreas or islet transplantation would improve the quality of life of the patients in avoiding daily insulin injections and dietary restrictions. Meanwhile, extended experimental work all over the world has shown that successful islet transplantation is possible in rodents and also in higher mammalians leading to prevention and, if done early, to reversing late complications such as diabetic retinopathy, neuropathy, cardiomyopathy, nephropathy and skeletal disorders. (1–11).

In principle, endocrine pancreas replacement has been attempted by either transplantation of vascularized pancreatic grafts or by transplantation of isolated islets of Langerhans as free grafts.

Clinical pancreas organ transplantation, according to the World Pancreatic

Table 1. Risk for a diabetic patient to develop secondary complications compared to the risk for age-matched non-diabetics. *Source*: Panzram, G. and Zebel-Langhennig, R.: *Med Praxis* **79**, 27–37 (1984).

Diabetic complications	Risk factor
Blindness	10–25
Nephropathy	15–20
Coronary heart disease	
Men	2–3
Women	5–6
Coronary heart death	2–3
Stroke	2–3
Gangrene	20

Transplant Registry in Minneapolis, has been performed in more than 2500 cases since 1966. In the era from January 1984 to June 1989, the success rate in terms of pancreatic graft survival has increased, but it is still not as effective as kidney grafting: the 4-year survival rate of pancreatic graft is now about 50% when simultaneously grafted with a kidney (n = 1104), about 35% when pancreas grafting is done after prior kidney grafting (n = 265) and finally only 10% in the case of pancreas grafting alone (n = 231). Another disadvantage of this approach is the lifelong strong immunosuppressive treatment of the recipient starting in most of the cases with a triple or even a quadruple regime using cyclosporine-A, glucocorticoids, azathioprine and antilymphocyte globulin, while frequent rejection crises, induced by the highly immunogenic exocrine tissue are usually treated by increased dosages of glucocorticoids, ALG and monoclonal antibodies, e.g. OKT3. The recently inaugurated treatment with a new immunosuppressive agent, FK 506, may be more potent and less toxic, but lifelong immunosuppressive treatment cannot be a solution for the young type I diabetic patient before end-stage renal disease.

Therefore, concurrent with a development of whole pancreas organ transplantation, islet transplantation has been pursued as an alternative approach for a variety of reasons: the ability to reverse experimental diabetes and to prevent or reverse its early complications on a par with vascularized pancreatic grafts; the ease and absence of serious morbidity; the ability of *in vitro* manipulation to prevent rejection without using immunosuppression or at least discontinue immunosuppression of the recipient; the elimination of possible complications due to the exocrine tissue; the ability to cryopreserve islet tissue for subsequent grafting (islet banking); the theoretical possibility to provide islet tissue from one pancreas for more than one diabetic recipient and the potential use of xenografts. The known details of 166 clinical islet allotransplantations in diabetic patients up to June 1984 have been summarized in previous reports of the International Pancreas and Islet Transplant Registry, held in Minneapolis. Since then registration of islet transplantation stopped and the recent pancreatic registry reports do not tabulate the cases of clinical islet transplantation. Since 1989 and in agreement with Dr Sutherland who runs the International Pancreas Transplant Registry in Minneapolis, our group in Giessen now keeps the International Islet Transplant Registry. This report summarizes the reported cases of clinical fetal and adult islet tissue transplantations in diabetic patients as reported to the former registry and an update of the new cases which were registered by January 1990.

Fetal islet transplantations

As listed in Table 2, 1545 allotransplants and zenotransplants of fetal islet tissue in human diabetics have been performed by January 1990. Most of these

Table 2. World Fetal and Adult Islet Transplant Registry, status by January 1990 (n = 1636; at 73 institutions).

Fetal (n = 1545)	n	Adult (n = 91)	n
U.S.S.R. (9 Instit.)[a]	n = 1000	Minneapolis	n = 23
China (30 Instit.)	n = 433	Geneva	n = 13
Szeged	n = 18	St Louis	n = 13
Denver	n = 16	Zurich	n = 8
Geneva	n = 13	East Berlin	n = 8
Stockholm	n = 12	Detroit	n = 7
Melbourne	n = 8	Miami	n = 5
East Berlin	n = 8	Pittsburgh	n = 3
Dallas	n = 6	Perugia	n = 3
Sydney	n = 5	Hannover	n = 2
Santa Barbara	n = 4	Edmonton	n = 2
Boston	n = 4	Giessen	n = 1
Madison	n = 3	Paris	n = 1
Belgrade	n = 3	Tel Aviv	n = 1
Shanghai/Toronto	n = 3	West Berlin	n = 1
Frankfurt/M.	n = 2		
Kansas	n = 2		
Albany	n = 1		
Bordeaux	n = 1		
Karlsburg	n = 1		
Minneapolis (Hen. County)	n = 1		
Rome	n = 1		

[a] Allo and Xeno.

were done in countries of the so-called Eastern Bloc, in particular the Soviet Union, China and Hungary. Only three institutions in countries of the Western Hemisphere have experience in more than ten cases. Much basic information according to donor tissue preparation, diabetic status of the recipients, effects of islet transplantation on metabolism and late complications are lacking, and therefore an assessment of the reported findings is extremely difficult. As shown in Table 3, 19 (1.2%) of the patients are reported to be off insulin therapy for periods of 2 days up to more than 45 months. C-peptide increase after the transplantation is reported in 243 (15.7%) cases. It has been generally accepted that relative changes in insulin requirements are not reliable enough to allow conclusion about the success of islet transplantation. It seems also unlikely that the xenogeneic fetal islet tissue was responsible for a reduction of insulin requirements and curative influence on secondary complications in non-immunosuppressed recipients claimed in some of the reported cases. On the other hand, recently an update of the 4 patients transplanted with fetal islet tissue at Santa Barbara indicated a detectable C-peptide secretory capacity persisting for one year in three cases. Four type I insulin-dependent diabetic men had received minced tissue from 6 to 12 pooled fetal pancreata cultured for 48

Table 3. Number and percentage of patients off insulin and with increased C-peptide levels after transplantation of adult or fetal islet tissue as reported to the registry.

	Adult tissue ($n = 91$)	Fetal tissue ($n = 1545$)
Off insulin	$n = 7$ (7.7%) 3 days to 17 months	$n = 19$ (1.2%) 2 days to ⩾45 months
C-Peptide increase	$n = 34$ (40%)	$n = 243$ (15.7%)

hours. Immunosuppressive therapy was not given. The tissue was transplanted under local anesthesia into the forearm muscle of the non-dominant arm or below the subcutaneous adipose tissue of the left lower quadrant of the abdominal wall. An increase in C-peptide secretion was documented following each procedure. The total insulin requirement showed a decrease of 71% to 100% at the time of maximum C-peptide secretion, which persisted in three cases as already mentioned. No increase in anticytoplasmic islet cell antibody titer was detected during the year of observation following transplantation. For the first time these well-documented studies show that transplantation of functioning fetal pancreatic insulin secreting tissue can be performed with minimal operative or immunologic risk to the recipient and insulin secretory capacity may persist for at least one year following implantation, without immunosuppressive treatment of the recipient at least when cultured fetal islet tissue is used.

Adult islet transplantation

Clinical transplantations of adult pancreatic islet tissue have been performed in 91 cases by January 1990 at 15 different institutions. Only three institutions have experience of more than 10 cases (Table 2). The clinical outcome is given in Table 3. Seven (7.7%) patients are reported as off insulin and this effect lasted from 3 days to a maximum of 17 months. An increase of C-peptide serum levels compared to the situation before islet grafting was observed in 34 (40%) cases. In brief, no long-term survival of allografted adult islet tissue has been demonstrated up to now. In this sense, islet transplantation at this time is without doubt clearly less efficient than pancreas transplantation. Although the concept of replacing only the required islets of Langerhans instead of the whole pancreas and thereby circumventing the problems associated with the acinar tissue remains very appealing despite remarkable advances in the area of experimental islet transplantation over the past two decades, successful clinical islet transplantation is still not a reality. A critical evaluation of all attempts of clinical application of islet transplantation on the basis of current knowledge indicates that almost all attempts have been performed prematurely using relatively unsophisticated techniques:

1. In particular, there might have been functional deterioration of islets during preservation of the donor pancreas before islet isolation.
2. Methods to provide adequate amounts of morphologically intact, viable and pure islets were not available until the last two years.
3. Deleterious effects on islets may have occurred between the time of isolation, purification, implantation and revascularization.
4. Islet transplantation was performed to inappropriate sites.
5. Microangiopathy of the recipient may result in impaired islet neovascularization.
6. An increased immunogenicity of isolated islets and an increased susceptibility to rejection has to be considered and almost no immunoalteration prior to transplantation was done.
7. Conventional immunosuppressive agents proved to be ineffective to prevent islet allograft rejection also in most of the experimental situations.
8. MHC identity seems not to guarantee prolonged islet allograft survival.
9. The inability to diagnose and consecutively start early treatment of acute rejection episodes has to be considered.
10. The likelihood of destruction of the grafted tissue by an autoimmune mechanism leading to insulitis and recurrence of diabetes.

As a result of recent innovations, the situation has impressively changed. With more defined techniques, various groups have demonstrated that it is possible to isolate 2000—4000 islets per gram pancreas even from human adult pancreas, thus amounting to 200 000—400 000 islets per pancreas. Using this new automated digestion technique and more effective purification methods, new cases of adult islet tissue transplantations in human type I diabetic patients were performed at six different institutions during the last two years (Table 4), with the exception of one case in St Louis, islets were obtained from one pancreas. Two transplants were performed in type II diabetic patients. In most of the cases strong evidence of endocrine function in terms of an increase of basal C-peptide levels and in some patients also of stimulated C-peptide was demonstrated. One patient transplanted at the institution in Paris has permanent endocrine function and is completely off insulin. The two cases transplanted at the University of Alberta in Edmonton suffered from intercurrent CM-virus infection probably transferred by the simultaneously transplanted kidney and finally C-peptide and insulin secretion stopped. In the three cases transplanted at the University of St Louis, and listed as currently functioning, their endocrine function has now also stopped. All these clinical trials were performed under conventional immunosuppressive treatment of the recipient. None of the various methods to immunomodulate islet tissue prior to transplantation, as has been proven so successfully in experimental studies, had been attempted up to now, to these clinical trials.

Table 4. Cases of adult islet transplantations performed in diabetic patients in 1988 and 1989 as reported to the registry.

Institution	Islet no.	Basal C-peptide (ng/ml) 1 wk post Tx	1 mo post Tx	Current function	Comments
Zurich	225 000	—	—	No	Seleno-dl-methionine
Paris	150 000	0.99	2.46	Off insulin	Hemochromatosis
Berlin	?	0.5—0.9	—	No	—
Edmonton	260 845	0.5	0.97	No	CMV/simult. kidney
	261 370	0.2	0.75	No	CMV/simult. kidney
St Louis	481 000	0.96	0.26	No	Presumed rejection Simult. kidney
	305 600	0.26	1.34	Yes	simult. kidney
	200 000	0.05	0.46	Yes	Simult. kidney
	750 000	?	?	Yes	Off insulin day 10—25 2 donors, simult. kidney
Perugia	588 000	0.3	?	No	Presumed rejection Simult. kidney
	180 000	1.8	2.0	Yes	Type II diabetes C-peptide before Tx Vascular prothesis
	?	?	?	No	Type II diabetes Vascular prothesis

Summary and future prospects

A surprisingly high number of fetal islet transplants have been reported by a few groups. There are indications that this kind of endocrine replacement therapy will not be neglected although not all questions seem to be adequately answered.

In most cases of adult islet transplantations, graft function, at least sufficient to allow withdrawal from insulin, was not always achieved. At a first glance these disappointing results seem to suggest that the prospects for clinical islet transplantation are bleak and the question arises as to whether islet transplantation shows any real prospect for clinical application. However, the application of more refined isolation and purification techniques in the recent clinical trials of adult islet tissue may provide encouraging aspects. There is now accumulating evidence of definite graft function, at least temporarily, which indicated that technical difficulties that have long been encountered in the isolation of islets have, at least in part, been overcome. Attention should be now focused on the improvement of islet purification techniques which appears to be a prerequisite for the application of islet immunoalteration. It remains to be determined whether approaches that have prevented rejection of islets in non-immunosuppressed or with short-term immunosuppressed rodents by eliminating or altering passenger leukocytes within the islet will facilitate human islet allograft acceptance under short-term immunosuppression, in the diabetic patient. If this goal could be achieved, transplantation of islets expressing histocompatibility antigens different from the recipient but immunoaltered will not be rejected as foreign tissue or recognized and consequently destroyed by the autoimmune mechanism. Even transplantation of islets derived from higher mammalians could become a clinical reality thus filling the gap between the limited number of donor pancreata available and the high number of potential.

With these new developments, transplantation of islets could be performed at an early stage of diabetes with reasonable expectation of success for preventing diabetic secondary complications without the risks currently encountered in vascularized pancreatic organ transplantation.

References

1. Lacy, P.E.: Islet transplantation. In: K.G.M.M. Alberti and L.P. Krall (eds), *The Diabetes Annual*, Vol. 3, pp. 189—200. Elsevier Science Publishers, Amsterdam (1987).
2. Scharp, D.W., Lacy, P.E., Santiago, J.V. *et al.*: Insulin independence after islet transplantion into type I diabetic patients. *Diabetes* **39**, 515—518 (1990).
3. Hering, B.J., Bretzel, R.G. and Federlin, K.: Current status of clinical islet transplantation. *Horm. Metabol. Res.* **20**, 537—545 (1988).
4. Stegall, M.D., Sutherland, D.E.R. and Hardy, M.A.: Registry report on clinical experience with islet transplantation. In: R. Van Schilfgaarde and M.A. Hardy (eds), *Transplantation of the Endocrine Pancreas in Diabetes Mellitus*, pp. 224—248. Elsevier Science Publishers, Amsterdam (1988).
5. Mintz, D.H.: The effect of FK 506 on human islet transplantation. Presented at the 10th Int. Workshop 'Immunology of Diabetes' and the 3rd Int. Workshop 'Lessons from Animal Diabetes', Jerusalem, March 18—24, (1990).
6. Warnock, G.L., Kneteman, N.M., Ryan, E.A. *et al.*: Continued function of pancreatic islets after transplantation in type-I diabetes. *Lancet* **8662**, 570—572 (1989).
7. Downing, R.: Historical review of pancreatic islet transplantation. *World J. Surg.* **8**, 137—142 (1984).
8. Bretzel, R.G.: Inseltransplantation und Diabetes mellitus. *Experimentelle Grundlagen und Klinische Versuche*, pp. 1—644. Pflaum, München (1984).
9. Sutherland, D.E.R.: Pancreas and islet transplantation. II. Clinical trials. *Diabetologia* **20**, 435—450 (1981).
10. Sutherland, D.E.R.: International human pancreas and islet transplant registry. *Transplant. Proc.* **12** (Suppl. 2), 229—236 (1980).
11. Sutherland, D.E.R.: Pancreas and islet transplant registry. *World J. Surg.* **8**, 270—275 (1984).

52. Prevention of rejection of islet allografts and xenografts without continuous immunosuppression of the recipients

PAUL E. LACY and DAVID W. SCHARP

The objective of transplanting islets into diabetic patients is to accomplish the transplants early in the course of diabetes with the hope that these transplants will prevent the development of the complications of diabetes such as blindness, renal failure and early onset of artherosclerosis. This objective places islet transplantation in a different setting as compared to transplantation of whole organs such as the heart, liver or kidney. The whole organ transplants are done in patients who are acutely ill and, in the case of heart and liver transplants are needed to preserve the life of the patient. In contrast, diabetes mellitus is a chronic disease requiring decades to develop the complications of this disease. Thus, the use of islet transplantation in diabetes requires an approach which would prevent rejection of the islet transplants without the need for continuous immunosuppression of the patients. The reason for this is that chronic administration of immunosuppressive drugs could lead to serious toxic side effects that could be more devastating than the complications of the disease itself.

The purpose of this presentation is to review the development of procedures which permit the successful transplantation of islet allografts in animals without the need for continuous immunosuppression. The effect of these procedures for immunoalteration of the donor islets will also be discussed with respect to prevention of rejection of islet xenografts. Finally, some comments will be provided with respect to the present status of transplantation of human islets in diabetic patients.

Prevention of rejection of islet allografts

The concept that has permitted the development of methods for prevention of rejection of islet allografts in animals is that passenger leukocytes carried along with the transplanted organ are responsible for initiation of the rejection of the allografts, whereas the paranchemal cells of the organ will not induce rejection. This passenger leukocyte concept was proposed by Snell in 1957 (1). The initial studies on prevention of rejection of islet allografts in rodents using this concept were first initiated in our laboratory and in the laboratory of Dr Kevin Lafferty.

We found that low-temperature culture of donor rat islets for one week, to alter or destroy passenger leukocytes, in conjunction with a single injection of antilymphocyte serum into recipient rats, would completely prevent rejection of islet allografts (2). Bowen and Lafferty (3) used high oxygen culture of aggregates of donor mouse islets to destroy passenger leukocytes and this approach prevented rejection of islet allografts in mice.

Subsequent to these initial studies many different methods have now been developed for alteration or destruction of passenger leukocytes in donor islets with resultant prevention of rejection of the allografts. Some of these methods include specific anitbodies to destroy passenger leukocytes in the islets (4, 5), ultraviolet irradiation to inactivate the antigen-presenting cells (6), methods to obtain pure isolated islet cells (7), methods for the formation of islets in culture devoid of passenger leukocytes (8), and utilization of small numbers of islets from several different strains of mice so that the specific passenger leukocyte content for each strain is below the critical level for initiation of rejection (9). These different methods for preventing rejection have been reviewed in detail in several different recent publications (10, 11, 12).

It is much easier to prevent rejection of islet allografts in mice than in rats. In mice, rejection can be prevented simply by pretreatment of the donor islets to destroy or alter passenger leukocytes in the islets. In contrast, in rats with a strong immune response to the donor animal, it is necessary not only to alter or destroy passenger leukocytes within the islets, but it also requires temporary immunosuppression of the recipient animals to prevent rejection. This temporary immunosuppression can be accomplished by a single injection of antilymphocyte serum at the time of transplantation or by the administration of cyclosporine A for 3 days, beginning at the time of transplantation. It is most probable that prevention of rejection of human islet allografts will also require procedures to alter or destroy the human islet antigen-presenting cells, as well as appropriate temporary immunosuppression of the recipient.

The sites for successful transplantation of islet allografts and isografts include the liver, spleen, kidney capsule, testes, and brain (11, 12). The sites that would appear to be most appropriate for implantation of human islet allografts would be the liver, spleen or kidney capsule. Each of these sites have certain advantages and disadvantages. Implantation of the islets in the liver is accomplished by injecting the islets into the portal venous system so they lodge in branches of the portal vein in the portal tracts of the liver. In order for this approach to be used in human islet transplants it requires that the preparation of islets be extremely pure in order to prevent intravascular thrombosis within the liver. Studies with rat islet allografts have indicated that the liver site provides an immunologic advantage with respect to induction of specific immune tolerance in the recipient animals which is not present when the islets are transplanted beneath the kidney capsule (13). From a functional standpoint, islets implanted in the liver, via the portal vein, would release insulin and have a direct effect on the liver cells as it does in normal circumstances where the insulin is released into the protal venous system from the islets in the pancreas. A disadvantage of this site is that some of the islets can become broken and pass through the liver and some may be entrapped in small thrombi and die before establishing a blood supply.

In the dog, the spleen can be used as a site of implantation since the islet grafts can be distributed by mechanical pressure on the spleen when they are injected, or they can be refluxed into the spleen via the splenic vein. The application of this approach to human islet allografts is fraught with difficulty because it would require an open operation and the spleen is not easily accessible for islet implantation and it is not possible to distribute the islets equally throughout the splenic pulp by massaging the spleen.

In rodents, the kidney capsule is a very effective site and can be used easily for the implantation of islet allografts or isografts. In constrast, we have not been able to establish either islet autografts or allografts in dogs when the canine islets are transplanted beneath the kidney capsule. Apparently, the capsule is different in the dog than in rodents and the question remains whether the kidney capsule could be used as a site for implantation of human islets.

It is apparent from studies in animals that these different sites have certain advantages and disadvantages for implantation of the islets. As the clinical trials on human islet allografts progress, it will be necessary to examine each of these three sites to determine the optimum site for implantation of human islets with respect to preservation of the islets transplanted, the optimum functional effect of the insulin secreted by the islets and the immunologic advantage of the site selected.

Prevention of rejection of islet xenografts

A critical problem in the future for the use of human islet allografts as a therapeutic approach to diabetes is the limited availability of human pancreases for isolation of islets. Thus, it is imperative that approaches be sought to attempt to prevent rejection of islets transplanted across a species barrier to that animal islets might be used for transplantation into diabetic patients. Studies have been initiated in this area and some fascinating results have been obtained.

Initially, studies were accomplished on prevention of rejection of islet xenografts transplanted across a closely related species barrier (rat to mouse). *In vitro* culture of donor rat islets at 24 °C for 7 days and a single injection of mouse and rat antilymphocyte sera at the time of transplanting the islets into the liver via the portal vein prevented rejection of rat islet xenografts in mice (14). As indicated earlier, this was the initial approach we had used for prevention of rejection of islet allografts in rodents. We have also found that low-temperature culture of the donor rat islets and treatment of the recipient mice for 7 days with an antibody to helper T lymhocytes (anti-L3T4) would produce indefinite survival of islet xenografts transplanted into the liver (15). In contrast, this same regimen simply prolonged the survival of rat islet xenografts when they were transplanted beneath the kidney capsule and did not achieve indefinite survival. These findings indicate an immunologic advantage to the intrahepatic site with respect to closely related islet xenografts. Recently, we have found that *in vitro* culture of rat islet xenografts in the presence of transforming growth factor beta and three injections of a monoclonal antibody to interferon gamma over a 2-week interval would produce indefinite survival of rat islets transplanted into the kidney capsule of mice (16).

Prevention of rejection of closely related islet xenografts without continuous immunosuppression does not solve the problem of a future source of animal islets for transplantation into diabetic patients due to the limited availability of non-human primates. Thus, the goal is to attempt to achieve indefinite survival of islet xenografts transplanted across a wide species barrier. Early studies on islet xenografts transplanted across a wide species barrier indicated that fish islets would survive and function for 1 to 2 days in rats following total irradiation of the recipients (17). Implants of embryonic chick pancreas in the liver permitted survival of diabetic rats but did not achieve normoglycemia in the recipients (18).

Recent studies using immunoalteration procedures on the donor islets have produced amazing results in prolonging the survival of islet xenografts transplanted across a wide species barrier. Low-temperature culture alone produced a marked prolongation of survival of xenografts of human islets transplanted into mice and the addition of a 7-day course of treatment with monoclonal antibodies to helper T lymphocytes in the recipients prolonged the survival even further (19). In studies in progress, we have found that low-temperature culture of human islets in conjunction with a single injection of mouse and human antilymphocyte sera produced a 60% survival of the human islet xenografts in mice at 100 days after transplantation.

Another approach for the prevention of rejection of islet xenografts transplanted across a wide species barrier is to use artifical membranes for encapsulation of the islets and separation of them from the immune system of the recipient. Microencapsulation techniques were developed several years ago and the initial findings provided encouraging results (20). In the interim many laboratories have attempted to use the microcapsules, and one of the deterring features is the biocompatibility of the capsules. Further intensive studies are needed to formulate biocompatible capsular membranes that will permit the rapid transport of glucose in one direction and insulin in the other and yet separate the islets from the immune system of the recipient.

The pig represents the ideal source of animal islets for possible human islet transplant, since pig insulin and human insulin are almost identical and pigs are readily available. Methods have been developed for isolation of pig islets (21) and further improvements in these procedures have been accomplished in several different laboratories. Thus, it is now possible to initiate studies on prevention of rejection of pig inlets in mice and then progress to larger animals as donors to develop procedures for the possible future use of pig islet xenografts for transplantation into diabetic human patients.

Adult islet transplants in human diabetes

Until recently, a major barrier for the transplantation of human islets has been the lack of methods which would permit the mass isolation of highly purified islets from a single human pancreas. In the last few years several methods have been developed which do provide massive numbers of islets from the human pancreas. Gray *et al.* (22) developed a collagenase technique which permitted the isolation of a larger number of human islets, however, the final preparation was not pure. Initially, we developed a maceration technique for separation of the islets in the human pancreas following collagenase digestion (23). A large number of islets could be obtained from the human pancreas, however, the purity of the final preparation was only 10—20% islet tissue. Recently, we have developed an automated technique for isolation of human islets which now permits the successful separation of several hundred thousand islets from a single human pancreas with a purity of 80—95% islet tissue (24). These purified islets can be maintained in culture for 7 days permitting an assessment of their functional capacity with respect to insulin secretion and quality control studies on possible bacterial contamination prior to transplantation.

The development of these new methods for isolating human islets has made it possible to initiate clinical trials on transplantation of islets into type I diabetic subjects. Mintz and his associates (25) have reported function of human islet allografts in diabetics for several months. These patients were not off insulin, but plasma C-peptide could be demonstrated in these individuals following islet transplantation and it was totally absent prior to the islet transplants. Clinical trials are in progress in our laboratory, using the automated method for isolating the human islets. Since this procedure results in an 80—95% purity of islet tissue in the final preparation, it is possible to use the umbilical vein for injection of the islets into the protal venous system of the recipient, and this operative procedure can be accomplished under local anesthesia. The recipients in this current clinical trial are diabetic patients who are already receiving immunosuppressive drugs for maintenance of their established kidney transplants. The only immunosuppressive agent added at the time of transplantation is a 7-day course of treatment with human antilymphocyte globulin and if rejection of the islets occurred, the rejection would not be treated. These studies are still in progress: however, the initial findings indicate that it is possible to achieve normal levels of C-peptide following transplantation of human islets, and in one patient normoglycemia and normal C-peptide levels were achieved in the absence of exogenous insulin for approximately 2 weeks before a rejection episode occurred.

We believe that the criteria to measure success of human islet transplantation should be, as a minimum, the absence of fasting and stimulated measurable plasma C-peptide prior to transplantation, the return of the fasting and stimulated levels to normal limits after transplantation and the patient remain normoglycemic in the absence of insulin therapy. It is important that these criteria be utilized to avoid misinterpretation of the findings.

Human fetal transplants in diabetic patients

The human fetal pancreas has an advantage over adult islets with respect to the ability of the cells to replicate. A disadvantage of the fetal pancreas is that the procedures which prevent rejection of adult islets in rodents are not successful with the fetal pancreas. Prolongation of survival has been achieved with rodent fetal pancreases: however, procedures and methods are needed in order to achieve the long-term survival that has been obtained with adult islets.

Several different laboratories have initiated studies on transplantation of cultured human fetal pancreases into type I diabetic subjects. To our knowledge it has not been demonstrated as yet in appropriate diabetic recipients with no measurable C-peptide prior to transplantation, that the transplants produced increasing amounts of C-peptide and achieved normal levels of C-peptide production and that the patients required no exogenous insulin therapy. Reports on the reduction of the amount of insulin therapy following fetal pancreas transplants have been made; however, it is difficult to interpret these findings since no data were presented on the absence of C-peptide prior to transplantation or an incremental gain in C-peptide following transplantation of the fetal pancreas.

It is most important that future studies and basic research be accomplished on the human fetal pancreas, since it would provide an available source of islet tissue and is needed for basic studies on elimination of passenger leukocytes, culture techniques for growth and differentiation of the fetal islets, and possible identification of islet precursor cells. Unfortunately, in the United States, a recent ruling by the government prohibits the use of fetal human pancreatic tissue for studies on these basic problems using funds obtained from the government. Guidelines have been provided to the government agencies which quite adequately safeguard the use of human fetal tissue in research and it is hoped that this moratorium will be lifted as soon as possible in order to permit the further exploration of the utilization of human fetal tissue for basic studies and possible transplantation into diabetic subjects in the future.

Summary and conclusions

Diabetes mellitus is a chronic disease requiring decades before diabetic complications such as renal failure, diabetic neuropathy, diabetic retinopathy and accelerated artherosclerosis occur. These complications are apparently due to the inability to maintain the blood sugar within normal limits at all times with present forms of therapy. If islet transplantation is to be used as a means of maintaining normoglycemia, then the transplants would have to be accomplished early in the course of diabetes to prevent the complications. Thus, the objective is to be able to transplant islets without continuous immunosuppression due to the toxic side effects of the immunosuppressive drugs during decades of administration. Methods have been developed for the prevention of rejection of islet allografts in rodents by destroying or altering passenger leukocytes in the islets with or without temporary immunosuppression of the recipients. These same methods for immunoalteration of the donor islets will also produce indefinite survival of islet xenografts transplanted across a closely related species barrier and marked prolongation of islet xenografts transplanted across a wide species barrier. Studies have also been accomplished on protecting islet xenografts from the immune system by encapsulation of the islets. These advances have stimulated the development of procedures for the mass isolation of human islets and the initiation of clinical trials on human islet allografts in diabetic patients. These islet transplants are in diabetic patients who are either receiving a kidney transplant or who have an established kidney transplant. The initial findings are mot encouraging. A subsequent phase of these trials is to attempt to transplant human islets without continuous immunosuppression by using procedures for immunoalteration of the donor islets with temporary immunosuppression of the recipients. The ultimate goal is to utilize animal islets as xenografts in diabetic patients and to establish the xenografts by procedures which do not require continuous immunosuppression of the recipients.

References

1. Snell, G.D.: The homograft reaction. *Ann. Rev. Microbiol.* **2**, 439–458 (1057).
2. Lacy, P.E., Davie, J.M. and Finke, E.H.: Prolongation of islet allograft survival following *in vitro* culture (24°C) and a single injection of ALS. *Science* **204**, 312–313 (1979).
3. Bowen, K.M. and Lafferty, K.J.: Reversal of diabetes by allogeneic islet transplantation without immunosuppression. *Aust. J. Exp. Biol. Med. Sci.* **58**, 441–447 (1980).
4. Faustman, D., Hauptfeld, V., Lacy, P.E. and Davie, J.M.: Prolongation of murine islet allograft survival by pretreatment of islets with antibody directed to Ia determinants. *Proc. Natl. Acad. Sci. (USA)* **78**, 5156–5159 (1981).
5. Faustman, D.L., Steinman, R.M., Gebel, H.M., Hauptfeld, V., Davie, J.M. and Lacy, P.E.: Prevention of rejection of murine islet allografts by pretreatment with anti-dendritic antibody. *Proc. Natl. Acad. Sci. (USA)* **81**, 3864–3868 (1984).

6. Lau, H., Reemtsma, K. and Hardy, M.A.: Prolongation of rat islet allograft survival by direct ultraviolet irradiation of the graft. *Science* **223**, 607—608 (1984).
7. Pipeleers, D., Pipeleers-Marichal, M., Gepts, W. *et al.*: Purified islet cell grafts are tolerated without immunosuppressive treatment in allotransplanted diabetic rats. *Abstract. Second Assisi Int. Symp.on Advanced Models for the Therapy of Insulin-Dependent Diabetes, Assisi, Italy* (1986).
8. Herge, O.D., Enriquez, A., Weinhaus, A.J., Marshall, S. and Serie, J.R.: Allotransplantability of neonatal rat islets in the BB/W rat. *Diabetes* **36** (Suppl.), 272 (1987).
9. Gotoh, M., Mati, T., Porter J. and Monaco, A.P.: Pancreatic islet transplantation using H-2 incompatible multiple donors. *Transplant. Proc.* **19**, 957—959 (1987).
10. Lafferty, K.J., Prowse, S.J., Simeonovic, C.J. and Warren, H.S.: Immunobiology of tissue transplantation: a return to the passenger leukocyte concept. *Ann. Rev. Immunol.* **1**, 143—173 (1983).
11. Lacy, P.E. and Davie, J.M.: Transplantation of pancreatic islets. *Ann. Rev. Immunol.* **2**, 183—198 (1984).
12. Lacy, P.E.: Islet transplantation. *The Diabetes Annual*, Vol. 4 (in press).
13. Kamei, T. and Yasunami, Y.: Demonstration of donor specific unresponsiveness in rat islet allografts: importance of transplant site for induction by Cyclosporin A and maintenance. *Diabetologia* **32**, 779—785 (1989).
14. Lacy, P.E., Davie, J.M. and Finke, E.H.: Prolongation of islet xenograft survival without continuous immunosuppression. *Science* **209**, 283—285 (1980).
15. Lacy, P.E., Ricordi, C. and Finke, E.H.: Effect of transplantation site and aL3T4 treatment on survival of rat, hamster and rabbit islet xenografts in mice. *Transplantation* **47**, 761—766 (1989).
16. Carel, J-C., Schreiber, R.D. and Lacy, P.E.: Transforming growth factor (TGF) beta decreases the immunogenicity of islet xenografts. Presented at the FASEB Meeting, New Orleans, March 1989.
17. Weber, C., Weil, R., McIntosh, R., Hogle, H., Warden, G. and Reemtsma, K.: Xenotransplantation of piscine islets into hyperglycemic rats. *Surgery* **77**, 208—215 (1975).
18. Eloy, R., Haffen, K., Kedinger, M. and Grenier, J.F.: Chick embryo pancreatic transplants reverse experimental diabetes in rats. *J. Clin. Invest.* **64**, 361—373 (1979).
19. Ricordi, C., Lacy, P.E., Sterbenz, K. and Davie, J.M.: Low temperature culture of human islets or *in vivo* treatment with L3T4 antibody produces a marked prolongation of islet human to mouse xenograft survival. *Proc. Natl. Acad. Sci. (USA)* **84** 8080—8084 (1987).
20. Lim, F. and Sun, A.M.: Microencapsulated islets as bioartifical pancreas. *Science* **210**, 908—910 (1980).
21. Ricordi, C., Finke, E.H. and Lacy, P.E.: A method for the mass isolation of islets from the adult pig pancreas. *Diabetes* **35**, 649—653 (1986).
22. Gray, D.W.R., McShane, P., Grant, A. and Morris, P.J.: A method for isolation of islets of Langerhans from the human pancreas. *Diabetes* **33**, 1055—1061 (1984).
23. Scharp, D.W., Lacy, P.E. Finke, E.H. and Olack, B.J.: Low-temperature culture of human islets isolated by the distention method and purified with Ficoll or percoll gradients. *Survey* **102**, 869—879 (1987).
24. Ricordi, C., Lacy, P.E. and Finke, E.H., Olack, B.J., Scharp, D.W.: Automated method for isolation of human pancreatic islets. *Diabetes* **37**, 413—420 (1988).
25. Alejandro, R., Mintz, D.H., Noel, J., Latif, Z., Koh, N., Russell E. and Miller J.: Islet cell transplantation in Tupe I diabetes mellitus. *Transplant. Proc.* **19**, 2359—2361 (1987).

53. Effect of islet transplantation on diabetic secondary complications

R.G. BRETZEL

Introduction

The organ lesions that develop in experimental diabetes mellitus are similar to those associated with diabetes mellitus in humans. In a series of experiments with syngeneic transplantation of fresh or cultured islets in spontaneous autoimmune and chemically induced type I diabetes and in a genetically determined dietary type II diabetes in rats, we could demonstrate a prevention or even reversal of renal, retinal, neural and cardiac lesions. Comparable studies with conventional insulin treatment of the animals proved the superiority of the islet transplantation approach. The bulk of our experiments was performed in the streptozotocin diabetes model of the rat (1—9).

Diabetic nephropathy

The renal lesions that develop in diabetic rats are similar in some respects to those associated with diabetes mellitus in humans. There is a progressive increase with the duration of the disease in mesangial matrix volume and in basement membrane thickness. Immunoglobulins and other macromolecules are non-specifically deposited within the mesangium and contribute to the mesangial enlargement. Tubular vacuolization (Armanni-Ebstein cells) and hyalinization of aterioles is present.

In a series of experiments with syngeneic transplantation of fresh or cultured islets we could demonstrate prevention and when transplantation has been performed not later than 3—6 months after onset of diabetes, there was even a reversal of these kidney lesions. Quantitative studies revealed a significant reduction of the number of affected glomeruli and of the mesangial enlargement and a rewidening of the capillary lumina. Signs of diabetic tubulopathy also disappeared. Electron microscopy showed a prevention of basement membrane thickening which took place to a large extent in non-transplanted diabetic controls.

In the context of our investigations, new markers of diabetic nephropathy were found. It turned out that structure related markers of glomerular basement membrane collagen metabolism as 7S-collagen and laminin P2 can be demonstrated in raised concentrations in the serum in diabetic rats. After normalization of the distrubed glucose metabolism by syngeneic islet transplantation, the serum concentration of these basement membrane antigens returned to normal. We found the same for the raised renal activity of collagen glucosyltransferase in diabetic rats. An increased urinary excretion of brush-border enzymes alanine aminopeptidase and alkaline phosphatase and a decreased urinary excretion of the enzyme, gammaglutamyltranspeptidase — both a sign of diabetic tubulopathy — could no longer be demonstrated after successful islet transplantation.

Diabetic cardiomyopathy

Studies in diabetic cardiomyopathy revealed a beneficial effect of successful islet transplantation with regard to biochemical and functional signs. The reduced utilization of carbohydrates found in diabetic rats, the decreased production of ATP and as a consequence, a reduced cardiac output became normal after syngeneic islet transplantation. Utilization of triglycerides by the heart muscle cells also normalizes following islet transplantation.

Diabetic retinopathy

Very recently a digestion technique to yield preparations of the retina was established in our laboratory. Streptozotocin diabetic Wistar rats developed retinal changes which are similar to those associated with diabetes mellitus in humans: microaneurisms, hyperplasia of mesodermal strands and pericyte migration as degenerative signs beginning after two to three months of diabetes. Furthermore, degeneration of occular capillaries including loss of intramural pericytes on single capillaries, omega-shaped capillary loopings and microthrombosis after 5—8 months of diabetes were demonstrated. The most striking feature which made quantification possible was the diffuse and selective diminution of pericyte density. Compared to normal control retinas, the pericyte number was significantly reduced in the diabetics one month after onset of diabetes and decreased further during the whole period of observation. Correspondingly, there was a steady increase in the E/P ratio which was approximately 1 : 1 in normal retinas.

For comparison 'early' syngeneic islet transplantation after one month of the disease and 'late' syngeneic islet transplantation (6 months after diabetes induction) was performed in 10 diabetic rats each. The retinas of islet transplanted rats showed no pathological changes except some equivocal microthrombosis in the early transplanted animals and several severe forms of capillary degeneration (strand formation) in the late transplanted animals. Quantitative analysis revealed an absolute prevention of pericyte loss as well as of endothelial proliferation in the early transplanted rats. Late transplanted rats showed a partial restoration of the decreased pericyte density still significantly different from normal controls. As a result, the increase in E/P ratio found in diabetic rats was completely prevented by early islet transplantation and significantly but not completely reversed by late islet transplantation.

Diabetic neuropathy

In another series of experiments, 7 groups of Lewis rats aged 10 weeks were studied over 12 months with onset of diabetes at 6 and 12 months. Comparisons were made among normal controls, untreated streptozotocin diabetics and streptozotoxin diabetics treated with syngeneic pancreatic islet transplantation at 1 month ('early transplantation') and 6 months ('late transplantation') of diabetes. Myelinated fibres and axonal area in the peripheral sural nerve were significantly less in the diabetic animals at 6 and 12 months as compared with age-matched normal controls. These peripheral nerve structural abnormalities resembled those associated with diabetes mellitus in humans.

The reduction in myelinated fibre and axonal area was prevented in early transplanted diabetic animals as the values were greater than untreated diabetics and not different from controls. The reduction in fibre area was also corrected in the diabetic animals which were transplanted 6 months after the induction of diabetes as the values were greater than untreated diabetics and not different from age-matched controls. Axonal area was also significantly increased in the late transplanted diabetics as compared with untreated diabetics but was not normalized. This pancreatic islet transplantation prevented as well as reversed peripheral nerve structural abnormalities in experimental diabetes.

Summary and conclusions

The effects of metabolically successful islet transplantation in diabetic rats on secondary complications of diabetes mellitus were as follows: early transplantation leads to prevention, late transplantation leads to arrest or in some cases even a reversal of diabetic retinopathy, nephropathy, cardiomyopathy and neuropathy. Furthermore, descriptive follow-up studies have demonstrated that diabetic cataract can be prevented but not reversed by successful islet transplantation. Other diabetic secondary complications which we did not investigate but were reported by other groups are skeletal disorders which can also be prevented by experimental islet transplantation.

A comparative investigation with conventional insulin treatment of diabetic rats proved that despite almost comparable good metabolic compensation, the renal and caridac changes cannot be prevented or reversed as successfully as by islet transplantation. In particular, semiquantitative analysis of the immunohistological appearance and the electron microscopic analysis of basement membrane thickness demonstrated the superior effect of iselt transplantation when compared to conventional insulin treatment.

References

1. Mauer, S.M., Sutherland, D.E.R., Steffes, M.W., Leonhard, R.J., Najarian, J.S., Michael, A.F. and Brown, D.M.: Pancreatic islet transplantation: effects on the glomerular lesions of experimental diabetes in the rat. *Diabetes* **23**, 748—753 (1974).
2. Mauer, S.M., Steffes, M.W., Sutherland, D.E.R., Najarian, J.S., Michael, A.F. and Brown, D.M.: Studies of the rate of regression of the glomerular lesions in diabetic rats treated with pancreatic islet transplantation. *Diabetes* **24**, 280—285 (1975).
3. Federlin, K., Bretzel, R.G., Schmidtchen, U.: Islet transplantation in experimental diabetes of the rat. V. Regression of glomerular lesions in diabetic rats after introportal transplantation of isogeneic islets. Preliminary results. *Horm. Metabol. Res.* **8**, 404—406 (1976).
4. Bretzel, R.G., Schneider, J., Zimmermann, I., Küppers, B., Weise, M. and Federlin, K.: Urinary excretion of alanine aminopeptidase and total proteinuria in experimental diabetes mellitus before and after islet transplantation. *Contr. Nephrol.* **24**, 153—164 (1981).
5. Bretzel, R.G., Menden, A., Richardt, M., Brocks, D.G., Draeger, K.E. and Federlin, K.: Renal collagen glucosyltransferase activity following islet transplantation in streptozotocin-diabetic rats. *Diabetologia* **21**, 428—429 (1981).
6. Bretzel, R.G., Breidenbach, Ch., Hofman, J. and Federlin, K.: Islet transplantation in experimental diabetes of the rat. VI. Rate of regression in diabetic kidney lesions after isogeneic islet transplantation. Quantitative measurements. *Horm. Metabol. Res.* **11**, 200—207 (1979).
7. Bretzel, R.G., Brocks, D.G., Timpl, R. and Federlin, K.: Reversal and prevention of nephropathy by islet transplantation in diabetic rats. In: E. Shafrir and A.E. Renold (eds), *Lessons from Animal Diabetes*, pp. 599—605. Libbey, London (1984).
8. Bretzel, R.G.: Inseltransplantation und Diabetes mellitus. *Experimentelle Grundlagen und Klinische Versuche*, pp. 1—644. Pflaum, München (1984).
9. Bretzel, R.G., Flesch, B.K., Hering, B.J. and Brendel, M., Klitscher, D., Brandhorst, H., Schelz, J., Münch, K.P. and Federlin, K.: Impact of culture and cryopreservation on MHC class II antigen expression in canine and porcine islets. In: K. Federlin, R.G. Bretzel and B.J. Hering (eds), *Methods in Islet Transplantation Research; Horm. Metabol. Res.* (Suppl.) ser. 25, 128—132 (1990).

54. Does pretreatment of islets of Langerhans with deoxyguanosine improve allograft survival without immunosuppression?

I.H. AL-ABDULLAH, M.S.A. KUMAR, M.S. AL-ADNANI and G.M. ABOUNA

Introduction

The immunogenicity of islets is attributed mainly to the presence of passenger leukocytes (dendritic cells, macrophages) (1, 2). These cells usually express an abundant of class II antigen (3, 4). Removal of these cells or of the antigens may result in prolongation survival of transplanted islets without continuous immunosuppression (5, 8). Several methods have been described to reduce islet immunogenicity prior to transplantation, such as the use of UV and gamma irradiation as well as pretreatment with anti-Ia and antibody to dendritic cells in the present of complement (5—8). Deoxyguanosine (dGuo) has been found to be toxic to lymphocytes and dendritic cells and effective in prolonging transplantation of the pretreated dGuo thymus without immunosuppression (9—12). This study was undertaken to investigate the efficiency of this agent on the attenuation of islet immunogenicity prior to transplantation into an MHC incompatible rat model.

Materials and methods

Animal model

Outbred Wistar and Hooded (PVG) rats were used for islet isolation and diabetic recipients respectively. The animals were kept in an air-conditioned quarter at constant temperature (22 °C) and allowed foor and water *ad libitum.*

Induction of diabetes. Male Hooded (PVG) rats were injected with streptozotocin (Sigma) i.v. 65 mg/kg body weight. Only rats with persistent elevation of blood glucose of > 20 mol/l, a loss of 12—15% of initial body weight and polyuria for 2 weeks were considered as potential recipients for islet transplantation.

Islet isolation and culture. Islets were isolated from male Wistar rats using a previously described method (13) with some modification using dextran gradients for islet purification (14). The isolated and purified islets were hand-picked and resuspended in CMRL—1066 + 10% FCS with PS and cultured at 37 °C, 5% CO_2 with or without deoxyguanosine for a total of 72 h before transplantation into diabetic Hooded (PVG) rats.

Pretreatment of islets with deoxyguanosine

Preliminary experiments showed that culturing islets for 48 h with dGuo followed by 24 h culture in fresh medium is the optimum time required to achieve functionally viable islets capable of reversing diabetes. In order to determine the dose required to achieve maximum graft survival, islets were cultured with various concentrations of dGuo using 1, 1.35, 1.5 and 2 μM dGuo per islet.

Islet transplantation

Fifty-one diabetic rats were transplanted intraportally with 1714 ± 177 (±SD) islets per rat. Post-transplant immunosuppression was not used. Eleven rats received islets cultured without dGuo (control) and 40 rats received islets cultured with dGuo (dGuo groups) where the concentrations of dGuo were 1.0, 1.35, 1.5 and 2 μM/islet. There were 11, 11, 11, and 7 recipients for each dGuo concentration, respectively.

Glucose monitoring and diagnosis of islet rejection

Transplanted rats were monitored initially daily for 10 days followed by twice a week for the remainder of the survival time. Islets were considered rejected when blood glucose levels were elevated on two consecutive days above 11 mmol/l (normal range: 4—6 mmol/l).

Histology

Liver slices and pancreas of transplanted normoglycemic rats were fixed in Bouin's fixative and processed for histology using hematoxylin-Eosin stain and peroxidase-antiperoxidase for insulin (Dako, Denmark).

Dendritic cells challenge

In order to investigate the mechanism of action of dGuo on the reduction of

Table 1. Effect of deoxyguanosine (dGuo) on islet allograft survival.

Deoxyguanosine concentration	Islet survival (%)	Islet survival time (days)
Control (without dGuo) ($n = 11$)	0	PNF[a], PNF[a], PNF, 6, 7, 8, 8, 8, 9, 9, 12
1 μM dGuo/islet ($n = 11$)	9	3, 7, 7, 7, 9, 9, 11, 11, 14, 252[a]
1.35 μM dGuo/islet ($n = 11$)	36	6, 7, 8, 10, 10, 12, 17, 230[a], 245[a], 288[a], >289
1.5 μM dGuo/islet ($n = 11$)	9	7, 7, 7, 8, 9, 10, 10, 11, 11, 17, >167
2 μM dGuo/islet ($n = 7$)	14.3	6, 7, 7, 8, 8, 10, >176

PNF = Primary non-function.
[a] Rats sacrificed for histological examination of the liver and pancreas.

islet immunogenicity, 3 transplanted normoglycemic rats were challenged with purified dendritic cells. Dendritic cells were purified according to a previously reported method (8) using donor strain splenocytes for isolation. The purified cells were suspended into 1 ml of TC 199 at 4.5×10^6 cells were injected i.v. Random blood glucose was monitored daily for 10 days and then twice a week for the remaining days of survival. Rats were then sacrified for histological examination of the liver and pancreas.

Statistical analysis

Data in the text are expressed as the mean ± SD. Mann-Witney U test was used to test for statistical significance between transplanted groups. Values of $p < 0.05$ were considered significant.

Results

Eight rats from the control group rejected the graft following normoglycemia for 6—12 days and 3 (27%) failed to restore normoglycemia which is described as a primary non-function (PNF) not attributed to technical error. However, islets pretreated with dGuo showed graft survival of 9, 36, 9, and 14% at 1, 1.35, 1.5 and 2 μM dGuo/islet, respectively (Table 1). The maximum graft survival was found at 1.35 μM/islet ($p < 0.01$ control). It thus appears that the effect of dGuo is dose dependent (Figure 1). Three rats from the 1.35 μM dGuo/islet group, when challenged with purified dendritic cells, failed to induce immunological rejection and the rats remained normoglycemic for >20 days of challenge. Histological examination of the liver showed no apparent lymphocyte infiltration of the graft (Figure 2).

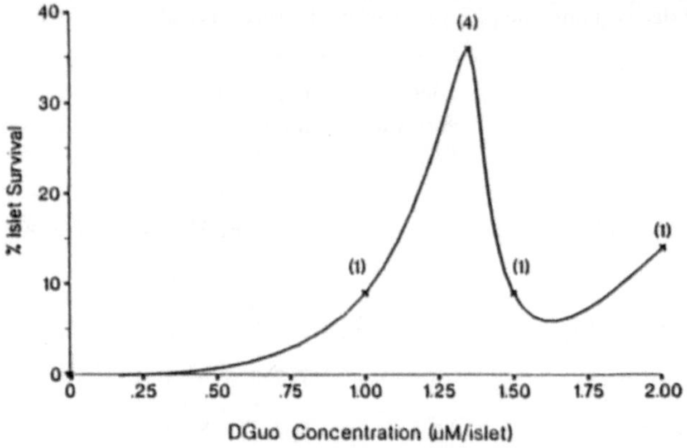

Fig. 1. Percentage of islet survival for control and dGuo-treated groups. Note the highest graft survival in the islets pretreated with 1.35 μM per islet prior to transplantation. Numbers in parentheses indicates number of the rats with long-term graft survival (>200 days).

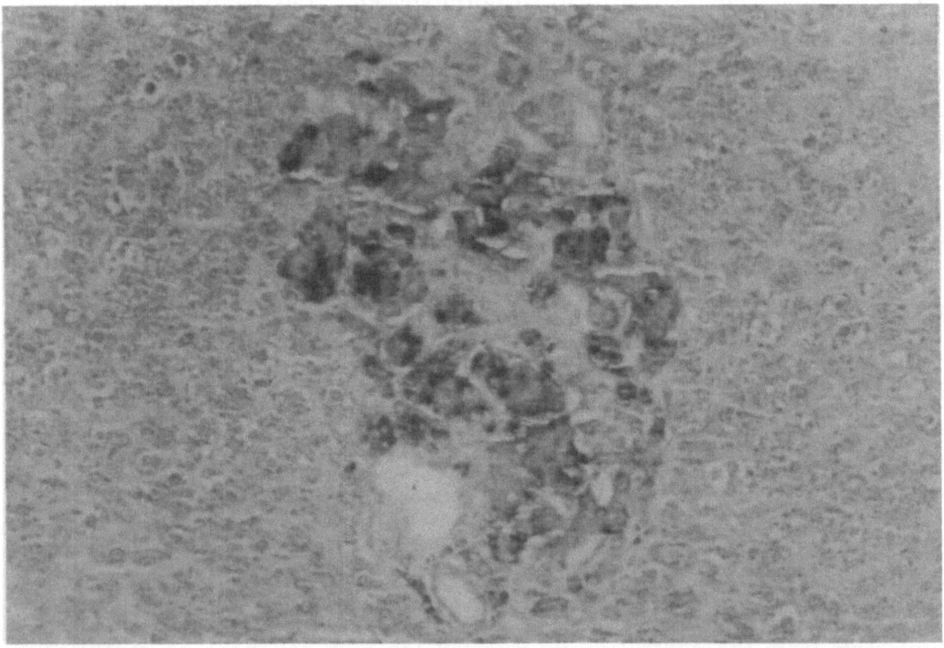

Fig. 2. Cross-sections of the liver slices taken from transplanted normoglycemic Hooded (PVG) (>200 days), showing normal islets which were pretreated with 1.35 μM dGuo/islet prior to transplantation. The normoglycemic animals were sacrificed 56 days after dendritic cells challenge. Note the positively stained islet cells in contrast to the surrounding negatively stained liver tissues (PAP, ×100).

Discussion

The use of deoxyguanosine to reduce islet immunogencity prior to transplantation was found to be effective in prolonging islet survival without immunosuppression. The effect seems to be dose dependent and the maximum graft survival was achieved when rats were transplanted with islets pretreated with 1.35 μM dGuo/islet. It is also equally important to mention that 3 (27%) of the control group failed to restore normoglycemia (which is described as primary non-function) while none of the rats treated with dGuo showed the same phenomenon. It is suggested that the dGuo pretreated islets may have affected surface membranes and in turn made the cells less susceptible to early graft rejection by activated lymphocytes and interleukin I (15, 16). It has been found that dGuo is toxic to activated lymphocytes, precursor T-lymphocytes and dendritic cells (12—18). The toxicity is thought to be due to an accumulation of deoxyGTP which; in turn, interferes with the DNA synthesis of pretreated cells (18). Hence it is possible that the pretreatment of islets with dGuo may have produced a similar action affecting some passenger leukocytes. It is suggested that pretreatment of premature islets isolated from fetal or newborn animals with dGuo could possibly be more effective in achieving higher graft survival. A previous study had reported that pretreatment of thymus with dGuo resulted in 100% graft survival without immunosuppression (9), while in this study the islets pretreated with dGuo resulted in 36% graft survival. Rejection was induced when animals transplanted with dGuo-pretreated thymus were challenged with dendritic cells (17). However in this study the 3 normoglycemic rats, that survived >200 days when challenged with dendritic cells, failed to induce immunological rejection and the rats remained normoglycemic for >40 days after dendritic cell challenge. Thus it would seem that the mode of action of dGuo on the attenuation of islet immunogencity may be different from that of thymus pretreated with dGuo (17, 18). Histological examination showed normal islets in the liver free from lymphocytes (Figure 2).

In conclusion, pretreatment of islets with dGuo prolonged islets survival without immunosuppression and is dose-dependent. It also demonstrated that pretreatment of islets with dGuo may prevent primary non-function.

Acknowledgements

This work was supported by Kuwait Foundation for the Advancement of Sciences, grant no. 86—10—02, and Kuwait University Medical Research Council, grant No. MT010.

We thank Mr Osama M. Hammad, Mrs Alice Babu and Mrs Lina Al-Zamamiri for their excellent technical and secretarial help.

References

1. Snell, S.D.: The homograft reaction. *Ann. Rev. Microbiol* **11**, 439—458 (1957).
2. Lafferty, K.J., Prowse, S.J. and Simeonovic, C.J.: Immunobiology of tissue transplantation: a return to the passenger leukocyte concept. *Ann. Rev. Immunol* **1**, 143—173 (1983).

3. Shienvold, F.L., Alejandro, R. and Mintz, D.H.: Identification of Ia-bearing cells in rat, dog, pig and human islets of Langerhans. *Transplantation* **41**, 364—372 (1986).
4. Lautenschlager, I., Inkinen, K., Taskinen, M., Charles, A. and Hayry, P.: Major histocompatibility complex protein expression on pancreas and pancreatic islet endocrine cell subsets. *Amer. J. Path* **135**, 1129—1136 (1989).
5. Faustman, D., Hauptfeld, V., Lacy, P. and Davie, J.: Prolongation of murine islet allograft survival by pretreatment of islets with antibody irected to Ia determinants. *Proc. Natl. Acad. Sci. (USA)* **78**, 5156—5159 (1981).
6. Faustman, D.L., Steinman, R.M., Gebel, H.M., Hauptfeld, V., Davie, J.M. and Lacy, P.E.: Prevention of rejection of murine islet allografts by pretreatment with anti-dendritic cell antibody. *Proc. Natl. Acad. Sci. (USA)* **81**, 3864—3868 (1984).
7. Lau, H., Reemtsma, K. and Hardy, M.A.: Prolongation of rat islet allograft survival by direct ultraviolet irradiation of the graft. *Science* **223**, 607—609 (1984).
8. James, R.F.L., Lake, S.P., Chamberlin, J., Thirdborough, S., Bassett, P.D., Mistry N. and Bell, P.R.F.: Gamma irradiation of isolated rat islets pretransplantation produces indefinite allograft survival in cyclosporine treated recipients. *Transplantation* **47**, 929—933 (1989).
9. Ready, A.R., Jenkinson, E.J., Kingston, R. and Owen, J.J.T.: Successful transplantation across major histocompatibility barrier of deoxyguanosine treated embryonic thymus expressing class II antigens. *Nature* **310**, 231—233 (1984).
10. Jenkinson, E.J., Franchi, L.L., Kingston, R. and Owen, J.T.: Effect of deoxyguanosine on lymphopoiesis in the developing thymus rudiment in vitro: application in the production of chimeric thymus rudiments. *E.J. Immunol* **12**, 583—587 (1982).
11. Jenkinson, E.J., Jhittay, P., Kingston, R. and Owen, J.T.T.: Studies of the role of the thymic environment in the induction of tolerance to MHC antigens. *Transplantation* **39**, 331-333 (1985).
12. Scharenberg, J.G.M., Rijkers, G.T., Spaapen, L.J.M., Toebes, E.A.H., Rijksen, G., Duran, M., Staal, G.E.J. and Zegers, B.J.M.: Different pathway for deoxyguanosine toxicity Tlymphocytes of various developmental stages. *Int. J. Immunopharmac.* **10**, 675—686 (1988).
13. Al-Abdullah, I.H., Kumar, M.S.A., Al-Adnani, M.S. and Abouna, G.M.: Transplantation of islets of Langerhans isolated by Trowell's T8 medium in outbred rats: effect of Cyclosporine. *Diabetes Res.* **13**, 29—34 (1990).
14. Van der Vliet, J., Meloche, R.M., Field, M.J., Chen, D., Kaufman, D.B. and Sutherland, D.E.R.: Pancreatic islet isolation in rats with ductal collagenase distention, stationary digestion, and dextran separation. *Transplantation* **45**, 493—495 (1988).
15. Lafferty, K.J. and Prowse, S.J.: Theory and practice of immunoregulation by tissue treatment prior to transplantation. *World J. Surg.* **8**, 187 (1984).
16. Kaufman, D.B., Rabe, F., Platt, J.L., Stock, P.G. and Sutherland, D.E.R.: On the variability of outcome after islet transplantation. *Transplantation* **45**, 1151—1153 (1988).
17. Benson, M.T., Buckley, G., Jenkinson, E.J. and Owen, J.J.T.: Survival of deoxyguansoine treated fetal thymus allografts is prevented by priming with dendritic cells. *Immunol.* **60**, 593—596 (1987).
18. Fairbanks, L.D., Taddeo, A., Duley, J.A. and Simmonds, H.A.: Mechanisms of deoxyguanosine lymphotoxicity. Human thymocytes, but not peripheral blood lymphocytes accumulate deoxy GTP in conditions simulating purine nucleoside phosphorylase deficiency. *J. Immunol.* **144**, 485—491 (1990).
19. Bowen, K.M., Prowse, S.J. and Lafferty, K.J.: Reversal of diabetes by islet transplantation: vulnerability of the established allograft. *Science* **213**, 1261—1262 (1981).

55. Current status of allogeneic bone marrow transplantation

RAINER STORB

Introduction

During the past two decades, bone marrow transplantation has been used with increasing success as treatment for patients with acute and chronic leukemias, malignant lymphomas, severe aplastic anemia, thalassemia major, congenital immunologic deficiency diseases, and inborn errors of metabolism. The International Bone Marrow Transplantation Registry estimated that, as of 1987, 20 000 transplants had been carried out, with more than 10 000 of them taking place between 1985 and 1987 and more than 80% being for patients with hematologic malignancies.

Initially marrow grafting was considered to be an experimental procedure appropriate only for end-stage or refractory patients, and disease-free survival following the procedure was only ≈ 15%. Experience has proven it now to be an effective treatment for patients with newly diagnosed hematologic disorders. Results in patients with acute non-lymphoblastic leukemia in first chemotherapy-induced remission have shown survival to be superior to that of patients given chemotherapy alone (50% versus 20%, respectively) (see Table 1). In patients with acute lymphoblastic leukemia in second or subsequent remission, 35—40% of those transplanted have achieved disease-free long-term survival whereas all of those receiving chemotherapy alone relapsed and died within 3.5 years. Similarly, in patients with chronic myelocytic leukemia in the chronic phase, long-term disease-free survival with marrow grafts is 50—60%; no cures have been seen with chemotherapy alone. In patients with aplastic anemia, survival with marrow grafting ranges from 60 to 80%, compared to 40 to 50% in patients treated with immunosuppressive therapy (antithymocyte globulin) and 20% with supportive therapy alone. Marrow grafting has resulted in disease-free survival of 70% in patients with thalassemia major and 50—60% in patients with severe combined immunodeficiency disease and other inborn errors.

Donor-recipient selection

To identify a marrow donor, histocompatibility typing is done to determine the

Table 1. HLA-identical marrow grafts for patients with leukemia and aplastic anemia.

Disease	5 years disease free		Grades II—I		Interstitial pneumonia (%)	Veno-occlusive liver disease (%)	Bacterial and fungal infections			Graft failure (%)	Secondary cancer (%)
							First 3 months[a]				
	Survival (%)	Relapse (%)	Acute GVHD (%)	Chronic GVHD (%)			Pre (%)	Post (%)	After 3 months (%)		
ANL	50	22									
1st CR	25	45	30—45	25—35	15—35	28					
2nd CR	30	30									
ALL											
1st CR	54	35									
2nd CR	35	45	35	25	15	7	20	12	20	1	5
3rd CR	30	58									
2nd Rel.	18	75									
CML											
Chronic phase	58	17									
Accel. phase	30	45	45	35	22	25					
Blast crisis	20	70									
AA											
Untransfused	82	—	30	40	6	< 1	20	12	20	10	1
Transfused	70	—									

[a] Before engraftment (pre) and after engraftment (post).

Abbreviations: ANL = acute non-lymphoblastic leukemia; ALL = acute lymphoblastic leukemia; CML = chronic myelocytic leukemia; AA = aplastic anemia; CR = complete remission; Rel. = relapse; Accel. phase = accelerated phase; GVHD = graft-versus-host disease.

alleles of the HLA-A, -B, -DR and -D loci. Most allogeneic transplants are carried out between HLA-identical siblings who have inherited the same haplotype of chromosome 6 from each parent. Identical (syngeneic) twins are completely matched at all genetic loci and are thus ideal donors for marrow grafts. Unfortunately, only 35% of all patients have a genotypically identical sibling or identical twin. Transplants using marrow from family members who are one HLA locus mismatched or who are only phenotypically matched have been carried out increasingly in the past few years. In this setting, the incidence of graft failure has increased but the risk of leukemic relapse has decreased, presumably due to a graft-versus-leukemia effect. As a result, survival in these patients is similar to that of recipients of HLA genotypically identical marrow. A small number of transplants have been carried out using marrow from unrelated phenotypically matched donors for patients with acute leukemia in end-stage disease. These patients appear to have an increased incidence of acute and chronic graft-versus-host disease (GVHD) but a decreased relapse rate, presumably due to the graft-versus-leukemia effect. The number of patients treated with unrelated marrow and the follow-up period are still small, but computerized registries of unrelated volunteer marrow donors are being set up in anticipation of expanded use of this procedure in the future.

Marrow grafting procedure

Donor

Multiple marrow aspirations are performed under general or spinal anesthesia from the anterior and posterior iliac crests. The marrow-blood mixture is sterilely collected in heparin, screened through wire mesh, and administered to the recipient by intravenous infusion. The volume of the transfused marrow average 750 ml in an adult. There is no permanent loss to the donor since marrow regrows quickly.

Recipient

In patients with hematologic malignancies, immunosuppressive therapy for graft acceptance as well as intense chemoradiotherapy to kill the malignant cells are required. A commonly used regimen is cyclophosphamide (CY) followed by a lethal amount of total body irradiation (TBI) given as a single dose or in several fractionated doses. In patients with severe combined immune deficiency, allogeneic marrow grafting can generally be carried out without preparation of the host by immunosuppressive agents. In patients with aplastic anemia, immunosuppressive therapy must be given for an allogeneic graft to be accepted, and CY is commonly used. In patients with non-malignant disorders and an active marrow (Wiskott — Aldrick syndrome, osteopetrosis, thalassemia major), CY has been used in combination with busulfan not only to provide immunosuppression but also to eradicate the affected marrow.

Recovery of the hematopoietic and immune systems

Marrow transplant recipients are usually severely pancytopenic for the first 3 to 6 weeks after grafting, and transfusion support is provided as necessary. Engraftment is evidenced by self-sustaining hematopoiesis, and chimerism is demonstrated by cytogenetic restriction enzyme polymorphism and red cell antigen marker studies.

Pronounced impairment of immunologic parameters is seen in all patients during the first 4 months, and serious infections with opportunistic organisms are observed. Supportive care includes prophylactic hyperalimentation (via right atrial catheters) and antibiotics. Both prophylactic granulocyte transfusions and protective environments (laminar air flow rooms with gut and skin decontamination) decrease the frequency of serious bacterial and fungal infections in the early granulocytopenic period. Herpes simplex or varicella-zoster virus infections are common but usually self-limited, and acyclovir is useful treatment.

Most troublesome are the interstitial pneumonias that typically occur between 30 and 100 days after transplantation. Their incidence is 40—50% in patients treated with TBI (mortality 15—35%) compared to 16% (mortality 6%) in patients treated with CY alone. About 20—40% of the interstitial pneumonias are of unknown origin, and it is believed that the radiotherapy is contributory. The change from single- to fractionated-dose schedule of TBI delivery has reduced the incidence substantially.

Approximately 60% of all pneumonias are associated with cytomegalovirus (CMV) and more than three-quarters of these are fatal. The use of CMV negative blood products in transplants where the donor and recipient are CMV negative has been effective prophylaxis, whereas immunoprophylaxis using CMV immunoglobulin has been controversial. There is no proven therapy for established CMV infection, although initial studies using an acyclovir derivative, ganciclovir, with CMV immunoglobulin look promising. Formerly, about 10% of all pneumonias were related to Pneumocystis carinii, but prophylaxis with trimethoprim-sulfamethoxazole has largely eliminated this problem.

The tempo and pattern of immunologic reconstitution demonstrates that patients without chronic GVHD generally return to normal immune function within the first year after transplantation, but chronic GVHD patients have a strikingly delayed return of function and often suffer recurrent bacterial infections, in particular pneumococcus.

Acute graft-versus-host disease

Human acute GVHD is caused by the infusion of immunologically active, genetically different bone marrow cells into a host who is immunologically impaired and incapable of rejecting the cells. Despite careful HLA matching and immunosuppressive therapy after transplantation, approximately 25—50% of allogeneic recipients develop evidence of significant acute GVHD. It has a case fatality rate of $\approx 50\%$ and is responsible for 10—25% of all deaths. In these HLA-identical matches, immunocompetent donor lymphocytes are thought to react to genetically determined 'minor' host histocompatibility antigens not detected by current tissue typing techniques. Acute GVHD is manifested by skin rash, liver abnormalities, diarrhea, infections, and profound deficiencies of immunologic function. Factors predictive of acute GVHD include increasing patient age and preceding pregnancy of the marrow donor; other factors which have been suggested are donor/recipient sex mismatch and certain donor or recipient HLA antigens. Death, often due to infection, is twice as likely among patients experiencing significant acute GVHD than among those with only mild or no GVHD.

Prevention of acute GVHD has been attempted most commonly with postgrafting immunosuppressive agents. In many patients, only 3—6 months of immunosuppressive therapy are needed for a state of graft—host tolerance to be reached, whereas omission of therapy has been proven to cause an unacceptably high incidence of acute GVHD in patients given unmanipulated marrow. To date, a combination of methotrexate and cyclosporine has been used most successfully to prevent acute GVHD.

Another method of attempting to prevent acute GVHD has been by depleting the donor marrow of T cells prior to infusing it into the host. This is accomplished through the use of monoclonal antibodies either to target lytic activities or for immunoadsorption, or by selective agglutination, or through E rosetting and elutriation. By reducing the number of donor T cells by 1—3 logs, most of the mature immune cells which cause GVHD are removed and the immune system is returned to a 'prenatal' state. The new stem-cell-derived T cells accept the host's antigenic environment as 'self' and thus are tolerant to it. To date, clinical studies have shown a significant decrease in acute GVHD in patients given T cell depleted marrow grafts. However, this has been achieved at the price of a substantial increase in graft failure, presumably caused by host immune cells which have survived the conditioning program and whose continued survival is possible with the absence of GVHD, and by increased relapse rates in patients with leukemia, presumably due to the absence of a graft-versus-leukemia effect. Since graft rejection and leukemic relapse almost uniformly result in death, no overall improvement in survival has been seen with T cell depletion. Nevertheless, the incidence of acute GVHD has decreased enough to suggest that this technique may be promising in the future if the risks of rejection and relapse can be lessened.

Graft rejection

Graft failure, or rejection, was once a serious problem in transplantation for aplastic anemia, occurring in 30—60% of all patients. Two factors were found to be predictive of rejection: positive pretransplant *in vitro* tests of cell mediated immunity of host against donor lymphocytes, and a low number of grafted donor marrow cells ($<3 \times 10^8$ cells/kg of recipient body weight). Immunity of recipient against donor is due to transfusion-induced sensitization; when transplantation is carried out before transfusions have been given, graft failure is rare and 80% of untransfused patients become long-term survivors.

Many programs have been utilized to decrease rejection in multiply-transfused patients, most involving more intensive immunosuppression. All contain CY, but other features vary, such as irradiation and the infusion of donor buffy coat cells. With all programs, rejection in multiply-transfused patients has decreased and long-term survival is 60—70%, but the risks of chronic GVHD and secondary malignancy seem to have increased. Thus, future emphasis should be placed on measures that avoid rather than overcome sensitization by blood transfusion. This is best done by transplantation before transfusion, or, if transfusions are unavoidable, by the use of red blood cells and platelets depleted of buffy coat.

Recurrence of leukemia

Leukemic relapse usually originates from host cells that survived the conditioning regimen of high dose chemoradiotherapy. Recurrent disease accounts for 17—75% of deaths in patients grafted for leukemia. To date, the program used most frequently to eradicate malignant cells prior to transplant in patients with leukemia has been the combination of CY and TBI. In the past, numerous chemotherapeutic agents have been used in addition to or in lieu of CY (etoposide, cytosine arabinoside, piperazinedione, BCNU, and others), but with only modest success. TBI is usually given in several fractionated doses rather than in a single dose, since a prospective comparison of the two schedules showed fractionated TBI to be better tolerated and to result in fewer long-term complications without any obvious increase in the risk of relapse. Several studies combining various chemotherapeutic drugs and radiation schedules have been underway at numerous transplant centers for the past several years, and it appears that the limits of tolerable non-hematopoietic toxicity have been reached. Further substantial improvements in relapse rates and survival cannot be expected using chemoradiotherapy.

In theory, agents which interact specifically with malignant cells could be used most efficiently in the eradication of those cells. This has been attempted with monoclonal antibodies directed against antigens expressed on malignant cells. Monoclonal antibodies injected *in vivo* concentrate on tumor cells; however, their anti-tumor effect is limited, partly because some tumor cells lack target antigens, and partly because some cells, though coated by antibody, are not destroyed by it. Attempts are being made to link antibodies to toxins such as the Ricin A chain for more effective tumor cell kill. Another approach has been to attach monoclonal antibodies to short-lived radioactive isotopes with short linear energy transfer, thus killing cells which express the target antigens; neighboring cells which are antigen negative may also be killed, however. If used for hematologic malignancies, this approach would ablate normal as well as cancerous cells, and subsequent 'rescue' by transplantation of normal marrow would be needed. Initial experiments in the canine model have shown promising results, and it is expected that refinements of this approach, particularly with the use of high energy beta emitting isotopes, will result in less toxic but more effective conditioning programs.

Graft-versus-leukemia effect

Some of the apparent cures seen after transplantation for hematologic malignancy may be the result of a graft-versus- leukemia effect directed at histocompatibility antigens and perhaps also at leukemia-associated antigens present on the patient's leukemic cells. This has been suggested by the fact allogeneic marrow recipients who experience acute or chronic GVHD and who live at least 5 months after grafting are significantly more likely than those without GVHD or those who received syngeneic marrow to still be in remission 2 years later. Similarly, recipients of T cell depleted marrow experience less G but have a higher incidence of leukemic recurrence than those given non-depleted marrow, and, as discussed above, the increase in relapse outweighs any advantage gained from the reduction in GVHD. It is possible that there are T cells in the donor marrow capable of eliminating residual leukemic cells in the host. Attempts at inducing GVHD for the purpose of decreasing the incidence of leukemic relapse, thus improving survival, have been unsuccessful to date, since increases in severe GVHD, infections, and other complications have offset the lessened incidence of relapse.

Animal experiments have indicated that certain cells in the transplanted marrow react specifically with surface antigens on leukemic cells while others react more broadly with histocompatibility antigens on host tissue. This suggests that a graft-versus-leukemia effect is distinguishable from GVHD, and that measures to prevent GVHD without increasing the incidence of leukemic relapse might be possible. Studies attempting to expand *in vitro* T cells sensitized to tumor antigens before infusing them into tumor-bearing hosts are also underway.

Toxicities related to conditioning regimens

Conditioning programs have been intensified to a point at which serious non-hematopoietic toxicity has been observed. Oral mucositis and diarrhea are frequent, but reversible. More serious has been veno-occlusive disease of the liver, a problem that has been particularly frequent in patients with underlying liver damage, and magnified by postgrafting cyclosporine. Acute myocarditis can be a problem in patients with previous exposure to anthracyclines. Leuko-encephalopathy can be a problem in children with ALL who had previous cranial radiotherapy. Total body irradiation is the cause of many complications, including idiopathic interstitial pneumonia, impairment of growth and sexual development in children, sterility, cataracts, and late-occurring secondary malignancies, although many of these complications appear to be less severe in patients who received fractionated-dose rather than single-dose TBI.

It is clear that current conditioning programs involving systemic exposure of patients to toxic agents have been pushed to their limit, and new regimens causing more specific destruction of malignant cells while sparing normal tissues need to be developed.

Chronic GVHD

Chronic GVHD is a late complication of allogeneic marrow transplantation, occurring in approximately 20—40% of patients surviving more than 180 days. This disorder resembles such autoimmune diseases as scleroderma, systemic lupus erythematosus, Sjogren's syndrome, lichen planus, and eosinophilic fasciitis. It develops 100—450 days after transplant, may persist for years if untreated, and affects target organs not generally involved by acute GVHD (oral mucosa, lacrimal glands, esophagus, serosal membranes, and muscles). Increasing recipient age at the time of transplant and the presence of acute GVHD are risk factors associated with a greater likelihood of developing chronic GVHD. Mortality is often the result of recurrent bacterial infections owing to the severe immunologic deficiencies of these patients. If untreated, the disease has a poor prognosis and most patients become disabled or die. With treatment, approximately 50% of the patients survive with Karnofsky performance scores of 100% and an additional 25% survive with scores of 80—90%. Early treatment is advisable to prevent disability and joint contracture formation. In about 50% of the patients, therapy can be discontinued after 9—12 months. Even with treatment, 25% of affected patients die, mainly with infections from encapsulated gram-positive bacteria due to their impaired immunologic status. Various trials comparing treatment with prednisone either alone or combined with procarbazine, CY, or azathioprine, showed prednisone given alone to be most successful at reversing the signs and symptoms of the disease and improving survival, whereas the combination of cyclosporine and prednisone has improved survival in thrombocytopenic patients with chronic GVHD.

Autologous marrow transplantation

Autologous marrow transplantation is of considerable current interest since it precludes the problems of donor unavailability and of GVHD. In this procedure, marrow is harvested and cryopreserved while the patient is in chemotherapy-induced remission. The marrow is treated before cryopreservation either with monoclonal antibodies plus complement, immunotoxins, or chemicals in attempts at removing clonogenic leukemia cells. In the event of subsequent relapse, a conditioning regimen of high dose chemoradiotherapy is administered and the stored marrow is reinfused to the patient. Evaluation of clinical trials is difficult, since relapses may be due either to failure of the preparative regimen or to infusion of tumor cells even though the marrow was collected while in remission.

Pilot studies have been reported with autologous marrow grafts for radiosensitive solid tumors, such as ovarian, testicular, and small-cell lung cancers, and neuroblastoma, usually after failure of other therapy. Results have been poor, with the exception of metastatic neuroblastoma, in which long-term disease-free survival and probable cures have been seen.

Outlook

Despite impressive improvements, a number of problems remain in the application of bone marrow transplantation. Host-versus-graft reactions can cause graft failure which is usually fatal, but successful engraftment can be accompanied by GVHD which is associated with life-threatening infections. These are interrelated problems, along with recurrence of the underlying disease for which the transplant was carried out. New approaches that will avoid GVHD without adversely affecting engraftment or the graft-versus-leukemia effect, and that will increase leukemic cell kill without increasing toxicity to non-hematopoietic organs, must be found. Perhaps more efficient use of chemoradiotherapy along with antibody isotope conjugates will bring about improved pretransplant conditioning programs. The use of recombinant human hematopoietic growth factors may result in a shorter period of post-transplant pancytopenia. It is possible that the transfer of genes into hematopoietic stem cells will find clinical application, conferring drug resistance and inhibiting or altering the function of genes involving in the generation of disease.

Acknowledgement

This work was supported by grants CA18029, CA18221, CA31787, CA18105, CA09515 and CA15704 awarded by the National Cancer Institute and by grant HL36444 from the National Heart, Lung and Blood Institute of the National Institutes of Health, U.S. Department of Health and Human Services.

Suggested reading

1. Gale, R.P. and Champlin, R. (eds): *Bone Marrow Transplantation: Current Controversies.* A.R. Liss, New York (1988).
2. Gale, R.P. and Champlin, R. (eds): *Progress in Bone Marrow Transplantation.* A.R. Liss, New York (1987).
3. Miescher, P.A., Jaffe, E.R., Van Rood, J. and Zwaan, F. (eds): *Seminars in Hematology XXI: Bone Marrow Transplantation I.* Grune & Stratton, Orlando (1984).
4. Storb, R.: Bone marrow transplantation. In: V.T. DeVita, S. Hellman and S.A. Rosenberg (eds), *Cancer: Principles and Practice of Oncology, 3rd edition*, pp. 2474—2489. Lippincott, Philadelphia (1989).
5. Thomas, E.D., Storb, R., Clift, R.A., Fefer, A., Johnson, F.L., Neiman, P.E., Lerner, K.G., Glucksberg, H. and Buckner, C.D.: Bone marrow transplantation. *New Engl. J. Med.* **292**, 832—843 and 895—902 (1975).

56. New approach to bone marrow transplantation in thalassemia

C. GIARDINI, G. LUCARELLI, M. GALIMBERTI, P. POLCHI, E. ANGELUCCI, D. GARONCIANI, S.M.T. DURAZZI, F. AGOSTINELLI, M. DONATI, C. GIORGI and M. FILOCAMO

The possibility of a cure of homozygous beta-thalassemia by bone marrow transplantation was first demonstrated by Thomas *et al.* in a 16-month-old patient transplanted on December 2, 1981 (1). Our experience was initiated on December 17, 1981 when a 14-year-old patient received a bone marrow transplant after preparation with cyclophosphamide and TBI without graft. Of four consecutive patients transplanted, 1 died, 2 rejected the graft and 1, transplanted on July 22, 1982, is alive and cured. We, therefore, transplanted 8 patients with various combinations of busulphan, cyclophosphamide and TBI before definitely adopting the regimen busulphan—cyclophosphamide in January 1983 (2, 3). In the recent report, we examine the results of marrow transplantation after preparation with busulphan and cyclophosphamide in 350 patients with thalassemia, aged 1 through 21 years.

Methods

Between January 1983 and February 1990, 350 patients between the ages of 1 and 21 received HLA-identical bone marrow transplantation for the treatment of beta-homozygous thalassemia: 336 received marrow from identical siblings and 14 from identical parents. All patients were prepared for transplantation with a modification of the regimen described by Santos *et al.* (4). Six patients received a total dose of busulphan of 16 mg/kg and 344 received a total dose of 14 mg/kg. This treatment was followed by a total dose of 200 mg/kg of cyclophosphamide. Details on the protocol for bone marrow transplantation in thalassemia used in Pesaro are reported elsewhere (5). Acute and chronic graft-versus-host disease was graded according to the Seattle criteria. Cytogenetic analysis and globulin chain synthesis examined by column chromatography were used to determine the graft. Liver biopsy was performed 15 days before transplantation. Grading system was established to record siderosis, chronic aggressive or chronic persistent hepatitis and protal fibrosis on liver biopsy. Three grades of severity (mild, moderate and severe) were identified (6). In evaluating the quality of chelation achieved, subcutaneous infusion of 20—40 mg of deferoxamine/kg for 8—12 hours a day at least 5 days a week initiated not later than 2 years after red-cell transfusions began, was considered to indicate good chelation. Failure to achieve this standard was categorized as poor chelation. Survival and event-free survival were evaluated by the product-limit method of Kaplan and Meier (7) and tested for *p*-value by the Mantel-Cox and Breslow statistics. Multivariate analysis were performed with the Cox proportional-hazard regression model (8).

Results

Table 1 reports the probabilities of survival, event-free survival and rejection for all 350 patients transplanted. In 161 patients transplanted after preparation to the transplant with the regimen used for all patients since June 1985 through March 1989, busulphan 14 mg/kg, cyclosphosphamide 200 mg/kg and cyclosporine alone (Protocol 6), age, number of transfusion received before the transplant, ferritine level, quality of chelation, hepatomegaly, splenomegaly, splenectomy, hemosiderosis, chronic aggressive hepatitis, chronic persistent hepatitis and portal fibrosis have been examined for their influence on survival and event-free survival. The results are summarized in Table 2. Three factors assessed at the time of transplantation were associated with significant reduced probability of survival and event-free survival: liver larger than 2 cm below costal rib ($p = 0.0001$), poor quality of chelation treatment ($p = 0.002$) and presence of portal fibrosis ($p = 0.01$). The 34 patients with none of the three factors were assigned to class 1 while the 33 patients that presented with all the three factors were assigned to class 3. The 100 patients with various association of only two of the three factors were assigned to class 2. Table 3 shows the probabilities of survival and event-free survival for these three classes. The probabilities for patients in class 1 were not significantly different from those in class 2 but significantly different when compared with those in class 3. The probabilities for patients in class 2 were significantly different from those in class 3. In March 1989 we modified the standard Protocol 6 as follows: busulphan 14 mg/kg, cyclophosphamide 120 mg/kg, ALG 10 mg/kg, cyclospo-

Table 1. Bone marrow transplantation in thalassemia.

Minimum follow-up	2 months
Maximum follow-up	7 years
Number of patients	350
Probabilities:	
Survival	82%
Event-free survival	73%
Rejection	12%

Table 2. Univariate analysis of risk factors (161 patients; Protocol 6; minimum follow-up, 1 year).

Significant	Not significant
	Age
Hepatomegaly ($p = 0.0001$)	Ferritine level
	No. of transfusions
Portal fibrosis ($p = 0.01$)	Splenomegaly
	Splenectomy
	Liver iron concentration
Chelation regular—irreg. ($p = 0.002$)	Hemosiderosis
	Hepatitis

Table 3. Bone marrow transplantation in 183[a] patients with thalassemia transplanted with Protocol 6 and divided into three classes of risk. (Input in class 3 stops in March 1989.)

Follow-up: minimum = 1 year, maximum = 3.5 years			
	Class 1	Class 2	Class 3
No. of patients	34	100	33
Probabilities:			
Survival	97%	86%	58%
Event-free survival	94%	83%	53%
Rejection	3%	6%	12%
	Survival		Event-free survival
Class 1 vs class 2	$p = 0.06$		$p = 0.08$
Class 1 vs class 3	$p = 0.0001$		$p = 0.0001$
Class 2 vs class 3	$p = 0.0004$		$p = 0.0003$

[a] Sixteen patients who did not have suitable liver biopsy have been excluded from the categorization into classes.

rine and short methotrexate (Protocol 12) for class 3 patients. For patients in class 1 and those in class 2, the standard Protocol 6 continued to be used.

Fourteen patients have been transplanted with Protocol 12 from March 1989 through March 1990. Actual survival and event-free survival are 100 and 79% respectively. This study is still under evaluation, but the rate of early transplant-related deaths already appears to be reduced. Table 4 reports the results obtained with Protocol 12 in 14 class 3 patients.

Table 4. Bone marrow transplantation in 14 class 3 thalassemic patients transplanted with Protocol 12. (Input initiated on March 1989.)

Follow-up: 2 to 12 months		
Survival	14/14	(100%)
Alive with return of thalassemia	3/14	(21%)
Event-free survival	11/14	(79%)

Conclusion

We conclude that patients with thalassemia who have an HLA-identical sibling or parent should be transplanted as soon as possible. If the results obtained with our Protocol 12 in class 3 patients are confirmed, thalassemic patients of all ages with a suitable donor can have access to the possibility of radical cure of their disease with bone marrow transplantation.

References

1. Thomas, E.D., Buckner, C.D., Sanders, J., Papayannopoulos, T., Borgna-Pignatti, C., Stefano, P., Sullivan, K.M., Clift, A. and Storb, R.: Marrow transplantation for thalassemia. *Lancet*, **2**, 8292 (1982).
2. Lucarelli, G., Izzi, T., Polchi, P., Manna, M., Agostinelli, F., Delfini, C., Galimberti, M., Porcelline, A., Moretti, L., Manna, A., Talevi, N., Nesci, S., De Biagi, M., Sparaventi, G., Andreani, M., Flippetti, A. and Stramigiolo, S.: Bone marrow transplantation in thalassemia. *J. Esp. Clin. Cancer Res.* **3**, 313 (1983).
3. Lucarelli, G., Polchi, P., Izzi, T., Manna, A., Sparaventi, G., Baronciani, D., Proietti, A. and Buckner, D.: Allogeneic marrow transplantation for thalassemia. *Exp. Hematol.* **12**, 676 (1984).
4. Santos, G.W., Tutschka, P.J., Brookmeyer, R., Saral, R., Beschorner, W., Bias, W.B., Braine, H.G., Burns, W.H., Elfenbein, G.J., Kaizer, H., Mellits, D., Sensenbrenner, L.L., Stuart, R.K. and Yeager, A.M.: Marrow transplantation for acute nonlymphocytic leukemia after treatment with busulphan and cyclophosphamide. *New Engl. J. Med.* **309**, 1347—1353 (1983).
5. Lucarelli, G., Galimberti, M., Polchi, P., Angelucci, E., Baronciani, D., Giardini, C., Politi, P., Durazzi, S.M.T., Muretto, P. and Albertini, F.: Bone marrow transplantation in patients with thalassemia. *New Engl. J. Med.* **322**, 417—421 (1990).
6. Muretto, P., Angelucci, E., Del Fiasco, S. and Lucarelli, G.: Reversal features of hepatic haemosiderosis and haemocromatosis in thalassemia after bone marrow transplantation. In: C.D. Buckner, R.P. Gale and G. Lucarelli (eds), *Advances and Controversies in Thalassemia Therapy: bone marrow transplantation and other approaches*, pp. 299—314, Vol. 309 of *Progress in Clinical and Biological Research.* Alan R. Liss, New York (1989).
7. Kaplan, E.L. and Meier, P.: Nonparametric estimation from incomplete observations. *J. Amer. Stat. Assoc.* **53**, 457—481 (1958).
8. Cox, D.R.: Regression models and life-tables. *J.R. Stat. (B)* **34**, 187—220 (1972).

57. Autologous bone marrow transplantation as treatment for bad-risk first remission acute lymphoblastic leukaemia

R.L. POWLES, C.L. SMITH and S. MILAN

Introduction

Treatment of poor-risk acute lymphoblastic leukaemia (ALL) with standard chemotherapy combinations is associated with a cure rate of less than 40% (1—3). We have therefore embarked on a programme of autotransplantation over the last six years. Transplantation was performed early in first remission, incorporating three approaches to improve the eradication of residual disease in both the patient and the re-infused marrow. Our first approach was to use melphalan and total body irradiation (TBI), a successful conditioning regimen for acute myeloid leukaemia (AML), (4, 5). Secondly, we investigated the use of purging the autografted marrow with a monoclonal antibody technique. In addition, patients were given maintenance chemotherapy with 6-mercaptopurine and methotrexate for two years after transplantation on the assumption that radical reducton of tumour load by the transplant procedure would improve the chances of chemotherapy eliminating minimal residual disease.

Patients and methods

Twenty-seven patients were accrued between January 1984 and November 1989. Eleven had common ALL, 10 had T-cell ALL, 4 had null-cell and 2 had Natural Killer cell ALL on phenotyping. All patients were transplanted in first remission. Those patients with common ALL were considered to have poor a prognosis either because of age (> 15 years) or high-presenting white cell count (> 200×10^9/l). The age range was 4—34 (median 18) years. All patients had UKALL X induction chemotherapy, consisting of vincristine, prednisone, asparaginase and duanorubicin, followed at 5 weeks by intensification with vincristine, cytosine arabinoside, VP16, prednisone and adriamycin (6). During this period, patients received prophylactic intrathecal methotrexate. Where possible, patients were autografted approximately 4—10 weeks after intensification, when full haematological recovery had occurred. The median time in autografting from first remission was 145 (18—483) days. Cranial irradiation of

24 Gray was given immediately prior to autografting. The patients were following up for a period of 0—5 years.

Bone marrow harvest

In the majority of patients the bone marrow was harvested immediately prior to myelo-ablative therapy. Because of the short conditioning period (single dose melphalan and single fraction TBI), cryopreservation was not necessary. The bone marrow was purged with the monoclonal antibody Campath 1 by a previously described technique (7) in 11 patients. The remaining 16 patients received unmodified marrow. The marrow harvested contained a median of 2.5 (1—4.5 × 10^8/kg) nucleated cells.

Marrow ablative therapy

Patients received 110 mg/M^2 melphalan, given as a bolus with intensive hydration. Single fraction TBI was administered 12 hours later at a rate of 4 cGy/min, up to a total dose of 10.5—11.5 G. Autologous marrow was infused 18—24 hours after melphalan administration.

Post-transplanted supportive therapy

Patients were nursed in protective isolation cubicles with filtered positive pressure ventilation until the neutrophil count exceeded 0.5 × 10^9/l. Sterile food was given and oral colistin, neomycin, nystatin and amphotericin were given as bowel decontamination. Broad spectrum antibiotics were used at fever greater than 38 °C and adjusted according to positive microbiological cultures and clinical findings. All blood products were irradiated with 15 Gy and patients with negative CMV antibody titres received CMV negative products.

Maintenance chemotherapy

Maintenance therapy was commenced when the neutrophil count exceeded 1 × 10^9/l and platelet count 100 × 10^9/l. Oral 6-mercaptopurine 50 mg/M^2 daily was given and oral methotrexate 10—15 mg/M^2 was introduced subsequently if peripheral counts remained adequate and both continued for 2 years. Patients were not randomized to receive maintenance chemotherapy, but 14 patients did not recover peripheral counts sufficiently to receive treatment (Table 1).

Table 1.

	Campath	No Campath
Maintenance[a]	5 (1)	13 (0)
No maintenance	6 (4)	3 (0)
Days to neutrophil > 500[b]	39 (18–56)	29 (15–55)

[a] Number of patients receiving maintenance chemotherapy in both the Campath-treated and the unpurged group. Toxic deaths indicated by parentheses.
[b] Median number of days for the neutrophil count to exceed 500 × 10^6 per litre with range indicated by parentheses.

Results

Of the 27 patients who received autografts, 4 have relapsed, all 4 relapsing within 7 months of autografting. Seventeen patients remain on a disease-free plateau between 1 and 5 years from autografting (Figure 1), giving an actuarial projected relapse rate of 18%.

Figure 2 shows a comparison of the relapse rate between patients receiving autografts in first remission, and a similar group of 42 poor-risk patients in first remission who received chemotherapy alone without autografting. Of these 42

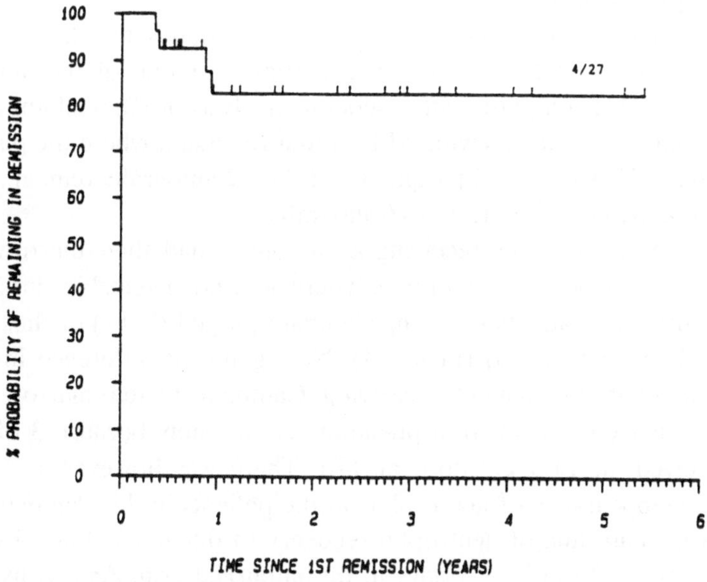

Fig. 1. The probability of remaining in survival of the poor-risk patients autografted in first remission ALL with numbers relapsing from the total population indicated.

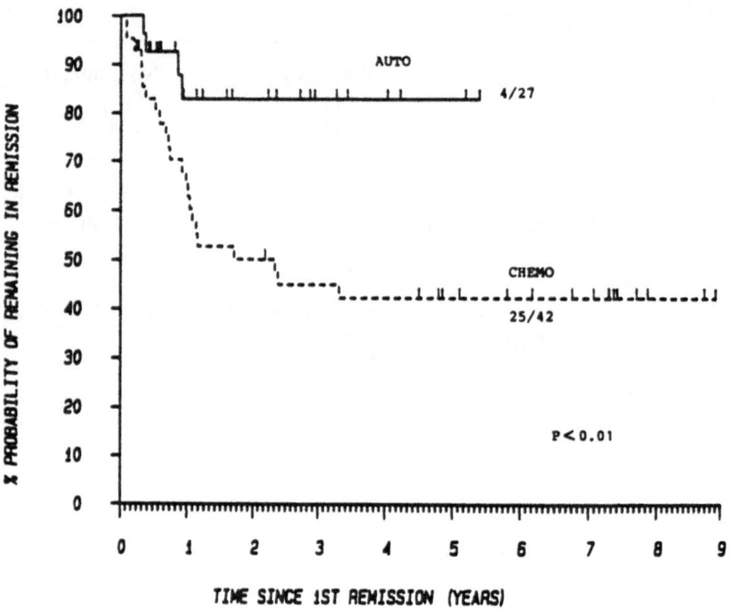

Fig. 2. The relapse rate of the autografted patients is compared with that of a similar population of poor-risk first remission ALL treated with chemotherapy alone.

patients treated with chemotherapy alone, 25 have relapsed. There is a significant difference between the autografted patients and those receiving only chemotherapy ($p < 0.01$).

Five of 27 patients receiving autografts died of transplant-related problems and Figure 3 shows that the expected actuarial cure rate of the autografted patients is 62%. This compares with a separate analysis of HLA sibling matched allografts in poor-risk patients with ALL in first remission where the plateau for expected cure is 37% (p = N.S.). Eighteen of the 27 autografts remain alive and disease free compared with only 7 of 16 allografts.

Eleven of the 27 patients receiving an autograft had their marrow purged with Campath 1 monoclonal antibody. There was no detectable difference in relapse rate between patients receiving Campath purged (2/11) or those receiving unpurged marrow (2/16) (Figure 4). No significant difference in survival was seen, although the patients receiving Campath-treated marrow had an increased incidence of death from pneumonitis, probably because 3 of these 5 patients received an 11.5 Gy dose of TBI. There was however, a significant delay in the reappearance of neutrophils in the patients in the Campath-treated arm, with a median time of neutrophil recovery to $0.5 \times 10^9/l$ at 39 (18—56) days, compared to 29 (15—55) days in the unpurged arm. As a consequence, there was a reduction in the number of patients in the Campath group who received maintenance chemotherapy (Table 1).

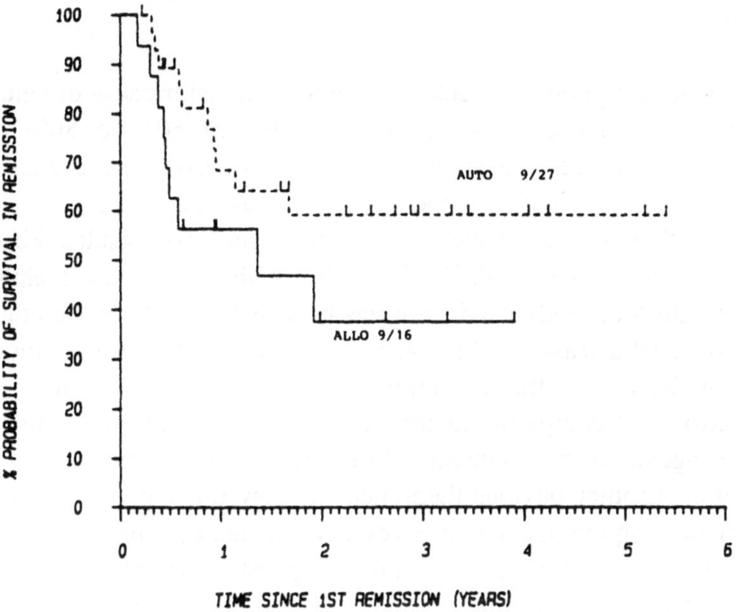

Fig. 3. The probability of survival in remission of the autografted patients is compared to that of a similar population of patients with poor-risk first remission ALL who were allografted. The number of patients that relapsed or have died from the total of each population is indicated.

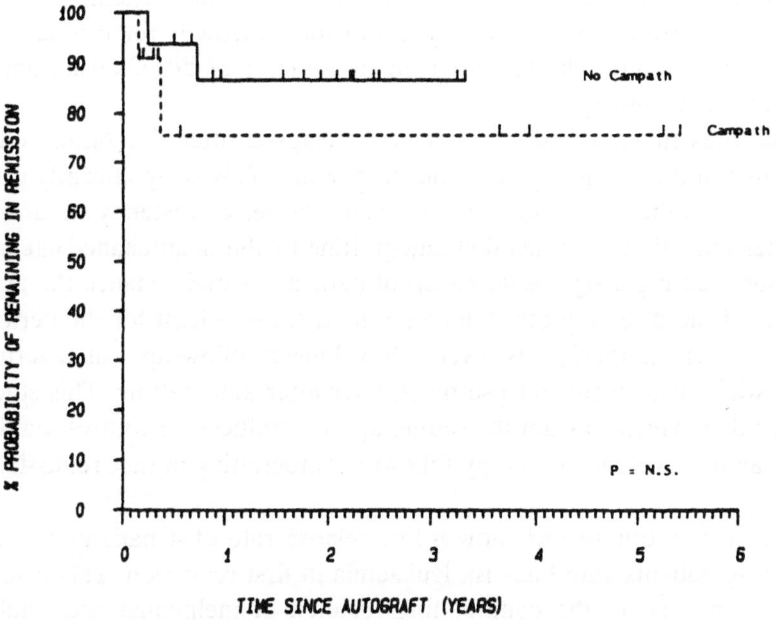

Fig. 4. The survival is compared between the patients autografted with unpurged or Campath purged marrow. Two of 11 patients receiving purged marrow relapse and 2 of 16 receiving unpurged marrow relapsed. There was no statistical significance between the two groups.

Discussion

Relapse of acute lymphoblastic leukaemia remains a major cause of failure after autografting with relapse rates reported of between 50 and 80% (8—12). Relapse may be from residual disease in the host or from re-inoculation from leukaemia remaining in the transplanted autologous marrow. Several different strategies are therefore available to attempt to improve results. Firstly, the conditioning regimen is crucial. We have shown that high dose melphalan in conjunction with total body irradiation has been shown to be more effective in destroying residual disease in AML (4, 5) and have used this as the rationale for extrapolating the use of this conditioning for ALL. However, there has not been a control trial comparing melphalan/TBI conditioning with other chemotherapeutic agents for first remission ALL and clearly this should be a priority for the future. Another obvious theoretical strategy for improving autografting results is by purging the marrow of residual leukaemic cells prior to re-infusion. We used Campath 1, a monoclonal antibody against all lymphoid cells, to purge the marrow. It was disappointing to find, therefore, that there was no evidence of reduction in relapse rate by the use of purging in our study, and in addition this technique had compromised the patients by causing a significant delay in neutrophil recovery. A third strategy for improving results is by the use of maintenance chemotherapy after the autograft. The rationale for this strategy is that whereas the residual disease remaining in bad-risk patients in first remission appears to too large to be cured by maintenance chemotherapy, the process of autografting whereby only 2% of the marrow is reintroduced to the patients, would reduce the tumour load by a factor of 50, allowing improved efficacy of chemotherapy.

In our present study no patients have relapsed after 7 months following autografting and there is a plateau out to 5 years. This is significantly different from our chemotherapy alone arm, in which relapses consistently occur up to 3 years after induction. It seems that autografting or the maintenance chemotherapy is either curing a significant group of patients or maintenance therapy may have altered the disease biology, holding the disease at least for the period that maintenance chemotherapy is given. Only longer follow-up will determine if patients will subsequently relapse much later after autografting. This study has produced data which warrant the setting up of a multicentre control trial for the use of maintenance chemotherapy following autografting in first remission bad-risk ALL.

In conclusion, our results show a low relapse rate of 4 patients in 27 after autografting patients with bad-risk leukaemia in first remission. This favourable result may be due to the conditioning regimen of melphalan and total body irradiation or may have been influenced by the use of maintenance chemotherapy post-autograft. Purging the marrow of residual leukaemia with Campath 1 did not improve these results and was shown to delay engraftment.

References

1. Hoelzer, D., Theil, E., Loffler, H., Bodenstein, H., Plaumann, L., Buchner, T., Urbanitz, D., Koch, P., Heimpel, H., Engelhardt, R., Muller, U., Wendt, F.-C. *et al.*: Intensified therapy in acute lymphoblastic and acute undifferentiated leukemia in adults. *Blood* **64**(1), 38—47 (1984).
2. Linker, C.A., Levitt, L.J., O'Donnell, M., Ries, C.A., Link, M.P., Forman, S.J. and Farbstein, M.J.: Improved results of treatment of adult acute lymphoblastic leukemia. *Blood* **69**(4), 1242—1248 (1987).
3. Gaynor, J., Chapman, D., Little, C., McKenzie, S., Miller, W., Andreeff, M., Arlin, Z., Berman, E., Kempin, S., Gee, T. and Clarkson, B.: A cause-specific hazard rate analysis of prognostic factors among 199 adults with acute lymphoblastic leukemia: The Memorial Hospital experience since 1969. *J. Clin. Oncol.* **6**(6), 1014—1030 (1988).
4. Helenglass, G., Powles, R.L., McElwain, T.J., Lakhani, A., Milan, S., Gore, M., Nandi, A., Zuiable, A., Perren, T., Forgeson, G., Treleaven, J., Hamilton, C. and Millar, J.: Melphalan and total body irradiation (TBI) versus cyclophosphamide and TBI as conditioning for allogeneic matched sibling bone marrow transplants for acute myeloblastic leukemia in first remission. *Bone Marrow Transplant.* **3**(1), 21—29 (1988).
5. Powles, R.L., Milliken, S., Helenglass, G., Treleavan, J., Pinkerton, R., Zuiable, A., Nandi, A., Aboud, H. and Millar, J.: The use of melphalan in conjunction with total body irradiation as treatment for acute leukaemia. *Transplant. Proc.* **21**(1), 2955—2957 (1989).
6. Pinkerton, C.R., Bowman, A., Holtzel, H. and Chessells, J.M.: Intensive consolidation chemotherapy for acute lymphoblastic leukaemia (UKALL × Pilot study). *Arch. Dis. Child.* **62**(1), 12—18 (1987).
7. Hale, G., Bright, S., Chimbley, G., Hoang, T., Metcalf, D., Munro, A.J. and Walmann, H.: Removal of T cells from bone marrow for transplantation: a monoclonal antilymphocyte antibody that fixed human complement. *Blood* **62**(4), 873—882 (1983).
8. Dicke, K.A., Jagannath, S., Walters, R.S., Horwitz, L.J. and Spitzer, G.: The role of autologous bone marrow transplantation in acute leukemia. *Ann. N.Y. Acad. Sci.* **511**, 468—472 (1987).
9. Gorin, N.C., Aegerter, P., Auvert, B. for the EBMTG: Autologous bone marrow transplantion (ABMT) for acute leukemia in remission: an analysis of 1322 cases. *Bone Marrow Transplant.* **4** (Suppl. 2), 3—5 (1989).
10. Kersey, J.H., Weisdorft, D., Nesbit, M.E., LeBien, T.W., Woods, W.G., McGlave, P.B., Kim, T., Vallera, D.A., Goldman, A.I., Bostsrom, B. *et al.*: Comparison of autologous and allogeneic bone marrow transplantation for treatment of high-risk refractory acute lymphoblastic leukemia. *New Engl. J. Med.* **317**(8), 461—467 (1987).
11. Preijers, F.W., De Witte, T., Wessels, J.M., De Gast, G.C., Van Leeuwen, E., Capel, P.J. and Haanen, C.: Autologous transplantation of bone marrow purged in vitro with anti-CD7 (WT1-) ricin A immunotoxin in T-cell lymphoblastic leukemia and lymphoma. *Blood* **74**(3), 1152—1158 (1989).
12. Simmonson, B., Burnett, A.K., Prentice, H.G., Hann, I.H., Brenner, M.K., Gibson, B., Grob, J.P., Lonnerholm, G., Morrison, A., Smedmyr, B. *et al.*: Autologous bone marrow transplantation with monoclonal antibody purged marrow for high risk acute lymphoblastic leukemia. *Leukemia* **3**(9), 631—636 (1989).

58. Conditioning regimens in bone marrow transplantation

R. STORB, F. APPELBAUM, C. BADGER, I. BERNSTEIN, C.D. BUCKNER, F.B. PETERSEN, P. MARTIN, J. HANSEN, C. ANASETTI, B. SANDMAIER, J. BIANCO, F. SCHUENING and E.D. THOMAS

The ideal conditioning regimen for marrow transplants both destroys the underlying malignant disease and abrogates host immunity sufficiently to prevent rejection of the graft without undue toxicity. Unfortunately, such a regimen does not exist. A commonly used regimen in Seattle includes the immunosuppressive and anticancer drug cyclophosphamide (CY), 60 mg/kg on each of 2 days, and 1200—1575 cGy of fractionated total body irradiation (TBI) given over 3 to 7 days (1—6). As shown in Table 1, this regimen is not sufficient to eradicate leukemia in all cases and, depending on the underlying disease and the disease stage, relapse rates ranging from 17 to 75% are seen. Moreover, the CY/TBI regimen is followed by a high incidence of graft failure in those

Table 1. Leukemic relapse and disease-free long-term survival after treatment with cyclophosphamide and 1200—1575 cGy total body irradiation followed by transplantation of marrow from HLA-identical siblings.

Disease	Disease phase	Long-term disease-free survival (%)	Relapse (%)
ANL	1st remission	50	22
	2nd remission	25	45
	1st relapse	34	31
ALL	1st remission	54	35
	2nd remission	35	45
	3rd remission	30	58
	2nd relapse	18	75
CML	1st chronic phase	58	17
	Accelerated phase	30	45
	Blast crisis	20	70

Abbreviations:
ANL = Acute non-lymphocytic leukemia.
ALL = Acute lymphocytic leukemia.
CML = Chronic myelocytic leukemia.

patients who are recipients of either T-depleted HLA-identical or non-T-depleted HLA-non-identical grafts (7—8). Finally, while inadequately serving its purpose, the CY/TBI regimen has at least a 10% mortality from associated toxicities.

Early results of recent uncontrolled trials have suggested advantages with newer regimens. One regimen has included busulfan (6.9—8.7 mg/kg over 4 days) and CY (49—67 mg/kg over 2 days) with 1200 cGy of fractionated TBI [9]. Disease-free survival at 18 months among 33 patients with advanced leukemia was 40%. Another program combined high-dose cytosine arabinoside (3 g/m^2 every 12 hours for 12 doses) with 1200 cGy of fractionated TBI with or without 60 mg/kg of CY in 29 patients with advanced leukemia [10]. Despite considerably early toxicity, 40% disease-free survival at 2 years has been seen. These results warrant confirmation in controlled trials comparing the new regimens to more established programs.

In another study, carried out in patients with ANL transplanted in first remission from HLA-identical sibling donors and using graft-versus-hosts disease prevention with methotrexate and cyclosporine, we evaluated CY combined with 6 × 200 cGY of TBI and compared results to those obtained with CY combined with 7 × 225 cGy of TBI (11). The patients given the lower dose of TBI had a significantly higher incidence of leukemic relapse (approximately 30%) compared to those given the higher dose of TBI (approximately 10%). Unfortunately, the benefit derived from the lower relapse rate in patients given more TBI was offset by an increase in the regimen-related toxicity, and survival of the two groups of patients was identical, close to 60% at 2 years. Despite the comparable long-term disease-free survival, the study is encouraging in that it suggests that the doses of irradiation needed to eradicate leukemia are not much in excess of 1600 cGy. Nevertheless, it would appear that for all approaches involving systemic chemotherapy and TBI, the limits of non-hematopoietic toxicity have been reached and, barring the development of new drugs, no quantum improvements can be anticipated from these regimens.

The most effective way to destroy leukemic cells would be use agents which interact specifically with them. Monoclonal antibodies directed against antigens expressed in leukemic cells would come closest to this ideal. Antibodies which are injected *in vivo* can concentrate on leukemic cells; however their antileukemic effect is weak, in part because some cells may lack target antigens and in part because some cells, although coated by antibody, may not be destroyed by it. Attempts to use antibodies linked to toxins, such as the Ricin-A chain, to more effectively kill leukemic cells have shown unexpected toxicities.

An alternative approach involves linking monoclonal antibodies to short-lived radioactive isotopes which deposit their energy within a very close radius. In this fashion, leukemic cells expressing the appropriate target antigens would be killed, as would be neighboring cells which may be antigen negative. Of course, normal marrow cells would also be ablated, and subsequent marrow 'rescue' would be needed.

We have carried out a number of studies in a preclinical model, the dog, using antibodies to which we have linked ^{131}iodine (12—16). Antibody labeling with ^{131}I is simple and can be performed without harming antibody immunoreactivity or avidity. ^{131}I can both be used for imaging and therapy. Our studies have included antibody 6.4, an IgG 2b antibody, which does not react with canine antigens and was used as control. Antibody 7.2, also an IgG 2b, reacts with a framework determinant of both canine and human Ia. Antibody S5, an IgG 1, reacts with canine and human CD44 lymphocyte adhesion molecules. Finally, antibody DM5, an IgG 1, reacts with a differentation antigen on canine myeloid cells.

Initial studies in dogs have shown the appropriate radiolabeled antibody to localize preferentially in marrow and spleen and, to a lesser extent, also in lymph nodes. Marrow to other organ ratios of isotope of 20 : 1 or better have been found. We have determined that fatal marrow ablation with an ^{131}I-labeled antibody was possible, and this effect could be reversed with marrow transplantation. The timing of marrow infusion in these studies is important. It can be estimated that if marrow is infused 7 days after treatment with 6mC of ^{131}I/kg, the new marrow would be exposed to no more than 30 cGy of radiation. This dose of radiation appears to be tolerable since previous work in the canine model has shown that newly infused autologous marrow can withstand up to 150 cGy of irradiation without impairing the ability of that marrow to engraft [17].

Combinations of TBI and radiolabeled antibodies are now being explored to condition dogs for T-cell depleted and DLA non-identical marrow grafts. We believe that refinements of this approach, particularly the use of high-energy beta-emitting isotopes with short linear energy transfers, will result in less toxic but more efficient conditioning programs. These programs would not only provide better eradication of leukemia but also carry the potential to ameliorate the problem of graft failure.

Acknowledgement

This work was supported by grants CA18029, CA18221, CA31787, CA18105, CA09515 and CA15704 awarded by the National Cancer Institute and by grant HL36444 from the National Heart, Lung and Blood Institute of the National Institutes of Health, U.S. Department of Health and Human Services.

References

1. Thomas, E.D., Storb, R., Clift, R.A., Fefer, A., Johnson, F.L., Neiman, P.E., Lerner, K.G., Glucksberg, H. and Buckner, C.D.: Bone marrow transplantation. *New Engl. J. Med.* **292**, 832—843 and 895—902 (1975).
2. Thomas, E.D., Buckner, C.D., Clift, R.A., Fefer, A., Johnson, F.L., Neiman, P.E., Sale, G.E., Sanders, J.E., Singer, J.W., Shulman, H., Storb, R. and Weiden, P.L.: Marrow transplantation for acute nonlymphoblastic leukemia in first remission. *New Engl. J. Med.* **301**, 597—599 (1979).
3. Appelbaum, F.R., Dahlberg, S., Thomas, E.D., Buckner, C.D., Cheever, M.A., Clift, R.A., Crowley, J., Deeg, H.J., Fefer, A., Greenberg, P., Kadin, M., Smith, W., Stewart, P., Sullivan, K., Storb, R. and Weiden, P.: Bone marrow transplantation or chemotherapy after remission induction for adults with acute nonlymphoblastic leukemia: a prospective comparison. *Ann. Int. Mied.* **101**, 581—588 (1984).
4. Johnson, F.L., Thomas, E.D., Clark, B.S., Chard, R.L., Hartmann, J.R. and Storb, R.: A comparison of marrow transplantation with chemotherapy for children with acute lymphoblastic leukemia in second or subsequent remission. *New Engl. J. Med.* **305**, 846—851 (1981).
5. Clift, R.A., Buckner, C.D., Thomas, E.D., Kopecky, K.J., Appelbaum, F.R., Tallman, M. Storb, R., Sanders, J., Sullivan, K., Banaji, M., Beatty, P.S., Bensinger, W., Cheever, M., Deeg, J., Doney, K., Fefer, A., Greenberg, P., Hansen, J.A., Hackman, R., Hill, R., Martin, P., Meyers, J., McGuffin, R., Neiman, P., Sale, G., Shulman, H., Singer, J., Stewart, P., Weiden, P. and Witherspoon, R.: The treatment of acute nonlymphoblastic leukemia by allogeneic marrow transplantation. *Bone Marrow Transplant* **2**, 243—258 (1988).
6. Sanders, J.E., Buckner, C.D., Thomas, E.D., Fleischer, R., Sullivan, K.M., Appelbaum, F.R. and Storb, R.: Allogeneic marrow transplantation for children with juvenile chronic myelogenous leukemia. Concise Report. *Blood* **71**, 1144—1146 (1988).
7. Martin, P.J., Hansen, J.A., Buckner, C.D., Sanders, J.E., Deeg, H.J., Stewart, P., Appelbaum, F.r., Clift, R., Fefer. A., Witherspoon, R.P., Kennedy, M.S., Sullivan, K.M., Flournoy, N., Storb, R. and Thomas, E.D.: Effects of in vitro depletion of T cells in HLA-identical allogeneic marrow grafts. *Blood* **66**, 664—672 (1985).
8. Anasetti, C., Amos, D., Beatty, P.G., Appelbaum, F.R., Bensinger, W., Buckner, C.D., Clift, R., Doney, K., Martin, P.J., Mickelson, E. Nisperos, B., O'Quigley, J., Ramberg, R., Sanders, J.E., Stewart, P., Storb, R., Sullivan, K.M., Witherspoon, R.P., Thomas, E.D. and Hansen, J.A.: Effect of HLA compatibility on engraftment of bone marrow transplants in patients with leukemia or lymphoma. *New Engl. J. Med.* **320**, 197—204 (1989).
9. Petersen, F.B., Buckner, C.D., Appelbaum, F.R., Clift, R.A., Sanders, J.E., Bensinger, W.I., Storb, R., Witherspoon, R.P., Sullivan, K.M., Bearman, S.I., Flournoy, N. and Thomas E.D.: Busulfan, cyclophosphamide and fractionated total body irradiation as a preparatory regimen for marrow transplantation in patients with advanced hematological malignancies: a phase I study. *Bone Marrow Transplant* **4**, 617—623 (1989).
10. Riddell, S., Appelbaum, F.R., Buckner, C.D., Stewart, P., Clift, R., Sanders, J., Storb, R., Sullivan, K. and Thomas, E.D.: High-dose cytarabine and total body irradiation with or without cyclophosphamide as a preparative regimen for marrow transplantation for acute leukemia. *J. Clin. Oncol.* **6**, 576—582 (1988).
11. Buckner, C.D., Clift, R., Appelbaum, F., Storb, R., Thomas, E.D. and Hansen, J.A.: An increased dose of total body irradiation decreased relapse in marrow allograft recipients with acute and chronic myeloid leukemia. *19th Annual ISEH Meeting, abstract.*
12. Appelbaum, F.R., Badger, C., Deeg, H.J., Nelp, W.B. and Storb, R.: Use of iodine-^{131}-labeled anti-immune response-associated monoclonal antibody as preparative regimen prior to bone marrow transplantation: initial dosimetry. *National Cancer Inst. Monogr.* **3**, 67—71 (1987).
13. Appelbaum, F.R., Brown, P.A., Graham, T.C., Sandmaier, B.M., Schuening, F.W. and Storb, R.: Characterization of malignant lymphoma in dogs and use as a model for the development of treatment strategies. In: S.J. Baum, G.W. Santos and F. Takaku (eds), *Recent Advances*

and Future Directions in Bone Marrow Transplantation (Experimental Hematology Today — 1987), pp. 31—35. Springer Verlag., New York (1988).

14. Appelbaum, F.R., Badger, C., Bernstein, I., Bianco, J., Brown, P., Eary, J., Press, O., Sandmaier, B., Schuening, F. and Storb, R.: Development of improved marrow transplant preparative regimens: use of antibody-radionuclide conjugates. In: G.L. DeNardo (ed.), *Biology of Radionuclide Therapy*, pp. 102—109. American College of Nuclear Physicians, Washington, D.C. (1989).
15. Appelbaum, F.R., Brown, P. Sandmaier, B., Badger, C., Schuening, F., Graham, T.C. and Storb, R.: Antibody-radionuclide conjugates as part of a myeloblative preparative regimen for marrow transplantation. *Blood* **73**, 2202—2208 (1989).
16. Bianco, J.A., Sandmaier, B., Brown, P., Badger, C., Bernstein, I., Eary, J., Durak, L., Schuening, F., Storb, R. and Appelbaum, F.: Specific marrow localization of an ^{131}I-labeled anti-myeloid antibody in normal dogs: effects of a "cold" antibody pretreatment dose on marrow localization. *Exp. Hematol.* **17**, 929—934 (1989).
17. Appelbaum, F.R., Graham, T., Sandmaier, B., Schuening, F. and Storb, R.: Sensitivity of newly transplanted marrow to further irradiation. *Transplant.* **45**, 813—814 (1988).

[illegible] Transplantation: Experimental [illegible], Springer-Verlag, New York (1989).

14. Appelbaum, F.R., Badger, C., Bernstein, I., Bianco, J., Brown, P., [illegible], Press, [illegible], Sandmaier, B., Schuening, F., [illegible] R.: Development of improved marrow transplant preparative regimens: use of antibody-radionuclide conjugates. In: [illegible] (1989).

15. Appelbaum, F.R., Brown, P., Sandmaier, B., Badger, C., Schuening, F., [illegible], and [illegible] marrow [illegible] transplantation. Blood 72: [illegible] (1988).

16. [illegible] Sandmaier, B. [illegible] Appelbaum, F.R.: [illegible] localization of an [illegible] labeled [illegible] marrow transplantation. Exp Hematol 17: [illegible] (1989).

17. Appelbaum, F.R.: [illegible] marrow transplantation [illegible]

59. The antileukaemic action of melphalan and total body irradiation in bone marrow transplantation

R.L. POWLES, C.L. SMITH, C. TILEY, M. FINDLEY and M. O'BRIEN

Introduction

We have previously reported that melphalan and total body irradiation (TBI) has a more powerful antileukaemic action than cyclophosphamide/TBI when used as conditioning for HLA-matched sibling allogeneic bone marrow transplantation for first remission acute myeloblastic leukameia (AML) (1, 2). To investigate whether this antileukaemic action is due to a direct effect of the conditioning programme or due to a more complicated indirect effect by factors such as graft-versus-host disease (GVHD), we have compared the antileukaemic action of melphalan/TBI in allografts to that of autografts for first remission AML. We have used two further groups of patients as controls for this investigation: a group with first remission AML who did not receive a bone marrow transplant, and a second group who were allografted using marrow purged of lymphocytes by the monoclonal antibody, Campath 1. The aim of purging was to irradicate GVHD and thus assess the role of GVHD in producing the favourable results we have seen with melphalan/TBI conditioning.

Patients and methods

One hundred and thirty patients with acute myeloblastic leukaemia in first remission have been included in the overall study and followed up for a period of up to 10 years.

Chemotherapy for first remission AML

When first remisison had been achieved, 44 patients received chemotherary consisting of medium dose cytosine arabinoside and 6-thioguanine given in short courses over a period of 4—6 weeks and then followed by a single dose of 10 mg/kg cytosine arabinoside infused over 24 hours and 1.5 mg/kg duanorubicin given as a single dose. No further chemotherapy was given from 3 months after diagnosis.

Melphalan/TBI sibling matched allografts

Following consolidation chemotherapy as for the chemotherapy alone group, 53 patients with AML in first remission received 110 mg/M^2 melphalan followed at 12 hours by single fraction total body irradiation to 10.5 Gy given at a rate of 4 Gy/min. All patients received cyclosporine prophylaxis for 6 months after transplantation to prevent graft-versus-host disease.

Melphalan/TBI autografts

Twenty-two patients in first remission AML, who had also received consolidation therapy as above, had marrow harvested, stored at 4 °C and then received 110 mg/M^2 melphalan and TBI, given as above. Their non-cryopreserved autologous marrow was reinfused 18—24 hours after melphalan. No further chemotherapy was given post-transplant.

Cyclophosphamide/TBI matched sibling Campath purged allografts

Eleven first remission AML patients, after receiving consolidation chemotherapy as above, received 60 mg/kg cyclophosphamide for 2 days followed by single fraction TBI as above. They received allogeneic bone marrow that had been purged by a previously described method using Campath 1 mouse monoclonal antibody to reduce T lymphocytes (3).

Results

Figure 1 shows the probability of remaining in remission for these four groups of patients. It can be seen that only 1 of 53 patients who received melphalan and TBI and an allograft, has relapsed. Ninety percent of these patients developed graft-versus-host disease of grade 1 or greater. For the other three groups of patients, it can be seen from Figure 1 that 5 of 11 patients who received Campath-treated marrow have relapsed, 9 of 22 melphalan/TBI autografts have relapsed, and 37 of 44 patients who received chemotherapy alone have relapsed. All of the later three groups of patients lie on actuarial probability curves that are essentially the same, and are significantly different from the melphalan/TBI allograft results.

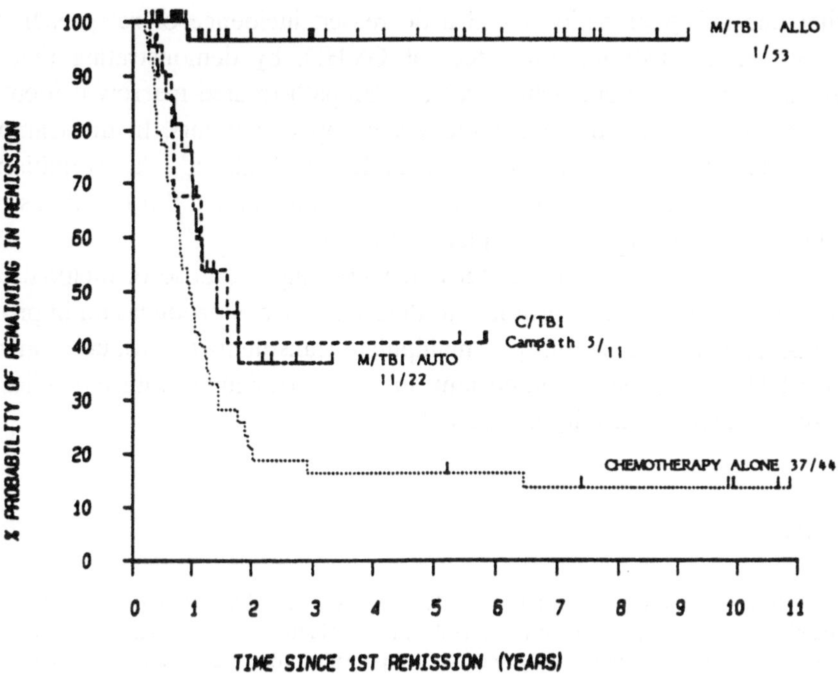

Fig. 1. The probability of remaining in survival for each of the four groups of patients, with the numbers of patients relapsed compared to the total in each group indicated.

Discussion

Patients in all four arms of this study received the same consolidation chemotherapy, with three of the arms proceeding to transplantation and the fourth having no further treatment. It was surprising to find that the results of the melphalan/TBI autograft arm were not substantially different from the chemotherapy alone arm, with no evidence that the melphalan/TBI conditioning had any effect on preventing relapse and improving survival. This was despite melphalan/TBI being so effective in the allogeneic group of patients. It is unlikely that these results are due to reinoculation of the host by residual leukaemia in the autografted marrow, as other groups (4, 5) have shown plateaux of cure at 40% in comparable patients. Marrow, likewise, was untreated and a similar number of cells to our study were reinfused. One can only conclude that melphalan/TBI has not irradicated residual host leukaemia remaining in the patient at the time of conditioning.

We have previously reported that graft-versus-host disease may be a factor in preventing leukaemic relapse when melphalan/TBI conditioning is given for allografting (2). We draw this conclusion from the results of a randomized trial comparing melphalan/TBI with cyclophosphamide/TBI where we found graft-versus-host disease was more prevalent in the melphalan/TBI group of patients and that this group of patients had a decreased incidence of relapse. In this report, we have illustrated the effect of GVHD, by demonstrating that the relapse rate for the patients who received Campath-treated marrow is identical to the autografting and the chemotherapy group of patients. In the Campath group of patients were GVHD was completely abolished, the conditioning regimen did not prevent relapse or improve outcome above those patients who did not undergo bone marrow transplantation.

We have now undertaken the study of increasing the dose of melphalan to 140 mg/M^2 in our autograft protocol to determine if this produces an improved antileukaemic action. The ability to manipulate transplants to produce controllable GVHD would be an important factor is designing future studies to successfully treat acute myeloblastic leukaemia.

References

1. Helenglass, G., Powles, R.L., McElwain, T.J., Lakhani, A., Milan, S., Gore, M., Nandi, A., Zuiable, A., Perren, T., Forgeson, G., Treleavan, J., Hamilton, C. and Millar, J.: Melphalan and total body irradiation (TBI) versus cyclophosphamide and TBI as conditioning for allogeneic matched sibling bone marrow transplants for acute myeloblastaic leukemia in first remission. *Bone Marrow Transplant.* **3** (1), 21–29 (1988).
2. Powles, R.L., Milliken, S., Helenglass, G., Treleavan, J., Pinkerton, R., Zuiable, A., Nandi, A., Aboud, H. and Millar, J.: The use of melphalan in conjunction with total body irradiation as treatment for acute leukaemia. *Transplant. Proc.* **21** (1), 2955–2957 (1989).
3. Hale, G., Bright, S., Chumbley, G., Hoang, T., Metcalf, D., Munro, A.J. and Walmann, H.: Removal of T cells from bone marrow for transplantation: a monoclonal antilymphocyte antibody that fixes human complement. *Blood* **62** (4), 873–882 (1983).
4. Burnett, A.K., Watkins, R., Maharaj, D., McKinnon, S., Tansey, P., Alcorn, M., Singer, C.R.J., McDonald G.A. and Robertson, A.G.: Transplantation of unpurged autologous bone-marrow in acute myeloid leukaemia in first remission. *Lancet* **ii**, 1068–1070 (1984).
5. Goldstone, A.H., Anderson, C.C., Linch, D.C., Franklan, I.M., Houghton, B.J. and Richards J.D.M.: Autologous bone marrow transplantation following high dose chemotherapy for the treatment of adult patients with acute myeloid leukaemia. *Brit. J. Haem.* **64** (3), 529–537 (1986).

60. Antifungal prophylaxis with fluconazole in bone marrow transplantation

R.L., POWLES, C.L. SMITH and S. MILLIKEN

Introduction

Fungal infection remains a significant cause of mortality and morbidity in patients receiving bone marrow ablative dosages of cytotoxic therapies. Candida species are well documented as major fungal pathogens in these patients (1). Prevention of fungal colonization reduces the risk of deep fungal infection. We have previously used an intensive regimen of oral polyenes as prophylaxis for fungal colonization in patients after high-dose chemoradiotherapy, but find that this has a high failure rate with greater than 6% of our patients having deaths attributable to deep fungal infection (2).

Fluconazole, a novel bistriazole antifungal drug, appears to be safe in man and highly effective in eradicating candida species (3). This aqueous preparation has the additional advantage, unlike polyenes, of being well absorbed orally in normal subjects (4). Our experience has been that fluconazole is also well absorbed in patients having chemoablative therapy, despite the potential for gastrointestinal damage from this high-dose chemotherapy (5).

Our study was an open comparative study to determine the efficacy, tolerance and safety of oral fluconazole compared with our standard regimen of oral polyenes when used for prophylaxis of fungal colonization and superinfection. All patients were having high-dose chemotherapy, with or without radiation, and bone marrow transplantation.

Patients and methods

Ninety-nine patients with leukaemia, lymphoma or myeloma were randomized to receive either oral fluconazole or polyenes, as shown: Fungal prophylaxis was commenced 1 week prior to high-dose melphalan, with or without autografting in the lymphoma and myeloma group of patients; or 1 week prior to conditioning for bone marrow transplantation in the leukaemic group of patients. Prophylaxis was continued for a least 4 weeks after the high-dose therapy or until the peripheral blood neutrophil count had exceeded $1 \times 10^9/l$, to a maximum of 8 weeks. Patients were considered to have failed prophylaxis if weekly fungal surveillance culture (month and genital swabs, blood, urinary and stool cultures) became positive or if the patients developed clinical evidence of fungal infection sufficient to require systemic amphotericin therapy. Patient groups were compared for compliance, tolerance and safety.

Patients who required systemic amphotericin therapy were stratified according to whether they received low-dose or high-dose therapy. Low-dose therapy was given for severe month infections and high-dose therapy if more extensive infection was present or systemic infection suspected.

Results

Forty-nine patients received fluconazole and 50 received oral polyenes. The median age was 41 (17—58) years. Sixty-eight patients were male and 31 were female. Underlying diseases are listed in Table 1.

Fluconazole 200 mg (2 capsules)
or

Amphotericin lozenges	10 mg 6 hourly
Amphotericin tablets	200 mg 6 hourly
Nystatin suspension	200 000 units 4 hourly
Nystatin tablets	500 000 units 12 hourly

The percentage of patients who did not have positive funal surveillance cultures during the prophylaxis peirod was 59% in those that received fluconazole and 46% in those who received polyenes, which was not significantly different. Likewisc, the percentage of those that remained free of evidence of clinical infection was 74% in the fluconazole group and 64% in the polyene group (Table 2).

Table 1. The number of patients in each treatment group as shown with the distribution of underlying diseases in each group.

	Fluconazole	Polyenes	Total
Multiple myeloma	23	20	43
Acute leukaemia	14	13	27
Hodgkin's disease	5	9	14
CGL	5	5	10
Other (rhabdomycosarcoma, medulloblastoma)	2	3	5
Total	49	50	99

Table 2. Patients in each treatment group who did not develop clinical or microbiological evidence of fungal colonization.

	Fluconazole	Polyenes	Significance
Culture negative	29 (59%)	23 (46%)	N.S.
No clinical infection	36 (74%)	32 (64%)	N.S.
Received amphotericin[a]	16 (33%)	24 (48%)	N.S.
Low does (<7 days)	9 (18%)	8 (16%)	N.S.
High does (>7 days)	7 (14%)	16 (32%)	N.S.

[a] Those patients receiving systemic amphotericin, either low dose for localized infection or high dose for suspected systemic infection are indicated for each treatment group.

Use of systemic amphotericin

Thirty-three percent of patients receiving fluconazole received systemic amphotericin as compared to 48% of those receiving oral polyenes, which was not statistically significant. However, 16 patients in the polyene group required high-dose systemic amphotericin, compared to 7 in the fluconazole group, but this also did not reach statistical significance. Low-dose amphotericin (0.25 mg/kg for 3 days) was given for localized clinical fungal infection such as mouth ulceration. High-dose amphotericin was given for suspected deep or systemic fungal infection at a dose escalated to 1 mg/kg over 72 hours.

Compliance

Two patients receiving fluconazole did not comply with treatment compared to 10 patients receiving polyenes ($p = 0.034$). Thirteen patients in the fluconazole group and 12 in the polyene group did not complete treatment as they were unable to take oral medication.

Toxicity

There were no clinically significant toxicities in either group. Liver function tests were analysed. There was no statistically significant difference in the elevation of alanine transaminase or gamma-glutamyl transaminase in the two groups. There was no effect upon engraftment in the fluconazole group as mean time to 0.5×10^9/l neutrophils was 25 (11–55) days compared to 33 (15–124+) days in the polyene group.

Discussion

Invasive fungal infection has become an increasing problem in heavily immunosuppressed patients. The incidence of fungal infection increases with the length of the neutropenic period (6). The prevalence of fungal infections may be related to more intensively immunosuppressive treatments, the use of broad spectrum antibiotics and the long-term use of indwelling intravenous and urinary catheters.

Deep fungal infections in bone marrow transplant recipients has an unknown incidence, largely because of the difficulties in obtaining a diagnosis antimortem. In a retrospective study of 160 autopsies, Martin *et al.* (7) found a 30% incidence of fungal infection. Fungal septicaemia in three series occurred in 18—28% of transplant recipients (8, 9, 10). Systemic fungal infection has been directly attributed to over 6% of deaths in our institution, a figure which has not decreased over the last 5 years (2).

The majority of fungal infections in immunosuppressed patients are candida species and less commonly aspergillus (1). Oral polyenes, which are the most commonly used prophylactic agents have been disappointing in preventing colonization and preventing fungaemia (1). Unlike oral polyenes, fluconzaole is well absorbed when given orally and is well distributed to body compartments (4). This systemic absorption would theoretically be advantageous in preventing invasion by fungal organisms.

We have found that oral fluconzaole was well tolerated, with significantly better compliance than oral polyenes when used as fungal prophylaxis in patients having marrow ablative therapy. Fulconazole is given conveniently as a single daily dose and no clinically significant toxicity was seen.

Fluconazole is equally as effective as oral polyenes in preventing fungal colonization, but in our severely immunosuppressed patients colonization was still prevalent.

More patients in the polyene group (32%) required high-dose systemic amphotericin for extensive candidal superinfection or suspected deep candidal infection than the fluconazole group (14%, $p = 0.064$). These findings suggest that systemic absorption of fluconazole may be advantageous in the prophylaxis of fungal infections in patients having intensive cytoreductive therapy, but because of the small numbers involved a statistical significance was not seen.

In conclusion, fluconazole is as efficacious as polyenes in preventing fungal colonization, is conveniently administered, with good compliance and can be given with safety in patients having high-dose chemoradiotherapy.

References

1. Meunier, F.: Prevention of mycoses in immunocompromised patients. *Rev. Infect. Dis.* **9**, 408—416 (1987).

2. Milliken. S.: Management of opportunistic fungal infections in the high risk patient. In: R.D. Richardson (ed), *Focus on Fluconazole*, pp. 39—45. Royal Society of Medicine Services International Congress and Symposium Series No. 153, published by Royal Society of Medicine Services Ltd.
3. Troke, P.F., Andrews, R.J., Brammer, K.W., Marriott, M.S. and Richardson, K.: Efficacy of UK-49, 858 (Fluconazole) against *Candida albicans* experimental infections in mice. *Antimicrob. Agents Chemother.* **28**(6), 815—818 (1985).
4. Humphrey, M.J., Jevons, S. and Tarbit, M.H.: Pharmacokinetic evaluation of UK-49, 858, a metabolically stable triazole antifungal drug, in animals and humans. *Antimicrob. Agents Chemother.* **28**(5), 648—653 (1985).
5. Milliken, S., Powles, R., Jones, A. and Helenglass, G.: Pharmacokinetics of oral fluconazole in autologous bone marrow transplantation recipients given TBI and high dose melphalan transplantation. *Transplant. Proc.* **21**(1), 3067 (1989).
6. Meyers, J. and Atkinson, K.: Infection in bone marrow transplantation. *Clin. Haematol.* **13**, 791—811 (1983).
7. Martin, D.H., Counts, G.W. and Thomas, E.D.: Fungal infections in human bone-marrow transplant recipients. In: Program and Abstracts of the 17th Interscience Conf. on Antimicrobial Agents and Chemotherapy, Abstract 406. American Society for Microbiology, New York (1977).
8. Meyers, J.D. and Thomas, E.D.: Infection complicating bone marrow transplantation. In: L.S. Young and R.H. Rubin (eds), *Clinical Approach to Infection in the Compromised Host*, pp. 507—551 Plenum Press, New York (1981).
9. Winston, D.J., Gale, R.P., Meyer, D.V. and Young, L.S.: Infectious complications of human bone marrow transplantation. *Medicine* **58**, 1—31 (1979).
10. Roger, T.R. and Barnes, R.A.: The management of infections in neutropenic patients. *Advanced Medicine* **23**, 246—256 (1987).

61. Mass islet isolation from the pancreas of higher mammals: a potential source for islet transplantation in diabetic patients

R.G. BRETZEL, B.J. HERING and K.F. FEDERLIN

Introduction

The isolation and purification of a sufficient mass of islets of Langerhans with preserved morphological and functional integrity is one of the prerequisites for a clinically successful islet transplantation in type I diabetic patients, besides solving a second problem which is the islet allo- and xenograft rejection. With a new automated ingestion-filtration method, modified according to the method developed by Ricodi *et al.* (1), we tried to isolate islets from canine, bovine and procine pancreas. The rational behind isolation of higher mammalian islets is to perform xeno-transplantations in type I diabetic patients with the final goal to prevent or even reverse secondary complications in these patients.

Material and methods

Key factors of the islet isolation process are an adequate intralobular disruption of the connective tissue stroma, a gentle dissociation without mechanical trauma to the islets and density-gradient purification. After digestion-filtration, we received crude preparations of isolated islets which were further processed by density-gradient purification using 'liquid' Ficoll. Recently, the purification procedure was further optimized by using the cell separator Cobe 2991. Various parameters were used to assess islet yield and islet purity. Meanwhile, qualitative and quantitative standards on islet isolation from large mammals were created in an international workshop held on September 20, 1989, in Minneapolis, chaired by Dr. C. Ricordi. These recommendations were developed by the groups of Edmonton, Giessen, Leicester, Milan, Miami, Oxford and St Louis and will be published in *Diabetes* this year. The parameters used by our group are islet yield and islet purity prior to and after density gradient centrifugation, assessment of the pellet volume, DNA content, total and per gram islet number and islet volume, mean islet diameter, insulin content and morphological analysis of the purity of the islets. Viability testing was performed by a microfluorometric viability test using fluorescene-diacetate and propidium iodate according to the method developed by London *et al.* (2). The endocrine function was assessed by testing the *in vitro* glucose-stimulated insulin secretion in a dynamic system (perifusion) and *in vivo* after transplantation into streptozotocin diabetic nude mice (porcine islets) or by autografting (canine islets).

Light microscopy and electron microscopy was done on representative probes during the islet processing and after transplantation.

Results

Dog pancrease

After pancreatectomy in Beagle dogs, 8 pancreata were processed with an average yield of 2055 ∓ 496 islets per gram pancreas. Intraportal autotransplantation of such an islet preparation resulted in an oral glucose test resembling that performed before pancreatectomy but with a slight delay of glucose assimilation when performed 6 weeks after autografting.

Human pancreas

Only a limited number of pancreata was sent to our laboratory. Thirteen pancreata were processed and an average of 2242 ∓ 594 islets per gram pancreas could be yielded.

The current risk to develop a type I diabetes mellitus in West Germany is about 7 cases per 100 000 inhabitants summing to an annual total number of about 4200 newly diagnosed type I diabetics. The prevalence of type I diabetes in children is reported to be 1 out of 2500 in our country. The annual risk of developing type I diabetes in Kuwait is reported as 5.6 per 100 000 inhabitants (LaPort *et al* (3)). Facing this gap between the limited number of available donor pancreata and the increasing number of potential islet recipients, we tried to isolate masses of islets from higher mammals with the aim to transplant immunoaltered or encapsulated xeno-islet grafts in type I diabetic patients. Therefore, we initially started with islet isolations from beef pancreata.

Beef pancreas

Table 1 gives the results of islet isolation and purification from 12 beef pancreata. The total number of isolated islets was quite reasonable to perform at least 2 : 1, probably also 1 : 1 ratio for transplantation. But, when we tested these preparations *in vitro* there was no insulin secretion when stimulated by a

Table 1. Results of studies on islet isolation from adult beef pancreata.

No. (*n* = 12)	Weight of processed pancreas sample (g)	Final pellet-volume (ml)	Insulin content-pancreas sample (U)	Insulin content of islet suspension (U)	Insulin recovery (%)	Total no. of isolated islets	No. of isolated islets per gram pancreas	Isolated islet-volume (μl)	Isolated islet-vol. per gram pancreas (μl)
$\bar{x}$	73.3	11.0	189.6	63.5	36.1	150 560	2098.8	114.1	1.60
± SEM	2.9	1.3	37.6	11.8	6.5	18 560	292.2	19.0	0.28

glucose challenge, despite normal morphological appearance, as tested by light microscopy and electron microscopy. Going through the literature, we found that glucose is not the natural stimulus for insulin secretion of adult ruminants, but fatty acids. With regard to xenografts in human diabetics, bovine pancreas may not be the ideal source for an islet bank. Therefore, we began to isolate islets from adult porcine pancreata.

Pig pancreas

More than 200 pig pancreata have been processed up to now. The yield of porcine islet isolations done consecutively in one of the last 10 cases is given in Table 2. There is now a reproducibly high number of islets per gram pancreas with a fairly high total islet volume. Sixty percent of the islets showed a diameter of 50—100 μm, 36.1% had a diameter of 100—200 μm. This is quite a good result which contributes to the relatively high isolated islet volume. Meanwhile, the purity of the islet suspension could be further augmented using the automated cell separator, Cobe 2991. The preserved viability of the isolated and purified porcine islets was assessed by *in vitro* assays using the micro-fluorometric viability test and glucose stimulated insulin secretion in a perfusion test system. Finally, transplantation of such a porcine islet preparation beneath the kidney capsule into diabetic nude mice resulted in a decrease of blood sugar which reached the normal range. When the grafts were removed by nephrectomy diabetes recurred.

Conclusions and prospects

With the use of widely automated and computer assisted methods for islet isolation and purification, it is now possible to perform mass isolation of islets from pancreata retrieved from slaughterhouse material on a day-by-day basis. The results of islet isolation from porcine pancreas provides good prospects of a

Table 2. Yield of adult porcine islets isolated from 10 consecutively processed pancreata.

Isolation No.	Weight of processed pancreas sample (g)	Volume of digest (ml)	Total islet count ($\times 10^3$)	No. of islet per gram pancreas	Islets belonging to diameter (μm) classes (%)				Isolated islet volume (μl)	Isolated islet volume/ g pancreas (μl)
					50—100	100—200	200—300	> 300		
1	42	4	110	2619	57	41	2	0	113	2.7
2	63	5	275	4365	55	41	4	0	325	5.2
3	55	18	284	5164	65	33	2	0	261	4.8
4	57	4	188	3298	49	42	8	1	348	6.1
5	66	10	196	2970	60	35	5	0	222	3.4
6	65	8	201	3092	59	38	3	0	204	3.1
7	72	6	233	3236	70	24	5	1	260	3.6
8	70	2	140	2114	65	32	3	0	139	2.0
9	65	8	155	2385	64	36	0	0	96	1.5
10	76	7	276	3632	56	39	5	0	324	4.3
Mean	63.1	7.2	206.6	3287.5	60.0	36.1	3.7	0.2	229.2	3.7
SEM	3.1	1.4	18.9	290.2	1.9	1.7	0.7	0.1	28.6	0.5

successful xenografting in human diabetic patients in the future. However, to reach this final goal another problem, the rejection of allografted or xenografted tissue, must be solved. New methods to immunomodulate higher mammalian islet tissue or to transplant encapsulated material which was recently shown give rise to the hope that prevention of diabetic secondary complications will be possible by a successful islet xenografting in the future.

References

1. Ricordi, C., Lacy, P.E., Finke, E.H., Olack, B.J. and Scharp, D.W.: Automated method for isolation of human pancreatic islets. *Diabetes* **37**, 413—420 (1988).
2. London, N.J.M., Contractor, H., Lake, S.P., Aucott, G.C., Bell, P.R.F. and James, R.F.L.: A microfluometric viability assay for isolated human and rat islets of Langerhans. *Diabetes Res.* **3**, 141—9 (1989).
3. LaPorte, R.E., Tajima, N., Akerblom, H.K., Berlin, N., Brosseau, J., Christy, M., Drash, A.L., Fishbein, H., Green, A., Hamman, R., Harris, M., King, H., Laron, Z. and Neil, A.: Geographic differences in the risk of insulin dependent diabetes mellitus: the importance of registries. *Diabetes Care* **8** (Suppl. 1) 101—107 (1985).

62. The relationship of eicosanoids and complement components to hyperacute xenogeneic rejection and its modification by the PAF-antagonist WEB 2086BS

DAVID M. SAUMWEBER, ROLF BERGMANN, CLAUS HAMMER and WALTER BRENDEL

Introduction

Experimental and clinical observations suggest that the xenograft rejection is based on two mechanisms. In animal species without natural antibodies, a mechanism similar to that in the allogeneic situation is responsible for the rejection. On the other hand, in species combinations where preformed natural antibodies (PNAB) directed against xenogeneic antigens are present, a hyperacute rejection is typical. The principle features of this hyperacute xenogeneic renal rejection (HXAR) are a rapid increase of arterial resistance, cessation of the organ's microcirculation within minutes, extravasation of blood and hematuria and cessation of urine production. Up to now, no reliable method to suppress this HXAR has been developed. Therefore, the major interest still lies either in the elimination of preformed antibodies or in blocking the major response of humoral mediators of which platelet-activating factor (PAF, PAF-acether) is supposed to be one. Recently, it was shown that PAF-acether does participate in transplant rejection. The first association with hyperacute rejection was suggested by Camussi *et al.* (1). In this reaction, PAF is regarded as a potent mediator of inflammatory reactions because of its broad range of biological activities. Commonly, the i.v. injection of PAF into different animal species is followed by hypotension, pulmonary hypertension, bronchoconstriction and increase of vascular permeability as systemic effects. The cellular sources of PAF are polymorphonuclear leukocytes (PMN), mast cells, platelets and endothelial cells. PAF is released from these cells when stimulated but also induces its own activation. Neutrophils and eosinophils participate in endothelial cell injury, e.g. by secreting proteases which destroy the basal membrane and activate the complement cascade. The close relationship between PAF synthesis and endothelial cell-dependent neutrophil adherence as well as the fact that PAF directly stimulates PMN activation and adhesion suggest that PAF may directly participate in transplant rejection (2, 3). The first evidence for PAF involvement in renal immune injury comes from the observation that PAF is released during hyperacute allograft rejection in kidneys. The participation of platelets and leukocytes in xenograft rejection provides the basis for the rationale of our trial to use PAF-antagonists in organ xenotransplantation.

This study evaluates the effect of the new synthetic PAF-receptor antagonist WEB 2086BS (8) in an *ex vivo* renal xenograft model with special interest on the mediator response.

Material and methods

Perfusion experiments

All experiments were conducted using landrace pigs of either sex weighing 20–28 kg.

The animals were anesthetized with hypnomidate/azaperon and ventilated mechanically with room air. A jugular venous catheter was inserted and isotonic saline was infused i.v. at 10 ml/min throughout organ preparation. Both kidneys were exposed through a midline laparotomy and the renal artery and vein were gently dissected free of adventitial tissue. After removal, the organs were flushed with 200 ml Eurocollins solution and immediately used for perfusion experiments with autologous porcine or xenogeneic human blood in a recirculating, continuously oxygenated system with constant flow of 16 ml blood per minute. During *ex vivo* perfusion, the perfusion pressure was measured continuously using a calibrated pressure transducer (Statham P23ID, GOULD Inc., U.S.A.) placed directly at the renal artery. The experiments were terminated after 60 min. Renal arterial and venous blood were sampled before and after the start of hemoperfusion at 5, 15, 30 and 60 min. Paired experiments were performed for each experiment, by assigning one kidney as the control and the other as the test (treated) kidney.

Preparation of human blood

Whole heparinized blood was collected from the animals who served as kidney donors and from volunteers not allowed to take any medication 1 week before blood donation. The blood was diluted with Ringer's to 30% hematocrit and always used within 30 min of collection. Eight experiments were performed using autologous porcine blood (group A) as well as seven experiments where the pig kidneys were perfused with xenogeneic human whole blood (group B). In a further seven experiments human blood (group C), identical to the corresponding test in group B, was used which was gently mixed with stock solutions of the compound WEB 2086BS (Boehringer Ingelheim/F.R.G.). The substance was dissolved in 0.1 *n* HCl and adjusted to pH 7.4 in the stock solution. The drug WEB 2086BS, a new type of triazolodiazepine, is one of the most potent PAF-antagonists without serious side effects and was used in a dosage of 300 mg per perfusion experiment.

Laboratory investigations

Blood samples were drawn from the circuit before and 5, 15, 30 and 60 min after the start of hemoperfusion. Blood was differentiated using a coulter counter (T 540, Coulter Diagnostics Inc., U.S.A.). All blood samples were centrifuged at 2500 rpm for 10 min and the plasma was stored at −70 °C in aliquots. The frozen plasma was thawed only once before it was used. The xenohemagglutinins in human plasma against pig erythrocytes (HA-assay) were titrated according to the methods described by Weir *et al.* (4). To study the activation of complement factors during the experiment, complement 4a (C4a) and complement 3a (C3A) were measured by radioimmunoassays based on the methods described by Hugli *et al.* (5) and Gorski *et al.* (6). The prostanoids TxB_2 and 6-keto-PGF_{1a}, the stable hydrolysis products of TxA_2 and prostacyclin, were measured by radioimmunoassays (7). The osmolalities of plasma and urinary samples were determined by freezing-point depression using a cryoscopic osmometer (Osmomat 030, GONOTEC/F.R.G.).

Statistical analysis

Results were expressed as means and SEM for groups and statistical comparisons were made using Scheffe's test. Results with $p < 0.05$ were considered to be statistically significant.

Results

Preformed natural antibody levels in human plasma

The levels of natural antibodies in human plasma were measured against pig erythrocytes by HA-assay in groups B and C. As shown in Table 1, PNABs were clearly detected at high levels prior to organ perfusion. After the start of hemoperfusion, the antibody level decreased dramatically to values of <4 within the first 15 min, persisting constantly low until the end of the experiment. No differences between both experimental groups using human blood perfusate could be detected.

Mediator release during hemoperfusion

In group B, the TXB_2 concentration in plasma increased from a prevalue of 0.238 ± 0.03 ng/ml to 0.521 ±0.16 ng/ml at 5 min of xenoperfusion. The concentrations in group A and group C were significantly lower compared to

Table 1. Titer of preformed hemagglutinins in groups B and C during hemoperfusion.

	Perfusion time (min)				
HA-assay group	0	5	15	30	60
Group B	128–512	<8	<8	<4	<4
Group C	128–256	<8	<4	<4	<4

that in group B at 5 min (group A, 0.25 ± 0.01 ng/ml; group C, 0.237 ± 0.04 ng/ml). After 15 min of auto- and xenoperfusion, no significant differences between the groups could be confirmed thought the concentration of TxB_2 was constantly higher in group B compared to the other groups until the end of the experiment (Figure 1). Five minutes of renal xenoperfusion in the non-treated

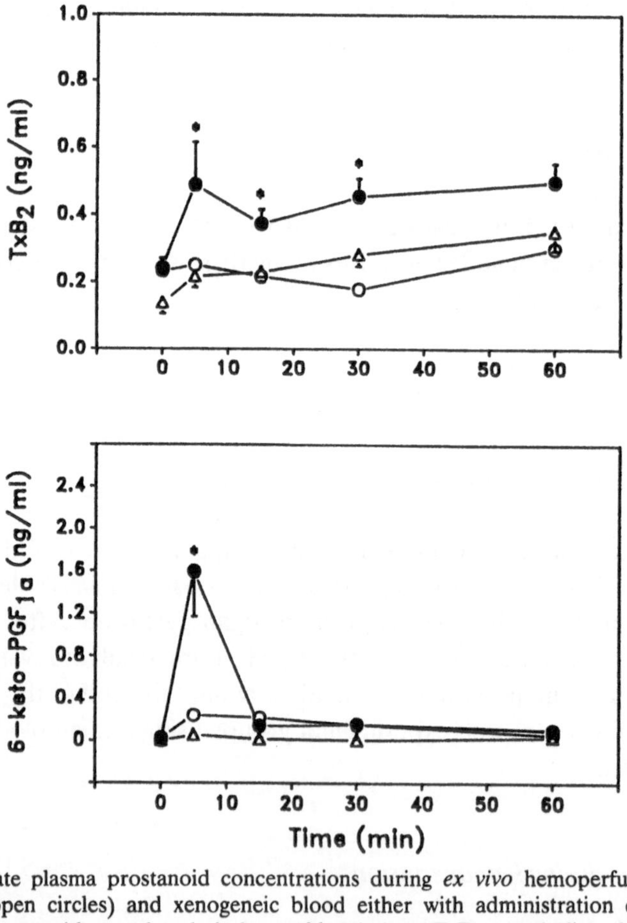

Fig. 1. Perfusate plasma prostanoid concentrations during *ex vivo* hemoperfusion with autologous blood (open circles) and xenogeneic blood either with administration of WEB 2086BS (open triangles) or without (closed circles). *Abbreviations*: TxB_2, metabolite of thromboxane A_2; 6-keto-PGF_{1a}, metabolite of prostacyclin. All values are expressed as means ± SEM. An asterisk indicates a significant difference (p <0.05) between autologous control and xenogeneic perfused groups.

group B led to a significant increase in 6-keto-PGF_{1a} levels to 1.083 ± 0.51 ng/ml compared to 6-keto-PGF_{1a} levels of 0.237 ± 0.073 ng/ml in group A and of 0.06 ± 0.04 ng/ml in group C. Later all groups showed similar concentrations of 6-keto-PGF_{1a} at prevalue levels in plasma samples during total perfusion time.

Plasma complement levels

Plasma samples were obtained in all groups and assayed for complement activation. As shown in Figure 2, C3a levels increased significantly in the plasma of group B and C immediately after start of hemoperfusion and remained at high levels during the experiment. Complement 4a showed a slight increase within the first 5 min of xenoperfusion and rose to the highest levels after 60 min in the non-treated group B, but clearly lower levels in group C. However, the C3a

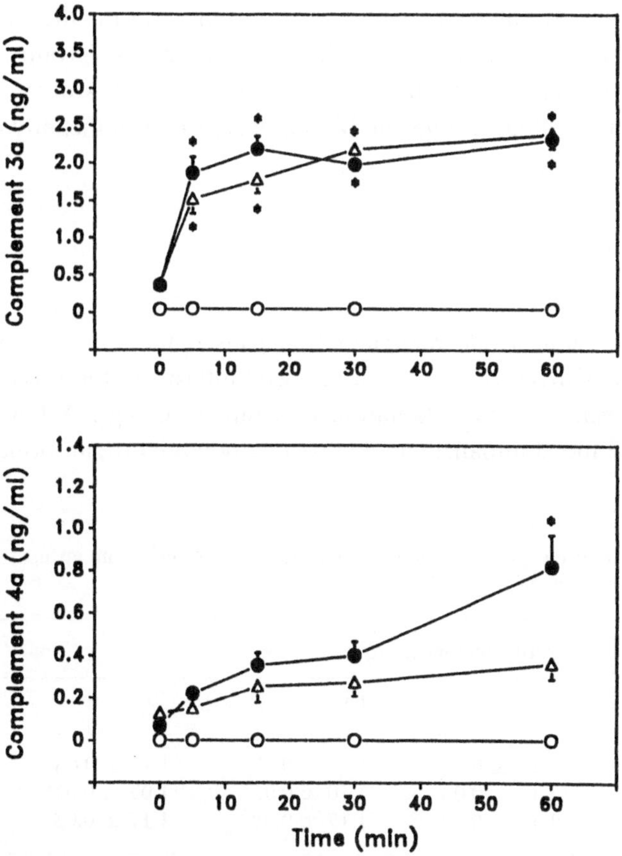

Fig. 2. Effect of auto- and xenoperfusion on activation of complement 3A (C3a) and complement 4a (C4a). See Figure 1 for abbreviations.

and C4a activity profile in group A did not change during autologous hemoperfusion and persisted at particularly low levels.

Renal hemodynamics

The renal perfusion pressure changed significantly between the non-treated (group B) and the WEB 2086BS treated (group C) experimental groups. As compared to the autologous perfused group A, the perfusion pressure increased in group B to about 29% but decreased in group C to about 36% within the first 30 min. These levels did not change during the whole perfusion time.

Kidney function

As an indicator of *ex vivo* kidney function the ratio between urine and plasma osmolality was determined (Table 2). Porcine kidneys perfused with autologous blood (group A) were able to concentrate constantly during the whole perfusion time. Xenoperfused but WEB 2086BS treated organs (group C) showed a similar behavior. However, the urine/plasma ratio of kidneys of group B perfused with untreated xenogeneic blood, decreased significantly during hemoperfusion.

Discussion

The success in clinical allotransplantation caused the situation of an extreme organ shortage. Currently, there is a renewed interest in the possibility of using xenogeneic organs for transplantation into human beings. A few experimental studies involve the chimpanzee or baboon as potential organ donor, but ethical

Table 2. Ratio of urine/plasma-osmolality during hemoperfusion in groups A–C. Data are expressed as the mean ± SEM.

	Perfusion time (min)			
U/P ratio group	5	15	30	60
Group A	1.13 ± 0.05	1.15 ± 0.07	1.17 ± 0.06	1.19 ± 0.07
Group B	1.16 ± 0.03	1.10 ± 0.02*	1.07 ± 0.01*	1.03 ± 0.01*
Group C	1.17 ± 0.02	1.17 ± 0.02	1.17 ± 0.03	1.17 ± 0.02

* Asterisks represent significant differences ($p < 0.05$) with respect to the autologous perfused group A.

as well as logistic problems do limit the availability of these scare species (10, 11). One way of avoiding this situation is suggested in using non-primate organ donors. Xenografting, which is defined as transplantation of organs or tissues between species of different zoological disparity, is classified into concordant and discordant transplantation. Grafts in closely related donor-recipient systems (concordant; e.g. baboon-man) are rejected within days, whereas xenografts in distantly related donor-recipient systems (discordant; e.g. pig-man) are destroyed rapidly within minutes. The hyperacute xenograft rejection occurring in discordant species combinations is thought so far to be primarily mediated by preformed anti-donor antibodies in the recipient, which react with antigens of the endothelium of the transplant after revascularization. In addition, the subsequent role of complement components, leukocytes, thrombocytes and vasoactive substances in mediating hyperacute graft rejection is implicated. Despite extensive experimental research reported by many authors (2, 9, 11), the general mechanism and the nature of the hyperacute rejection process *per se* is not yet fully understood. In animal experiments, the local intravascular release of platelet-activating factor (PAF) during HXAR of renal grafts has been demonstrated suggesting that this mediator may be in part responsible for graft rejection (1). The cells capable of synthesizing PAF can be divided into those involved in inflammatory processes and those belonging to shock target organs, e.g. the kidney or vasculature. Recently, specific antagonists to PAF have become available (12, 13, 14). The novel substance WEB 2086BS derived from triazolodiazepines has been reported to possess a PAF-antagonistic activity *in vitro* and *in vivo* (8). Our experimental purpose was to clarify the involvement of mediators (eicosanoids, PAF) and complement fractions in an *ex vivo* model of renal xenotransplantation very close to the clinical situation of discordent organ transplantation from non-primates to man and the possibility to bias the xenogeneic response by a specific PAF-antagonist. The study showed that the eicosanoid response during xenoperfusion in group B was markedly higher in PGI_2 compared to TxA_2, as indicated in Figure 1. The comparison of their release shown in this study may suggest a more important response of PGI_2 compared to TxA_2. Furthermore, the reaction in releasing PGI_2 and TxA_2 seemed to be related with the action of PNABs in this discordant transplantation model and not with a situation of pre-existing ischemia after perfusion with Eurocollins solution. This can be clearly implicated by consideration of the release of eicosanoids in the autologously perfused kidneys which were extremely low. A comparable low release of PGI_2 and TxA_2 could be found in group A and in the xenogeneic perfused but WEB 2086BS treated group C, indicating that the vasoactive lipid mediator PAF must be involved in the eicosanoid release in group B. The presence of TxA_2 may be related to thrombocyte interaction during xenoperfusion. On the other side, TxA2 as well as PGI_2 can be released by endothelial cells from the transplanted organ itself during xenoantibody mediated hyperacute rejection (1). In addition, the role of

PGI_2 release during xenoperfusion may be multifold. Prostacyclin is known to have a cytoprotective effect (15). It is difficult to prove this effect in this experimental study. The fact that PGI_2 was produced at high concentrations during xenoperfusion in group B but at extremely lower concentrations in groups A and C might indicate a possible response of prostacyclin acting in cytoprotection of xenogeneic perfused tissue.

Participation of humoral factors such as antibodies, complement and the coagulation system has been described in HXAR (16). It was suggested that antibodies and the complement system participate in the induction of this kind of rejection. In our study, complement levels of C3a and C4a were determined. These two anaphylatoxins are split products from Complement 3 and Complement 4 and will provide a direct index of their activation. The activation of C3a during the complement cascade indicates an unspecific response whereas C4a is a result of activation of the classical complement cascade by antibody-antigen interaction. Our results indicated a significant activation of C3a in group B and group C which could not be detected in the autologously perfused group A. This demonstrates the activation of the alternative complement pathway in both xenoperfused groups. By contrast, the measurement of C4a showed a significant activation in group B at high levels, but clearly lower levels in group C suggesting that the PAF-antagonist WEB 2086BS might influence the activation of the classical complement pathway in this discordant system (Figure 2). As a direct index of ex vivo kidney function the urine/plasma ratio for osmolality was measured. The data listed in Table 2 demonstrate that kidneys of group B loose their function during the experiment. In contrast, autologous perfused kidneys (group A) and kidneys treated with the PAF-antagonist were able to concentrate at all time.

In conclusion, the results described in this paper show that this discordant renal *ex vivo* xenograft model between pig and man is characterized by an almost immediate fixation of performed natural antibodies and complement activation, by major release of the arachidonic acid metabolities TxA_2 and PGI_2, by deterioration of the 'graft' hemodynamics and finally by the impairment of kidney function. One step in the pathogenesis of this HXAR might be the release of platelet-activating factor (PAF) acting as a trigger. This can be suggested from our results when the specific PAF-antagonist WEB 2086BS was used. It is conceivable that a causal relationship exists between the graft damage mediated by antibodies and complement, and the release of vasoactive lipid mediators (TxA_2, PGI_2, PAF, etc.) including vasoconstriction and the release of vasoactive lipid mediators (TxA_2, PGI_2, PAF, etc.) inducing vasoconstriction and microthrombosis resulting in graft failure. The results suggest that a polydirectional treatment with various specific and potent mediator antagonists might add to delay hyperacute rejection of xenografts for a clinical useful long-term xenograft survival.

Acknowledgements

The authors thank Dr H.M. Brecht (Boehringer Ingelheim, F.R.G.) for supplying us with WEB 2086BS, Mrs Bärbel Lorenz for expert technical assistance, and Mrs Lydia Rieder for typing the manuscript.

References

1. Camussi, G., Niesen, N., Tetta, C., Saunders, R.N. and Milgrom, F.: Release of platelet-activating factor from rabbit heart perfused in vitro by sera with transplantation alloantibodies. *Transplantation* **44**, 113—118 (1987).
2. Ito, S., Camussi, G., Tetta, C., Milgrom, F. and Andres, G.: Hyperacute renal allograft rejection in the rabbit. *Lab. Invest* **51**, 148—161 (1984).
3. Braquet, P., Touqui, L., Shen, T.Y. and Vergraftig, B.B.: Perspectives in platelet-activating factor research. *Pharmacol. Rev.* **39**, 97—145 (1987).
4. Weir, D.M. (ed.): *Handbook of Experimental Immunology*, pp. 720—744. Blackwell Scientific, Oxford, Edinburgh (1967).
5. Hugli, T.E. Vallota, H.E. and Müller-Eberhard, H.J.: Purification and partial characterization of human and porcine C3a anaphylatoxin. *J. Biol. Chem.* **250**, 1472—1478 (1975).
6. Gorski, J.P.: Quantitation of human complement fragment C4a in physiological fluids by competitive inhibition radioimmune assay. *J. Immun. Methods* **47**, 61—73 (1981).
7. Conzen, P., Habazettl, H., Gutmann, R., Hobhahn, J., Goetz, A., Peter, K. and Brendel, W.: Thromboxane mediation of pulmonary hemodynamic responses after neutralization of heparin by protamine in pigs. *Anesth. Analg.* **68**, 25—31 (1989).
8. Weber, K.H. and Heuer, H.O.: Hetrazepines as antagonists of platelet-activating factor. *Med. Res. Rev.* **9**, 181—218 (1989).
9. Miyagawa, S., Hirose, H., Shirakura, R., Nakata, S., Naka, Y. *et al.*: The mechanism of discordant xenograft rejection. *Transplant. Proc.* **21**, 520—521 (1989).
10. Reemtsma, K.: Xenografts. *Transplant. Proc.* **21**, 517—518 (1989).
11. Auchincloss, H.: Xenogeneic transplantation. *Transplantation* **46**, 1—20 (1988).
12. Braquet, P.: BN 52021 and related compounds; a series of highly specific PAF-acether receptor antagonists. *Prostaglandins* **30**, 687—690 (1985).
13. Shen, T., Hwang, S., Chang, M., Doebber, T., Lam, M., Wu, M. and Wang, X.: The isolation and characterization of kadsurenone from haifentent (piper futokadsura) as an orally active specific receptor antagonist of platelet-activating factor. *Int. J. Tissue Reac.* **5**, 339—345 (1985).
14. Terashita, Z., Tsushima, S., Yoshioka, Y., Nomura, H., Inada, Y. and Nishikana, K.: CV-3988, a specific antagonist of platelet-activating factor (PAF). *Life Sci.* **32**, 1975—1977 (1983).
15. Araki, H. and Lefer, A.M.: Role of prostacyclin in the preservation of ischemic myocardial tissue in the perfused cat heart. *Circulation Res.* **47**, 757—763 (1980).
16. Adachi, H., Rosengard, B.R. and Hutchins, G.M.: Effects of cyclosporine, aspirin, and cobra venom factor on discordant cardiac xenograft survival in rats. *Transplant. Proc.* **19**, 1145 (1987).

63. Antibody-induced rejection of established pig proislet xenografts in CD4$^+$ T cell depleted diabetic mice

J. DENNIS WILSON, CHARMAINE J. SIMEONOVIC and RHODRI CEREDIG

Introduction

The xenotransplantation of pancreatic islet tissue between phylogenetically disparate species has generally been restricted to the use of immunoincompetent athymic nude mice as transplant recipients (1, 2). Such studies have bypassed the immunological problems of graft rejection. Studies in our laboratory have investigated the mechanism(s) of rejection of fetal pig proislet (pancreatic islet precursor) xenografts in CBA/H (H-2^k) mice. This analysis was carried out in two ways: (i) using Cyclosporine A (CsA) immunosuppression and (ii) using *in vivo* administration of mAbs to CD4 and CD8 T cell subsets. CsA immunosuppression prevented the rejection of pig proislet xenografts only for the duration of CsA treatment (3). The normal mechanism of rejection of pig proislet xenografts was therefore shown to be CsA-sensitive, suggesting a role for T cells in the rejection process. To identify which T cell subpopulation was involved in the rejection process, transplant recipients were depleted of CD4 or CD8 T cells via the *in vivo* administration of anti-CD4 (GK1.5)(4) mAb or anti-CD8 (49—11.1)(5) mAb, respectively. Only treatment with anti-CD4 (GK1.5) mAb resulted in the histological survival of developing pig islet tissue at 2 weeks post-transplant (6). Thus, the rejection of pig proislet xenografts in mice was shown to be CD4$^+$ T cell-dependent. In addition, the survival of pig proislet xenografts extended beyond 6 weeks post-transplant without additional mAb treatment (3, 7). This finding indicated that, unlike CsA immunosuppression, *in vivo* anti-CD4 mAb therapy can result in proislet xenograft survival far beyond the period of treatment. The GK1.5 mAb dose determined the duration of CD4$^+$ T cell depletion and the extent to which the survival of pig proislet xenografts was prolonged (7). We have also demonstrated long-term survival and function of pig proislet xenografts in initially CD4$^+$ T cell-depleted, streptozotocin-induced diabetic mice (8, 9). Diabetic recipients in which normoglycemia had been restored following pig proislet xenotransplantation failed to reject their long-term functioning grafts following challenge with pig peripheral blood lymphocytes, MHC-identical to the grafted tissue (8, 9). These findings suggested that such animals were xenograft-tolerant. The present study examines the susceptibility of these established xenografts to humoral rejection mechanisms and identifies a possible mechanism responsible for xenograft tolerance.

Methods

Pig proislets (pancreatic islet precursors) were prepared by collagenase (6 mg/ml) digestion of fetal pig pancreas (dd haplotype (10), 66—73 days of gestation) followed by culture of the digested tissue for 5 days of gestation) followed by culture of the digested tissue for 5 days at 37½C in 10% CO_2, 90% air (6,7). Diabetes was induced in CBA/H ($H\text{-}2^k$) mice by intravenous streptozotocin (250 mg/kg) (8, 9). Diabetic mice received injections of GK1.5 mAb (4.2—5.4 mg protein 9/0.5 ml/injection) i.p. on days −1, 1, 3, 7 and 10 or −1, 1, 3, 7, 10, 14, 17 and 21. One half or three quarters of a fetal dd pig pancreas equivalent of proislets was transplanted beneath the kidney capsule on day 0 (8, 9). Non-fasting blood glucose levels were measured using a Beckman Glucose Analyzer 2 (Beckman, Fullerton, CA). The criterion for reversal of diabetes was the restoration of blood glucose levels to within the normal range (6.5—10.1 mmol/l). Pig peripheral blood lymphocytes (PBL) were prepared from EDTA-whole dd pig blood by centrifugation at 550 g for 30 min at 18½C through Ficoll-Paque (Pharmacia) (9). Anti-pig antibody levels in sera were monitored and quantitiated by single colour flow microfluorimetry (FMF) (9) Freshly isolated dd pig PBL were incubated with graded dilutions of sera and bound antibodies were revealed using FITC-labelled sheep anti-mouse Ig (Silenus). Hyperimmune anti-dd PBL serum was prepared in normal CBA/H mice which received 7 injections of 5×10^6 dd pig PBL i.p. over 10 weeks (9). Anti-pig Ig was semipurified from hyperimmune serum by ammonium sulphate precipitation followed by dialysis into PBS. Ig isotypes in hyperimmune serum and sera from transplanted mice were analysed using sheep red blood cell (SRBC) coupled rat anti-mouse IgG_1 IgG_{2a}, IgG_{2b}, IgG_3, IgA and IgM mAbs (Serotec mouse mAb isotyping kit; MMIT RCI) in a rosetting assay (11); 0.05% methyl violet (11) was used to facilitate identification of pig lymphocytes.

Results

Normoglycemia was achieved in 7/12 recipient mice by 37—94 days post-transplant; the remaining 5/12 animals either remained diabetic for the duration of the study or showed temporary reversal of diabetes (8). At 106—146 days, 6 of the 7 animals with long-term functioning grafts received two injections of 5×10^6 followed by 5×10^7 dd pig PBL i.p. over 3 weeks. All mice remained normoglycemic indicating that the PBL injections failed to stimulate xenograft rejection. FMF analysis of sera from these mice (± PBL) showed a strong anti-pig antibody response with staining titres of 2.6—14.4 × background (9). Parallel studies in acutely $CD4^+$ T cell-depleted CBA/H mice showed that the anti-pig antibody response was $CD4^+$ T cell-dependent (9). These findings indicated that (i) the anti-pig antibody produced in xenografted mice was insufficient to induce xenograft rejection and (ii) $CD4^+$ T cell recovery was well established (9). To determine whether established proislet xenografts were susceptible to antibody-mediated damage, hyperimmune CBA/H anti-dd pig PBL serum or semipurified Ig was administered (0.5 ml injection) i.p. to 6/7 host mice. All grafts were rejected, as indicated by the return of diabetes in host animals and by histological appearance. Histological examination of these grafts at 8—12 days after transfer of hyperimmune serum/Ig showed extensive graft destruction often with small amounts of damaged or intact islet tissue remaining. Sera taken from these mice at 8—17 days post-hyperimmune serum or Ig showed anti-dd pig staining titres of 42—50 × background (9). $CD4^+$ T cell depletion immediately prior to administration of semi-purified hyperimmune Ig did not alter the kinetics of rejection. These studies demonstrated that established pig proislet xenografts were susceptible to antibody-mediated destruction and that the process of antibody-mediated rejection following passive transfer of hyperimmune Ig was $CD4^+$ T cell-independent. Comparison of Ig isotypes in hyperimmune serum and sera from transplanted mice showed significant qualitative differences in IgG. At 7 days post-final PBL challenge, sera from transplanted mice contained only 23.5 ± 8.0% of the IgG_{2a} content of hyperimmune serum, 44.9 ± 47.7% of IgG_{2b}, 53.1 ± 23.4% of IgG_3 and 70.2 ± 6.2% of IgG_1. At 10—12 days post *in vivo* administration of hyperimmune serum of Ig, the IgG_{2b} content of sera from xenografted mice showed a significant > 4-fold increase to 98.7 ± 14.1% of that in hyperimmune serum and the IgG_3 content increased 1.6-fold to 83.6 ± 30.7%; there were no significant changes in IgG_1 and IgG_{2b} levels. These data suggest that IgG_{2a} may be the active component of hyperimmune serum responsible for mediating xenograft destruction.

Discussion

This study indicates that the mechanism of preventing xenograft rejection by anti-CD4 treatment *in vivo* involves not only initial $CD4^+$ T cell depletion but also qualitative modulation of a $CD4^+$ T cell-dependent anti-pig antibody response. We propose that more than one mechanism involving $CD4^+$ T cells is involved in proislet xenograft rejection. The first, operating early after transplantation is antibody-independent and involves $CD4^+$ T cells acting as effector cells in the rejection reaction (7). The second mechanism may act at later times and may be antibody-dependent, possibly directed at antigens on vascular endothelium (12). Such a late-acting mechanism may explain the chronic rejection of adult human islet xenografts in initially CD4$^+$ T cell-depleted mice (13). The presents study suggests that in animals carrying long-term, functioning pig proislet xenografts, the CD4$^+$ T cells that have regenerated in the presence of the xenograft are partly tolerant of pig xenoantigens. This is in contrast to the situation where mouse adult islet allografts have been successfully grafted to CD4$^+$ T cell-depleted recipients; in this instance, priming with mouse spleen cells resulted in graft rejection (14, 15) indicating absence of tolerance induction and suggesting that different rejection mechanisms may operate for islet tissue allografts and xenografts (7). We postulate that xenograft tolerance may result from dysfunction of Th1 or Th2 CD4$^+$ T cells that recover in initially CD4$^+$ T cell-depleted hosts, giving rise to altered regulation of B cell function (antibody production).

References

1. Korsgren, O., Sandler, S., Landstrom, A.S., Jansson, L. and Andersson, A.: Large-scale production of fetal porcine pancreatic islet-like cell clusters. *Transplantation* **45**, 509—514 (1988).
2. Tuch, B.E., Grigoriou, S., and Turtle, J.R.: Growth and hormonal content of human fetal pancreas passaged in athymic mice. *Diabetes* **35**, 464—469 (1986).
3. Simeonovic, C.J., Ceredig, R. and Wilson, J.D.: Mechanism of rejection of fetal pig proislet xenografts in mice. *Transplant. Proc.* **21**, 2728—2729 (1989).
4. Dialynas, D.P., Quan, Z.S., Wall, K.A., Pierres, A., Quintans, J., Loken, M.R., Pierres, M. and Fitch, F.W.: Characterisation of the murine T cell surface molecule, designated L3T4, identified by monoclonal antibody GK1.5: similarity of L3T4 to the human Leu-3/T4 molecule. *J. Immunol.* **131**, 2446—2451 (1983).
5. Hogarth, P.M., Edwards, J., McKenzie, I.F.C., Goding, J.W., Liew, F.Y.: Monoclonal antibodies to the murine Ly-2.1 cell surface antigen. *Immunology* **46**, 135—144 (1982).
6. Wilson, J.D., Simeonovic, C.J., Ting, J.H.L. and Ceredig, R.: Role of CD4$^+$ T cells in the rejection by mice of fetal pig proislet xenografts. *Diabetes* **38**, 217—219 (1989).
7. Simeonovic, C.J., Ceredig, R. and Wilson, J.D.: Effect of Gk1.5 monoclonal antibody dose on survival of pig proislet xenografts in CD4$^+$ T cell-depleted mice. *Transplantation* (in press).
8. Simeonovic, C.J., Ceredig, R. and Wilson, J.D.: Reversal of diabetes in CD4$^+$ T cell-depleted mice by xenotransplantation of pig proislets. *Transplant. Proc.* **21**, 3811—3812 (1989).
9. Simeonovic, C.J., Wilson, J.D. and Ceredig, R.: Antibody-induced rejection of functioning pig proislet xenografts in CD4$^+$ T cell-depleted diabetic mice. *Transplantation* (in press).
10. Kirkman, R.L., Colvin, R.B., Flye, M.W., Leight, G.S., Rosenburg, S.A., Williams, G.H. and Sachs, D.H.: Transplantation in miniature swine. VI. Factors influencing survival of renal allografts. *Transplantation* **28**, 18—23 (1979).
11. Parish, C.R. and McKenzie, I.F.C.: A sensitive rosetting method for detecting subpopulations of lymphocytes which react with alloantisera. *J. Immunol. Methods* **20**, 173—183 (1978).
12. Jooste, S.V., Colvin, R.B., Soper, W.D. and Winn, H.J.: The vascular bed as the primary target in the destruction of skin grafts by antiserum. I. Resistance of freshly placed xenografts of skin to antiserum. *J. Exp. Med.* **154**, 1319—1331 (1981).
13. Ricordi, C., Lacy, P.E., Sterbenz, K. and Davie, J.M.: Low-temperature culture of human islets of in vivo treatment with L3T4 antibody produces a marked prolongation of islet human-to-mouse xenograft survival. *Proc. Natl. Acad. Sci. USA* **84**, 8080—8084 (1987).

14. Shizuru, J.A., Gregory, A.K., Chao, C.T.B. and Fathman, C.G.: Islet allograft survival after a single course of treatment of recipient with antibody to L3T4. *Science* **237**, 278–280 (1987).
15. Hao, L., Wang, Y., Gill, R.G. and Lafferty, K.J.: Role of the L3T4$^+$ T cell in allograft rejection. *J. Immunol.* **139**, 4022–4026 (1987).

64. Occurrence of malignancies in immunosuppressed organ transplant recipients

ISRAEL PENN

Prolonged or intensive immunosuppressive therapy used in organ transplantation is associated with certain complications: side effects peculiar to each of the agents, an increased incidence of infections, and an increased risk of certain cancers. In this report we provide data concerning the problem of malignancies based on data sent to the Cincinnati Transplant Tumor Registry (CTTR) up to March 1990.

Incidence of tumors

The CTTR has data on 4997 post-transplant malignancies that occurred in 4692 recipients, of whom 4333 received kidney transplants, 207 heart, 71 liver, 60 bone marrow, 13 pancreas, 5 heart-lung, 2 abdominal organ clusters, and 1 pancreatic transplant. Cancers commonly seen in the general population (carcinomas of the lung, breast, prostate, colon and invasive uterine cervical carcinomas) showed no increase or even a decrease. Only 2 types of neoplasm, commonly seen in the general population, were encountered in significant numbers among transplant patients. Excluding lip cancers the percentage of non-melanoma skin cancers was no different from that observed in the general population (36% vs 32% of tumors), but the incidence of squamous cell carcinomas (SCCs) was markedly increased (see below).

The only other common tumor in the general population seen also in transplant patients was *in situ* carcinoma of the uterine cervix (3% vs 3% of tumors). If non-melanoma skin cancers and *in situ* carcinomas of the cervix were excluded, as they are from most cancer statistics, we then observed a variety of tumors in transplant patients that were uncommon in the general population (1, 2): lymphomas 21% vs 5%; lip cancers 6% vs 0.3%; Kaposi's sarcoma (KS) 6% vs a negligible incidence; carcinomas of the vulva and perineum 4% vs 0.6%; carcinomas of the kidney 5% vs 2%; sarcomas (excluding KS) 1.7% vs 0.5%; and hepatobiliary tumors 3% vs 1%.

Clinical features of post-transplant tumors

The tumors affected a relatively young group of people whose average age at the time of transplantation was 40 years (range 3 months to 80 years) (1). Forty-eight percent were under 40 years of age at the time of transplantation. Sixty-five percent were male in keeping with the 2 : 1 ratio of male to female patients who undergo renal transplantation (1).

The incidence of cancer increased with the length of follow-up after transplantation. A study of 3846 Australian renal transplant recipients showed an incidence of 3% at 1 year, 14% at 5 years and 49% at 14 years (3). These startling figures should be interpreted with caution as most tumors were skin cancers (which are very common in Australia) and the number of 14-year survivors was relatively small. Nevertheless, they stress the need to follow transplant patients indefinitely.

As the length of follow-up of organ transplant recipients has increased it became evident that certain tumors appeared at fairly distinct intervals after transplantation (1). In contrast with other known oncogenic stimuli in man, which often take 15—20 years or more before they cause clinical lesions, cancers were diagnosed a relatively short time after transplantation. KS was first to appear at an average of 20 (range 2—225.5) months after transplantation. Lymphomas appeared at an average of 34 (range 1—196.5) months after transplantation. Carcinomas of the vulva and perineum appeared at the longest time after transplantation at an average of 103 (range 9—241.5) months. Including all tumors the average time of their appearance was 61 (range 1—298.5) months.

Cancers of the skin and lips

The most common tumors (38%) affected the skin and lips (Table 1). Their incidence varied with the amount of sunshine exposure (1, 3). In regions with limited exposure, there is a fourfold to sevenfold increase, but in areas with copious sunshine there is an almost 21-fold increase over the already high incidence seen in the local population. In addition, lip cancers are increased 29-fold in incidence as compared with controls (4). Almost all the increase was in SCCs (see below), but an Australian study also showed a fivefold increase in malignant melanomas (3). The incidence of skin cancers increased with the length of follow-up after transplantation as demonstrated by an Australian study of 3846 renal transplant recipients of whom 11% had cancers at 5 years, 29% at 10 years and 43% at 14 years.

Skin cancers in transplant patients showed some unusual features compared with similar lesions in the general population (1). Basal cell carcinomas (BCCs) outnumber squamous cell carcinomas (SCCs) in the general population by 5 to

Table 1. 4997 de novo malignancies in organ allograft recipients.

Type of tumor	No. of tumors[a]
Cancers of skin and lips	1891
Lymphomas	726
Carcinomas of the lung	259
Carcinomas of uterus (cervix 215; body 31; unknown 3)	249
Kaposi's sarcoma	201
Carcinomas of colon and rectum	188
Carcinomas of the kidney (host kidney 145; allograft kidney 14; unknown 7)	166
Carcinomas of breast	157
Carcinomas of the vulva, perineum, penis, scrotum	140
Carcinomas of the head and neck (excluding thyroid, parathyroid and eye)	136
Metastatic carcinoma (primary site unknown)	118
Carcinomas of urinary bladder	111
Leukemias	110
Hepatobiliary carcinomas	88
Carcinomas of thyroid	65
Carcinomas of prostate gland	61
Sarcomas (excluding Kaposi's sarcoma)	59
Cancers of stomach (2 carcinoid tumors)	56
Testicular carcinomas	52
Ovarian cancers	41
Miscellaneous neoplasms	123

[a] There were 4692 patients of whom 288 (6%) had two or more distinct tumor types involving different organ systems. Of these, 15 patients each had three separate types of cancer and 1 had four.

1, but the opposite was true in transplant recipients in whom SCCs outnumbered BCCs by 1.8 to 1. In the general population SCCs occur mostly in people in their 60s and 70s but the average age of transplant patients was 30 years younger. In addition, the incidence of multiple skin cancers in this worldwide collection of patients (present in at least 41%) is remarkably high and is similar to that seen only in areas of copious sunlight. Several individuals each had more than 100 skin cancers. SCCs were more aggressive in transplant recipients than in the general population. Metastases to lymph nodes occurred in 120 of the 1891 patients (6.3%) of which 81% were from SCCs and only 13% from melanomas. In addition, 5.2% of the skin cancer patients died of their malignancies with 63% of deaths being caused by SCCs and only 31% by melanomas. In contrast, most lymph node metastases and deaths from skin cancer in the general population are caused by melanomas.

Some conditions that are common in transplant patients can closely resemble skin cancers (1). They include warts, hyperkeratoses and keratoacanthomas. If there is any suspicion of malignancy one should biopsy any questionable lesions. Lip cancers may also pose diagnostic problems as they frequently are atypical, and appear as superficial ulcers that do not have an indurated base and rolled everted edge. Occasionally two superficial lip cancers may occur simultaneously. It is advisable to biopsy all lip ulcers which persist for more than a month except during the early post-transplant period when herpetic ulcers are common.

Non-Hodgkin's lymphomas

Of a total of 726 lymphomas in the CTTR (Table 2) only 20 (3%) were cases of Hodgkin's disease whereas it comprises 14% of lymphomas in the general population (1, 2). Similarly, myeloma comprised only 29 cases (4%) compared with a 21% incidence among lymphomas in the general population (1, 2). The bulk of the post-transplant lymphomas (677) were non-Hodgkin's lymphomas (NHLs) which made up 93% of the lymphomas compared with only 65% in the general population (1, 2). The high incidence found in the CTTR is confirmed by two epidemiologic studies that show that the incidence of NHLs is increased 29- to 49-fold above that observed in age-matched controls (5).

Table 2. Most common immunosuppressive measures used.

Agent	No. of patients
Prednisone	4605
Azathioprine	4182
Antilymphocyte globulin (ALG)	1211
Cyclosporine	1131
Splenectomy	649
Local irradiation of the homograft	636
Cyclophosphamide	204
Actinomycin	188
Monoclonal antilymphocyte antibodies	114
Total body irradiation	53
Thoracic duct fistula	39
Methotrexate	20

Morphologically most NHLs were classified as immunoblastic sarcomas, reticulum cell sarcomas, microgliomas or large cell lymphomas (1). Of those studied immunologically, 86% arose from B lymphocytes, 13% were of T cell origin and 1% were of null cell origin. Fifty-one percent involved multiple organs or sites while 49% were confined to a single organ or site. Post-transplant NHLs differed from their counterparts in the general population in several respects (1). Whereas extranodal involvement occurs in from 24 to 48% of NHL patients in the community at large, it was present in 70% of NHLs in transplant patients. In the general population about 1% of NHLs affect the brain parenchyma, whereas in organ transplant patients 29% involved the central nervous system (CNS), usually the brain, in which the lesions were frequently multicentric in distribution. Spinal cord involvement was rare. Another notable feature was that in 65% of patients with CNS involvement the lesions were confined to the brain, whereas in the general population cerebral lymphomas are frequently associated with involvement of other organs.

The clinical presentation of NHLs was extremely variable (6, 7). Some patients were completely asymptomatic or presented with a picture resembling infectious mononucleosis. Other presenting features included fever, night sweats, upper respiratory infection, weight loss, diarrhea, abdominal pain, lymphadenopathy and tonsillitis. Tonsillar enlargement was sometimes so massive that emergency tracheotomy was necessary. As the gastrointestinal tract was frequently involved a quite common presentation was acute perforation of an intestinal lesion causing peritonitis. Less commonly gastrointestinal bleeding or intestinal obstruction was the major feature. At times patients presented with lung lesions, a renal mass or prostatic obstruction. Occasionally the presentation imitated allograft rejection and the diagnosis was made when an atypical lymphoblastic infiltrate was found in a biopsy specimen. Some patients presented with disseminated sepsis and multiple organ failure and the diagnosis was only made at autopsy examination.

A possible CNS lymphoma should be suspected whenever a transplant patient develops neurologic symptoms (1). A thorough work-up is necessary and may include examination of the cerebrospinal fluid, computerized axial tomography, electroencephalography, radionuclide brain scan, cerebral angiography and magnetic resonance imaging. Such tests help to exclude other causes of neurologic symptoms in these patients such as hypertensive encephalopathy, meningitis, brain abscess or intracranial bleeding.

Kaposi's sarcoma

The frequent occurrence of Kaposi's sarcoma (KS) in transplant patients stands in stark contrast with its incidence in the general population in the United States (before the Acquired Immunodeficiency Syndrome (AIDS) epidemic started) where it comprised only 0.02—0.07% of all cancers (1). The high incidence of KS in this worldwide collection of patients is comparable to that seen in tropical Africa where it occurs with greatest frequency, and where it makes up 3—9% of all tumors. It is remarkable that the number of transplant patients with KS (201) in the CTTR exceeds those with carcinomas of the colorectum (188) or breast (157) (Table 1). Apart from individuals with IDS, who are frequently afflicted by KS, there is probably no other series in which the number of KSs exceeds either of these two common cancers, except possibly in tropical Africa where KS occurs frequently and colon cancer is rare. An epidemiologic study shows a

400—500-fold increase in incidence of KS in renal transplant recipients compared with controls of the same ethnic origin (1).

KS affected males to females in a 2 : 1 ratio, similar to that seen in transplant patients having other cancers, but far less than the 9 : 1 to 15 : 1 ratio seen with KS in the general population (1). KS was most common in transplant patients who were Arabic, Jewish, black or of Mediterranean ancestry. Fifty-nine percent had non-visceral KS confined to the skin, conjunctiva, or oropharyngolaryngeal mucosa and 41% had visceral disease, affecting mainly the gastrointestinal tract and lungs, but other organs were also affected.

The physician should suspect KS whenever a transplant patient presents with reddish blue macules or plaques in the skin or oropharyngeal mucosa, or apparently infected granulomas that fail to heal (1). If the diagnosis is confirmed, a comprehensive work-up including CT scans of the chest and abdomen and upper and lower gastrointestinal endoscopy is needed to exclude any internal visceral involvement.

Carcinomas of the uterus

Carcinomas of the cervix occurred in 13% of women with post-transplant malignancies (Table 1). *In situ* lesions comprised at least 77% of cases. As mentioned above, the CTTR shows no difference in incidence from the general population. This finding is in contrast with two epidemiologic studies showing a 14—16-fold increased incidence in transplant patients. This suggests that many cases are being missed. Every post-adolescent female organ transplant recipient should have regular pelvic examinations and cervical smears to detect this disorder at an early stage.

Carcinomas of the vulva and perineum

The increased incidence of carcinomas of the vulva, perineum, scrotum, penis, peri-anal skin or anus in the CTTR (Table 1) is in keeping with an epidemiologic study showing that the incidence in renal transplant recipients is increased 100-fold compared with controls (4). Females outnumbered males by 2 : 1 in contrast with most other post-transplant cancers where males outnumbered females by more than 2 : 1.

One-third of patients had *in situ* lesions. A disturbing feature is that patients with invasive lesions were much younger (average age 42 years) than their counterparts in the general population, whose average age is usually between 50 and 70 years. Some transplant patients gave a history of condyloma acuminatum or, less frequently, herpes genitalis prior to the development of the malignancy (1). Female patients sometimes exhibited a 'field effect' with cancerous involvement not only of the vulva but also the vagina and/or uterine cervix (1).

Hepatobiliary tumors

An epidemiologic study shows a 30-fold increased incidence compared with controls (5). Most cases in the CTTR (Table 1) were hepatomas and a substantial number of patients gave a preceding history of hepatitis B infection (1).

Influence of immunosuppressive agents

The mot commonly used immunosuppressive agents are listed in Table 2. It appears that cancer is a complication of intense immunosuppression *per se* rather than being related to the use of any particular agent (1). However, certain agents appear to have modified the picture described above.

The pattern of malignancies seen after treatment with cyclosporine was somewhat different from that seen with so-called conventional immunosuppressive therapy (CIT), consisting of azathioprine (or cyclophosphamide) and prednisone, sometimes supplemented by antilymphocyte or antithymocyte globulin (8). Analysis of 1151 tumors that occurred in cyclosporine-treated patients showed a disproportionately high incidence of lymphomas (27% vs 11%) and KS (8% vs 3%) compared with 3846 CIT tumors. In addition there was a lower incidence of skin cancers (27% vs 41%), uterine cervical carcinomas (2% vs 5%) and carcinomas of the vulva and perineum (1% vs 3%) in the former group compared with the latter.

Allowance must be made for the fact that only 400 of the 1131 cyclosporine-treated patients (20 had more than one tumor) received cyclosporine only or cyclosporine with prednisone, and the remainder also received azathioprine or cyclophosphamide or both. When these cases are separated out (Table 3) we note a preponderance of lymphomas, KS, and renal tumors in the cyclosporine/prednisone group (group C) compared with the azathioprine/cyclophosphamide group (group A). In addition we still see a preponderance of skin cancers, carcinomas of cervix, and carcinomas of the vulva and perineum in group A compared with group C patients. The patients who received both types of immunosuppressive therapy (group B) displayed a pattern of malignancies intermediate between those seen in groups A and C.

A disproportionately high incidence of lymphomas was also seen in patients treated with monoclonal antibodies (OKT3; 64.1; Camplus; T_{12}). Of 114 tumors 74 (65%) were lymphomas and 7 (6%) were KS. As these agents were not used alone but in combination with two or more other agents the high incidence of lymphomas and KS probably are a reflection of very intensive

Table 3. Cancers after cyclosporine (excluding patients given azathioprine or cyclophosphamide).

Cancer	Group A[a] (%) (3846 tumors)	Group B[b] (%) (745 tumors)	Group C[c] (%) (406 tumors)
Skin and lip cancers	**41**	30	22
Lymphomas	11	27	**28**
Carcinomas of cervix	5	1	2
Carcinoma of vulva/perineum	**3**	1	0.5
Kaposi's sarcoma	3	7	10
Renal tumors	3	3	**6**

[a] Group A (3561 patients): Patients treated with azathioprine or cyclophosphamide or both with prednisone.
[b] Group B (731 patients): As above with the addition of cyclosporine.
[c] Group C (400 patients): Patients treated with cyclosporine only or with cyclosporine and prednisone.
Note: Some patients in each of the groups also received other treatments such as ALG, splenectomy, local irradiation of the graft, monoclonal antibodies, etc.

immunosuppressive therapy. A disproportionately high number of recipients of extrarenal organs developed lymphomas and KS after treatment with cyclosporine or monoclonal antibodies or both (as well as with some other agents) reflecting the need to save lives by reversing rejection of organs such as the liver and heart whereas with severe rejection of kidney allografts we are likely to discontinue immunosuppression and return the patient to dialysis.

Acknowledgement

The author wishes to thank his many colleagues throughout the world who have generously contributed data concerning their patients to the CTTR. Supported in part by grant number 6985 from the Veterans Administration.

References

Owing to space limitations and the vast number of papers on the subject only a few references are cited. Many others can be obtained from the articles cited.

1. Penn, I.: In: E. Pimental (ed.), *CRC Critical Reviews in Oncogenesis*, pp. 27—52. CRC Press Inc., Boca Raton, Florida (1989).
2. Silverberg, E., Boring, C.C. and Squires, T.S.: *Cancer statistics, 1990. CA* **40**, 9—26 (1990).
3. Sheil, A.G.R., Flavel, S., Disney, A.P.S. and Mathew, T.H.: Cancer development in patients progressing to dialysis and renal transplantation. *Transplant. Proc.* **17**, 1685—1688 (1985).
4. Blohme, I. and Brynger, H: Malignant disease in renal transplant patients. *Transplantation* **39**, 23—25 (1985).
5. Kinlen, L.: Immunosuppressive therapy and cancer. *Cancer Surveys* **1**, 565—583 (1982).

6. Hanto, D.W., Gajl-Peczalska, K.J., Frizzera, G., Arthur, D.C., Balfour, H.H. (Jr), McClain, K., Simmons, R.L., Najarian, J.S.: Epstein-Barr virus (EBV) induced polyclonal B-cell lymphoproliferative diseases occurring after renal transplantation. Clinical, pathologic, and virologic findings and implications for therapy. *Ann. Surg.* **193**, 356–369 (1983).
7. Starzl, T.E., Nalesnik, M.A., Porter, K.A., Ho, M., Iwatsuki, S., Griffith, B.P., Rosenthal, J.T., Hakala, T.R., Shaw, B.W. (Jr), Hardesty, R.L., Atchison, R.W., Jaffe, R. and Bahnson, H.T.: Reversibility of lymphomas and lymphoproliferative lesions developing under cyclosporine-steroid therapy. *Lancet* **1**, 583–587 (1984).
8. Penn, I. and Brunson, M.E.: Cancers following cyclosporine therapy. *Transplant. Proc.* **20** (Suppl. 3), 885–892 (1988).

65. Transmission of cancer with donor organs

ISRAEL PENN

Tumor transplantation in animals is an important field of cancer research. Inbred strains frequently are used to avoid histocompatibility differences between the donor of the cancer cells and the recipient, as these will cause rejection of the grafts. Where incompatibility exists it is necessary to use a modified recipient animal, either a congenitally immunodeficient one such as the 'nude' mouse which will even accept xenografts of human cancer cells, or one that has been made immunodeficient by immunosuppressive therapy.

Transplantation of cancer cells between humans was studied extensively by Southam (1). It proved to be unsuccessful except in recipients who had advanced malignancies and who demonstrated severe impairment of immune reactivity (2). Transplantation of neoplasia into healthy humans is, fortunately, extremely rare; otherwise, the surgeon who accidentally pricks a finger in the course of doing a cancer operation might be at risk. A unique case has been reported of transplantation of malignant melanoma from a daughter to her healthy mother, who eventually died of the malignancy (3). Presumably there was a close histocompatibility match which permitted growth and dissemination of the tumor in the recipient. In organ transplantation, despite the frequent occurrence of significant histocompatibility differences, immunosuppressive therapy may permit the survival of cancer cells inadvertently transplanted with an allograft obtained from a donor with cancer. The cells may multiply, invade surrounding structures and even disseminate widely (4—10). The present report deals with patients reported to the Cincinnati Transplant Tumor Registry up till March 1990.

Clinical material

We have data on 135 patients (4—10) who received organs from donors with cancer, excluding most donors with primary malignancies confined to the brain as these seldom spread outside the central nervous system (11). There were 128 renal allograft recipients, 3 cardiac, 3 hepatic and 1 pancreatic allograft recipient. One hundred and fourteen organs were obtained from 81 cadaver donors of which 51 were single-organ donors and 30 were multiple-organ donors from which 63 organs were used for transplantation. Of these, 28 donors each provided 2 organs, 1 provided 3, and 1 provided 4 organs. In addition there were 18 living related donors, and 3 were unrelated living donors, of whom 2 provided 'free' kidneys removed during operations for cancer.

Donor data

All allografts obtained from cadavers appeared grossly normal and free of cancer. One donor had been treated 5 years previously for carcinoma of the colon and had no tumor at autopsy examination. After transplantation, primary renal carcinomas developed in 2 recipients, but we cannot determine whether these had been present in the donors or had developed *de novo* at a later period. At the time that the organs were harvested, all the other cadaver donors had cancers, many of which were widely disseminated. The most common were carcinomas of the lung (26), kidney (19), malignant melanoma (6), breast (4), and hepatobiliary (4). In all there were 85 tumors among the 81 donors, including 3 brain tumors in donors with other malignancies. One of these donors who died of an astrocytoma, also had a renal carcinoma of one kidney and was the father of the recipient. The contralateral kidney was transplanted and the patient had no evidence of neoplasia when she died of unrelated causes 14 years later.

The cause of brain death was misdiagnosed in 10 donors (involving organs transplanted into 17 recipients). The diagnosis was either primary brain tumor or cerebral hemorrhage in the case of 3 donors with choriocarcinoma, 3 with renal cell carcinoma, 2 with bronchial carcinoma, 1 with malignant melanoma, and 1 with a primary carcinoma of unknown origin.

The 21 living donors had been treated for cancer within 5 years before nephrectomy or were found to have neoplasia at the time of donation, or developed evidence of it within 18 months after the procedure. They had a total of 22 malignancies of which the most common were carcinomas of the kidney in 7 and of the colon in 3.

One allograft was a 'free' kidney, removed from a patient as treatment for a hypernephroma. The organ was deliberately transplanted into a recipient dying of uremia, during the early era of transplantation when very few cadaver donors were available. The patient died 15 weeks after transplanation and at autopsy the cancer was found to have invaded adjacent structures.

Several months after transplantation a donor developed an anaplastic carcinoma at the nephrectomy site. The recipient manifested an identical tumor in the allograft and died of widespread metastases 10 months after transplantation.

Malignancy in recipients

In an extensive autopsy study Muiznieks *et al.* (12) found that patients with head and neck carcinomas had a 5% incidence of renal metastases, while those with bone, uterine, visceral and soft tissue sarcomas had a 10% incidence. In the present series of 135 patients, 64 (47%) had evidence of malignancy that involved the allograft. The actual incidence is higher if we exclude some donors who had neoplasms that were most unlikely to spread to the organs used for transplantation. One had had an *in situ* carcinoma of the cervix removed 2 years previously. One had a large basal cell carcinoma of the neck and 2 had had successful excisions of carcinomas of the colon and tongue, respectively, 5 years previously. The neoplasms were discovered from days after transplantation, when several renal allografts were removed for varying reasons, through various periods of time up to 38 months after transplantation. In the case of the recipients who did not show evidence of malignancy we presume that the allografts were free of cancer or that transmitted malignant cells failed to survive after transplantation.

In the 64 patients who developed post-transplant malignancies the tumors, in most instances, were histologically identical to those in the original donors. Fifty-seven (89%) received organs from cadavers and 7 received organs from living donors (11%). In 24 of the 64 recipients (37%) the malignancy was confined to the allograft. The original malignancies in the donors were 19 carcinomas of the kidney, 2 breast cancers, and 1 each of carcinoma of the thyroid gland, an oat cell carcinoma, and an anaplastic carcinoma. In 14 instances the tumors were discovered either at recipient autopsy or at the time of transplant nephrectomy, performed for rejection or for technical problems, while the other 10 (all renal tumors) were noted at the time of harvesting. The 10 renal tumors, 5 from related living donors and 5 from cadavers, were small and were treated by wide excision before transplantation in 7 patients. Nephrectomy 2—10 days after transplantation was performed in 2 patients because final biopsy reports indicated that the suspicious nodules were indeed malignant. In the case of the tenth kidney the initial biopsy report was equivocal. Re-exploration of the allograft 3 months after transplantation showed an increase in size of the nodule; a partial nephrectomy was performed and the diagnosis of carcinoma was confirmed. No recurrences were observed among the 10 patients in a follow-up of 13—186 (average 92) months.

Five patients (8%) had local spread of the neoplasms, 1 being the individual mentioned above, into whom a hypernephroma had been deliberately transplanted. The second patient, whose kidney allograft was obtained from a donor with bronchial carcinoma, died from infection 17 months after transplantation and the tumor was discovered at autopsy examination. Several months after transplantation the third patient developed a large mass in and adjacent to the transplant kidney (the donor had a carcinoma of the bronchus), which was treated by transplant nephrectomy, discontinuation of immunosuppression, and chemotherapy. A year later the patient has no evidence of residual tumor. The fourth patient, whose donor had a cerebellar medulloblastoma, treated by ventriculo-atrial shunting, was diagnosed as having tumor at 5 months post-transplantation and was treated by transplant nephrectomy, chemotherapy, and discontinuation of immunosuppressive therapy and was well 12 months later. The fifth patient, whose donor had a malignant melanoma, had a transplant nephrectomy for chronic rejection 44 months after transplantation when tumor in and around the allograft was discovered. The residual tumor underwent rejection after transplant nephrectomy and discontinuation of immunosuppressive therapy and was well on dialysis 124 months later.

Thirty-five patients (55%) had widespread metastases. Only one had received an allograft from a living donor. Cadaver donors with primary carcinoma of the lung (8 cases), choriocarcinoma (6 cases), malignant melanoma (6 cases), and carcinoma of the kidney (5 cases) were the major source of the organs that transmitted the tumors. One of the patients who received a kidney from a donor with widespread choriocarcinoma had cancer cells in the kidney but no histologic proof of dissemination, the diagnosis of which was based on high levels of human chorionic gonadotropin (hCG).

Twenty-seven of the recipients with metastases died of neoplasia. However, 7 patients had complete remissions following treatment. In 5 of them regression following reduction of the tumor burden by nephrectomy and cessation of immunosuppressive therapy (7, 10). Presumably their depressed immune systems were able to recover and to reject the cancers. In the other 2 patients these measures were supplemented by radiotherapy in one and chemotherapy in the other. In addition to these 7 patients, another patient is currently alive with tumor after undergoing transplant nephrectomy and discontinuation of immunosuppressive therapy. Although removal of the allograft and discontinuation of immunosuppression has been successful in some patients it is disappointing that the neoplasms in 11 other recipients failed to regress and caused a fatal outcome despite discontinuation of immunosuppression (11 patients), graft nephrectomy (9 patients), cytotoxic therapy (4 patients), immunotherapy (2 patients) and local radiotherapy (2 patients). Presumably the immune systems of these patients were unable to cope with widespread and extensive metastases which caused the fatal outcomes.

While transplant nephrectomy and discontinuation of immunosuppression is an option in kidney allograft recipients who can be returned to dialysis it cannot be utilized to any extent in recipients of heart or liver transplants. Of 8 extrarenal allograft recipients, only 1 is currently alive and well at 9 months whereas the other 7 all are dead from metastatic tumor.

Prevention of tumor transplantation

Most of the experience with transmitted malignancies was accumulated in the early years of transplantation, when the risks of grafting organs from donors with malignancy into immunosuppressed recipients were not appreciated. Today such hazards rarely occur because the transplant surgeon has learned some valuable lessons (4—8, 10, 13).

Every effort must be made to avoid transmitting cancer from donors to recipients. Each donor must be carefully screened for possible neoplasms. Measurement of chorionic gonadotrophin levels may be necessary in female donors in the child-bearing age group, who die of cerebral hemorrhage, because of the possibility that this disorder may have been caused by metastases from an undiagnosed choriocarcinoma, as occurred in several patients in this series (13). The need for caution is increasingly important now that we are harvesting multiple organs from a single donor. This does not mean that every potential donor with cancer must be rigidly excluded (6). Exceptions are those with low grade skin cancers, or with primary brain tumors which rarely spread outside the central nervous system. However, one must be certain that brain malignancies originated there since, in some instances autopsy examinations, performed after organ harvesting, have shown that the apparent brain cancers were actually metastases from occult primary neoplasms. We should also avoid using donors with brain tumors, which have been treated with ventriculoperitoneal or ventriculoatrial shunts, or have had craniotomies, as these open pathways for neoplastic dissemination. Thus, 3 patients who received grafts of the kidneys, pancreas and heart from a donor with a cerebellar medulloblastoma, treated with a ventriculoatrial shunt, developed widespread metastases, which were fatal in 2 of them.

Kidneys being harvested should be carefully examined (6). If a suspicious nodule is found, it should be biopsied and a prompt frozen section examination obtained. If cancer is diagnosed, the neoplasm should be widely excised and the kidney transplanted as was done successfully in several patients in this series. All such patients must be carefully followed for long periods for signs of recurrence. However, the kidney should not be transplanted if the malignancy is large or excision gives inadequate margins.

When a kidney has been transplanted from a cadaver donor in whom a later autopsy reveals a previously unsuspected, but widespread cancer, the surgeon should promptly remove the allograft as there is at least a 47% chance that it contains tumor cells (6). Sometimes the patient refuses to have the allograft removed, or the surgeon decides to leave it in place. In such an event the patient must be carefully evaluated at frequent intervals. Besides clinical examination, computerized axial tomography or magnetic resonance imaging may be performed and serum chorionic gonadotrophin levels measured in cases where the donor had choriocarcinoma. If a transplanted cancer becomes apparent at a later date, the allograft should be removed, immunosuppressive therapy discontinued, and the patient placed on regular dialysis. If necessary residual tumor can be treated with radiotherapy, chemotherapy, or immunotherapy with agents such as Interferon or Interleukin-2. If the tumor undergoes complete remission, further renal transplantation should be delayed until the patient has been free of cancer for at least 1 year.

The danger of inadvertently transmitting tumors from donor to recipients needs to be viewed in perspective. Most reported cases occurred in the pioneering era of transplantation, when the risks were not fully appreciated. Many tens of thousands of solid organ transplants have been performed, but only a handful of transmitted malignancies have occurred. Nowadays, with careful selection of donors, inadvertent transplantation of cancer has become a rare event.

Acknowledgement

The author is grateful to numerous colleagues working in transplant centers throughout the world for their generous contribution of data concerning their patients. Supported by a grant from the Veterans Administration.

References

1. Southam, C.M.: Host defense mechanisms and human cancer, *Ann. Inst. Pasteur.* **107**, 585 (1964).
2. Eilber, F.R. and Morton, D.L.: Impaired immunologic reactivity and recurrence following cancer surgery, *Cancer* **25**, 362 (1970).
3. Scanlon, E.F., Hawkins, R.A., Fox, W.W. and Smith, W.S.: Fatal homotransplanted melanoma. A case report, *Cancer* **18**, 782 (1965).
4. Penn, I.: *Malignant Tumors in Organ Transplant Recipients*, Springer-Verlag, New York (1970).
5. Penn, I.: Transplantation of kidneys containing primary malignant tumors, *Transplantation* **16**, 674 (1973).
6. Penn, I.: Transmission of cancer with donor organs, *Transplant. Proc.* **20**, 739 (1988).
7. Wilson, R.E., Hager, E.B., Hampers, C.L., Corson, J.M., Merrill, J.P. and Murray, J.E.: Immunologic rejection of human cancer transplanted with a renal allograft, *New Engl. J. Med.* **278**, 479 (1968).
8. Wilson, R.E. and Penn, I.: Fate of tumors transplanted with a renal allograft, *Transplant. Proc.* **7**, 327 (1975).
9. Martin, D.C., Rubini, M. and Rose, V.J.: Cadaveric renal homotransplantation with inadvertent transplantation of carcinoma, *J. Amer. Med. Assoc.* **192**, 82 (1965).
10. Zukoski, C.F., Killen, D.A., Ginn, E., Matter, B., Lucas, D.O. and Seigler, H.F.: Transplanted carcinoma in an immunosuppressed patient, *Transplantation* **9**, 71 (1970).
11. Hoffman, H.J. and Duffner, P.K.: Extraneural metastases of central nervous system malignancies, *Cancer* **56**, 1778 (1985).
12. Muiznieks, H.W., Berg, J.W., Lawrence, W., Jr and Randall, H.T.: Suitability of donor kidneys from patients with cancer, *Surgery* **64**, 871 (1968).
13. Baquero, A., Penn, I., Bannett, A., Werner, D.J. and Kim, P.: Misdiagnosis of metastatic cerebral choriocarcinoma in female cadaver donors, *Transplant. Proc.* **20**, 776 (1988).

66. Long-term experience with surgical repair for transplant renal artery stenosis

M. P. POSNER, A.L. KING, K. B. BROWN and H.M. LEE

Introduction

Hypertension, with or without accompanying renal dysfunction, is common following renal transplantation. The etiology is multifactorial and includes acute or chronic rejection, recurrence of original renal pathology in the transplanted kidney, underlying native renal disease, immunosuppression which includes cyclosporine, and main or branch renal artery stenosis (1—4). Our interest in the problem of transplant renal artery stenosis (TRAS) and its surgical repair is long standing (5—8). Herein we report our experience with this surgical entity over the past three decades.

Patients and methods

Between 1962 and 1989, 1054 kidney transplants (KT) have been performed at our center: 802 were from cadaver (CD) donors and 252 from living (LD) donors. In the time period before 1983, the majority of kidneys were preserved using pulsatile hypothermic perfusion. Since that time, most CD kidneys and LD kidneys have been stored at 4 °C on ice after *in-situ* perfusion with either Eurocollins (1983—87) or UW Solution (1988—89). The mean total preservation time for CD KTs has been approximately 30 hours. Standard techniques of implantation developed by the senior author (H.M.L.) have been used for all kidney transplants, with emphasis upon end-end arterial anastomosis in the early period of the study, and gradual favoring of end-side anastomosis in later years (since 1980). Attempts at keeping anastomosis time and total warm ischemic time to less than 30 minutes have been successful in almost all cases.

Postoperative care has been uniform and has included liberal use of sonography and nuclear perfusion scanning to rule out technical problems. Over the last 6 years, with the advent of cyclosporine (CyA) as part of our immunosuppressive regimen and its attendant nephrotoxicity, percutaneous core needle biopsy has frequently been used to confirm acute rejection.

Our post-transplant immunosuppressive protocol has evolved over the study period as follows: azathioprine and steroids, 1962—74; azathioprine, steroids, rabbit ATG, 1974—82; cyclosporine and steroids, 1983—84; azathioprine, steroids, rabbit ATG, delayed addition of cyclosporine, 1985—87; azathioprine, steroids, rabbit ATG or OKT3, delayed cyclosporine, 1987—89. 'Conventional' immunosuppression was given to 835 patients (prior to 1983) and 219 patients received an immunosuppressive regimen which included CyA (1983—89). Rejection episodes were treated initially with high-dose pulse methylprednisolone and if steroid resistant, patients were given either rabbit ATG or more recently, OKT3.

Our approach to the renal transplant patient who develops new onset (high diastolic) hypertension, or worsening of existing hypertension, with or without an audible bruit, where other etiologies (i.e. rejection, technical problems, CyA nephrotoxicity) have been satisfactorily excluded, has included the aggressive use of contrast angiography. Acute renal dysfunction in this setting has contributed to the urgency of evaluation.

Hemodynamically significant transplant renal artery stenosis was defined as greater than or equal to 50% narrowing of the lumenal diameter of the transplant renal artery. Criteria for repair included; (a) hypertension refractory to medical management (3 or more medications), (b) deterioration of renal function or (c) both, in the presence of a hemodynamically significant transplant renal artery stenosis. Intrarenal changes on arteriography suggesting chronic rejection were a deterrent to aggressive surgical intervention, and in recent years prompted biopsy confirmation. All patients meeting these strict criteria were subjected to repair of their renal artery stenosis. One patient underwent unsuccessful percutaneous transluminal angioplasty, which was subsequently salvaged by surgical repair. Renins were obtained in most of the patients, but were found to be useful only in the setting of 'three kidney' hypertension (native kidneys still *in situ*) where the decision to remove the native kidneys simultaneously was in question. Approximately 60% of the patients who came to repair had been previously bi-nephrectomized.

Postoperative results were classified as: excellent (cure) — hypertension relieved, renal function stabilized or improved; good (improved) — hypertension easier to control (less medications), renal function stable; poor (failure) — hypertension unchanged, renal function stable or worse. Follow-up was complete in over 90% of patients undergoing repair, with a range of 7 months to 20 years (mean 50 months). Results are reported as of each patient's longest follow-up interval.

Results

Hemodynamically significant TRAS meeting criteria for repair was discovered in 57 patients (5.4%). Four of these represented 'recurrence' following previous transplant renal artery stenosis repair. Forty CD KTs (5.2%) and 13 LD KTs (5.2%) developed symptomatic transplant renal artery stenosis. Of 219 KT patients receiving CyA as part of their immunosuppressive regimen, only 4 (1.8%) developed renal artery stenosis versus 53/835 (6.3%) of KT patients receiving conventional immunosuppression.

Presentation of symptomatic transplant renal artery stenosis occurred from 1 to 144 months following KT. Fifty percent developed the lesion in the first 6 months post-transplant, 30% between 6 and 12 months, 10% in the second year following transplantation and 10% from 2 to 12 years after KT.

Fifty-seven repairs were carried out in 53 patients using a variety of surgical techniques: 18 (31%) vein patch repair; 34 (60%) saphenous vein bypass; and 5 (9%) resection and end-end reanastomosis. The one patient who was salvaged after unsuccessful percutaneous angioplasty was treated by saphenous vein bypass with good postoperative outcome. Three (5.3%) restenoses occurred, all under path repairs, all successfully reoperated. One patient developed progression of a polar artery stenosis which became symptomatic and was repaired successfully.

At operation, four types of stenosis were encountered. The most commonly found lesion consisted of a long smooth narrowing in the donor artery beginning 1 cm distal to the anastomosis. Next most common was a sharp, short stenosis in the donor artery as well, followed by narrowing or kinking at the anastomosis, and external kinking of the donor or recipient artery, or both, being the least common.

Outcome following repair of transplant renal artery stenosis is illustrated in Table 1. Eighty-four percent of patients experienced good—excellent results (49% 'cure', 35% improved). One patient (1.7%) died with a functioning graft in the postoperative period of overwhelming sepsis, and 4 patients (7%) required transient hemodialysis postoperatively.

Ten patients developed deterioration of renal function despite satisfactory anatomical repair of transplant renal artery stenosis, and grafts were lost 2—24

Table 1. MCV TRAS Series, 1990.

		Outcome				
Type of repair	*n*	Excellent	Good	Poor	Mortality	Morbidity
Vein patch	18 (31%)	9 (50%)	5 (28%)	4 (22%)	0	1
S/V bypass	35 (60%)	17 (50%)	12 (35%)	5 (15%)	1	3
Reanastomosis	5 (9%)	2 (40%)	3 (60%)	0 (0%)	0	0
Totals	57 (100%)	28 (49%)	20 (35%)	9 (16%)	1 (1.7%)	4 (7%)
		84%				

months postoperatively. All had either angiographic or biopsy evidence of ongoing chronic rejection.

Although the number of rejection episodes per patient in the first 3 months did not correlate with either the development of arterial stenosis or outcome of repair, angiographic evidence of chronic rejection was, nevertheless, highly predictive of poor outcome following surgical repair. The quality of pre-repair renal function was likewise predictive of outcome. Whereas only 19/27 (70%) of patients with preoperative serum creatinine greater than 2.0 mg/dl obtained improvement, 97% (29/30) of patients with serum creatinine less than 2.0 mg/dl were improved following surgical intervention. This distinction may well reflect undetected, ongoing chronic rejection, in those patients with abnormal renal function who failed to improve.

No correlation between previous bi-nephrectomy, simultaneous bi-nephrectomy, donor source or age, recipient age or total preservation time, and development of, or outcome following repair of, transplant renal artery stenosis could be ascertained.

Discussion

The incidence of transplant renal artery stenosis has been reported in the range of 1—30% (1—3, 7—14), with the average of multiple series being 5—10% (14). This is consistent with our reported incidence of 5%. The suggestion has been made that it occurs more frequently following cadaveric renal transplantation, however our results do not confirm this (7). To a great extent, following exclusion of multiple other (more common) etiologies of post-transplant hypertension, the discovery of transplant renal artery stenosis depends upon how aggressive one is with angiographic investigation, which does carry a small but significant nephrotoxic risk (5, 8). It is clear that one cannot depend on the presence of a bruit overlying the kidney to lead one to angiography, since no more than 75% of clinically significant stenoses were heralded by a bruit (7). The risk of transplant renal artery stenosis going undetected and/or untreated includes not only the complications attendant to untreated hypertension, but ultimate deterioration of transplant renal function, either secondary to the hypertension, or due to sudden, subtle occlusion of the transplant renal artery (8). In recent years, we have found Duplex scanning to be of some utility in leading one to angiographic confirmation of transplant renal artery stenosis (15).

There seems to be no unified etiology for the development of transplant renal artery stenosis. Possibilities include atherosclerotic changes in the recipient vessels, trauma to donor/recipient arteries during implantation, imprecise surgical suture technique, flow disturbances, external factors (i.e. fibrosis, kinking), perfusion injury and angulation (2). Most series have suggested an immune mediated mechanism, since the majority of lesions found at surgery are confined to the donor artery (2, 3, 6, 8, 9—13). Our results corroborate this idea, and moreover suggest that the incidence has diminished since our patients have been receiving CyA as a part of their immunosuppressive regimen.

Reported results of surgical intervention for transplant renal artery stenosis have for the most part included small series, but in general suggest a favorable outcome following repair in the range of 75—85%, with minimal morbidity and low mortality (2, 3, 9—13). This is in contrast to recent reports of percutaneous transluminal angioplasty for transplant renal artery stenosis demonstrating only 50—60% clinical success rates, with reasonably high recurrence rates over the short term, and with unacceptable graft loss secondary to the intervention (16, 17). Moreover, repeat PTA for recurrence has been largely unsuccessful (17).

In summary, our results suggest that aggressive surgical therapy aimed at relief of transplant renal artery stenosis, is justified and durable, in those patients with hemodynamically significant symptomatic transplant renal artery stenosis when there is no evidence of intrarenal vascular changes consistent with ongoing chronic rejection.

References

1. Margules, R.M., Belzer, F.O. and Kountz, S.L.: Surgical correction of renovascular hypertension following renal allotransplantation. *Arch Surg.* **106**, 13—16 (1973).
2. Lacombe, M.: Arterial stenosis complicating renal allotransplantation in man: a study of 38 cases. *Ann. surg.* **18** (3), 283—288 (1975).
3. Dickerman, R.M., Peters, P.C., Hull, A.R., Curry, T.S., Atkins, C. and Fry, W.J.: Surgical correction of posttransplant renovascular hypertension. *Ann. Surg.* **192** (5), 639—644 (1980).
4. Kahan, B.D.: Cyclosporine. *New Engl. J. Med.* **321** (25), 1725—1738 (1989).
5. Smellie, V.A.B., Vinik, M. and Hume, D.M.: Angiographic investigation of hypertension complicating human renal transplantation. *Surg. Gynecol. Obstet.* May, 963—968 (1969).
6. Lee, H.M., Linehan, D., Pierce J. and Hume, D.M.: Renal artery stenosis and gastrointestinal hemorrhage in human renal transplantation. *Transplant. Proc.* **4** (4), 681—683 (1972).
7. Lee, H.M., Madge, G.E., Mendes-Picon, G. and Chatterjee, S.N.: Surgical complications in renal transplant recipients. *Surg. Clin. North Amer.* **58** (2), 285—304 (1978).
8. Ende, N., Currier, C.B., Johnson, K.H., Lee, H.M., Williams, M. and Wombolt, D.G.: Unusual vascular findings in transplanted kidneys. *Human Pathol.* **13** (3), 272—278 (1982).
9. Doyle, T.J., McGregor, W.R., Fox, P.S., Maddison, F.E., Rodgers, R.E. and Kauffman, H.M.: Homotransplant renal artery stenosis. *Surgery* **77** (1), 53—60 (1975).
10. Schacht, R.A., Martin, D.G., Karalakulasingam, R., Wheeler, C.S. and Lansing, A.M.: Renal artery stenosis after renal transplantation. *Amer. J. Surg.* **131**, 653—657 (1976).
11. Morris, P.J., Yadav, R.V.S., Kincaid-Smith, P., Anderton, J., Hare, W.S.C., Johnson, N., Johnson, W. and Marshall, V.C.: Renal artery stenosis in renal transplantation. *Med J. Australia* June, 1255—1257 (1971).
12. Lindsey, E.S., Garbus, S.B., Golladay, E.S. and McDonald, J.C.: Hypertension due to renal artery stenosis in transplanted kidneys. *Ann. Surg.* **181** (5), 604—610 (1975).
13. Eslami, H., Ribot, S., Brief, D.K., Alpert, J., Brener, B., Frankel, H.J., Goldblat, M. and Parsonnet, V.: Stenosis of the renal artery in human kidney transplantation. *J. Med. Soc. N.J.* **74** (3), 215—220 (1977).

14. Smith, R.B. and Ehrlich, R.M.: The surgical complications of renal transplantation. *Urol. Clin. North Amer.* **3** (3), 621–647 (1976).
15. Reinitz, E.R., Goldman, M.H., Seas, J., Rittgers, S.E. and Lee, H.M.: Evaluation of transplant renal artery blood flow by doppler sound spectrum analysis. *Arch. Surg.* **118**, 415 (1983).
16. Meakins, J.L.: Percutaneous transluminal dilatation for post-transplantation renal artery stenosis. *CMA Journal*, **123**, 711 (1980).
17. Mollenkopf, F., Matas, A. and Veith, F.J.: PTA for transplant renal artery stenosis. *Transplant. Proc.* **15**, 1089 (1983).

67. Lymphoproliferative disorders after liver transplantation (OLT): a recent experience

T.G. HEFFRON, J.C. EMOND, J.R. THISTLETHWAITE, X.M. ROGIERS, M.D. YANG, K.L. KING and C.E. BROELSCH

Introduction

Lymphoproliferative disorders (LD) have been recognized as a complication after organ transplantation. Past incidence has varied by immunosuppressive regimen and varies from 1 to 5%. It has been suggested that the recent use of lower doses of cyclosporine (Cy) might result in a lower incidence of this complication. To assess this, we reviewed our experience with LD in 230 patients receiving OLT since 1985.

Post-transplant lymphoproliferative disorders is a generic term to describe proliferation of B-lymphocytes that occur in immunosuppressed transplant recipients (1).

Materials and methods

Two hundred and thirty patients received 289 grafts between 1985 and 1989. All patients were managed using standard protocols based on cyclosporine and steroids +/− azathioprine (AZA) (Table 1). Cyclosporine was started 24 hours postoperation accepting therapeutic whole blood, HPLC levels 150—200, early postoperation and levels of 60—100 optimal after the first week. Solumedrol was tapered to 0.3 mg/kg in the first week with continued reduction throughout the first year (Table 2).

Biopsy proven rejection was treated by Solumedrol pulse therapy (500 mg

Table 1. Liver transplantation: the University of Chicago experience, 1985—89.

	Patients	Grafts
Children	112 (49%)	138 (48%)
Adults	118 (51%)	151 (52%)
Total	230	289

Table 2. Immunosuppression: liver.

Cyclosporine:	Starting 24 hours post-operation Whole blood HPLC 150—200 in first week Levels 60—100 optimal after first week
Solumedrol:	Tapered to 0.3 mg/kg in first week by POD7 with continued reduction
Imuran:	OR5 mg/kg Maintenance dose 1 mg/kg

bolus IU × 3 days). OKT3 treatment was used for failed treatment with Solumedrol. (D3 T-cells + OKT3) serum levels (100 mg/ml) were monitored to optimize successful therapy.

Results

Six liver transplant recipients (2.6%) who developed lymphoproliferative disorders included 4 children (3.6%) and 2 adults (0.9%). Median time of onset was 3 months. Sites of origin were tonsils and adenoids ($n = 1$), ethmoid sinus ($n = 1$), cervical lymph nodes ($n = 1$), and 3 in the liver graft ($n = 3$) (Table 3).

One lesion in an adult presented as a biliary stricture 3 months after transplantation, resulting from a periportal monoclonal B-cell lymphoma. He was treated with cessation of immuno-suppression. Four months after transplantation he developed Roux Y anastamotic breakdown and a spontaneous transverse colon perforation (both Bx. + for CMV) and, subsequently, expired due to sepsis. Five of 6 OLT patients (83%) with LD also had positive cultures for CMV. Twenty-two percent of patients without LD receiving OLT had positive cultures of CMV (Table 4).

All LD were of B-cell origin; 5 monoclonal and 1 polyclonal. Rejection treatment was required in 4 (67%), OKT3 in 2 (33%), and CMV infection

Table 3. Lymphoproliferative disorders after liver transplantation.

Case	Age/sex	Primary site	Time (months) after transplant
1	4 years/male	Nasopharynx	6
2	8 months/male	Liver explant	2
3	1 year/male	Ethmoid sinus	24
4	11 years/female	Cervical lymph node	9
5	56 years/male	Periportal mass (liver tx)	3.5
6	62 years/female	Liver biopsy	3.5

Table 4. Lymphoproliferative disorders after liver transplantation.

Case	Treatment	Alive	Rejection	OKT_3	CMV
1	Immunosuppression	No	No	No	Yes
2	Immunosuppression chemotherapy (CHOP)	No	Yes	Yes	No
3	Immunosuppression	Yes/2 years	Yes	No	Yes
4	Immunosuppression	No	Yes	Yes	Yes
5	Immunosuppression	No	Yes	No	Yes
6	Immunosuppression	No	No	No	Yes

occurred in 5 (83%). Comparative frequencies in other OLT patients were 78, 15 and 22% (Table 5).

One pediatric patient with polyclonal LD 9 months after transplantation responded promptly to reduction in immunosuppression and is asymptomatic after 2 years. Four of 5 patients with monoclonal LD were treated by reduction in immunosuppression and 1 by chemotherapy (CHOP). Only 1 presented late (24 months). All 5 died within 4 months of diagnosis associated with positive CMV culture and multiple septic complications (Table 4).

Discussion

These results demonstrate that LD continues to be a risk despite the modifications in the use of cyclosporine.

Median time of onset in our series (3 months) was much earlier than that reported in previous series. Besides its earlier presentation, LD had a more virulent course with death in 5 of 6 cases and no response to reduction or cessation of immunosuppression and/or surgery or chemotherapy. This differs from a large previous study in which 43% of patients had complete regression of lesions followed by various treatments (2).

It has been suggested by previous studies that lower doses of immunosuppressive agents (Cy) might result in a lower incidence of LD. In one study,

Table 5. Comparison of LD and non-LD patients.

	LD (%)	University of Chicago liver transplant experience (%)
Rejection	67	78
OKT_3	33	15
CMV	83	22

lymphomas occurred with large doses but when immunosuppression was reduced, no lymphomas were observed. Measured quantitative parameters of immunosuppression (mean cyclosporine level), number of days of T cell suppression, were higher in patients with lymphomas than in patients who were tumor free in this study (3, 4).

LD can be regarded as a complication of immunosuppression *per se* rather than as a side effect of any specific agent. The association of CMV and sepsis supports this and suggests a context of global immune failure.

Conclusion

LD, after liver transplantation, continues to be a risk despite modifications in cyclosporine. In our series LD are characterized by an even earlier appearance after transplantation with a virulent course unresponsive to therapeutic measures, including reduction or cessation of immunosuppression. The association of CMV and sepsis suggests a context of global immune failure.

References

1. Frizzera, G., Hanto, D.W., Gajl-Peczalska, K.J. *et al.*: Polymorphic diffuse B-cell hyperplasias and lymphomas in renal transplant recipients. *Cancer Res* **41**, 4262–4279 (1981).
2. Penn, I.: Cancers following cyclosporine therapy. *Transplantation* **93**, 32–35 (1987).
3. Braumbaugh, J., Baldwin, J.C., Stinson, E.B. *et al.*: Quantitative analysis of immunosuppression in cyclosporine heart transplant patients with lymphoma. *Heart Transplant.* **4**, 307–311 (1985).
4. Starzl, T., Porter, K. *et al.*: Reversibility of lymphomas and lymphoproliferative lesions developing under cyclosporine/steroid therapy. *Lancet* **1**, 583 (1984).

68. Experience with Kaposi's sarcoma in recipients of renal transplants in Tunisia

T. BEN ABDALLAH, A. EL-MATRI, C. KECHRID, R. BARDI,
F. BEN HAMIDA, F. EL-YOUNSI, H. BEN MAIZ, F. BEN AYED,
Y. GORGI and H. BEN AYED

Introduction

Kaposi's sarcoma (KS) is a rare tumor but its incidence is higher following renal transplantation and especially among people of Arab, Jewish and Mediterranean ancestry. We report 3 cases among 120 recipients of renal transplants followed-up for at least 3 years.

Materials and methods

In Tunisia, from 1979 to 1986, 4 transplanted patients developed Kaposi's sarcoma; 3 of them were followed-up by our team. All received cadaveric kidneys under triple immunosuppressive therapy (azathioprine, corticosteroids and cyclosporine A). All had at least one acute rejection and had been treated with methylprednisolone pulses and antilymphocyte globulin. Evaluation included physical examination and skin biopsy, chest X-ray, gastroscopy, colonoscopy, bronchoscopy and ultrasonography. Laboratory assessment included: HLA-A, -B and -DR typing in all cases and T-lymphocyte subsets (in 2 patients), CMV, anti-HIV antibodies, Hbs antigen and tuberculine and candida skin tests (Table 1).

Table 1. Immunologic data on patients with Kaposi's sarcoma

Patients	Age	Sex	HLA-DR	T-lymphocyte subsets	Ratio CD4/CD8*
No. 1	34	M	A2–11/B14–44 DR 2–4	TL 43% CD3 40%	1.14
No. 2	32	M	A2–26/B51–49 DR 4		
No. 3	36	F	A30/B18–50 DR37–4	TL 40% CD3 39.4%	1.06

* Immunologic data were mainly a decrease of the ratio CD4/CD8 with increase of CD8.

Results

The patients with Kaposi's sarcoma were 2 males and 1 female, aged 34, 31 and 36 years. The mean duration from transplantation to the appearance of Kaposi's sarcoma was 15, 23 and 11 months. They were HIV negative, CMV positive and had negative tuberculine and candidine skin test. Hbs test was positive in two cases.

At the beginning, patients 1 and 3 had only skin lesions mainly on the limbs, but patient 2 had, from the onset, a generalized sarcoma also involving lymph nodes, lungs, stomach, liver, colon and rectum. In all cases diagnosis was confirmed by pathology (Table 2).

In Case 1, where KS was localized to the skin, immunosuppressive therapy was decreased and chemotherapy was commenced with Vinblastine. At 34 months, renal function decreased progressively, serum creatinine increasing from 110 to 250 μmol/l. After a stable period, skin lesions became smaller but KS extended to trachea, bronchi and stomach. However, the patient is still living.

In Case 2, with a generalized KS, immunosuppression was decreased and Vinblastine added. Blood creatinine increased slightly, but the patient developed a CMV and pseudomonas lung infection and died 2 months after diagnosis.

In Case 3, immunosuppressive therapy was decreased but without the addition of chemotherapy. Serum creatinine remained stable after 34 months of follow-up and there has been a partial regresion of skin lesions.

Table 2. The outcome of Kaposi's sarcoma.

Patient	Skin lesion	Visceral KS	Decrease of immunosuppression/ add Vinblastine	Renal function	Outcome of patients
No. 1	Partial regression	Secondary extended	Yes/Yes	Decreased	Living 34th month
No. 2	Partial regression	Primarily visceral	Yes/Yes	Decreased	CMV + pseudo-lung infection, death 2nd month
No. 3	Partial regression	No	Yes/No	Stable	Living 34th month

Discussion

In our center, the incidence of Kaposi's sarcoma is 8.3%, as in other reported series of Arab recipients (3); 400—500 times more than in the general population. In our center, there were 2 males and 1 female while in the literature, the sex ratio is 2 : 1. The interval between transplantation and diagnosis was 16.6 months while in the literature, it ranges between 1 and 72 months.

In our center, the disease was generalized in 2 cases and only cutaneous in 1. In the literature, 2 out of 3 cases are benign skin KS, usually widespread to limbs and sometimes the face and trunks (2). In one-third of cases, the disease is generalized, cutaneous and multivisceral, involving gastrointestinal tract (50%), lymph nodes (10%), liver, spleen, pancreas, lungs and adrenal glands.

The diagnosis is usually clinical but confirmed by pathology. Staging must be done to discover visceral involvement and associated diseases. Disturbance of cellular immunity is usual. It consists of cutaneous anergy to skin tests, decrease of T lymphocytes, decrease of the CD4/CD8 ratio, with increase of CD8, as occurred in 2 of our cases.

Viral factors may play a role in the pathogenicity and the relationship between KS and CMV and Epstein Barr disease is still unclear.

In our experience, immunosuppression was reduced in all cases and Vinblastine was added in the generalized form of disease, but it is usually advised to cease immunosuppression if this is associated with infection.

The outcome depends on the localization of the sarcoma. The prognosis is good in localized skin disease and bad when it is generalized and specially when associated with infection.

Conclusion

We confirm that KS has a higher incidence in transplant recipients having Mediterranean ancestry, especially adult males. Generalized KS is usually rarer but its prognosis is poor. Reduction in immunosuppression may be sufficient to induce skin lesions to regress but, in generalized KS, cessation of immunosuppression is required despite the risk of graft rejection.

References

1. Penn, I.J.: Kaposi's sarcoma in immunosuppressed patients. *Clin. Lab. Immunol.* **12**, 1—10 (1983).
2. Harwood, A.R., Osoba, D., Hofstader, S.L. *et al.*: Kaposi's sarcoma in recipients of renal transplants. *Amer. J. Med.* **67**, 759—765 (1979).
3. Al-Sulaiman, M., Haleem, A. and Al-Khader, A.: Kaposi's sarcoma in post renal transplantation. Recent aspects of the use of cyclosporin in renal transplantation. *Proc. of a Workshop Cairo, April 15—16*, pp. 103—107 (1986).

69. Urological complications in 510 consecutive renal transplants

H. ABDUL KARIM, M.S.A. KUMAR, M. SAMHAN, P. JOHN,
I.M. HASSAN, S. ABDUL BASIT, E.M. PHILIPS and G.M. ABOUNA

Introduction

Renal transplantation is a successful and widely accepted treatment for patients with end-stage renal disease. Improved surgical techniques and potent immunosuppressive drugs have led to improved graft survival in both living related or cadaveric kidney transplantation. However technical problems, including urological complications and lymphocele formation continue to contribute toward the morbidity and mortality of renal transplant recipients. In previously reported series, urological complications occur in 10—13%, and lymphocele formation in 0—22% of renal transplant recipients (1—4). Recent developments in ultrasonic and computed tomographic scanning techniques have led to an earlier and more accurate diagnosis, which is crucial in preventing irreversible renal damage secondary to chronic obstruction (4). We report our experience with urological complications in 510 consecutive renal transplants carried out in a single center over the last 11 years.

Patients and methods

Between March 1979 and March 1990, 510 renal transplantations have been carried out in Kuwait, of which 407 were from living donors and 103 from cadaver donors. Most of the cadaveric kidneys were imported from North America and Europe (6).

The selection of recipients and living donors are based on our previously described protocols consisting of strict ethical, legal and medical criteria (6). The surgical technique of renal transplantation was a standard procedure. Transplantation was carried out either in the right or left iliac fossa. After meticulous retroperitoneal dissection, renal vein was anastomosed end-to-side to the iliac vein and the renal artery end-to-end to the internal iliac artery or end-to-side to the common iliac artery. In small children, the vascular anastomoses were carried out directly to the aorta and the inferior vena cava. The ureter was implanted into the bladder by a modified Politano—Leadbetter technique performed through a cystotomy on the anterior surface of the bladder. Through a small incision in the bladder mucosa a submucosal tunnel was created on the right or left posterolateral aspect of the bladder close to the trigone. The transplant ureter was trimmed to its final length and the tip carefully tailored and spatulated, brought through the submucosal tunnel which was anastomosed to the bladder mucosa using polyglycolic acid (dexon) sutures. In few selected cases, a temporary ureteric stent was used for 10—15 days. The cystotomy was closed in three layers; the mucosa was closed with a continuous suture using dexon and the muscle in two layers using interrupted silk sutures. At the end of surgery a vacuum drain was left *in situ* alongside the vessels and ureter which was removed at a variable time after surgery according to clinical circumstances, but usually on the second post operative day. During operation, the wound was washed with an antibiotic-containing solution and after careful hemostasis it was closed in layers. The Foley catheter was removed 20 days after surgery.

A baseline radionuclide renal scan was obtained within 24 hours of the operation and a baseline ultrasonography was obtained within 2—3 days, and both were repeated at each episode of functional impairment of the transplant kidney. Prophylactic immunosuppression was either conventional with azathioprine and prednisone or more recently with triple therapy consisting of azathioprine, prednisone and cyclosporine. Antirejection therapy was according to our previously described protocol using pulse doses of intravenous methylprednisolone daily for 3—5 days and, in steroid-resistant cases, intravenous infusion of ATG or OKT3 (7).

All urological complications were diagnosed promptly by radionuclide radioisotope study and ultrasound examination of the transplanted kidney and were treated appropriately.

Results

Twenty (3.9%) of the 510 renal transplant recipients developed urological complications of which 17 were seen in living-donor transplantations and 3 in cadaver kidney transplantations. Table 1 shows the recipient data and clinical presentation in these 20 cases.

The complications were mainly of three types. They were lymphoceles causing ureteric obstruction in 10 recipients, urinary leak due to injury to the ureter, kidney, urinary bladder or urethra in 8 and intrinsic ureteric obstruction in 2.

Lymphoceles were seen in 10 recipients and were causing ureteric obstruction in all the cases. In 2 cases they additionally caused obvious swelling at the site of the transplantation wound. In 6 cases the lymphoceles were drained percutaneously under ultrasonic guidance and a fine silastic catheter was left *in*

Table 1. Patient data and clinical presentation.

	Living donor transplantation	Cadaver kidney transplantation
Total no. of recipients	407	103
No. of recipients with urological complications	17 (4%)	3 (3%)
Mean age of the recipients in years (range)	39 (11–66)	46 (40–52)
Male to female ratio	15 : 2	2 : 1
Clinical presentation		
Transplant dysfunction due to urinary obstrction	11	3
Peroperative bladder injury	2	–
Urine leak through the wound	2	–
Swelling over the transplant site	2	–

situ for 3–4 days. In 3 recipients the lymphocele was cured with this procedure while, in the remaining 3, lymphocele recurred and required surgical intervention. Seven recipients – in 3 of whom percutaneous drainage was not successful – required either intraperitoneal drainage or excision of the lymphocele.

Urine leak was seen in 8 recipients. The causes of urine leak were: rupture of a rejecting kidney causing calyceo-cutaneous fistula in 1 recipient of living donor kidney, sloughing of ureter in 2 cadaveric kidney recipients, ureteric injury at the site of ureterovesical anastomosis in 1, and improper closure of the urinary bladder in 4 (from the cystotomy suture line in 2 and from the ureterovesical anastomosis in 2).

Intrinsic ureteric obstruction was seen in 2 recipients. In one it was due to ureteric stenosis at the site of ureterovesical anastomosis and, in the other, to pelvi-ureteric junction obstruction.

The urine leak and ureteric obstruction were dealt appropriately. Table 2 gives details of the urological problems seen, management and its outcome. All the grafts recovered and continue to function normally. There were no patient deaths or graft losses due to urological complications in this series.

Discussion

Renal transplantation is increasingly becoming a common procedure in the treatment of patients with end-stage renal disease because of improved results both in living related and cadaver kidney transplantation. This has been made possible by improved surgical techniques and more effective immunosuppressive agents. However urological complications continue to contribute significantly toward morbidity and mortality (8). There are two main factors which contribute toward urological complications: surgical techniques and immunosuppression, particularly the use of steroids. The incidence of urological

Table 2. Urological complications in 20 renal transplant recipients: management and outcome.

Type of complication	No. of recipients	Management		Outcome
Lymphocele	10	Percutaneus drainage	3	All have recovered with normal graft function
		Marsupialization	4	
		Excision	3	
Ureteric				
Ureteric injury	2	Excision and re-implantation		
Ureteric stenosis	1	Excision of stenotic segment and re-implantation		Normal graft function
Ureteric necrosis	2	Anastomosis of pelvis of transplant kidney to be native ureter		
Pelvi ureteric obstruction	1	Permanent indwelling double 'J' catheter		Obstruction relieved; normal graft function
Calyceo-cutaneous fistula (ruptured kidney)	1	Temporary nephrostomy drainage		Complete healing and closure of fistula; normal graft function
Urinary bladder				
Injury	1	Repair of bladder and Foley catheter drainage		Complete healing of bladder; normal graft function
Urine leak from suture line	1	Prolonged bladder drainage through Foley catheter		
Urethral injury	1	Temporary suprapubic drainage of bladder		Normal graft function

complications are reported to be 0.9—29.6% (1, 3, 4, 5, 8). The need for careful dissection of the kidney and ureter in the donors is well recognized. It is important that the ureteric blood supply be protected as far as possible since excessive skeletonization of the ureter is likely to result in ischemia and subsequent urological problems such as ureteric stenosis and ureteric necrosis. An equally important factor is meticulous ureterovesical anastomosis for which a variety of techniques have been advocated. With the introduction of cyclosporine and low-dose steroids, there are reports of a significant fall in urological complications (8).

In our current series of 510 consecutive renal transplants the incidence of urological complications is around 4%. Most of the complications included either urine leak or urinary obstruction due to lymphoceal and in one case urethral injury.

Lymphoceles which occurred between 10 and 180 days after transplantation accounted for 2% of urological complications. The causes of lymphocele are thought be due to either extensive retroperitoneal dissection or lymphatic leak from the transplant kidney (2, 9). In the current series, 70% of the lymphoceles occurred in recipients requiring extensive retroperitoneal dissection. The management of lymphoceles in our center is initially by percutaneous drainage under ultrasonic guidance, and if this method fails, surgery is carried out either to drain the lymphocele into the peritoneal cavity or, in a few cases, to excise the lymphocele sac completely.

Thirty percent of lymphoceles have been successfully treated by percutaneous drainage without major surgical intervenation.

Urinary obstruction, when recognized, must be managed aggressively if function is not be irretrievably lost. Apart from lymphoceles, the other causes of urinary obstruction are ureteric stenosis, pelvi-ureteric obstruction and uretral injury accounting for less than 1%. The major problem of urine leak is infection which may ultimately result in graft loss or patient death.

Urological complications in renal transplantation can be minimized by meticulous dissection of kidney and ureter in the donor and, in the recipient, by avoiding extensive retroperitoneal dissection, and the use of the Politano—Leadbetter technique for ureter ovesico anastomosis. Foley catheter drainage of the urinary bladder and vacuum drainage of extravesical tissue for 48—72 hours should also be practised. Early diagnosis of urological complications, when they occur, is essential to prevent irretrievable renal function. Urgent drainage procedures with revisional surgery if necessary should be carried out to prevent graft loss.

References

1. Bennett, L.N., Voegeli, D.R., Crummy, A.B. *et al.*: Urologic complications following renal transplantation: role of interventional radiologic procedures. *Radiology* **160**, 531—536 (1986).
2. Burleson, R.L. and Marbarger, P.D.: Prevention of lymphocele formation following renal allotransplantation. *J. Urology* **127**, 18—19 (1982).
3. Jaskowski, A., Jones, R.M., Murie, J.A. *et al.*: Urological complications in 600 consecutive renal transplants. *Brit. J. Surg.* **74**, 922—925 (1987).
4. Santiago-Delpin, E.A., Baquero, A. and Gonzalez, Z.: Low incidence of urologic complications after renal transplantation. *Amer. J. Surg.* **151**, 374—377 (1986).
5. Zaontz, M.R., Hatch, D.A. and Firlit, C.F.: Urological complications in pediatric renal transplantation: management and prevention. *J. Urology* **140**, 1123—1128 (1988).
6. Abouna, G.M., Kumar, M.S.A., White, A.G., *et al.*: Renal transplantation in the Middle East: experience with 250 transplants. *Dialysis and Transplant.* **16**(2), 81—84 (1987).
7. Kumar, M.S.A., White, A.G., John P., *et al.*: Antilymphocyte infusion in the treatment of acute allograft rejection. In: *Current Status of Clinical Organ Transplantation*. ed: G.M. Abouna, pp. 49—56. The Hague. Martinus-Nijhoff, 1984.
8. Mundy, A.R., Podestar, M.L., Bewick, M., Rudge, C.J. and Ellis, F.G.: The urological complications of 1000 renal transplants. *Brit. J. Urol.* **53**, 397—402 (1981).
9. Nghiem, D.D., Schulak, J.A. and Corry, R.J.: Decapsulation of the renal transplant as a mechanism of lymphocele formation. *Transplant. Proc.* **14**, 741—742 (1982).

70. Preservation of the kidney and other organs into the nineties

G. KOOTSTRA, R. WIJNEN and J.G. MAESSEN

Workers on organ preservation are scarce. Although their achievements were vital to the development of clinical transplantation some 20 years ago, the enormous empirical success of simple cold storage seemed to make them superfluous. However, at the beginning of the third decade after the initial steps in clinical transplantation, they suddenly presented some exciting results that again arouse interest among transplant physicians and surgeons.

The first decade

From 1968 to 1978 investigators were in search for an adequate clinical preservation method. The definitive establishment of kidney transplantation in clinical medicine and the rapidly increasing numbers of transplantations pressed investigators to focus on the development of simple and safe, universally applicable techniques. The introduction of tissue typing for matching donor and recipient, allowed the development of large organ exchange programs. On behalf of the transport of organs a preservation time of 24—48 hours was necessary. Prolongation of preservation time was therefore the major topic in preservation research in those years. In the meantime, new boundaries were explored. Limitations to the maximum preservation time of tissues were determined. Because most experimental achievements were empirical in nature, exciting ideas like organ banking and organ freezing could be frankly discussed, falsely suggesting that implementation might take place in the near future (1, 2).

In the next decade from 1979 to 1988 the excitement for the results of preservation research subsided. Cold storage with Eurocollins solution (3), a simplified version of a cold storage solution developed by Geoffry Collins (4) in the late sixties, was generally accepted as a convenient technique in everyday transplantation practice. Preservation of kidneys up to 48 hours and of liver and pancreas up to 8 hours was simple and safe with this solution. The eternal controversy between machine preservation and simple cold storage became rather academic. In its simplicity and reliability cold storage had won the game.

There were still other factors responsible for a reduced interest in preservation research. The introduction of cyclosprine caused a revolution in rejection treatment. Transplant physicians became primarily interested in the evaluation of various treatment schedules including steriods, cyclosporine and monoclonal antilymphocyte antibodies. New insights arose on the pathophysiology of rejection. New T cell receptors were isolated and the important role of cytokines was recognized. An overwhelming amount of papers concerning these subjects dominated international congresses and transplantation journals (5).

Furthermore, as a result of the considerably increased success rate of kidney transplants, the interest in the transplantation of other organs was renewed. Clinical liver, pancreas, heart and heart-lung transplantation programs were successfully developed in many transplantation centers. As a result, a new phenomenon came in view: the multiple organ donor. It was undoubtedly this particular phenomenon that became the most important impetus for the revival of preservation research in our decade.

The Nineties

A major drawback for a widespread use of non-renal transplants is still a limited preservation time. Using Eurocollins, liver and pancreas can be stored up to 8 hours. The maximum preservation time for hearts or heart-lung preparations is even less with the Bretschneider solution (6). A large number of other preservation techniques are in use with similar or worse results (7). However, for a proper use of multiple organ donors, a single flush solution would by far be preferable.

At the end of the eighties a new solution was introduced, the University of Wisconsin (UW) solution, which is the hallmark of a new decade in preservation research. It was initially designed for pancreas preservation, and specifically to reduce post-transplant oedema and thus the risk for thrombosis (8). UW proved to be very effective in prolonging liver and pancreas perservation, and currently in the clinical setting preservation times of 18 hours for both organs are generally applied. This has made liver and pancreas transplantation a semi-elective procedure. There is evidence that UW is at least as good as Eurocollins (9) for kidney perservation and therefore nowdays UW is the solution of choice in multiple organ donors (MOD's) with the exception of preservation of the heart.

Cold storage

At present, three cold storage preservation solutions are in general use: Eurocollins, UW and HTK. Eurocollins is effective in kidney preservation and in short-term (up to 8 hours) liver and pancreas preservation. It is simple and inexpensive. It effectively flushes out the blood from the organ, and provides good core cooling. The high potassium content is assumed to save high-energy phosphates by decreasing the load on the cellular membrane pumps, while the osmotic activity of glucose prevents cell swelling. The solution is buffered by 60 mmol/lu bicarbonate-phosphate. In fact, its only drawback is the restricted preservation time for liver and pancreas. In the University of Wisconsin (UW) solution, glucose is replaced by the trisaccharide raffinose and the colloid hydroxyethylstarch to provide a better prevention of cell swelling. Lactobionate was added as an anion, which gives in the experimental setting better results than chloride. UW is expensive. It has a high viscosity and therefore its flush-out and core-cooling properties are considered less prominent than with Eurocollins, although no hard data are available to substantiate this. Cardiac arrhythmias have been reported which are probably caused by adenosis during reperfusion before transplantation (9, 10).

The HTK (custodiol R) solution is derived from the so-called Bretschneider solution which is currently in use for myocardial protection during open heart surgery (12). HTK is supposed to be an excellent flush-out solution. The perfusion resistance for Eurocollins perfused kidneys is higher than for those perfused with HTK. Apparently, a better equilibrium of the extracellular space is reached (13, 14, 15). The strong buffer capacity of HTK by the Histidine-HCL buffer of 180/18 mmol is claimed to be especially important during anaerobiosis (15). In a preliminary report of a study in which 215 kidneys were preserved with HTK, an immediate function of 74% was obtained (16). A prospective trial, in cooperation with the Eurotransplant organization, is planned (16).

Other possible future developments

Organ preservation has always been associated with cooling. Cooling decreased the rate of the cellular metabolism and thus the metabolic need for oxygen and a number of other metabolites. From a conceptual point of view, a complete metabolic arrest might be the ultimate and unlimited method of organ preservation. However, at 4 °C metabolism is still going on albeit at a lower level (17). Thus, there is still a need for metabolic support. Limitations to current preservation techniques might result from inadequate substitution of the artificial environment of the isolated organs. Perhaps we will learn in the near future from cell culture specialists which amino acids or spore elements or other substances are essential to support cellular metabolism at low temperatures.

Although cooling at 4°C is convenient it may not be the ideal storage temperature. To avoid membrane phase transitions which occur at preservation temperatures below 10 °C and which become irreversible after a certain period of time, it may appear better to cool down organs to a level between 10 and 20° (18). Alternatively, intermittent rewarming of organs during preservation time may prevent membranes from becoming physically damaged. Experimentally, it has already been shown that intermittent rewarming considerably prolongs maximum preservation time (19).

Apart from the attention to storage conditions, more attention will have to be paid in the next decade to potential pre-existing damage of the organs and the transition from storage to blood perfusion during and following implantation. In the past few years the important role of ischemia-reperfusion injury to the eventual function of donor organs following implantation has been recognized. Although the mechanism of reperfusion injury to tissues with ischemic or preservation damage is incompletely understood, the induction of reactive oxygen metabolites and the increased influx of calcium ions are undoubtedly involved. Many studies have already clearly demonstrated that it is possible to reduce or prevent reperfusion injury by the use of calcium blockers and scavengers of reative oxygen metabolites (20). Still, a widespread use of these drugs in clinical medicine has not yet been established. For a proper evaluation of the effectiveness of these drugs, large multicentred studies are needed to irradicate the intercurrent effects of the variations in surgical and preservation techniques and the effects of rejection prevention treatment. New developments in the manipulation of the inflammatory reaction in response to reperfusion injury may be expected. The beneficial effect of changing neutrophil behavior has demonstrated that treatment of reperfusion injury is still possible after the very first moment of reperfusion itself (20).

Although continuous perfusion preservation (machine preservation) is at present in use in only a limited number of transplant centers it might become an important option for improved preservation of organs in special cases. Continuous perfusion has the advantage that it allows the delivery of oxygen and nutrients, the removal of waste products and better control of physical parameters (21). Probably, it is the best approach to achieve control of cooling and (intermittent) rewarming, and drug treatment of ischemically damaged kidneys.

Organ shortage

To conclude this brief summary of possible developments in organ preservation in the near future we have to consider that despite our research investments with exciting and promising data, the major culprit to the expansion of organ transplantation in the next decade, has remained undiscussed: shortage of donor organs. The only way to alleviate this problem, in my view, is a proper and more effective use of all possible donors at hand, including non-heart-beating donors (22).

Against the backgroud of this concept, the focus of our research program in

Maastricht has been switched from prolongation of preservation time to more fundamental research concerning the impact, prevention and treatment of possible ischemic damage in organs from non-heart-beating donors. The capacity of kidneys to recover from ischemic damage is substantial. When we subjected canine kidneys to 90 minutes of *in situ* warm ischemia, no animal survived after immediate contralateral nephrectomy. When this contralateral nephrectomy was delayed for 5 weeks, the animals survived with adequate renal function. Studies of the energy metabolism showed that despite 90 minutes of ischemia the metabolic integrity of the cells remained intact. The non-functional state seemed to result from temporary and reversible membrane instability (17, 23, 24). The intention of our current research efforts is to reduce this period of initial non-function following reperfusion using drugs to prevent the effects of reperfusion injury and by influencing the inflammatory response, as pointed out earlier.

In our clinical transportation program kidneys from non-heart-beating donors were used from 1981 onward. In a retrospective analysis of 28 non-heart-beating donors that were harvested during the first seven years of our program, good results could be reported (25). The mean first warm ischemia time, denoted as the time between cardiac arrest and start of the cold perfusion, was 28 minutes, ranging from 0 to 110 minutes. One-third of the kidneys were machine perfused whereas the others were simply stored on ice using Eurocollins. Twenty-one percent of all kidneys showed immediate function. In 61% of

Table 1. Composition of the three preservation solutions in use in Europe in 1990.

	Eurocollins	UW	HTK
Na^+	10	30	15
K+	115	115	10
Ca^{++}	—	—	0.015
Mg^{++}	—	5	4
Cl^{-1}	15	—	50
SO^4	—	5	—
Substrates	198 Glucose	100 Lactobionate 30 Raffinose	2 Tryptophan 1-α-Ketoglutarate 30 Mannitol
Buffer	43 HPO_4^- 15 $H_2PO_4^-$	20 HPO_4^- 5 $H_2PO_4^-$	180 Histidine 18 Histidine-HCl
Pharmaca	—	Adenosine, glutathione, allopurinol, insulin, bactrim	—
Colloid	—	50 g/l Hydroxyethyl starch	—
Osmolarity	406	325	310

all cases good renal function was obtained following temporary postoperative hemodialysis. Acute tubular necrosis was the main cause of delayed function. Eighteen percent of the grafts never reached an adequate functional state. Despite the high incidence of delayed function, no difference was found in 1, 2, and 3 year patient and graft survival between the non-heart-beating donor kidney recipients and a control group of heart-beating donor kidney recipients. Similarly, no differences in creatinine clearances were found at 3, 6, and 12 months following transplantation.

In the near future the Dutch law will be adjusted in a way that it will be permissible to introduce a double-balloon-triple-lumen catheter into the femoral artery of a potential, non-heart-beating donor to start cooling of the organs as soon as possible. Actual harvesting of the organs will only take place if permission of the relatives is obtained. The combination of this juridical breakthrough and the developments in prevention and treatment of organ preservation damage will make the non-heart-beating donor an important source of organs in our next decade in which the need for transplant organs will become more urgent than ever before.

References

1. Pegg, D.E.: *Organ Preservation.* Churchill Livingstone, Edinburgh and London (1973).
2. Pegg, D.E. and Jacobsen, Ib.A.: *Organ Preservation II.* Churchill Livingstone, Edinburgh, London and New York (1979).
3. Dreikorn, K., Horsch, R. and Röhl, R.: 48- to 96-hour preservation of canine kidneys by initial perfusion and hypothermic storage using Eurocollins solution. *Eur. Urol.* **6**, 221 (1980).
4. Collins, G.W., Bravo-Shugarman, M. and Terasaki, P.D.: Kidney preservation for transportation. Initial perfusion and 30 hours' ice storage. *Lancet* **2**, 1219 (1969).
5. Morris, P.J. and Tilney, N.L.: *Progress in Transportation.* Churchill Livingstone, Edinburgh (1985).
6. Bretschneider, H.J.: Myocardial protection. *Thorac. Cardiovasc. Surg.* **28**, 295 (1980).
7. Fragomeni, L.S., Bonser, R.S. and Jamieson, S.W.: Cardiopulmonary transplantation: a current practice. *Transplant. Int.* **1**, 103—108 (1988).
8. Wahlberg, J.H., Southard, J.H. and Belzer, F.O.: Development of a cold storage solution for pancreas preservation. *Cryobiology* **23**, 477—483 (1986).
9. Ploeg, R.J.: Kidney preservation with UW and Euro-Collins solution: a clinical comparison. *Transplant. Proc.* (in press).
10. Prien, Th., Diel, K-H., Zander, J., Hachenberg, Th. and Buchholz, B., Bradyarrythmia with University of Wisconsin preservation solution. *Lancet* **i**, 1319—1320 (1989).
11. Belzer, F.O., Sollinger, H.W., Glass, N.R., Miller, D.T., Hoffman, R.H. and Southard, J.H.: Beneficial effects of adenosine and phosphate in kidney preservation. *Transplantation* **36**, 633—635 (1983).
12. Groenewoud, A.F., Isemer, F.E., Stadler, J., Heidecke, C.D., Florack, G. and Hoelscher, M.: A comparison of early function between kidney grafts protected with HTK solution versus Euro-Collins solution. *Transplant. Proc.* **21**, 1243 (1988).
13. Kallerhoff, M., Hoelscher, M., Kehrer, G., Klaess, G. and Bretschneider, H.J.: Effects of preservation conditions and temperature on tissue acidification in canine kidneys. *Transplantation* **39**, 485 (1985).

14. Hoelscher, M., Kallerhoff, M., Klaess, G., Helmcher, U. and Bretschneider, H.J.: Successful dog kidney preservation for 4 hours of warm ischemia or 48 hours of cold ischemia using the HT buffer solution Bretschneider. *Transplantation* (in press).
15. Kallerhoff, M., Hoelscher, M., Kehrer, G., Klaess, G. and Bretschneider, H.J.: Effects of preservation conditions and temperature on tissue acidification in canine kidneys. *Transplantation* **39**, 485—489 (1985).
16. Groenewoud, A.F.: Personal communication.
17. Maessen, J.G., van der Vusse, G.J., Vork, M. and Kootstra, G.: Potentiation of ischemic injury during hypothermic storage in donor kidneys: role of energy metabolism. *Transplant. Proc.* **20**, 854—857 (1988).
18 Kruuv, J., Glofcheski, D. and Cheng, K.H.: Factors influencing survival and growth of mammalian cells exposed to hypothermia I. Effects of temperature and membrane lipid perturbers. *J. Cell. Physiol.* **115**, 1979 (1983).
19. Rijkams, B.G., van der Wijk, J., Donker, A.J.M., Sloof, M.J.H. and Kootstra, G.: Functional studies in 6 days surgical preserved canine kidneys. *J. Urol.* **127**, 163—165 (1982).
20. Hearse, Jan Willem: Personal communication.
21. Belzer, F.O., Ashby, B.S. and Dumphy, J.E.: 24- and 72-hour preservation of canine kidneys. *Lancet* **2**, 536 (1967).
22. Kootstra, G., Ruers, T.J.M. and Vroemen, J.P.A.M.: The non-heartbeating donor: contribution to the organ shortage. *Transplant. Proc.* **18**, 1410—1412 (1986).
23. Maessen, J.G., van der Vusse, G.J., Vork, M. and Kootstra, G.: The stunned kidney: postischemic renal failure and adenine nucleotide homeostatis (submitted).
24. Maessen, J.G., van der Vusse, G.J., Vork, M. and Kootstra, G.: Assessment of nucleotides, nucleosides and oxypurines in human donor kidneys. *Transplant. Proc.* **20**, 889—890 (1988).
25. Vromen, M.A.M., Leunissen, K.M.L., Persijn, G.G. and Kootstra, G.: Short and long-term results with adult non-heart-beating donor kidneys. *Transplant. Proc.* **20**, 743—745 (1988).

71. Clinical experience with liver preservation

ROBERT D. GORDON and SATORU TODO

The modern techniques for liver preservation evolved from work over many years in Thomas Starzl's lab in Denver, Sir Roy Calne's lab in Cambridge, and Folkert Belzer's laboratory in Madison. In 1963 Marchioro, working in Starzl's laboratory, reported the first systematic attempt to preserve organs by continuous hypothermic perfusion, using the cadaver as the perfusion chamber and providing flow and oxygenation with a mechanical heart-lung machine (1). The method was used clinically in the mid-60's before brain death became a condition of organ donation. Cadavers with no heart beat could be effectively and quickly cooled with this technique. This experience provided the basis for the *in situ* cooling techniques that are now in standard use for modern multiple organ procurement.

Brettschnieder, also working in Starzl's laboratory, in 1968 reported that the liver could be perfused continuously *ex vivo* using a perfusate containing whole blood and orthotopically transplanted as long as one or two days later (2). Oxygenation was provided by a single membrane oxygenator in a hyperbaric chamber. The method was used clinically on several occasions but was eventually abandoned because of its complexity and dangers.

Ackerman and Snell (3) and Merke *et al.* (4) popularized cooling of cadaveric kidneys with cold electrolyte solutions infused into the distal aorta. Until 1976, techniques for preserving the liver either severely limited the acceptable time of cold ischemia or were too complicated for use in outlying hospitals. In 1977, Benichou, again in Starzl's laboratory in Denver, showed that the liver could tolerated much more cold ischemia induced with Ringer's lactate than previously realized and that further increase in storage time could be obtained with Collins or plasma-like solutions (5). Wall, working in Cambridge, showed the same thing with a plasma-like solution brought to Cambridge from Holland (6). The methods used in these studies allowed safe preservation for as long as 8 to 12 hours. These studies demonstrated the feasibility of donor liver retrieval from distant sites. Prior, to this it has been necessary to bring the donor to an operating room adjacent to the recipient.

All that was left was to standardize the surgical procedure for multiple organ retrieval. Starzl's landmark paper in 1984 provides us with a detailed description of what is now, with some additional modification (especially for pancreas retrieval), the basis of methods presently in general use of multiple organ procurement (7).

The modified versions of the solution described by Collins in 1969 or a plasma based solution similar to one described by Schalm, also in 1969, have until recently been the most commonly used preparations for preservation of the solid organs. However, the development of a new liver preservation solution by Jamieson, working in Belzer and Southland's laboratory at the University of Wisconsin, now permits the liver to be stored safely well beyond the previous 8 hour limit (10—12).

Belzer and Southard have recently described the principles behind the development of the UW solution (13). These include (a) prevention of hypothermic cell swelling, (b) prevention of intracellular acidosis, (c) prevention of extracellular space expansion, (d) preservation of cellular energy stores, and (e) prevention of oxygen free radical injury. The liver cell plasma membrane is more permeable to glucose and the liver contains higher glycogen stores than the kidney. Liver glucokinase is active at high glucose concentrations and is not inhibited by glucose-6-phosphate. As a result, the liver has a higher capacity to metabolize glucose than the kidney and preservation solutions rich in glucose would not be effective in preventing cell swelling or acidosis.

UW solution contains no glucose. Rather, it contains three impermeants: (a) lactobionate, a large molecular mass anion, (b) raffinose, a large molecular mass saccharide, and (c) hyroxyethyl-starch which provides in UW solution are glutathione (a reducing agent), allopurinol (to inhibit xanthine oxidase and free radical production), and adenosine (to stimulate ATP synthesis after reperfusion).

We began using UW solution for clinical liver preservation in Pittsburgh in October, 1987 and reported out initial clinical experience in 1989 (14). In this report, we compared our experience with 185 cadaveric liver grafts preserved 4 to 24 hours with UW solution to 180 grafts preserved for 3 to 9 hours using conventional preservation with Eurocollins solution. Despite the much longer average preservation time for the grafts preserved in UW solution, the UW preserved grafts had higher graft survival rates, equal patient survival rates, a lower rate of primary non-function, a reduced need for retransplantation, and a lower incidence of hepatic artery thrombosis. We observed no correlation between storage time out to 24 hours and early postoperative liver function abnormalities (Figures 1 and 2).

With this experience accumulated, we have continued for the last two years to use UW solution as the preservation fluid of choice for storage of liver allografts. Nearly all liver grafts have been procured as part of a multiple organ procurement. Whenever we are requested not to use UW solution for the *in situ* flush, it can be used as a final flush through the portal vein and hepatic artery on the back table after the liver has been removed from the donor. Thus, even

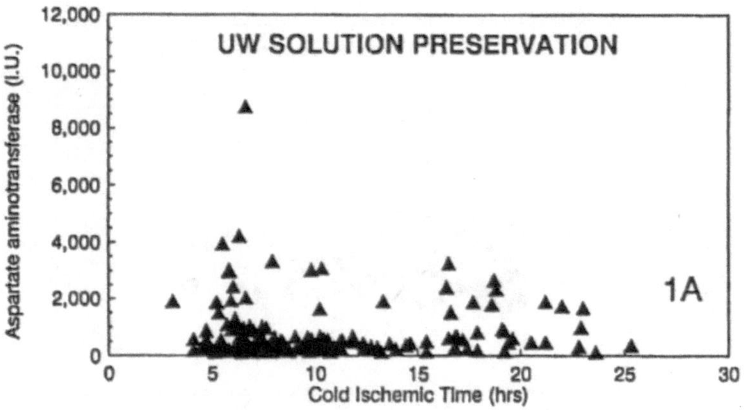

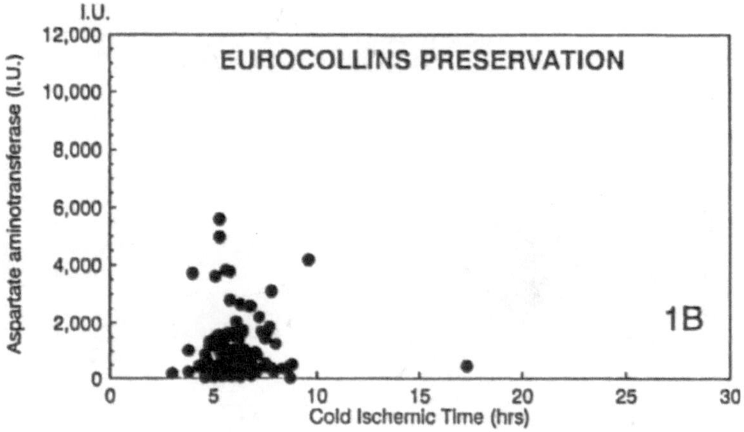

Fig. 1. Scatter plot for early postoperative peak alanine aminotransferase (ALT) versus cold ischemia time (in hours) for human liver allografts preserved in UW solution (1A) compared to those preserved in Eurocollins solution (1B). (Adapted from reference (14).)

when another team instists on *in situ* aortic flush with another solution such as Ringer's lactate or Collins type solutions, it is still possible to preserve the liver in UW solution.

In addition to the practical benefits of an increase in the safe storage times for liver preservation, an important additional benefit of preservation with UW solution may be better protection of the hepatic microvasculature. Ueda has demonstrated remarkable preservation of renal microvasculature in kidneys preserved in UW solution (15). Improved preservation of the hepatic microcirculation may explain the reduced incidence of hepatic artery thrombosis seen in our clinical experience with livers preserved in UW solution.

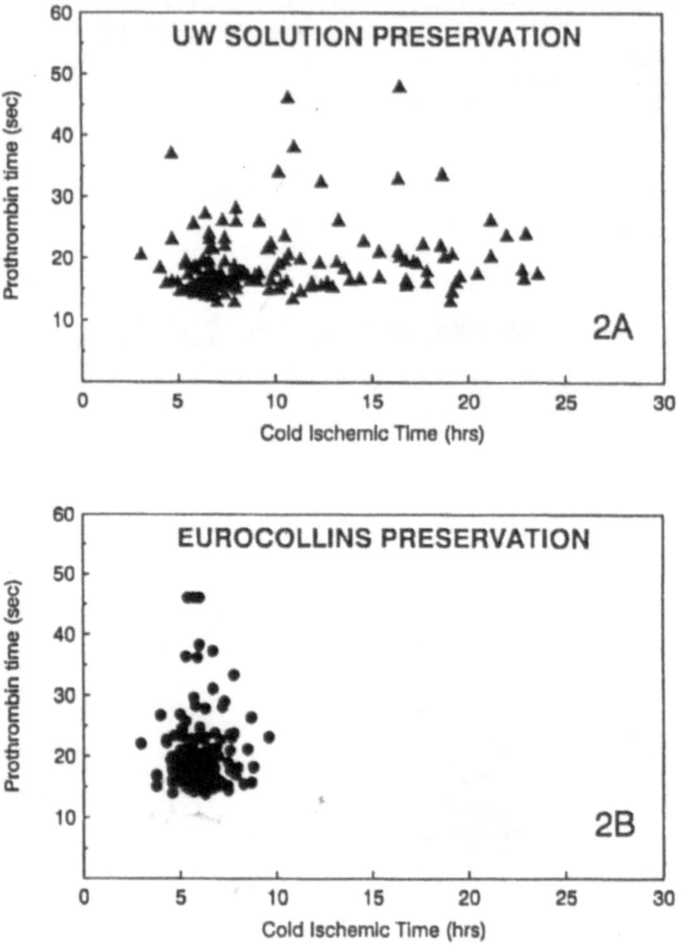

Fig. 2. Scatter plot for early postoperative peak prothrombin time (seconds) versus cold ischemia time (in hours) for human liver allografts preserved in UW solution (2A) compared to those preserved in Eurocollins solution (2B). (Adapted from reference (14).)

Acknowledgement

This work was supported by research grants from the Veterans Administration and Projct Grant No.DK29961 from the National Institute of Health, Bethesda, MD.

References

1. Marchioro, T.L., Huntley, R.T., Waddell, W.R. and Starzl, T.E.: Extracorpeal perfusion for obtaining postmortem homografts. *Surgery* **54**, 900—11 (1963).

2. Brettschneider, L., Daloze, P., Huguet, C. *et al.*: The use of combined preservation techniques for extended storage of orthotopic liver homografts. *Surg. Gynecol. Obstet* **126**, 263—274 (1968).
3. Ackerman, J.R. and Snell, M.E.: Cadaveric renal transplantation. *Brit. J. Urol.* **40**, 515—512 (1963).
4. Merkel, F., Jonasson, O. and Bergan, J.J.: Procurement of cadaver donor organs: evisceration technique. *Transplant. Proc.* **4**, 585—589 (1972).
5. Benichou, J., Halgrimson, C.G., Weil, R. III *et al.*: Canine and human liver preservation for 6 to 18 hr by cold infusion. *Transplantation* **24**, 407—411 (1977).
6. Wall, W.J., Calne, R.Y., Herbertson, B.M. *et al.*: Simple hypothermic preservation for transporting human livers long distances for transplantation: Report of 12 cases. *Transplantation* **23**, 210—216 (1977).
7. Starzl, T.E., Hakala, T.R., Shaw, B.W., Jr *et al.*: A flexible procedure for multiple organ procurement. *Surg. Gynecol. Obstet.* **158**, 223—230 (1984).
8. Collins, G.M., Bravo-Sugarman, M. and Terasaki, P.I.: Kidney preservation for transportation: initial perfusion and 30 hours' ice storage. *Lancet* **2**, 1219 (1969).
9. Schalm, S.W., Terpstra, J.L., Drayer, B. *et al.*: A simple method for short-term preservation of a liver homograft. *Transplantation* **8**, 877 (1969).
10. Jamieson, N.V., Sundberg, R., Lindell, S. *et al.*: A comparison of cold storage solutions for hepatic preservation using the isolated perfused rabbit liver. *Cryobiology* **25**, 300 (1984).
11. Jamieson, N.V., Lindell, S., Sundberg, R. *et al.*: An analysis of the components in UW solution using the isolated perfused rabbit liver. *Transplantation* **46**, 512—516 (1988).
12. Jamieson, N.V., Sundberg, R., Lindell, S. *et al.*: Preservation of the canine liver for 24—48 hours using the simple cold storage with UW solution. *Transplantation* **46**, 517—522 (1988).
13. Belzer, F.O. and Southard, J.H.: Principles of solid organ preservation by cold storage. *Transplantation*, **46**, 673—676 (1988).
14. Todo, S., Nery, J., Yanaga, K. *et al.*: Extended preservation of human liver grafts with UW solution. *J. Amer. Med. Assoc.* **261**, 711 (1989).
15. Ueda, Y., Todo, S., Imventarza, O. *et al.*: The UW solution for canine kidney preservation. *Transplantation* **48**, 913—918 (1989).

72. Management of the organ donor

YOOGOO KANG

The successful outcome of transplantation depends on the function of the donor organs. Proper management of organ donation includes the anticipation of potential donors, the confirmation and declaration of brain death without unnecessary delay, and care of donors that includes an understanding of the pathophysiologic changes that occur with brain death.

Definition of brain death

One of the difficulties in donor management has been the evolving definition of brain-death criteria. A modern definition of brain death was developed in 1968, when Harvard Medical School outlined a criteria (1). This group considered irreversible coma to constitute brain death, and suggested certain clinical tests to confirm the absence of function in the brain hemisphere and brain stem. The silence of electrical activity in the brain was considered important. However, this criteria was considered to be too strict, and the University of Minnesota developed a new set of guidelines in 1971 that stressed the importance of clinical signs rather than of electrophysiologic findings (2). This new outline was followed by a similar set of guidelines developed by the National Institute of Neurological and Communicative Disorders and Stroke (3). The most current brain-death criteria are found in a 1981 guideline designed by the President's Commission for the Study of Ethical Problems in Medicine and Biomedical Research (4). This guideline defined cardiopulmonary death as the irreversible cessation of circulation and respiration as determined by repeated examination. Neurologic death was defined as the irreversible cessation of all brain functions, including those of the brain stem. The guideline stressed that irreversibility should be established by the presence of a recognizable cause of coma, a brain injury that has no potential for recovery, and clinical signs of brain death that persist after repeated examination. In addition, confirmatory tests are required in children and in all patients with drug or metabolic intoxication or hypo-*thermia. The clinical criteria for brain death, however are not specified in this* guideline. These criteria are found in the United Kingdom code, which places more emphasis on clinical examination of patients, rather than on complicated laboratory tests (5). The prerequisite conditions of the UK code specify that patients should be comatose without hypothermia, without the effects of central nervous system depressants, and without metabolic or endocrinic causes. The cause of the coma should be established. Patients should be apneic and dependent on ventilatory support without the effect of muscle relaxants. Confirmatory clinical signs include fixed and dilated pupils, and the absence of corneal, vestibulocular, gag, and cough reflexes. These patients should not exhibit motor response to the stimulation of cranial nerves, although spinal reflex-related movement may be intact. An apnea test is considered to be the most essential clinical test, and apnea should not initiate respiratory movement. To test for apnea, the patient is ventilated with 100% oxygen for several minutes (6). Ventilation is stopped while apneic oxygenation is performed by the insufflation of oxygen via a nasal cannula (6 l/min) and monitored by pulse oximetry. During the apneic period, arterial blood gas is drawn repeatedly to measure $PaCO_2$. Although respiratory movement should occur when $PaCO_2$ reaches 40 mmHg, when apean persists even when $PaCO_2$ is greater than 60 mmHg, the patient is considered to be brain dead and ventilation is resumed (7). More specific confirmatory tests are used for children under 5 years of age and for patients with drug intoxication, a coma of metabolic origin, or with hypothermia.

Electroencephalography or evoked potential monitoring is one of the confirmatory tests, but isoelectric EEG does not confirm brain death. One definite confirmatory test is the demonstration of the absence of cerebral blood flow by angiography, a radionuclide computerized tomographic scan, or a magnetic resonance test.

Management of brain-dead donors

Once brain death is declared, the concepts underlying medical management shift from patient care to donor care. The primary goal is to maintain the donor's physiologic condition to minimize potential ischemic injury to donor organs. The donor's physiologic changes that occur in brain-dead donors are illustrated in Figure 1. Brain injury is frequently associated with brain edema that results in an excessive release of endogenous catecholamines. This increased catecholamine level leads to hypertension, bradycardia, dysrhythmia, and myocardial ischemia caused by catecholamine-induced coronary vasoconstriction (8). Progressive brain edema results in brain herniation and cessation of the cerebral cortex and brain stem functions. The absence of brain stem function is followed by myocardial depression, vasomotor paralysis, and diabetes insipidus, and the donor becomes poikilothermic with the absence of the temperature control center function. These physiologic changes are com-

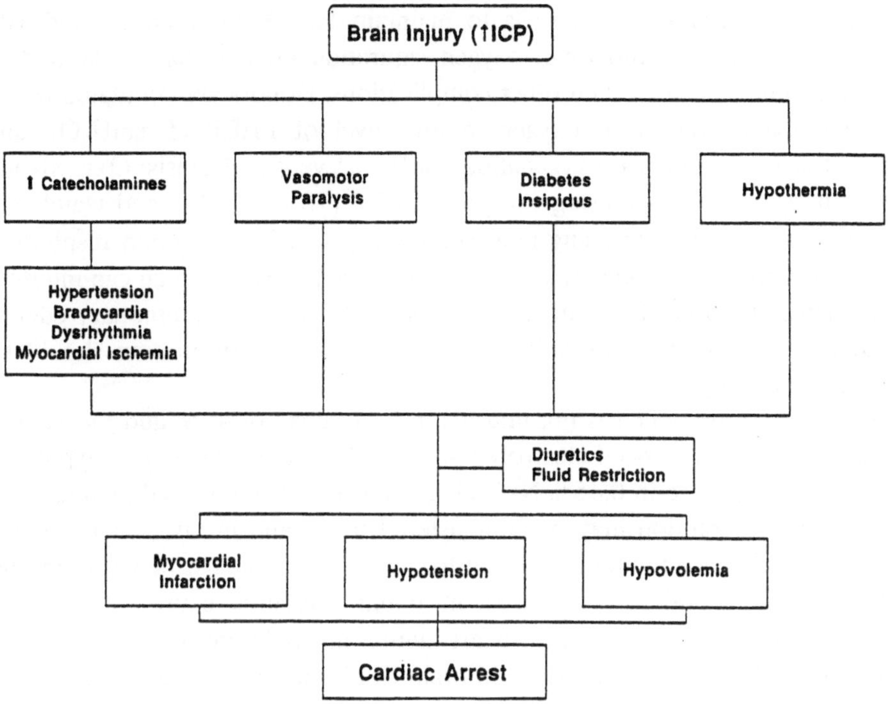

Fig. 1. Physiologic changes in brain-dead donors.

pounded by fluid restriction and diuretic therapy given to protect the brain from swelling, which results in hypovolemia and hypotension. All these insulting factors, such as hypovolemia, hypothermia, dysrhythmia, and myocardial ischemia, lead to cardiac arrest.

Therefore, the medical care of donors should include general supportive care, cardiopulmonary support, and the treatment of complications. General supportive care is essentially the same as that used with patients in the intensive care unit, and is crucial in minimizing the incidence and severity of complication. Organ donors require invasive hemodynamic monitoring, including the use of a radial arterial catheter, measurements of central venous pressure and pulmonary capillary wedge pressure, and frequent measurements of cardiac output. Urine output and body temperature should also be monitored. Laboratory tests include measurements of hemoglobin, electrolytes, arterial blood gas tensions and the acid-base state, and the blood glucose level. Donors should be turned frequently and a tracheal toilet should be performed to prevent atelectasis and pneumonia. Nasogastric suction is continued to prevent aspiration pneumonitis. Normothermia (> 35 °C) is maintained by infusing warmed fluids, by attaching a heated humidifier to the inspiratory limb of the ventilator, by using a warming blanket and heating lamps, and by raising the room temperature. Aseptic technique is essential.

The goal of pulmonary care is to maintain $PaCO_2$ between 70 and 100 mmHg and arterial hemoglobin oxygen saturation greater than 95%, and to avoid respiratory acidosis and other complications. Donors are ventilated with a sufficient concentration of oxygen, a low level of PEEP (5 cmH_2O), and frequent signs to improve oxygenation and to prevent atelectasis. Oxygenation can be improved by increasing FIO_2 and PEEP (10 cmH_22O), and ventilation can be improved by increasing tidal volume (up to 20 ml/kg) and respiratory rate (up to 20/min). However, a high intrathoracic pressure, which can interfere with splanchnic blood flow should be avoided. Pneumonia, pulmonary edema, atelectasis, aspiration pneumonia, pneumothorax, and hemothorax should be treated accordingly.

A blood volume deficit is not unusual in brain-dead donors, and this should be replaced with a balanced electrolyte solution (lactated Ringer's). A hypotonic solution (5% dextrose in 0.45% NaCl) is the most commonly used maintenance fluid. A colloid solution may be administered to expand intravascular volume, and red blood cells may be transfused to maintain hematocrit between 25 and 35%. However, moderate increases in filling pressures caused by volume expansion may lead to congestive heart failure and pulmonary edema because of a decrease in cardiac compliance in brain-dead donors (9). Therefore, central venous pressure should be maintained at less than 10 cmH_2O.

The goal of hemodynamic management is to maintain systolic blood pressure between 100 and 120 mmHg. To meet this goal, the donor's cardiovascular system is continuously supported as indicated by cardiac output and filling pressures. The need for pharmacologic support is not unusual. Generally, dopamin hydrochloride (2—10 μg/kg per min) is given to improve cardiac contractility. Dobutamine hydrochloride and isoproterenol hydrochloride may be given to increase cardiac output, but the vasodilating effects of these drugs may decrease blood pressure. Doses of all vasopressors should be carefully titrated, since donors have high levels of catecholamines. Alpha-vasoconstrictors such as phenylephrine hydrochloride and norepinephrine bitartrate are avoided (10), since these agents may decrease splanchnic blood flow and increase the afterload of the depressed myocardium. Donors do not respond to centrally acting chronotropic drugs, such as atropine sulfate. Therefore, direct-acting agents such as epinephrine or isoproterenol are preferred to restore heart rate. Hypertension should be avoided because it may cause pulmonary edema, decrease organ blood flow, and increase oxygen consumption of the heart. Ten percent of potential donors develop cardiac arrest and require resuscitation (11). The goal of cardiopulmonary resuscitation is to restore circulation within 15 minutes using the standard guidelines except that no intracardiac injection of medication is given when donation of the heart is anticipated.

The goal of renal care is to maintain urine output greater than 80 ml/h. When urine output is not adequate, fluid is given to maintain central venous pressure close to 10 cmH_2O. Furosemide (40—200 mg) and mannitol (12.5—

25 g) may be administered to increase urine output. Dopamine (<5 μg/kg per min) may be given to promote urine output and protect renal function. Diabetes insipidus is anticipated in 38–87% of donors because of inappropriate secretions of antidiuretic hormone. Treatment of diabetes insipidus consists of fluid replacement and the administration of antidiuretic hormone. A hypotonic solution (0.45% NaCl) is given to maintain adequate intravascular volume, and potassium (15 mEq) is supplemented. Hypoglycemia may be seen in a high urine output state, and it should be corrected. Pitressin tannate is given (0.5–1 unit/h) as a supplemental hormone. A synthetic hormone (Desmopressin acetate, 0.5–2 μg/8–12h) may be preferred since it has a less potent vasopressor effect than does pitressin (12).

In brain-dead animal models, serum levels of triiodothyronine, insulin, and cortisol are found to be low and the administration of triiodothyronine improves cardiac function (13). Triiodothyronine was reported to improve cardiac function and to reduce the requirement for inotropes in human donors (14), but its effectiveness requires further investigation.

Other medical management is directed to the treatment of abnormalities in electrolyte imbalances and the acid-base state, and to the treatment of coagulopathy, and infection. Many types of electrolyte imbalance may be seen: hypernatremia, hypokalemia, hypophosphatemia, and hypomagnesemia. Ionized hypocalcemia may be seen when the donor requires a large volume of blood transfusion and metabolic acidosis in hemodynamically unstable donors. Major coagulation problems are associated with dilutional problems that occur when the donor suffers from trauma. Some degree of disseminated intravascular coagulation has been reported to occur in 80% of donors. Antifibrinolytic therapy is not recommended, because of the potential occurrence of hypercoagulability.

Intraoperative management of donors

The intraoperative care of donors is a continuation of intensive care. Blood products and other necessary fluids should be available to maintain normovolemia. Although donors do not perceive surgical stimulation as pain, they require anesthetics. Inhalation anesthetics (e.g. isoflurane) are frequently used to suppress spinal sympathetic responses (15), and narcotics may be added when the circulatory system does not tolerate these potent inhalation anesthetics. Muscle relaxants are given frequently, since spinal reflex-related involuntary movement may be seen and tension of abdominal wall may make surgical procedures difficult.

Frequently, a long midline incision is made from the suprasternal notch to the pubis and all organs are then skeletonized. After systemic heparinization (300 units/kg), the aorta is cannulated and preservation solution is infused.

Then the organs are swiftly removed in the following sequence: heart and lung, liver, pancreas, kidney, and other tissues. Once cardiac arrest is induced, all cardiopulmonary support and monitoring can be terminated. These organs are hypotermically preserved in Wisconsin solution and are then transported to the location of the recipients, where one hopes they find a second life.

References

1. Beecher, H.K., Adams, R.D. and Banger, A.C.: A definition of irreversible coma. Report of the Ad Hoc Committee of the Harvard Medical School to examine the definition of brain death. *J. Amer. Med. Assoc.* **205**, 337 (1966).
2. Mohandas, A. and Chou, S.N.: Brain death: A clinical and pathological study. *J. Neurosurg.* **35**, 211 (1971).
3. A collaborative study: An appraisal of the criteria of cerebral death: A summary statement. *J. Amer. Med. Assoc.* **237**, 982 (1976).
4. Report of the medical consultants on the diagnosis of death to the President's Commission for the Study of Ethical Problems in Medicine and Biomedical and Behavioral Research: guidelines for the determination of death. *J. Amer. Med. Assoc.* **246**, 2184 (1981).
5. Diagnosis of brain death (Statement issued by the honorary secretary of the Conference of Medical Royal Colleges and their facilities in the U.K. on 11.10.76). *Brit. Med. J.* **1187** (1976).
6. Darby, J.M., Stein, K., Grenvik, A. and Stuart, S.A.: Approach to management of the heartbeating 'brain dead' organ donor. *J. Amer. Med. Assoc.* **261** 2222 (1989).
7. Belsh, J.M., Blatt, R. and Schiffman, P.L.: Apnea testing in brain death. *Arch. Int. Med.* **146**, 2385 (1986).
8. Novitzky, D., Rose, A.G. and Cooper, D.K.C.: Injury of myocardial conduction tissue and coronary artery smooth muscle following brain death in the baboon. *Transplantation* **45**, 964 (1988).
9. Wicomb, W.N., Cooper, D.K.C., Lanza, R.P., Novitzky, D. and Isacs, S.: The effects of brain death and 24 hours storage by hypothermic perfusion on donor heart function in the pig. *J. Thorac. Cardiovasc. Surg.* **91**, 896 (1986).
10. Slapak, M.: The immediate care of potential donors for cadaveric organ transplantation. *Anesthesia* **33**, 700 (1978).
11. Emery, R.W., Cork, R.C., Levinson, M.M. *et al.*: The cardiac donor: a six-year experience. *Ann. Thorac. Surg.* **41**, 356 (1986).
12. Richardson, D.W. and Robinson, A.G.: Desmopresin. *Ann. Int. Med.* **103**, 973 (1985).
13. Novitzky, D., Wicomb, M.N., Cooper, D.K.C., Rose, A.G., Fraser, R.C. and Barnared, C.N.: Electrocardiographic, hemodynamic and endocrine changes occurring during experimental brain death in the chacma baboon. *Heart Transplant.* **4**, 63 (1984).
14. Novitzky, D., Cooper, D.K.C. and Reichart, B: Hemodynamic and metabolic responses to hormonal therapy in brain-dead potential organ donors. *Transplantation* **43**, 852 (1987).
15. Wetzel, R.C., Setzer, N., Stiff, J.L. and Rogers, M.C.: Hemodynamic responses in brain dead organ donor patients. *Anesth. Analg.* **64**, 125 (1985).

73. The role of the National Kidney Foundation in cadaveric transplantation in Saudi Arabia

S. ASWAD, S. TAHA, M. BABIKER and A. QAYUM

Introduction

The number of chronic renal failure patients in the Kingdom of Saudi Arabia (KSA) has increased over the years. At the end of 1989, this number reached 2100 patients (Figure 1). It is gratifying to note that in answer to this evident need there has been a proportionate increase in the number of dialysis facilities to the present total of 76 centers.

The first kidney transplant with a living related donor (LRD) was performed in 1979 in Riyadh. Since then, the total number of LRD transplants undertaken in Saudi Arabia has reached 497 cases.

With the increase in number of renal failure patients came the realization that living-related donation was not the answer to the problem. It was imperative to

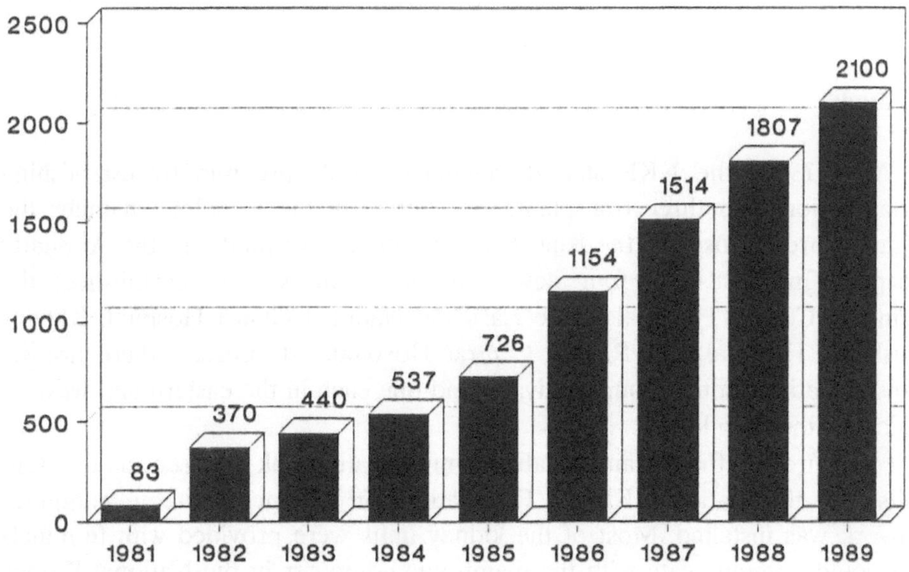

Fig. 1. Annual increase in dialysis patients.

look for other sources of grafts. The first step taken in this direction was to collaborate with other international agencies to supply the centers in the Kingdom with kidneys. Though the number of kidneys brought from abroad was small, some patients benefited from this and the need was partially met. The second step was establishing a local cadaveric program. However, being one of the conservative Islamic countries, religious aspects had to be clarified and support of the religious scholars had to be obtained.

In 1982, the Senior Ulama Commission (Religious Council) gave a declaration allowing organ donation from both live and dead donors. This was followed by the decision of the high Islamic Council, meeting in Amman, Jordan in 1986, of acceptance of the brain-death concept. After these very important landmarks, a clear policy was made to regulate kidney transplantation from cadavers.

The National Kidney Foundation (NKF) was established in 1986 to fulfill this policy. One of the main objectives of the NKF is to encourage local kidney donation and transplantation.

To achieve these objectives, NKF has used every means of professional and public education and advertising through the media. Donor cards, posters and stickers were distributed in large numbers all over the Kingdom. Television, radio and newspapers have been utilized to educate people about the benefits of kidney donation and to clarify religious, social and medical aspects of the program.

Intensive care unit (ICU) facilities are available in almost every hospital of the Kingdom and it is estimated that the annual number of brain death cases in these ICU is more than 300, thus making a high potential for cadaver organs.

Methods

In April 1987, the NKF started implementing its program by establishing collaboration with three transplantation centers in the Kingdom, namely: the Armed Forces Hospital, the King Faisal Specialist Hospital and the Al-Shatty Hospital. In 1988–89, four new transplant centers were established: the Damman Central Hospital in the East, the National Guard Hospital, Khamis Mushayat Hospital and Riyadh Central Hospital. At present, there are six transplantation centers: four in Riyadh and one each in the eastern and western regions of the Kingdom.

To ensure an efficient and reliable communication link between the different units and the National Kidney Foundation, an advanced remote computer network was installed. Most of the kidney units were provided with terminals that could communicate with the mainframe computer in the National Kidney Foundation. This main computer network played an important role in data collection, matching and organ distribution. Among the 2000 patients undergoing dialysis in Saudi Arabia, we have a transplant waiting list of 300 patients on the NKF computer.

To ensure effective communication between the NKF transplant centers and ICU's where brain deaths are located, a coordination system network was established (Figure 2).

Finally, the NKF played an important role in the collection and analysis of scientific data and supplied special forms to all transplant centers to be filled in and returned to the NKF directly, to be entered in the computer system. These forms help the Foundation to put out a statistical annual report about all transplantations and organ retrieval activity in the country.

Results

In the three years since this program was implemented, 357 brain-death cases were reported to the NKF from 46 hospitals and organs were harvested from 82 of these. Of the brain-death cases, 195 were Saudians and 162 were foreigners living in Saudi Arabia. Of all the brain-death cases, 87.1% were male and 12.9% female. Of the 82 cases from which organs were removed, 35 (42.6%) were Saudians and 47 (57.4%) non-Saudians and 92.3% were male and 7.7% were female. Age range of both brain-death and harvested cases shown in Figures 3 and 4.

During the 3-year period, the total number of kidneys being coordinated through the NKF was 176, of which 164 were harvested locally and 12 were

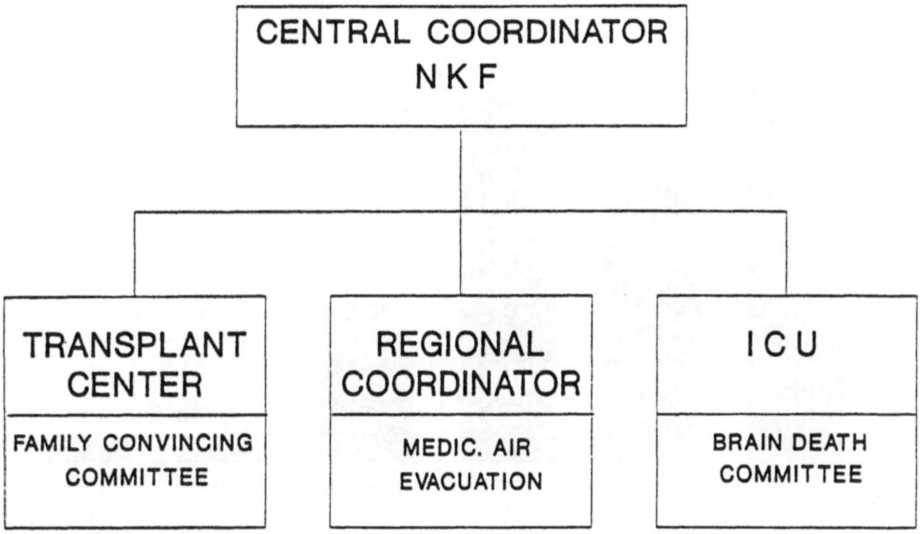

Fig. 2. Coordination system.

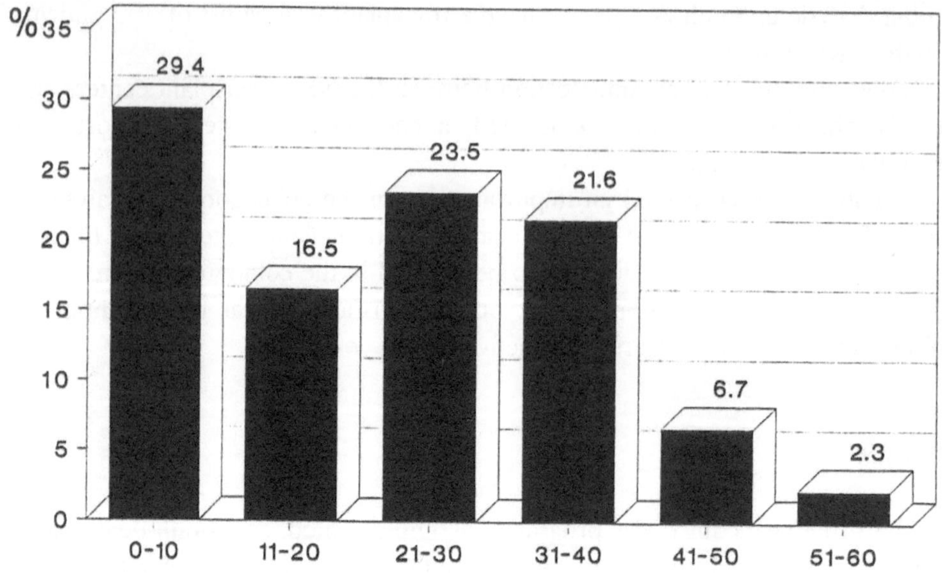

Fig. 3. Age range in brain-death cases.

brought from outside. Failure to harvest kidneys were: family refusal (60%), medical reasons (22%), inability to locate the family (14%) and other reasons (4%). The 164 harvested kidneys were transplanted in the various centers shown in Table 1. Two kidneys were not usable for medical reasons. Of the 162

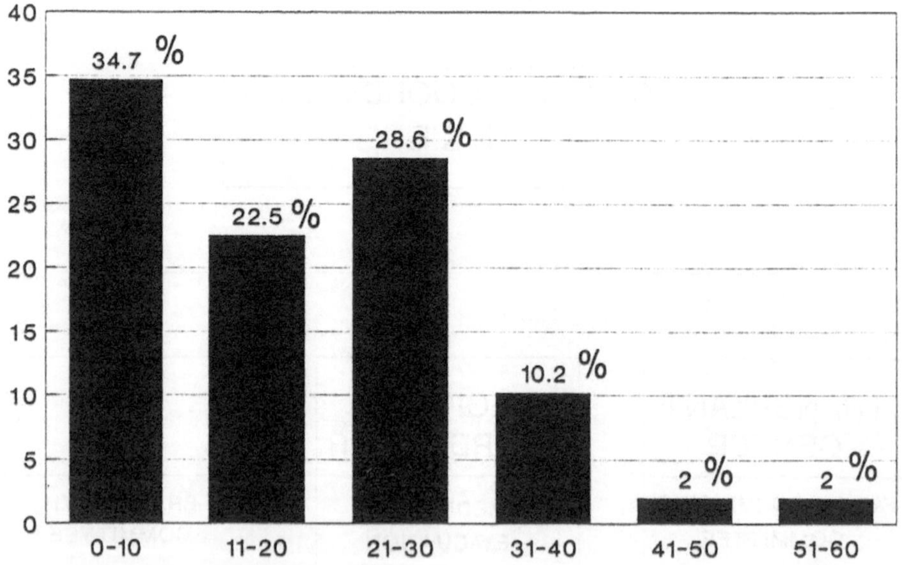

Fig. 4. Age range in harvested cases.

Table 1. Transplant centers and number of kidneys harvested.

	No. of kidneys
1. Riyadh Armed Forces Hospital	66
2. King Faisal Specialist Hospital	44
3. Al-Shatty Educational Hospital	37
4. Al Dammam Central Hospital	4
5. National Group Hospital	9
6. Khamis Mushayat Hospital	2

patients transplanted from the harvested kidneys, 154 (95%) were Saudians. In addition to kidneys, we succeeded in getting the consent of the family in four cases to harvest the hearts and also one pair of corneas.

After 3 years of the program, 76.6% of the 162 transplanted patients were doing well with functioning grafts, 16% had non-functioning grafts while 7.4% of the transplanted patients have died.

Discussion

When it was established in 1986, the National Kidney Foundation was a unique organ procurement organization, the first of its kind in the Middle East. Later, however, other countries have started similar organizations. In Kuwait, some 22 cadaveric kidneys have been harvested from local cadavers while in Egypt only 8 cadaveric donors have been reported.

In order to understand the achievements of the NFK in Saudi Arabia in comparison to other similar international organizations, one must take into consideration the short period of its existence and the enormous difficulties it encountered in a deeply religious Islamic country. At the present time, the six transplant centers in Saudi Arabia are performing 12 transplants PMP per year from locally harvested kidneys and from live donors. This is small in comparison to 46 PMP in Catalonia or 31 PMP in Spain, for example. While we clearly need more cadaver donors, the results so far obtained in an Islamic country such as Saudi Arabia, within the space of only 3 years, is very encouraging. As mentioned earlier, the annual number of brain-death cases on record is 300, of which so far, only 30% were reported to the NKF and of these, 23% became actual donors. In order to meet the current annual need of nearly 400 patients now on the transplant waiting list in Saudi Arabia, we clearly need to have access to some 200 cadaver donors. It is hoped that, with time, more people in the Kingdom will become aware of the humanitarian efforts being exerted by the Foundation and of their responsibility as citizens to help save the lives of others so that these goals might be reached.

References

1. Abouna, G.M., Kumar, M.S.A., White, A.G. *et al.*: Experiences with 130 consecutive renal transplants in the Middle East. *Transplant. Proc.* **16**, 114–117 (1984).
2. Abouna, G.M.: Personal communication (1990).
3. Combined report on regulr dialysis and transplanted in Europe: *Annual Report on European Dialysis and Transplantation*, p. 41. Springer-Verlag, London (1987).

74. The position of the Transplantation Society on commercialization in organ transplantation

J.R. BATCHELOR

When the Transplantation Society was formed, clinical transplantation was virtually confined to kidney allografting, and this was carried out at a limited number of pioneer centres. At that time, the Society was like many scientific societies in which the chief activity was the holding of meetings at which scientific papers were read. However, transplantation is not just a subject of great biological interest. Over the past three decades, the scope and amount of clinical transplantation has grown to a such an extent that it has become a major enterprise, involving patients, their families, those who carry out the transplants and look after the patients, the wider public, and governments. Indeed, the very success of transplantation has been a factor in creating problems. Thoughtful members of the Society have recognized the development of these problems, and have shown courage and humanity in that they have led the Society to take a wider view of its functions than those of an ordinary scientific society. As well as providing a forum for scientific discussions, the Society has declared publicly that it is also concerned with the maintenance of proper ethical standards in clinical transplantation.

I will start by making a self-evident but important point. The rules and guidelines of the Society are entirely separate from the laws of any country; naturally, the first duty of all of us is to obey the law of the land in which we reside. These laws, which of course differ from country to country, have something to say about what is not permissible for transplanters and patients, and they carry legal penalties if there is any infringement. The Transplantation Society has no legal powers; its guidelines carry no sanctions except that of expulsion from the Society membership.

During the 1980s, when the buying of kidneys from living donors came to their attention, the Council of The Transplantation Society published a statement in the *Lancet* (September 28, 1985, pp. 715—716) entitled 'Commercialization in transplantation: the problems and some guidelines for practice'. This is the most recently published statement of the position of the Society, and those of you who are in any doubt should consult this document. I believe it is worth emphasizing that the Society considers that the interests of us all are best served by the widespread establishment of effective, publicly supported, cadaver donor programmes. The Society also considers that the establishment of such programmes should be a stated objective in countries where they do not already exist.

During the past five years a number of those engaged in transplantation have pointed out difficulties in adhering to the guidelines of 1985. The most acute difficulties are apparent in countries where there is no effective cadaver organ donor programme. In such countries, if no live related donor is available, there is a stark choice between death, continuation on dialysis for an indefinite period, or transplanation with an organ from an unrelated, living donor. Even continuation on dialysis for an indefinite period may be an impractical option because of economic reasons.

The question has therefore arisen: 'Should the guidelines of the Transplantation Society be modified in any way, taking into account the special difficulties being experienced by countries without cadaver donor programmes?' Before embarking on a debate of the issues involved in this question, the Society needs information. As president of the society I therefore asked Dr. R.A. Sells of the U.K. and Dr. Abdullah Daar of Oman to carry out a fact-finding mission. They did so earlier this year and compiled a report. Their report will go to the Society's Ethical Sub-Committee which will formulate advice for the Council.

In summary then, the position of the Transplantation Society on commercialization in organ transplantation is as laid down by the Council in the statement in the *Lancet* (1985). However, it is recognized that there are great difficulties for countries in which cadaver donor programmes are not in effective operation. There is a debate in progress on the many and complex issues involved, which cannot be hurried.

75. Ethics and transplantation: an analysis of 'rewarded gifting'

JOHN B. DOSSETOR

First of all, I must state that I completely abjure all third-party entrepreneurial traffic of human organs in the market place as being unethical. Other aspects I will offer in debate, but not rampant commercialism.

Are ethics and technology linked?

Does Western technology transfer Western bioethics? Western health care technology springs from forces released in Europe at the Renaissance in the fifteenth and sixteenth centuries which have had accelerating evolution ever since. Although grounded in Judeo-Christian religious traditions, the Renaissance challenged the traditionalism of medieval Europe with respect to sources of authority for those who govern (politics), or regulate conventional religious expression (the medieval church and the Protestant movement), or dictate orthodoxy of scientific belief (Galenic medicine). New political thought championed the concept of egality (of men, but not women), individual worth, rights to privacy, and a return to democracy — the latter having been lost when the Greco-Roman culture became imperial. In philosophy, the rights of individuals (men and women) to think freely and independently was expressed through Hobbes, Locke, J.S. Mill, Rousseau and the authors of the Declaration of American Independence.

The events whereby this liberation of thought was linked to progress in scientific discovery seemed to many, including this author, to have a cause and effect relationship. They evolved into the scientific technologies of modern medical science. Transplantation medicine is but an example of this.

Although most persons were very slow to abandon the dogma of religion as the basis for their view of the world, a growing proportion, especially scientists, did do so. They adopted a variety of ethical systems: (a) 'Natural Law' philosophy, or (b) rational secular humanism, based on the philosophy of a 'social contract' between members of a given society.

Many nowadays hold that 'social contract' philosophy, because it allows for too many options and too much flexibility, also fails to provide consensus on what constitutes the good life and the actions which pertain to it. It has failed to establish sufficient moral authority. The same is argued for Natural Law philosophy, based on an intuitive examination of Nature and the natural world.

This means that both (a) the coercive force of religious dogma, and (b) rational arguments based on of the 'social contract', or Natural Law, seem to have failed. If that is so then one's last hope would seem to be resolution of conflict by a process of peaceable negotiation, and to base moral authority on such negotiated agreement. This is the state which now exists in the West: negotiated moral agreement, grounded in widely accepted ethics principles, many of which stem from differing religious traditions, it is essentially non-sectarian and pluralistic — and medical technology is practised within its ethical boundaries. It is the ethics of liberal democracy.

Despite this, conflict still arise between those who hold a broad liberal ethic based on full personal autonomy for all men and women and those who hold to more restrictive ethics codes, usually directly grounded on divine revelation. When such conflicts can be examined by the techniques of science — as in the confrontation between Darwinian Evolutionists and the Creationists, or the medieval church and the cosmology of Galileo — the scientific position usually comes to predominate. But such is *not* the case when scientific technology cannot be brought to bear on a conflict — as in the conflict in the West over the moral status of the fertilized human ovum or the moment of its human ensoulment.

Of particular interest are situations which arise when new technology such as organ transplantation is transferred from Western to non-Western cultures. Some would argue that because liberal individualistic free-thinking fostered Western science, importation of Western technology should carry Western ethics standards with it. The weakness of this argument is obvious from the history of how Western countries used power derived from their technology in the past, when it was transferred. Regrettably, the history is one of rampant exploitation, greed, and human enslavement, coupled with a denial to others of ethical status accorded by the innovators to themselves. Thus, though there may be a link in the West between liberalized individualized ethics and scientific *creativity*, there is no evidence for a link between science and ethics when Western technology comes to be *applied.*

So the answer to the first question 'Are ethics and technology linked?' would seem to be 'No'. Thus, Western transplant technology when introduced into a predominantly Islamic society, as in the Middle East, is under the ethical dictate of Islam (1, 2), and the same technology, on introduction into the society of India, might equally be largely under the ethical dictates of Hinduism (3, 4).

But before accepting this conclusion one needs to examine a pre-emptive question: 'Is there, in fact, a universal ethical system which is shared both by all religious traditions as well as the principles of secular rational humanism?'

Is there a universal code of ethics?

The answer to this question is also 'No'. It would be much simpler if there was. One would have to do no more than learn the code and have everyone agree to abide by its guidelines and rules. However, we do all share a universal ethic in a very broad sense:

- It is wrong to kill the innocent.
- It is right to promote the welfare of others.
- Justice acknowledges that every person has instrinic value, or worth.
- Self-determination (autonomy) is a fundamental component of personal freedom, when so doing brings no harm to others or society.

All cultures might agree on such principles. But a universal code would also have to have at its base some measure of agreement on such questions as:

- Is there sanctity to human life? What is sanctity?
- Do we have full ownership of our own bodies or are they ours by stewardship from a Divine Being?
- Is there a God, and if so by what process or by whom has God's divine nature been revealed?

Surely, a universal code of ethics would mandate that all cultures would have to agree at least on these three questions, as well. It requires no more than a simple glance at history to convince us that there is no such agreement.

We remain quite divided, even as members of a single profession or discipline, on the principle and rules which we should use to resolve our dilemmas. Some of us have absolutes; others absolutism is abhorrent. Presumably we might all subscribe to such general ethical principles as the Geneva 1948 Declaration of the World Medical Association which states (5):

> 'I solemnly pledge myself to consecrate my life to the service of humanity; I will practice my profession with conscience and dignity; the health of my patient will be my first considerations of religion, nationality, race, party politics or social standing to intervene between my duty and my patient; I will maintain the utmost respect for human life, from time of conception; even under threat, I will not use my medical knowledge contrary to the laws of humanity.'

But so such broad principles give us enough common ground to resolve the dilemmas which we face in transplantation today? I submit they do not. These principles are not detailed enough to support the view that we have a universal system or code of ethics.

The same observation may be made, too, I believe, concerning the oath of a Muslim Physician adopted by the Islamic Medical Association in 1977 (6).

Can we solve the central crisis in transplantation ethics in the Middle East and in the Indian Subcontinent?

What is the central question to 'rewarded gifting'? I have considered and rejected the following:

(*For recipients*)

- Is it ethical for the rich to victimize the poor when the rich are in need of organs?
- Is it ethical to buy organs regardless of the sum involved?

(*For physicians*)

- Is it ethical for physicians to operate on normal persons to remove healthy organs for the benefit of others?
- Is it ethical for physicians to be involved in 'rewarded gifting'?

(*For donors*)

- Should societies prevent the poor from enriching themselves by selling a kidney, if they and their families are in great need?
- Are there overwhelming religious and ethical prohibitions against selling one's kidney to save another's life?

Let me state what I deem to be the crucial question and then examine methodologies for possible resolution. The crucial question is:

> 'Can *society safely enable* persons to *express their autonomy* in such a way as willingly to give up a kidney for *adequate reward*?'

To many the immediate answer quite simply is 'No — absolutely not.' To others, myself included, the immediate answer is 'Probably no; conceivably yes; but let us debate it and see. . . .'

Each of us could make our commentary on this question but before I give mine on methodology, let me analyze the question further.

First the question recognizes the right of society to overrule both physician decision-making AND personal decision-making, *even* when their actions would do nothing but good to others. Societies claim the right to prevent fully competent persons from possibly doing harm to themselves as a consequence of coercive persuasion by others.

Society has interests in protecting its members from possibly being victims as a consequence of their own needs. Note that the word society implies that this is NOT primarily a MEDICAL decision. To me, it simply is not part of a physician's duty to resolve a societal issue of this sort. It is the duty of physicians to insist that jurists, theologians, politicians, consumer groups and others know the problem and act to resolve it; physicians obviously have a right to be involved, too.

The question recognizes that persons have elements of autonomy which can only be expressed if they are fully informed of all consequences, short term and long term, both as regards (a) *their own health* and (b) the ways in which *the reward is best handled.* The reward cannot be 'adequate' if unsophisticated persons do not know how to handle it. How best to conserve the benefit of the reward is a large part of the issue of informed consent, in this question. Those who assume permissive authority also have to accept responsibility for ongoing post-operative financial advice for investment safeguards, in my view.

So much for the question; What about the answer? I see this evolving from a process which is part philosophical and part pragmatic.

Firstly, as there is no universal ethic system that can do the job, these issues must be resolved within each culture, for itself. I see no way out of that conclusion. All attempts to avoid that conclusion 'smell' to me of unacceptable 'ethic imperialism'.

Secondly, except for cultures which have a more or less universally accepted religious basis for all issues of medical ethics, the solution should come from consensus of appropriate decision-makers by applying their variously balanced ethical principles, NOT by predetermined moralistic decree.

Thirdly, if consensus is the name of the process, then crucial attention must be paid to the composition of the group of consensus negotiators.

Fourthly, if consensus cannot be achieved by application of principles, the process becomes more pragmatic — a process of negotiated agreement on moral issues. There is nothing to be ashamed of here. It is simply a recognition of lack of consensus on moral principles, at that time (7). This process of negotiated moral agreement has similarities to the tradition of moral reasoning formerly known in Europe as 'casuistry'. Thus, it might be that there would be no moral consensus on the practice of 'rewarded gifting' and yet complete acceptance that cadaveric organ procurement is the ultimate best answer. A negotiated moral agreement' might then consist of a 3—5 year agreement on how to proceed with (a) a *temporary* acceptance of rewarded gifting; (b) commitment to a full research project on the psycho-social and financial outcome for live unrelated kidney donors in respect to the 'adequacy of their reward'; (c) a determination by all parties actively to promote cadaveric organ procurement by every means (including money from recipients from the rewarded gifting program); and (d) a resolve to renegotiate all the moral issues involved after 3—5 years.

Some would judge the suggestion of 'negotiated moral agreement' as a compromise of moral principles. I would vigorously maintain that it need not be so.

In conclusion, transplantation in the Middle East and the Indian sub-continent takes place in a context of wide disparities of wealth and health care opportunity. In many countries there is no governmental security against the evil victimizing and degrading effects of poverty and illness, unlike for most people in many Western and some Middle East countries. Cultures with differing religious beliefs place different values:

- on practices relating to the body — live or dead — and its organs, for this life or an after-life;
- on the value and extent of acceptable altruistic self-sacrifice for one's family; one's soul, or one's reincarnation;
- on what defines the limits of legitimate self-determination in situations of great personal need.

The situation in more complex when transplantation ethics arches between two cultures. It would seem that transcultural or intercultural issues should be 'on-hold' until intra-cultural issues are resolved. They should be placed 'on-hold' by international legislation, in my view.

I believe we have an almost worldwide consensus on (a) the use of cadaveric organs in transplantation, and, (b) that priority should be given to resolving ethical and financial aspects of maintaining brain-dead bodies for cadaveric transplantation, but I also believe the transplantation community will be judged by how it obtains societal answers to the crucial question stated above. I hope it will be by negotiated moral agreement if consensus on moral principle cannot be achieved. The least successful way, in my view, is an attempt to resolve it by decree.

References

1. Rispler-Chaim, V.: Islamic medical ethics in the 20th century. *J. Med. Ethics* **15**, 203—208 (1989).
2. Rahman, A., Amine, C. and Elkadi, A.: Islamic Code of Medical Professional Ethics. In: Robert M. Veatch (ed.), *Cross Cultural Perspectives in Medical Ethics*, pp. 120—125. James Bartlett (1989).
3. Srikanta Murthy, K.R.: Professional ethics in ancient Indian medicine. *Indian J. Hist. Med.* **18**, 45—49 (1973).
4. Oath of Initiation (Caraka Samhita): *Med. Hist.* **14**, 295—296 (1970).
5. *The Declaration of Geneva.* Adopted by the World Medical Association at Geneva, Switzerland, September 1948.
6. *The Oath of a Muslim Physician.* Convention Bulletin of the Islamic Medical Association, October 1977.
7. Engelhardt, H.T.: *Foundations of Bioethics*, pp. 39—44. Oxford Univ. Press (1986).

76. Moral, ethical and medical values sacrificed by commercialization in human organs

G.M. ABOUNA

Introduction

Recent advances in organ transplantation have created a situation where there is a widening disparity between organ demand and organ supply, which has led to a flourishing international trade in human organs, particularly in those areas of the world where cadaver organs are not available and where there is marked disparity in wealth, such as India and the Far East on the one hand and the Middle East on the other. As a consequence, a new and deplorable kind of medical practice has emerged where human kidneys are brought from the poor and the destitute for transplantation into wealthy clientele with soaring profits for brokers, private hospitals and physicians, as Dr Vas and Dr Colabawalla have emphasized elswhere in this book. This unfortunate situation also illustrates the plight of so many renal failure patients in the Middle East and elsewhere who are driven to the market place out of desperation because cadaver organs have not yet been made available to them in their own countries. Indeed, since 1986, nearly 500 patients from the Arabian Gulf countries have received purchased kidney transplants in India, Egypt and, more recently, Iraq. Trading in human organs has also taken place in Europe and the Americas, albeit on a smaller scale, and recently in England where some of the physicians involved in this practice were duly reprimanded.

It is not surprising that such practices have alarmed both the medical profession and the public and have been rightly condemned by international medical societies and organizations, including the international, the European, the American and more recently the Middle East Societies for organ transplantation (1, 2). However, in order to get around this professional and public outcry and in an attempt to make this abhorrent practice less disagreeable, a new and more attractive label was recently introduced. It is called 'rewarded gifting' (3, 4) which is not only a contradiction in terms, since a gift by definition is never given for a reward, but in our view and from our experience it is only another more subtle form of trading in human organs and has the same negative impact on many of our moral, medical and ethical values.

Observations on paid transplantation in the Middle East

Between 1986 and 1990, 72 patients were seen and treated at the Kuwait Transplant Center, one of the largest referral centers in the Middle East, after returning from abroad where they had received paid renal transplants. Another 40–50 patients who also received purchased kidneys abroad were followed by their referring nephrologist in Kuwait. Of these, 55% received their kidney grafts in India, 30% in Iraq, 9% in Egypt and the remainder in the Far East. Most of the patients who went to India were transplanted in private hospitals in Bombay from poor donors, supplied by the hospital or by brokers. The 21 patients transplanted in Iraq were done at the Al-Khayal Hospital which is now the busiest private hospital in the Middle East for paid kidney transplantation which purportedly uses the system of 'rewarded gifting' as described by Dr Reddy of Madras (3). As we have reported earlier, a large number of serious medical, social, moral and linguistic problems were observed (5).

The medical outcome for these patients leaves much to be desired. Within the first 6 months of transplantation, 11 patients (15.2%) died and 28 grafts (36.3%) were lost as a result of complications, many of which are avoidable today. Another 15 recipients (21%) were 'rescued' from possible death and/or loss of their grafts by extraordinary and intensive effort at our center for treatment of a multitude of technical, immunologic and medical problems including a variety of communicable diseased, such as hepatitis, malaria, TB and HIV infections (Table 1). Four patients from Kuwait and an estimated 24 others from the Arabian Gulf became HIV positive with many of them developing AIDS disease.

While it is easy to rationalize that paid organ donation may be one way of coping with organ shortage, especially in the current poor health care and

Table 1. Recipients of paid kidney transplants abroad, and those patients 'rescued' by the Department of Organ transplantation, Kuwait University, between February 1986 and April 1990.

Serious problems within first 6 months			
Problem		Number of recipients	%
Patient death		11	15.2
Graft loss		28	36.3
Serious complications (rescued)		15	21
Type of complication 'rescued':			
Vascular	(2)	Ureteric	(5)
HIV infection	(4)	Wound disruption and sepsis	(6)
TB + nocardia + malaria	(4)	Severe rejection	(6)
Septicemia + Hepatitis	(4)		

economic environment of countries like India and the Middle East, we believe this to be a flawed, short-sighted, and self-defeating approach to a complex problem. From our observations, paid organ donation in all its forms seriously sacrifices many of our medical, moral and ethical values, including those related to the donor, the recipient, the local transplant programs, the medical profession, society and the international transplant community. I will now consider each of these areas separately.

The Donor

It is generally agreed that in organ transplantation from living donors, there are three fundamental principles which cannot be violated: first, the removal of an organ from the donor must not impair the health, life or functional integrity of that donor; second, the consent to donate must be voluntary and without pressure or coercion; and, third, the donor should be fully informed of all the possible consequences and risks of the procedure.

From our observations and from the type of environment where paid living donors are sought, most or all of these basic principles have not been fulfilled. Most of the donors come from a section of the society where their health and nutrition are already compromised by poverty and economic hardship. A major surgical operation such as nephrectomy and the removal of a healthy organ is likely to further impair the health and functional integrity of these individuals. A truly voluntary and non-coerced consent is also unlikely in the circumstances of these individuals. The mere placement of a thumb imprint on a consent form is no proof of volunterism. The desperate financial need of the donor is an obvious and clear economic coercion for, as has been admitted by Reddy and his colleagues: 'All donors have only one thing in common, great financial need and most of them come from the lower strata of society' (3, 6). A truly informed consent is equally unlikely because this involves an in-depth discussion of the nature of the procedure and the likely hazards and complications that may follow. Given the educational and literacy levels from which these donors generally come, it is doubtful that this important principle can ever be met.

There are other problems and injustices arising out of this practice. Exploitation of the donor by the hospitals, by the physicians and by the recipients has been common. The mere renaming of this practice by the label of 'rewarded gifting' does not remove this possibility. There are many reports of donors who have been cheated by the hospital and by the recipient, and of donors not given the full sum of money promised to them before harvest which is often less than 10—15% of the costs charged to the recipient. It has been recently reported that with the rapidly increasing number of poor people in India wanting to sell their kidneys, the market price for a kidney is falling considerably. Also, many of these donors are known not to receive optimum care during operation and after discharge. Surgery is often carried out in badly equipped hospitals and the patients discharged at the earliest possible time to cut costs and increase profits. After-care and follow-up of the donor, if any, is negligible or limited (5, 7).

The recipient

Many of the recipients who receive paid kidney transplants do so out of desperation because of lack of cadaveric organs in their own countries. Like the situation with the donor, the recipients have neither the free choice nor a properly informed consent for the procedure. They are at the mercy of the hospital and the physicians regarding costs, choice of donor and the quality of evaluation and investigation. Many of the recipients of Kuwait had to pay exorbitant charges which are continuing to rise and when these are compared to the local currency and living costs, they are astronomical. Four to five thousand Kuwaiti dinars (US$15 000—20 000), the average costs of having a transplant in the private hospital in Baghdad and other Indian hospitals in Bombay, is the equivalent of the earnings of a physician in those countries for a few years.

Exploitation of the recipients goes further. They are required to bring with them expensive medications including cyclosporine and antilymphocyte globulin in excessive quantities. They are kept in the hospital for the shortest possible time and in many cases they are discharged with the wounds opened or in the midst of rejection and other serious complications. The philosophy is obvious: once payment is made, get rid of the patient as soon as possible to cut costs and increase profits. The pretransplant evaluation of the donor has been minimal and unacceptable (again to cut costs). Many hospitals, including those in Iraq, Egypt and in Bombay, do not carry out tissue typing. Screening of the donor for communicable disease is inadequate or non-existent and it is so wonder that patient and graft losses are high, that so many patients have become HIV positive and that many more have developed other communicable diseases like malaria, tuberculosis and hepatitis (Table 1).

The local transplantation programs

There is considerable evidence to indicate the marketing in human organs will eventually deprecate and destroy the present willingness of members of the public to donate their organs out of altruism and charitable deed. Indeed, why should anyone donate his or her organs freely when others are selling them at a price? Why should a living-related donor, especially if he is rich, go through an operation to give away one of his kidneys when he can go to India, Egypt, Iraq or elsewhere and buy a kidney for his relative quite cheaply? Again, why should any government within the Middle East put great effort and expense in developing a cadaver procurement program when kidneys can be bought elsewhere with little more than the cost of a television set.

Our experience in Kuwait has indeed shown that all of these possibilities did take place. About 66% of the recipients who went abroad to buy a kidney had potential living-related donors and half of these had already been evaluated and were found to be suitable for donation, but when they heard they could go to India or Iraq and buy a kidney, they disappeared. They were seen again with their relative upon their return to our center, often with a profound feeling of guilt and remorse, especially when the kidney was lost or the patient died from complications. The two sons of a recipient who died with AIDS following a paid transplant in India wept with shame for not giving him one of their kidneys.

Some of the senior officials in the Ministry of Health of Kuwait were reluctant to invest in a national program of organ procurement even though the country had already enacted an excellent cadaver transplant law (Law No. 55 for 1987), because they did not consider that there was enough pressure or need to go through such an effort when it was much easier to write a cheque for their citizens to buy a kidney abroad. Consequently, very few cadaver organs could be obtained in spite of the fact that the annual death rate from trauma in that country was among the highest in the world (200 persons/million population).

Finally, the negative impact on the development of a cadaveric program does not only affect renal transplantation, but more specifically, the transplantation of other more life-saving organs such as the liver and the heart. Indeed, because an active program of cadaver organ procurement received no support from the appropriate authorities in Kuwait, not only did the number of renal failure patients on dialysis continue to escalate, but many patients with liver failure who could have been transplanted locally either died or if, fortunate, received a transplant in the West at prohibitive costs.

The medical profession

Paid organ donation in all its forms has become a lucrative business in which medical decisions are controlled more by the market forces than by acceptable professional codes of conduct and medical ethics. Examples of exploitation of donor and recipient by the hospitals and by the physicians have been reported (5, 7). As is stated by Dr Colabawalla and by Dr Vas of India elsewhere in this book, there have been many instances of false documentation of donor's age and health status, of fee-splitting among physicians and of unnecessary consultations and excessive billing. It is in the nature of things that when a medical service is carried out solely for profit, and where there are a large number of patients who are in desperate need of that service, there is often the temptation and the opportunity for deception, exploitation and corruption with least regard to many of the most cherished moral and ethical values of the medical profession and society. The other aftermath is that when the public knows that the medical profession is engaged in the buying and selling of human organs, they become disillusioned and distrustful and many who would be donors no longer wish to participate in a system in which there is corruption, exploitation and unjust distribution of organs which favors the rich and the influential.

Society

In his recent testimony to the American Congress, Arthur Caplan rightly pointed out,

> 'What is truly distinctive about transplantation is not technology or cost, but ethics. Transplantation is the only area in all of health care which cannot exist without the participation of the public. For it is the individual citizen, who while alive or, in the case of vital organs, after death who makes organs and tissues available for transplantation. If there were no gift of organs or tissues, transplantation would come to a grinding halt' (8).

Paid organ donation, under whatever label, will drown all voluntary donation by the public and all serious effort of initiating cadaver organ procurement programs in countries like India, the Far East and the Middle East. In other words, by accepting paid organ transplantation, not only will we be compromising our ethics but we will lose the very battle which we are fighting to win, i.e. making more cadaver organs available.

We often hear from protagonists of organ sale such dramatic statements as 'Buy or let die' (3) and that there is nothing wrong with this practice since the rich recipient is restored to better health and the donor receives financial benefits and thus there is some sharing of the wealth. This is both misleading and deceptive for what happens in practice is not sharing of wealth but a sharing of health by the rich recipient at the expense of poor donor. The past President of the Indian Society of Nephrology, Dr Chugh, had stated in 1988: 'If the current trend of selling human kidneys continues at the present rate, most of the poor people of India will be minus one kidney by the year 2000.' Indeed, according to the reputable journal *The Times of India*, there are already colonies and villages of poor people in India where most of their inhabitants have sold one of their kidneys.

If the human body can be treated like ordinary goods to be sold for known and predetermined rewards, we are inviting corruption is society and an unjust and unfair system of organ access and distribution, for the rich will always be on the receiving end and the poor on the giving one. On the other hand, there is great advantages to the public and to society to treat all human organ and tissue as true gifts, as Thomas Murray, Editor of *Medical Humanities Review*, had noted when he said

> 'Gifts help create and sustain initimate personal relationships. In the face of impersonal bureaucracies, gifts to strangers affirm a number of vital social values including our solidarity with others in our community and our vision of human development, individual and social, which requires more than the thin relationship established by markets and contacts.'

It is sometimes argued that an individual should be free to sell his organs just as he sells his labors and why should there be any objection. This argument, if taken to its conclusion, may easily be used to justify a return to allowing individuals to sell themselves into slavery, which is clearly unacceptable. If an individual is forced to have to sell part of his body at a price dictated by the market forces, it is surely against the autonomy and the dignity of the human individual as well as the many fundamental religious and cultural beliefs of all civilized societies. Another possible negative impact on society is the potential criminal consequences which the sale of organs for profit is likely to bring, just as drug trafficking has brought with it. There are already many press reports from different parts of the world where women and young children have been abducted, have disappeared or have been sold for their organs.

The international transplant community

In transplantation, it is very important that we should have one code of ethics regardless of the geography or culture where this statement is being given, especially when the countries of the world are getting so much closer together. For if that were not the case, a person from Germany, U.S.A., or U.K. who knows he cannot buy a kidney in his own country because of local ethical or legal codes against the sale of organs, can do so by going to India or the Far East. In this way he can easily flout the legal and the ethical standards laid down in his country and by his society, and indeed this is what is happening today. In Kuwait, for example, many patients left to buy a kidney in India and elsewhere since the Islamic Code of Ethics and Kuwait Law No. 55 for 1987 prohibit the buying and selling of human organs.

Another reason for having one standard of ethics throughout the international transplant community is clearly to do with the fact that the people and the medical profession in India, the Far East and elsewhere, will consider it an insult if they are relegated a second rate standard of ethics by condoning organ sales in their country while the West prides itself of having a different and higher standard of conduct. In a recent letter to the President of the Transplantation Society, signed by three leading Indian transplant physicians, it was rightly stated that:

> 'The concept of either rampant commercialization or of "Rewarded Gifting" has been rejected by the West. ... If that be so, then advocating it for

countries like India opens the transplantation society to a justifiable criticism of having dual standard of ethics. We, as Indians, feel that a "second rate" standard of ethics is unacceptable.' (Colabawalla, July 1990, Personal communication)

Conclusions and recommendations

The sale of human organs, in all its form, is one of the evils of current technological advances. It is damaging to the cause of transplantation as well as to the many cherished moral, religious and ethical values and beliefs of civilized society. Indeed, the Judeo-Christian and the Islamic religious condemn the sale of human organs (9). Organ sale has a serious negative impact on organ donation through altruism and volunterism by the public and also on the establishment of cadaver procurement programs by national governments. It leads to exploitation of both donors and recipients by private hospitals and physicians. It deprecates many of the fundamental professional and moral values of society by demeaning the dignity and the autonomy of the human individual. It promotes an unjust system of organ access and distribution controlled by market forces which favors the rich at the expense of the poor. It invites social and economic corruption, exploitation and even criminal dealings in the acquisition of organs for profit.

Table 2. Legislation required and morally acceptable incentives for procurement of organs.

LEGISLATION

1. Legalized removal of organs from cadavers upon the diagnosis of brain and/or cardiac death
2. Introduction of presumed consent laws as in some European countries, and now in Singapore
3. Legal prohibition of all paid donation — to remove the negative feedback effect on cadaver donation

INCENTIVES

1. *Exemptions from 'standard' financial obligations*
   - A. Funeral costs
   - B. Taxes on income or inheritance
   - C. Loss of income from disability during and after donation in case of living genetically or emotionally related donors
2. *Providing needed support*
   - A. To the bereaved family of the donor, e.g. widow's pension
   - B. Family relief grant
   - C. Free medical care to donor (in living genetically or emotionally related)
3. *Insurance plans for donor's family*

   Government-sponsored life insurance payable upon death and donation to be made available to all who wish to donate their organs after death

Since all these negative developments are the consequences of non-availability of cadaver organs and the poor socioeconomic conditions in the countries of the East, where organ sales are most rampant, the solution to this problem must lie in the creation of appropriate conditions for voluntary organ donation and the introduction of the necessary reforms by local governments for the establishment of national programs of cadaver organ procurement. In the current environment of India, the Middle East and the Far East, the key to achieving this goal is by a combination of legislation and creative and morally acceptable incentives (Table 2), many of which were outlined by us at the previous Congress of the Middle East Society for Organ Transplantation held in Ankara in 1988 (7) and later also by Dr Monaco (10).

We strongly believe that in view of the profound negative feed back effect of organ sales on voluntary and legitimate organ donation, it is imperative that all forms of paid organ donation be made illegal in all countries of the world, if the efforts to create local cadaver procurement programs are likely to succeed. Here, I believe, national and international transplant societies as well as the World Health Organization have a vital responsibility.

References

1. Ruling of the Council of the Transplantation Society: *Transplantation* **41**, 1 (1986).
2. Middle East Society for Organ Transplantation: Resolution condemning the sale of organs. *Second Int. Congress of MESOT, Kuwait*, March 12, 1990.
3. Reddy, K.C., Thiagarajan, C.M., Shunmugasundaram, D. *et al.*: Unconventional renal transplantation in India. *Transplant. Proc.* **22**(3), 910—911 (1990).
4. Sells, R. and Daar, A.: Unrelated renal transplantation. *Transplant. Rev.* **4**, 128—140 (1990).
5. Abouna, G.M., Kumar, M.S.A., Samhan, M. *et al.*: Commercialization in human organs — a Middle Eastern perspective. *Transplant. Proc.* **22**(33), 918—921 (1990).
6. Thiagarajan, C.M., Reddy, K.C., Shunmugasundaram, D. *et al.*: The practice of unconventional renal transplanation at a single center in India. *Transplant. Proc.* **22**(33), 912—914 (1990).
7. Abouna, G.M.: Organ transplantation in the Middle East — problems and possible solutions. In: M. H. Haberal (ed.), *Recent Advances in Nephrology and Transplantation*, pp. 233—242. Haberal Educational and Research Foundation, Ankara, Turkey (1990).
8. Caplan, A.L.: Testimony to the Subcommittee on Health and the Environment of the United States Congress. April 20, 1990 (personal communication).
9. Al-Awadi, A.A., Al-Mathour, K., Saif, A. *et al.: Proc. Symp. on Islamic Views on Current Medical Practice* (Arabic Text) held under the auspices of the 'Islamic Organization for Medical Sciences,' Kuwait, April 1987.
10. Monaco, A.P.: Transplantation — the state of the art. *Transplant. Proc.* **22**(33), 896—901 (1990).

77. Commerce and trade in human organs

B.N. COLABAWALLA

In this brief review, I shall offer some observations on the issues of commerce in human organs, with specific reference to India.

This commerce in India is exemplified by the trading in relation to live, unrelated donors for kidney transplantation. The scenario is, in essence, not very different from that seen in other countries where this nefarious trade prevails. Let me, though, clarify that the vast majority of colleagues involved in transplanation programs in India strongly condemn this. There are, though, some who openly advocated it in the projected belief that it is necessary at this point in time. But the vast majority on that side of the fence are involved in surreptitious deals, for reasons not difficult to imagine! There is then a conflict of value systems which needs to be analysed. The issues not only involve professions but impinge on society and the international community.

Leaving aside for the moment the wider aspects of philosophical or theological ethics, there are some secular aspects to be considered. There is a general concensus today that certain norms have to be observed in transplantation procedures. For one, removal of any donor organ or tissue must not impair health, life or functional integrity of the donor. Most of those donors come from a strata of society where their health and nutrition are already compromised due to economic stringency. Hence, removal of their organs is likely to further impair health and functional integrity. Many of these donors may not have been adequately investigated for transmissible diseases and hence pose a danger to the recipient. In this context, it is worth noting that of late some reports have documented the occurrence of AIDS in recipients who have received kidneys from this category of donor.

The next requisite is that the donation must be based on detailed and well-informed voluntary and uncoerced consent. Informed consent is not achieved merely by a cursory discussion and a perfunctory appending of the donor's signature or merely even his thumb impression in many instances to a document. Such informed consent involves an in-depth discussion on the nature of the procedure, and likely complications, rare as they may be, in a language comprehensible to the donor and involving his family members too. Given the social and literacy levels from which these donors generally come, it is doubtful if these criteria can be fulfilled.

As for voluntary and uncoerced consent, what can be a greater coercion than dangling a large sum of money before a poor donor? Any voluntary aspect then is thrown out of the window.

Finally comes the question of exploitation. The most lurid is that by the broker. He thrives on the gullibility of the illiterate or on the economic stringency of the weaker sectors. How much of the brokerage lands in the donor's pocket is a matter of guesswork. The next individual to exploit the situation — admittedly out of necessity — is the rich recipient. It is argued that a little redistribution of *wealth* occurs thereby. May I suggest it is a redistribution of *health* from the poor — who can ill afford it — to the rich! The social inequity in this proposition is evident. The next group to exploit is the institutions and professionals. Many of these insitutions are abominably ill-equipped for transplantation procedures and are aided and abetted by the professionals.

Impacts on society

There is an argument that there is a shortage of donor organs and why should we then not utilize whatever is available irrespective of other considerations? It is also postulated that an individual is free to donate his kidney for a price, much as he may sell his labour or other services, and hence why should society object? There are grave dangers in such propositions to the value systems of social structure. It immediately puts the value systems of an individual in need and his methods of fufilling and need versus the value system of organized society. The freedom of an individual to behave as he likes is always circumscribed by the needs of the greater good of social morality. The replacement of the ethical concept of 'intrinsic value' of the human organism by that of a concept of 'extrinsic value' of the body or its parts makes the human body or its parts a 'saleable and marketable commodity' with a price structure dictated by market forces. Whatever the circumstances of an individual, we in society have to concede that he should never be compelled to sell something, and certainly not one of his organs! It is against the grain of maintaining a human being's autonomy and dignity.

There are then dangers of extortion, blackmail and even criminalization, all of which have occurred.

Effects on transplant programmes

The deleterious effect on existing transplantation programmes is becoming evident. There are families today who are proposing to 'buy' the kidney rather than to donate one from a family member. Then, again, cadaver donation programmes are hampered; the graver danger is that commercialization may creep into these programmes.

There is an international dimension to this program. International cooperative and exchange of organs has been hampered by the intrusion of commercialization. Today kidneys, donors and recipients are carted by air from one country to another for a price. An advertisement in a German paper offered an 'Asian transplantation holiday' package deal. The International Commission of Health Professionals (ICHP) has recorded that recipients are from richer countries whilst the donors are from poorer countries.

Many of us in India, as individuals and groups, are trying to evolve strategies to combat this evil. Our effort are directed towards:

(i) raising social conscience and awareness about the immorality of this commerce;
(ii) inducing government to legislate against trading and trafficking in human organs;
(iii) bringing in statutory controls over institutions where transplantations can be performed;
(iv) accelerating the pace of cadaver donation programmes and transplantation.

Nonetheless, this still leaves us with the bottom line, viz. the dilemma of organ shortage.

It is then for international groups such as we have today and other such bodies to formulate guidelines on whether unrelated donors should be accepted, and if so, in what set of circumstances and with what forms of control to separate it from the nexus of commercialization. I for one am groping for an answer.

At this point, I would like to refer to the recently floated concept labelled as 'Rewarded Gift'. It seems to me to be a contradiction in terms as I did not realize that a 'gift' needs a 'reward'. I suggest that this concept needs a very critical analysis as it seems to be a terminological subterfuge for commerce with a stamp of approval.

Finally, it must be realized that the onus is not entirely on countries where this commerce prevails, but also on countries from which potential recipients originate.

78. Some ethical concerns in organ transplantation

C.J. VAS

Organ transplantation [OT] is no longer a futuristic concept. It is a matter of reality — a day-to-day affair for many medical practitioners and an urgent necessity for some of our patients. OT has helped millions of people all over the world and will help many more. It has truly proved to be a boon for humanity.

Medical advances in this day and age have ameliorated the condition of very many patients with intractable disorders involving the kidney, heart, pancreas, blood and brain. It is well to recall that OT has been current since 1982 when blood transfusions were first started and later found useful during World War I. Programmes of OT have progressed in most countries from those of blood to skin, fascia, tendon and bone, cornea, blood vessels, kidney, heart, pancreas, lungs and bones marrow. In the field of reproductive medicine, we have artificial insemination, *in vitro* fertilization with embryo transfer and gamete intra-fallopian transfer (GIFT). In the last three to five years, tissue transplants — preferably called implants, into the central nervous system have also come into fashion. These have raised a hue and cry for much of the implant tissue was obtained from aborted foetuses — some of whom were created, or co-created, for this specific purpose. An American economist, Mr E. Thorne, writing in the *Wall Street Journal* of August 19, 1987, had this to say:

> 'Clearly, human beings have become useful to each other in ways never before possible. In the U.S. last year, . . . (organs) were tranplanted at a total cost of nearly $1 billion.
>
> 'A transplant industry based upon fetal-tissue technology could dwarf the present organ-transplant industry. Fetal-cell implants have the potential to offer relief to several million Americans, including one million with Parkinson's disease, 2.5 million to 3.0 million suffering from Alzheimer's disease. . . .'

In the U.S. alone, this could be a multi-billion dollar industry and one can imagine its magnitude if the 'market' is extended to include the rest of the advanced and developing world. Can one think of the colossal expenditures internationally, the most unimaginable corruption and unethical conduct that is likely to occur if we are to only go by our present experience?

It is common knowledge that evil often follows good. We have, for instance, the momentous splitting of the atom that altered the ways of our world and also destroyed Hiroshima and Nagasaki! Our understanding and progress in the field of genetics has already done so much for the benefit of humankind but we are confronted with female foeticide, cloning of humans, the artificial production of chimeras and interspecies crossing or fertilization. We are now faced with the prospect of treating Parkinson's disease, albeit at an experimental level, with brain implants of adrenal or neural tissue obtained from the patients themselves — a matter of no serious ethical concern. However, foetal cerebral or nigral tissue has been preferred as implants. This raises many ethical difficulties because the needed tissue is now obtained not from spontaneously aborted foetuses as was initially done but rather from foetuses obtained after elective or induced abortions. The slippery slope has now taken us further down — with women prepared to have themselves artificially impregnated with the sperms of relatives, even their own fathers, in an attempt to 'harvest' immunologically acceptable foetal tissue at a subsequent deliberately induced abortion. Simply put, an illegitimate creation of a human for a cold-blooded killing. How do some see it? We have the statement of the President of the American Parkinsons Association, reported in the *New York Times* of August 17, 1987: '. . . the majority of people with the disease couldn't care less about the ethical issues — they just want something that works.' This has also been the experience of many neurologists, including myself.

Turning to OT, there is ample evidence of unethical and criminal conduct in many parts of the world and understandably, the World Health Assembly of the WHO had little option but to appeal to all national governments to enact legislation to prevent commercial trafficking in human organs for transplantation, as it did on May 15, 1989.

In a Congress of the Middle East Society for Organ Transplantation it would be quite incongruous for me to detail basic principles of medical ethics or to merely enumerate the evils of organ transplantation which are well known to us all and have been dealt with in two other papers relating to this subject (1, 2). I must address myself, however, to the requirements of the organizers, and to Prof. G.M. Abouna in particular, who have me in their debt for their kind invitation to participate in this volume and their gracious hospitality. I need to give of my experience and views and those of the International Commission of Health Professionals for Health and Human Rights based in Geneva, on the problems of buying and selling of human organs in the Third World, and India in particular, with a special emphasis on the possible ways and means of preventing the horrifying aftermath of modern technological advances.

Blood transfusions

Naive as it may sound, blood transfusions are still the most common form of

OT and probably the most important as they are essential for almost any form of surgical procedure and certainly for OT. But as blood is a regenerative tissue or organ, no ethical problems arise, especially as blood donation is a voluntary exercise, except in some areas of the developing world where the need is exceedingly great and the supply never seems to keep up with the demand. Blood is considered the very nectar of life and parting with it is mistakenly believed to give rise to a weakening of the human body. Many will, therefore, refuse to donate blood even for their loved ones out of sheer ignorance. They would rather buy the required amount of blood from habitual or professional donors, or from laboratories which sell blood commercially. As can be well imagined, this commercially available blood is often of poor quality and a source of sexually transmitted diseases, hepatitis and now, AIDS.

Reports about professional blood donors continue to appear from time to time in the Indian communication media. Recently, it was found that some professional blood donors may donate as many as 5—6 units of blood every week for a price of Rs. 64 (US$ 3.25) per unit and that such donors are encouraged by Blood Bank personnel who stand to get a 'cut' or commission from the transaction. A daily tabloid (*Mid-Day*) revealed on December 4, 1989, that there were 22 blood donors at one center (Parel) in Bombay who had AIDS and the same periodical stated on December 10, 1989, that 2000 odd professional donors existed in Bombay and that 'most of them are now HIV virus carriers'. In the same report, it was confidently stated that one AID's carrier had donated a kidney in New Delhi 3 months earlier and that another carrier, had 3 months earlier, 'almost donated' a kidney in Bombay.

It is because of this commerce in blood that ethical considerations arise. These will hopefully disappear with education of the public and the establishment of many more voluntary blood banks which will refuse to buy or receive, check or dispense blood from professional donors. Nevertheless, the indigent professional donors will not be deterred by such measures. Ways and means will be found for donating blood for some form of reward or compensation, whatever it be called. Rigidly enforced methods for the detection of transmissible infectious diseases need to be implemented despite the considerable expenditure involved and the inadequate financial resources available. When is this moment to be? How many more recipients of blood are to be infected with hepatitis or the deadly AIDS virus? We are already aware of 10 patients in the Middle East who have been reported to have contracted AIDS after receiving kidney transplants in India. Urgent action is warranted on the part of health professionals and institutions as well as governmental and para-governmental authorities.

Kidney transplants

Kidney transplantation is the commonest form of transplant, after that of blood and corneas, and is the area of greatest concern in the field of ethics and human rights. In most countries, kidneys have been collected from both cadavers and live donors. It was reported in 1985 that in Europe, live donors accounted for only 10% of the total whereas in the U.S.A., 30% of organs were obtained from live donors. The positive is, however, quite different in most parts of the third world, as for instance in India, where exceedingly few cadaver transplants have been performed largely because brain-death criteria have not yet been legally accepted or recognized. The vast majority of kidney transplants have been from unrelated live donors (URLD) and related live donors (RLD) only form a small group.

In India, Bombay is reported to be the major centre for kidney transplants. Whereas it was reported in March 1987 that kidney transplantation was performed in 15 centres all over India, it is now known that in Bombay alone there exist probably some 15 centres which include major hospitals and small poorly equipped nursing homes. We have two other hospitals in Bombay which have restricted themselves to undertaking kidney transplants from related donors only where there is not question whatever of any commercial consideration. Moreover, it was reported in March 1987 that 10 transplants were done weekly in the city of Bombay, but it is now estimated that in the northern suburbs of Bombay alone, 11 kidney transplants on an average are conducted weekly in nursing homes.

It was reported that 1000 kidney transplants were probably performed in India during 1988 and of these about 56% involved patients from abroad: the Middle and Far East, Europe and America. It is suspected that the figures had not changed substantially during 1989. As donors were also comparatively easy to find in India for whatever reason, it was learnt that some were dispatched to West Germany, the United Kingdom and the United States of America.

In end-stage renal disease, where a kidney transplant appears to be the only satisfactory mode of treatment, a RLD is preferred. To achieve this, indirect pressure is at times exerted on members of extended or joint families to 'voluntarily' donate a kidney without apparent commercial exploitation. Some instances are on record where 'business and financial pressures' have been exerted on comparatively poor relatives to act as donors for their next-of-kin. A case has also been described where the wife of a donor has for a year or more, demanded large sums of money from her brother, who was the recipient, for alleged ill health of the donor — her husband. If such examples were exceptional, it would be understandable. Unfortunately, they are not.

Reliable information regarding payments and incentives to kidney donors is not difficult to collect from the many brokers and agents involved in this nefarious transplantation business. It is reliably reported that donors of kidneys are paid between Rs. 20 000 and Rs. 80 000 (US$ 1000—4000) but the prices are apparently falling as the volunteers are many. To make matters worse, there have also been incidents reported where monies promised have only been delivered under threat of physical violence.

Even the hardened observer may well be surprised at the number of individuals who volunteer to donate one of their vital non-regenerative organs — the kidney — often to a totally unknown person in need of one. The reason is quite simple: it is money that is wanted. There is, for a poor person, no other means of getting such huge sums of money so easily and, for a person in urgent need, future consequences are of no matter.

Where human subjects are concerned there is the important requirement of voluntary informed consent. Ethical guidelines have been internationally proclaimed and accepted; but in India the grave danger of illiteracy creates a serious barrier where the signature or thumb impression on a form of voluntary informed consent can make this a document of legal hypocrisy. This has reached such proportions that in some large hospitals the management is opposed to kidney transplantation from non-related living donors. This can seriously affect the number of tranplants effected, as against those needed, and some are therefore waiting patiently for the commencement of cadaveric transplant programmes.

The increasing need for transplants requires considerable national resources, for few individuals are financially able to cope with the costs especially in developing nations. Consideration of the economic structure of any country, makes it obvious that the allocation of scarce resources will present a dilemma for society, administrators and governments. Distributive justice is essential, based on equity and decency.

Since organs such as kidneys are in such short supply, some health professionals and ethicists question the mortality and the underlying basis of the ban of the sale or buying of human organs. It is pointed out that blood was sold until recently in the U.S.A. and is still openly sold in many developing countries. Similarly, they ask why should there be a ban on the buying and selling of kidneys? Human semen is as yet sold in the U.K. and in many other countries. In such circumstances, it is indicated that the sale of body tissues or parts as commodities, which may be considered as a desecration of the human body, is not an argument acceptable to all. It was suggested that a more 'secular' argument would point to:

(a) the obligations of the medical profession to the donor and the recipient;
(b) the harm or injustice that may result from commerce in human tissue.

Moreover, it was suggested that dangers of cross-infection to recipients of paid 'donations,' as well as such risks as AIDS to donors, of militate against the buying and selling of human organs.

Another concern that is deserving of attention revolves around the fact that it is mainly the poor and the down-and-out that will come forward to sell their organs. The 'quality' therefore, is sure to suffer. Commerce will also then not be restricted to the confines of any one country but will follow the well-trodden paths of international trade, i.e. from the poor to the affluent countries. This has indeed happened, as is shown by the movement of donors from Turkey, India and some Latin American countries to Europe and North America. The commercial trafficking of kidneys in India has reached such proportions that it led Prof. K.H. Chugh, President of the Indian Society of Nephrology in 1987, to state: 'If this is allowed to continue like this, most of the poor people in India will be minus one kidney by the year 2000.'

Some proponents of organ commerce, and they are not a few, advise that those against it should refrain from the buying and selling of human organs but permit others to participate in an open market. One is reminded of the infamous Dred Scott decision of Chief Justice Roger B. Taney who in 1857 commented that no one who objected to slavery was obliged to own slaves!

At an international congress held during August 1989 in Ottawa, Canada, on the theme of 'Ethics, Justice and Commerce in Transplantation: A Global View', some delegates apparently made a fervent appeal for international acceptance, on ethical, grounds, of a supposed Indian practice labelled 'rewarded gifting' i.e. a process of purchase of kidneys through a non-profit-making agency. Subsequent to the Ottawa congress, Dr John B. Dossetor, one of the organizers, circulated for comment an article entitled: 'Kidney donation in the developing world (India)'. In it, he enumerated two manifestations of commercialism which were identified in Ottawa. These were: (a) rampant commercialism through entrepreneural organ brokers; and (b) 'rewarded gifting' wherein the donor's interests were safeguarded to some extent by the very institutions providing the kidneys. I must add that this practice has apparently been discussed or introduced in a southern State but does not exist elsewhere in India. Dr Dossetor went on to warn his readers not to be beguiled by the euphemism and stated that both practices were commercial transactions and condemned by Western countries as being 'victimization of the poor, a form of corporeal prostitution, resonant with the undertones of slavery'.

In the course of the article, Dossetor claimed that 'there are special conditions in India which make it difficult to apply Western ethics' and that it 'is clearly up to Indian citizens to obtain consensus on what is ethically acceptable in that culture'. His concerns devolved around the fact that India was a poor and populous country, inhabited largely by poor people and some rich, devoid of social policies relating to health care, unemployment benefits, old age pensions; with a high infant and child mortality; and, if I may add, a high incidence of maternal mortality, malnutrition, starvation, chronic illnesses such as tuberculosis and Hansen's disease and a myriad other acute bacterial and viral ailments. Nevertheless, the life expectancy of the Indian citizen has gone up to 52 years since the country gained independence in 1947. Surely, such progress is not due to the acceptance of second-rate ethical standards and the Malthusian dictum of the survival of the fittest but rather to the significant developmental, social and political measures undertaken by a succession of governmental, para-governmental and non-governmental organizations and Indian society in general. Moral and ethical standards have been fast declining in India, as elsewhere. Corruption is rife. Serious attempts are, however, being made to stem the rot and these need to be supported with the promotion of a high standard of conduct, ethics and morality rather than by diluted standards of ethics, be they from West or East, North or South.

For international acceptance of the alleged Indian practice of rewarded gifting, Dr Dossetor advises the implementation of ethical guarantees and monitoring by physicians, local professional and institutional regulatory bodies, and ethical supervisory groups. He also advocates Indian legislation to outlaw rampant or 'for-profit commercialism' and to impose on professional licensing and regulatory bodies the responsibility of monitoring approved programmes, presumably of 'rewarded gifting'. But for what purpose are all these recommendations made? For unrelated live donor (URLD) transplant programmes to be facilitated until such time as cadaveric kidney transplant programmes are initiated! It appears to be that Dr Dossetor has not only got his priorities wrong but that he is also unaware of the Indian reality.

The practice of OT in Bombay, and probably also in other parts of India, has often been associated with a number of defects, i.e. a lack of genuine informed consent from donors leading to theft, coercion of donors with relatively large financial incentives — a form of bribery, refusal to pay assured monies after surgery in lieu of organs 'donated'; medical negligence and malpractice with respect to both donors and recipients; use of poorly equipped nursing homes and hospitals by inexperienced health professionals; commercial trafficking by health personnel and administrators, nursing homes and hospitals, agents or touts and taxi drivers who ferry patients arriving at airports to selected OT centres for a price.

Advertisements appear in newspaper requesting donations to meet the costs of a kidney transplant, with costs inflated at times by 100%. Some of these advertisements have on occasion been so worded as to attract communal and caste sympathies, which is something that we are trying hard to suppress at a national level.

Involvement of the criminal element of the Indian society in organ transplantation has already occurred from personal experience and newspaper reports such as the *Times of India* (February 3, 1990) announcing that a kidney mafia existed in Bombay and was behind the deaths of 3 young men from Kerala.

The former Minister of Health, Ms S. Kharpade, stated in both Houses of Parliament in February and August, 1989, that the Government of India was actively considering enactment of legislation on organ transplantation to curtail rackets in the sale of human organs. She went on to also state that no precise information was available about the extent of trading in human organs, the institutions or individuals involved.

At the present time, the reputation and standing of the medical profession in India, or at least the metropolitan cities, is in serious doubt. A media statement read: 'Not all doctors are imbued with the spirit of the noble profession. The machinations of a few have reduced the calling to a conspiracy aimed at exploiting the lay and gullible.' A quick perusal of daily newspapers over the past three months may give an impression of 'doctor bashing' having arrived in India but this may not be quite so. We find submissions in Courts of Law alleging negligence against four public and private hospitals in Bombay, authenticated reports of excessive charges in New Delhi and Bombay, alleged illegal private practice by full-time medical staff in Kanpur hospitals, direct advertising by non-allopathic medical practitioners and indirect advertising by practitioners of allopathic or Western medicine, tall claims for cure of asthma, epilepsy and AIDS in the dailies, doctors accused of rape being arraigned before Courts and others falsely accused of rape by newspapers who later offer no defence before the Press Council, provision of substandard drugs at governmental health centres with the probable connivance of personnel belonging to governmental departments in two northern states, the evils accruing from professional blood donors such as AIDS and hepatitis, excessive reports of foetal distress necessitating Caesarean sections, performance of banned sex determination tests leading to female foeticide which led to the *Sunday Daily* (June 11, 1989) stating: 'Though the Government of Maharashtra has banned the use of sex determination (SD) tests, the problem still persists with unscrupulous doctors having dived underground to continue with their money spinning venture and making a mockery of the Law', etc. The list seems endless.

Reports are available in abundance of violations of existing Medical Codes of Conduct. These include actions such as 'fee-splitting' by some specialists with general practitioners in some cities to the extent of 40—60%, leading to unnecessary consultations, investigations and operations as well as excessive billing; false certification, dishonesty, negligence and incompetence, failure in obtaining genuine informed consent, employment of touts or agents, etc. Whereas the communication media carry many such reports, there seems to be little that is done to correct it. Against such a background, some ask what does it matter if there is commercial trafficking in human organs where the rich get the organs they want, and the poor the money they so sorely need and will never see otherwise. In such circumstances, should the medical or health personnel and their institution not profit? One is reminded that corruption begins in microscopic proportions! 'Rewarded gifting' of organs for transplant is the thin end of the wedge, or the beginning of the descent on the slippery slope of ethical conduct.

Whereas these evils are reported from India, other countries are also involved: Lack of informed consent in China before the insertions of IUDs, alleged stealing of kidneys and commerical trafficking in human organs in the United Kingdom, alleged killing of patients in a Vienna hospital by three nursing orderlies, a 43-year-old American woman pregant again in the hope of having a child who will in the future be a marrow donor for a sibling with leukemia, etc. — and all these culled from the media in the past three months only.

These reports need to be seen in the light of the role of the Medical Council of Indian (MCI) and the Medical Council in the various Indian States. Dr P.S. Jain, Secretary of the MCI, was reported (*The Times of India*, January 20, 1990) as stating that the Medical Council Act of 1954 was sought to be amended in 1972 but the amendment was put into cold storage. The amendment was intended to make a contravention of the code of medical ethics a cognizable offence; and to enable the establishment of an inspectorate to take action against offenders against medical ethics. Meanwhile, he stated that 'the object of the MCI is to monitor the profession but since this offence is not cognizable, we cannot take any action unless a complaint is made to us. So far no such complaints have been forthcoming.' Well before this was said, the Sunday *Mid-Day* (June 18, 1989) reported a case in a southern State of a surgeon who undertook minor surgery in a nursing home while drunk. Things apparently went wrong during the operation and the patient died. The surgeon was exonerated of the offence by the State Medical Council on the basis of an 'error of judgement'. A subsequent appeal to a Court by an aggrieved husband resulted in the surgeon being found guilty and fined, along with the anaesthetist who owned the nursing home and assisted the surgeon. This example needs no elaboration.

I am inclined to believe that Dr Dossetor's code of ethical conduct is that of 'situation ethics' which to me often changes with the wind. For myself, I would much prefer a set of ethical rules which remain consistent in a variety of circumstances. In relation to OT, whether one be a believer in a Divine Being or a secular humanist, the human body is paramount and needs to be protected and preserved almost without qualifications. Given this important consideration and the frailty of human nature among health personnel and the public, at least in India, I see no reason whatever for the ethical acceptance of a carefully monitored form of commerce, i.e. 'rewarded gifting' which is nothing but a subterfuge. Indeed, the promotion of such an idea is a great disservice to the people of India who are seriously trying to cleanse the Indian environment. Many Indians have said that there is no law which does not have a loophole. Let us all lend our shoulder to the wheel and demand the legalization of brain death in 1990 itself and the establishment of cadaver donor organ transplant programmes and the prohibition of commerce of any kind in OT.

With the URLD transplant programme conducted, by and large, unethically by international and even Indian standards, it is imperative that well-regulated cadaveric transplant programmes must be urgently initiated. For this to be achieved, the kidneys must be viable and the donors must truly be cadavers. This requires a widespread update on the concept and criteria of brain death in the minds of the medical personnel and the public which has not yet been achieved, but this omission is likely to be remedied hopefully in the near future.

We need to be vigilant, however, that the criteria of brain death are scrupulously and rigidly applied in a consistent manner at all ages of patients. Or else, we may be faced with the prospect of a subject being officially declared dead in one State but alive in another, as has indeed happened elsewhere. Moreover, human nature being what it is — liable to 'slippery slope' judgements, and being aware of criminality and psychopathy — the unjustifiable declaration of brain death or its determination in anticipation of the event among moribund or terminally ill patients, because of significantly better transplant results, is so patently criminal and yet, tempting. So much so, that two different teams of health professionals are required for the determination of brain death and the performance of transplant procedures in most countries. This is a principle that should not be abandoned in any circumstances, as it will also allay much anxiety in the minds of the public.

The International Commission of Health Professionals

This commission (ICHP) — aware of international concerns relating to health professionals, patients and the international community — commenced its involvement in the subject of organ transplantation in October 1988. At that time, a subcommittee was charged with the responsibility of documenting the many problems, collating data on infringement of human rights and internationally accepted codes of ethics and, finally, with submitting proposals that would assist in the international maintenance of human rights and the upholding of a high standard of conduct and ethics. On the basis of the information collected, the ICHP submitted to the Commission of Human Rights of the United Nations during its 41st Session in Geneva held in August 1989, a memorandum on infringements of human rights in OT and indicated some recommendations for implementation by national governments.

A similar report was also presented in Ottawa by Dr Rosalie Bertell, Chairperson of our subcommittee on organ transplantation, at the International Congress on 'Ethics, Justice and Commerce in Transplantation: A Global Issue' referred to earlier. This report consisted of data only recently collected, relating to trafficking in human organs and body parts for transplantation. It should be pointed out that the data were collected from newspaper reports which appeared reliable, information presented by ICHP Commissioners and other non-governmental organizations.

The information revealed that organ recipients were affluent or had access to money and were largely from Europe, North America, the Middle East and Singapore but some small numbers were identified from the developing countries like India, Pakistan and some from Latin America. The donors who were indigent, came mainly from Latin America, Asia and Turkey. Most of the transplant operations were performed in the donor's country but some of the donors were transported to Europe or North America for surgery.

The data also revealed that true voluntary informed consent was not always obtained, especially in relation to children, the mentally incompetent or the victimized. In some cases, even the intelligent and educated were not specifically informed of the intention of the doctors to remove a kidney, or of the short-and long-term consequences of such a procedure. Indeed, there was a report which showed that donors were moved from one institute to another, when an administrator questioned the donors to satisfy himself that voluntary informed consent had indeed been obtained. As this was not so, the donors were transferred to another institute under the care of the same physician. Very occasionally, it had also been claimed, that their organs had been 'snatched' under anaesthesia in hospitals and nursing homes, but the evidence for such stories has been deficient, and, at times, such claims have in reality represented attempts at extortion or blackmail of health professionals.

As so often happens, it is the poor, needy and uneducated who suffer. In some countries, it is alleged that children have been sold or abducted; later, fattened and sacrificed for their organs. Adults have been lured with sums of money usually beyond their reach or comprehension, but not large enough in terms of hard cash even in poor countries. Some of these poor individuals have willingly given up their organs but later been cheated of the promised money at the time of discharge from hospital.

On many occasions health professionals engaged in kidney transplant activities have not been sufficiently experienced and have undertaken the procedures in nursing homes or small hospitals, far too ill-equipped for such work. Unfortunately, also, there appears little control over such centres and their proliferation.

It is exceedingly difficult to document such information that will stand up in a Court of Law, but attempts should nevertheless be made in a coordinated manner towards this end.

Furthermore, it was found that entries of birth dates were occasionally falsified to ensure that the donors did not appear to be the minors that they were. Travel documents were falsified and no records kept, or at any rate, made readily available for inspection. There was undoubted evidence of financial incentives and monies paid to donors and 'agents' who procured the donors.

At the recent Ottawa Conference, suggestions of trafficking in children's organs were refused on the basis that hard evidence did not exist and that allegations made by prominent individuals in some countries were withdrawn without explanation. Such accounts were described as 'rumour mongering' and also as a tool of the old 'cold war' where one country was said to spread disinformation about another. We are all aware that the absence of hard evidence, acceptable in a Court of Law, does not indicate that an offence has not been committed.

There is little doubt that there is need for an international, independent, non-governmental body to probe into these allegations and innuendoes as they undoubtedly represent infringements of human rights and codes of medical ethics.

We, in ICHP, would suggest: that there should be international cooperation in ensuring that birth records are not falsified; that determination of death be made competently and records maintained; that there be a truly international consensus on the acceptance of brain death; that there be no commercialization of organ transplantation; and that the national registries be established for such activities where all the relevant data are stored and available for scrutiny.

Our international community needs to be alerted and initiated to discuss the meaning of illegal trafficking in human organs, to establish lists of health professionals competent in the performance of organ transplantation; and, we also need to know in which medical institutions these operations can be safely done according to legislation that has a large measure of international support.

If I may again quote Mr E. Thorne: 'allowing the human tissue industry to develop without humane, universally accepted guiding principles may lead to terrible abuses of human rights while also denying to many the transplant miracle.'

The ICHP has for its objective the promotion and preservation of human rights in the field of health and medical ethics worldwide. As no other international organization with these specific aims exists, ICHP wishes to be supportive of any group or organization with this objective in the field of OT and, if need be, we are ready to initiate it internationally. We need, however, your help and that of many others around the world. In this way, we can ensure that medical ethics and human rights will be upheld; that our time and age will not see the concept of the survival of the fittest extended to the survival of the richest with justice to none.

When all is said and done, what do we do about those who continue to go their own way? There are those who do not heed the advice and the principles of the international community; those who believe that all is fair in the business of life and death. What shall we do about them? They need to learn. They need to be taught the right way. Is it time again for another Nuremberg Doctors Tribunal and Trial?

It will be recalled that in the Nuremberg Doctors Trial of 1946, all the 23 accused pleaded innocence. In the words of the late Dr F.C. Redlich, 'the testimony provided the most ignominious evidence of cruel suffering and annihilation of victims.' This trial gave us the Nuremberg Code which led to the Declaration of Helsinki in 1964, but the problems are still with us. The form and guise has changed.

The ICHP has taken a first step in this direction. Consultations, study and reflection have commenced. We need the advice and support of all those who believe in humankind, human dignity, medical ethics and human rights. We appeal to you to help and associate with us in the task ahead.

References

1. Vas, C.J.: Invited Address at Silver Jubilee Celebrations and Annual Conference of the Kuwait Medical Association, 'Organ Transplantation — An Overview' (1989).
2. De Souza, E.J. and Vas C.J.: Problems of transplantation (with reference to the Indian Scene). *Arzt und Krist* **3**, 165—170 (1989).

References

1. [illegible] Seven Selected [illegible] and Annual Conference of the Kuwait Medical Association: Organ Transplantation — An Overview (1989).
2. [illegible] and Vas, C.J.: Problems of [illegible] in India [illegible]

79. Islamic view on organ transplantation

MOHAMMED ALI ALBAR

Introduction

Islam is a religion that differs from many other religions. It encompasses the secular with the spiritual, the mundane with the celestial. It provides a code of life. Man is the vicegerent of God (Allah) on earth. 'Behold thy Lord said to the angels: I will create a vicegerent on earth' (1). He fashioned man in due proportion and breathed into him something of His spirit (2). Not only Adam was honored by Allah, but his progeny also, provided they trod on the right path. 'We have honored the progeny of Adam, provided them with transport on land and sea; given them for sustenance things good and pure; and conferred on them special favors above a great part of our creation (3).

Human life begins at the time of ensoulment, which is stated in the sayings of the Prophet to be the 120th day from the moment of conception (4). Prior to that moment the embryo has a sanctity, but not reaching that of a full human being. The life ends with the departure of the soul (or spirit), a process which cannot be identified by mortals except by the accompanying signs; the most important of which is the cessation of respiration and circulation.

The sanctity of the human body, however, is not lessened by the departure of soul and declaration of death. The human body whether living or dead should be venerated likewise. The Prophet Mohammed (PBUH) rebuked a man who broke a bone on a deceased which he found in a cemetery. The Prophet said 'The sin of breaking the bones of a dead man is equal to the sin of breaking the bones of a living man (5, 6).

The dead body should be prepared for burial as soon as possible, in order to avoid putrefaction which occurs rapidly in hot climates. Cremation is not allowed. Due respect and reverence should be given to the funeral. The Prophet himself stood in veneration for the passing by funeral of a Jew, at a time when Jews were his bitter enemies. One of the companions of the Prophet exclaimed: 'It is the funeral of a Jew', the Prophet answered, 'Is it not a human soul?' (7).

Historical Background

Organ transplantation is not a novelty of the twentieth century. Indeed, it was known in one form or another even in prehistoric eras. Ancient Hindu surgeons described methods for repairing defects of the nose and ears using autograft from the neighboring skin, a technique which remains to the present day. Susruta Sanhita, an old Indian medical document written in 700 B.C., described elegantly the procedure which was emulated by the Italian Tagliacozzi of the sixteenth century and by the British surgeons working in India late in the seventeenth and eighteenth centuries (8).

Teeth transplantation was practised in ancient Egypt, Greece, Rome, Pre-Columbian North and South America. The Arab surgeons were experts at this technique one thousand years ago (9, 10).

At the time of the Prophet Mohammed (PBUH) (560—632 AD) one of his companions called Qatada bin Nooman lost his eye during the battle of Ohod. The Prophet replanted it back and it became the best of his two eyes (11). In the battle of Badir the Prophet (PBUH) replaced the arm of Muawath bin Afra and the hand of Habib bin Yasaf (12, 13).

Muslim jurists sanctioned transplantation of teeth and bones, which has been practised by Muslim surgeons for a millennium. Imam Nawawi (631—671 A.H./1233—1272 A.D.) discussed fully the subject of bone and teeth transplantation in his voluminous reference textbook of jurisprudence Al-Majmooh (14) and his concise textbook *Minhaj Attalibin* (15). Al Imam Asshirbini commented on this subject in his book *Mughni Al-Muhtaj* (16). Zakaria Al-Qazwini (600—682 A.H./1203—1283 A.D.) advocated the use of the porcine bone graft as they take much better than other xenografts and function more efficiently (17), despite the fact that Muslims consider the pig and its products untouchable. Jurists allowed the use of porcine material in medicine provided there was no other or equal alternative.

Some Islamic principles and rules that are related to organ transplantation

1. Islam considers disease as a natural phenomenon. It is not caused by demons, stars or evil spirits. Indeed, disease is not even caused by the wrath of God or any other celestial creature. Diseases and ailments are a type of tribulation which expiates sins. Those who forebear and endure in dignity are rewarded in this world and the Day of Judgement.
2. Man should seek a remedy of his ailment. The Prophet (PBUH) told the Muslims to seek remedy and treatment (18). He ordered his cousin Saad ibn Abi Wagas to seek the medical advice of Al-Harith ibn Kaledah, a renowned physician of his time (18).
3. The prophet (PBUH) declared that there is a cure for every illness, though we may not know it at the time (19).
4. We are encouraged to search for such a cure (20). New modalities of treatment should be searched for and applied if proved successful.

5. The Prophet ordered Muslims to be compassionate to every human being. He also said 'All mankind is the family of Allah; those who best serve his family are best loved by God.'
6. The human being should always keep his dignity even in disease and misfortune. The human body, living or dead, should be venerated likewise.
7. However, doing postmortem or donating organs from a cadaver does not mean mutilation of the corpse or an act of disrespect. The harm done, if any, by removing any organ from a deceased should be weighed against the benefit obtained by, and the new life given to, the recipient. The principle of saving human life takes precedence over whatever assumed harm that would befall the corpse.
8. In the case of a living donor, the principle of doing no harm 'premium non nocere' is invoked. The donor cannot give one of his vital organs, which would end his life. It is an act of homicide or suicide, both of which are considered among the most abominable and detestable crimes in Islam. Donation of an organ whose loss would unusally cause no harm or a minimal increased risk to the health or life of the donor is acceptable. It invokes the principle of accepting the lesser harm when faced with two evils. The harm done by the disease, which can kill a human life, is not to be compared to the harm incurred by donation.
9. Organ transplantation is a new modality of treatment that can save many human lives and improve the quality of life to many others. Islam encourages search for cure and invokes Muslims not to despair, for there is certainly a cure for every ailment, albeit we may not know of at the present time.
10. Donation of organs is an act of charity, benevolence, altruism and love for mankind. God loves those who love fellow humans and try to mitigate the pains and sorrows of others and relieve their misfortunes.
11. Good intention: any action carried out with good intention and which aims in helping others is respected and indeed encouraged, provided no harm is done.
12. The human body is the property of God, however man is entrusted with his body, as well as with other things. He should use it in the way prescribed by God as revealed by His messengers. Any misuse will be judged by God in the Day of Judgement, and transgressors will get their punishment. Suicide is equated in Islam with homicide. Even cremation of the corpse is not allowed. The only accepted dignified way is burial of the corpse, which should be done as soon as possible. Donation of organs is not an act of transgression against the body. On the contrary, it is an act of charity and benevolence to other fellow humans, which God loves and encourages.
13. The human organs are not a commodity. They should be donated freely in response to altruistic feelings of brotherhood and love for other fellow men.

Islamic jurists' fatwas (decrees) regarding organ transplantation

Muslim surgeons practised autograft transplantation which they learned from other nations, especially Indians. They also practised teeth and bone grafting from both animal and human sources (i.e. xenografts and homografts) for a millennium, after obtaining the consent of the jurists.

In the twentieth century, the Muslim jurists sanctioned blood transfusion, though blood is considered as 'Najas', i.e. dirt. The Fatwa of the Grand Mufti of Egypt No. 1065 date June 9, 1959, is an example of Islamic jurists attitude to new modalities of treatment (21).

The majority of the Muslim scholars and jurists belonging to various schools of Islamic law invoked the principle of priority of saving human life and hence gave it precedence over any other argument. Skeikh Hassan Maamoon (the Grand Mufti of Egypt) also sanctioned corneal transplants from cadavers of unidentified persons and from those who agree to donate after their death (Fatwa No. 1087, dated April 14, 1959) (22). His successor, Skeikh Hureidi, extended the Fatwa to other organs in 1966 (Fatwa No. 993). Skeikh Khater, the new Grand Mufti of Egypt, issued Fatwa (Decree) allowing harvesting of skin from unidentified corpses in 1973 (24). Grand Mufti Gad Al-Haq sanctioned donation of organs from the living provided no harm is done and provided it is given freely in good faith and for the sake of God loving and human fraternity. He also sanctioned cadaveric donors provided there is a will of testament or the consent of the relatives of the deceased. In the case of unidentified corpses, an order from the Magistrate should be obtained prior to harvesting organs (Fatwa No. 1323, dated December 5, 1979). The Saudi Grand Ulema Fatwa No. 99, 1982, addressed the subject of autografts which was unanimously sanctioned. It also sanctioned with a majority of votes donation of organs both by the living and the dead, who gave a will of testament or the consent of the relatives (26). The Kuwaiti Law No. 7, 1983, reiterated the previous Fatwas and pointed out that the living donor should be over 18 in order to accept his informed consent.

The subject of 'brain death' was not addressed in all these Fatwas. It was discussed for the first time in the Second International Conference of Islamic Jurists held in Jeddah, in 1985. No decree was passed then, until further studies and consultations were obtained. In the Third International Conference of Islamic Jurists held in Amman in 1986, the historical resolution (No. 5) was passed with a majority of votes, which equated brain death to cardiac and respiratory death (27). Death in the true Islamic teachings is the departure of the soul, but since this cannot be identified the signs of death are accepted.

This decree paved the way for extension of organ transplant projects which were previously limited to living donors. Campaigns for organ donations from brain-dead persons were launched both in Saudi Arabia and Kuwait. The unfortunate high incidence of motor vehicle accidents in the Gulf area provide many cases of brain death. This tragedy should be averted by issuing and pursuing stricter traffic laws and other means. Meanwhile it is a great pity to waste such candidate cadavers without trying to save the life of many others who need these organs.

The Islamic League Conference of Jurists held in Mekkah Al-Mukaramah (December 1987) decree No. 2, 10th session, did not equate cardiac death with brain death. In fact, it did not recognize brain death as death. However, it sanctioned all the previous Fatwas on organ transplantation. This decree had little publication in the media, and the authorities in Saudi Arabia seem to ignore it. Cardiac and kidney transplants from brain-dead individuals continued without any hinderance from the jurists.

The most detailed Fatwa on organ transplantation was that of the Fourth Conference of the International Jurists held in Jeddah, February 1988 (Resolution No. 1). It endorsed all previous Fatwas on the organ transplantation, clearly rejected any trading or trafficking of organs and stressed the principle of altruism (28).

The jurists started to discuss new subjects related to organ transplantation viz: (a) transplantation of the nervous tissues as a modality for treating Parkinsonism or other ailments, (b) transplantation from anencephalics, (c) transplantation of tissues from embryos spontaneously, medically or electively, (d) left over pre-embryos from IVF projects (29).

New frontiers are opened and the jurists are keeping pace with tremendous advancements in medicine and new technology.

References

1. Glorious Quran, Sura 2, Verse 30.
2. Glorious Quran, Sura 3, Verse 9.
3. Glorious Quran, Sura 17, Verse 70.
4. Al-Bokhari, M.I.: *Sahih Al-Bokhari*, Vol. 4, p. 135. Matabi Asshab, Cairo, Egypt (1378H; 1958).
5. Abu Dawud: *Sunan Abi Dawud*, Vol. 3, pp. 212—213. Dar Al-Hadith, Homs, Syria (no date mentioned).
6. Ahmed ibu Hanbal: *Musnad Ahmed*, Vol. 6, p. 58. Commented by Ahmed Shakir. Dar Al-Maarif Publishing Co., Cairo, Egypt (no date mentioned).
7. Al-Bokhari, M.I.: *Sahih Al-Bokhari, Kitab Al-Ganayiz*, Vol. 2, p. 107. Matabi Asshab, Cairo, Egypt (1378H; 1958).
8. Bollinger, R. and Stickel, D.: Historical aspects of transplantation. In: D. Sabiston (ed.), *Textbook of Surgery*, 13th ed. pp. 370—380. Saunders Co., Philadelphia; London, Igaku-Shoin (International edition).
9. Guthrie, D.A.: *A History of Medicine*, p. 12. Lippincot Co. (1946).
10. Peer, L.A.: *Transplantation of Tissues*. Williams and Wilkins, Baltimore (1955).
11. Hawa, S.: *Arrasul* (*The Messenger*), 2nd ed. Vol. 2, p. 97. Assharikah Al-Mutahida, Beirut (1971).
12. Asshibani, A.R. (Ibu Addaiba): *Hadaiq, Al-Anwar Wa Matali Al-Asar Fi Sirat Annabi Al-Mokhtar*, 2nd edn, Vol. 1, p. 244. Ministry of Endowment, Qater (no date mentioned).

13. Al-Khafaji, A.S.: *Naseem Arriyadh*, Vol. 3, p. 111. Dar Al-Fikir, Beirut (no date mentioned).
14. Al-Nawawi, M.S.: *Al-Majmooh Shareh Al-Mohazab*, Vol. 1, p. 293. Commented by M. Al-Mutteei. Al-Fajalah Press, Cairo (no date mentioned).
15. Al-Nawawi, M.S.: *Minhaj Attalibin*, Vol. 1, p. 1909. Dar Al-Fikir, Beirut (1978).
16. Asshirbini, M.: *Mughni, Al-Muhtaj Limarifat Alfaz Al-Minjah* Vol. 190, p. 191. Dar Al-Fikir, Beirut (no date mentioned).
17. Al-Qazwini, Z.: *Ajayib Al-Makhologat* (*Wonders of Creatures*), 3rd ed., p. 422. Dar Al-Afaaq Al-Jadidah, Beirut (no date mentioned).
18. Ibn Al-Qayim, M.: *Zad Al-Ma'ad Fi Hadiy Khir Al-Ibad*, Vol. 3, p. 78. Mustafa Al-Babi Al-Halabi, Cairo (1970).
19. Al-Bokhari, M.I.: *Sahih Al-Bokhari, Kitab Attib.*, Vol. 7, pp. 148—182. Matabi Asshab, Cairo (1378H; 1958).
20. Al-Qushairi, M.: *Sahih Muslim Bishareh Al-Nawawi*, Vol. 14, pp. 191—200. Dar Al-Fikir, Beirut (1972).
21. Dar Al-Ifta Al-Misryah: *Al-Fatawa Al-Islamiyah*, Vol. 7. p. 2495. Fatwa of Sheikh Hassan Maamoon (No. 1065, dated June 9, 1959), Ministry of Endowment, The Supreme Islamic Council, Cairo (1982).
22. *Ibid.*: Vol. 7, p. 2552.
23. *Ibid.*: Vol. 6, pp. 2278—2282.
24. *Ibid.*: Vol. 7, pp. 2505—2507.
25. *Ibid.*: Vol. 10, pp. 3702—3715.
26. Saudi Grand Ulema: Fatwa No. 99 dated 6/11/1402 H (August 25, 1982), *Majalat Al-Majma Al-Fiqhi* (*Journal of Fiqh Academy*) **1**, 37 (1987).
27. Fiqh Academy: *Fiqh Academy Book of Decrees*; p. 34. Decree No. 5, 3rd Conference of Islamic Jurists held in Amman (October 11—16, 1986). Jeddah Fiqh Academy (1988).
28. *Ibid.*, pp. 55—58.
29. Fiq Academy and Islamic Organization of Medical Sciences: *Seminar on New Issues in Organ Transplantation*, Kuwait, October 1989.

Index of subjects

ABO imcompatible transplantation, 203, 301
Acute rejection, 8
  bone marrow, 420
  cardiac, 341
  liver, 255
  renal, 136, 148, 175, 195, 206, 228
Acquired immunodeficiencies (AIDS), 546, 561, 566
Acute tubular necrosis (ATN), 194
Acute leukemia, 429
Alloreactive T cell, 11
Allograft rejection, cellular and molecular mechanism, 5
Antibodies
  idiotype-antiidiotype, 59
  highly sensitised patients, 51, 302
Antifungal prophylaxis, 447
Antilymphocyte globulin, 75, 83, 102, 170, 390
Anti-rejection therapy, 169, 190, 212, 218, 227, 248
Autologous marrow transplantation, 423, 439
Autotransfusion, 315

B lymphocytes, 6, 148, 168
Biliary atresia, 264
Biopsy, fine needle, 43
Blood transfusion
  donor specific transfusion, 67
  in transplantation, 65
Bone marrow transplantation, 415, 425, 429, 437, 443, 447
  acute lymphoblastic leukemia, 429
  autologous marrow, 423, 429
  conditioning regimen, 437, 443
donor-recipient selection, 415
  graft rejection, 420
  graft-versus-host disease, 419, 422
  grafting procedure, 417
  immunosuppression, 418
  infection prophalayis, 447
  leukemia, 420
  thalassemia, 425
toxicity of conditioning regimens, 422
Brain death, 2, 526

Cancer, *see* Malignancy
Cluster operation, 323
  indications, 326
Commercialization in organ transplantation, 539, 545, *see also* Ethics
Complement, 461, 463
Chronic graft rejection, 175, 228
Cyclophosphamide, 444, 437
Cyclosporine
  assay, 159, 191
  blood levels, 73, 102
  bone marrow transplantation, 426
  cadaver renal transplantation, 189, 87
  combined pancreas and kidney transplantation, 384
  liver transplantation, 255
  living donor renal transplantation, 93
  pancreas transplantation, 386
  toxicity, 105
  triple therapy, 226
  withdrawal, 101
Cytomegalovirus (CMV), 79, 340, 347
Cytotec, 178
Cytotoxic antibody, 29, 51, 59, *see also* Preformed antibody

Deoxyspergualin, 123
Deoxyguanosine, 409
Diabetes (IDDM)
  cardiomyopathy, 406
  Dopamine, 528, *see also* Islet transplantation
  nephropathy, 405
  neuropathy, 407
  pancreas transplantation in non-uremic, 365
  recurrence of diabetes, 387

retinopathy, 405
secondary complication, 405
Donors organs
kidney donors, 233
management, 525
selection, 233
specific blood transfusion, 135
specific bone marrow infusion, 141
DR antigens, 12, 17

Ethics in transplantation, 539, 545, 555, 559, 573

Fine needle aspiration biopsy, 43, 218
FK 506
islet transplantation, 390
liver transplantation, 260, 274
pancreas transplantation, 129
pharmacological monitoring, 120
toxicity, 117
Fluconazole, 447
Fungal infections, 450

Graft rejection
bone marrow, 420
islet cell, 390, 397, 409
kidney, 175, 190, 228, 229
liver, 301
pancreas, 365
xenografts, 397, 398, 459
Graft survival
heart-lung, 342
kidney, 228, 163, 167, 189
liver, 270, 258
lung, 334
pancreas, 361, 366, 373, 377, 384
Graft versus host disease
acute, 419
chronic, 422, *see also* Bone marrow transplantation

Heart-lung transplantations, 337
donor selection, 338
immunosuppression, 340
surgery, 338
post-operative management, 340
Heart graft rejection, 345
cytoimmunology, 346
infection in, 347
rejection, 347
Hepatic encephalopathy, 266, 279
Hepatoblastoma, 310
History of transplantation, 1, 5
HLA matching
bone marrow transplantation, 416, 438, 444
highly sensitised patients, 29
kidney transplantation, 176, 225, 250
organ transplantation, 17
pancreas transplantation, HTK solution, 515
Hyperacute rejection, 459

IDDM. *see* Diabetes
Immunological mechanism and transplantation, 5, 11, 141
Immunosuppression
ATG, 390, 83
Azathioprine, 2, 170, 386
Deoxyspergualin, 123
cyclosporine, 101, 189
FK 506, 109, 129, 260, 274
OKT 3, 83, 91
quadruple therapy, 71
rejection, *see* Anti-rejection therapy
sequential combination, 83
triple therapy, 78, 101
malignancy, 475
methotrexate, 430
prednisone, 101, 340
Induction of tolerance, 141
Infections
bacterial, 19, 363, 347, 230
fungal, 447, 345
viral, 9, 347, 340, 230
International pancreatic registry, 353
International islet cell registry, 389
International tumor registry, 475, 485
Interleukins, 5
Irradiation, 377
Islet transplantation
adult islet, 392, 401
CD4+ T-cell, 469
deoxyguanosine, 409
fetal islet, 390, 402, 469
immunogencity, 397
isolation, 453
mammals islet, 453
prevention xenograft rejection, 399
prevention allograft rejection, 397
registry, 389
secondary diabetic complication, 405, *see also* Diabetes
xenograft, 469
Islam and organ transplantation, 573, *see also* Ethics

Kaposis sarcoma, 479
Kidney
cadaver, 83, 228
commercialization in, 545, 559, 555, *see also* Ethics
HLA matching, 85

in pediatric recipients, 225, 228
indications, 226
Kaposis sarcoma in, 501
living related, 168, 241, 225, 233
living unrelated, 217, 241, 168
preservation and procreument, 511, 525
transplantation in Kuwait, 224, 233
transplantation in Turkey, 136, 203
transplantation in Iran, 247
transplantation in Saudi Arabia, 531
transplantation in Tunisia, 501
urological complications, 505
Kidney donors, long term surveillance, 233

Leukemia, 420, 429, 443, *see also* Bone marrow transplantation
Liver transplantation, 254, 280, 313
acidosis, 320
anaesthesia, 279
blood loss and management, 313
blood transfusions, 313
coagulation, 285, 315
hepatobiliary malignancy, 307
hyperkalemia, 319
hypocalcemia, 319
immunology, 301
in adult, 289
in children, 263
indication for, 264
intraoperative management, 281
living related, 299
Lymphoproliferative disorders, 498
malignancy, 307, 323
metabolic disorders, 267
reduced size, 295
risk factors, 289
split, 295
techniques, 256
Living related donor renal transplantation, 203, 235, 175
Living related donor for pancreatic transplantation, 383
Lung transplantation, 329
donor selection, 330
immunosuppression, 330
post operative management, 334
recipient selection, 329
surgical technique, 331
Lymphocyte function, 5, 11
Lymphocyte crossmatch in renal transplantation, 39
Lymphomas, 477, 255
Lymphocele, 508

Major histocompatibility antigens, 11, 18, 303, 367
liver and, 303
pancreas grafts and, 354, 367
Malignancy in organ transplantation, 307, 475, 485, *see also* Immunosuppression
Melphalan, 444
Mercaptopurine, 2
Methylprednosolone, 75, 227, 248, 341, 170
Monoclonal antibody, 141

Nephrectomy, 227
simultaneous native nephrectomy with transplantation, 227
Nephropathy, diabetic, *see* Pancreas transplantation
Non-Hodgkin's lymphoma, 478

OKT 3, 75, 83, 91, 94, 102
Organ preservation
collins, 339
composition of solution for, 515
future of, 513
kidney, 511
liver, 257, 519
pancreas, 511
UW, 511, 519
HTK, 515
Organ procurement
brain death, 2, 525
donor maintenance, 526
ethical consideration, *see* Ethics
legal aspects, *see* Ethics
non-heart-beating cadaver, 515
operation, 529

Pancreatic drainage, *see* Pancreas transplantation
Pancreas transplantation, 353, 359, 365, 371, 377
donor of, 359, 371
duodenum, 377
kidney transplantation and, 372
living related, 383
pancreas islet transplantation, 389
post-operative management, 372
registry report, 354
spleen and, 377, *see also* Diabetes
Passenger leukocyte, 2
Pediatric cadaver donor renal transplantation, 201, 211
en-block transplantation, 211
single organ transplantation, 201, 211
Pediatric renal transplantation, 225, 228
Platelet-activating factor-antagonist, *see* WEB 2086 BS
Post-transplantation

care, 257
complications, 229
Preformed antibody, 29, 51, 301, 461

Radiation, whole body, 443, 437
Renal transplantation
artery stenosis and, 491
HLA matching, 225, 250
in children, 225, 228
in living unrelated, 247
in cadavic, 228
in living related, 227, 235, 247
indications, 226
Kaposi's sarcoma in, 501
urological complications in, 505

Sandimmune, *see* Cyclosporine
Sensitized patients, *see* Highly sensitized patients
Splenectomy, 203, 205

Suppressor cells, 6, 146, 150

T-cells, 11, 168, 148
Thoracic duct drainage, 2, *see also* History
Tissue culture, *see* Islets transplantation
Tissue typing, *see* History and major histocompatibility antigens
Tolerance, 141
Transplantation, *see* Individual organ
Tumor, *see* Malignancy

University of Wisconsin (UW) Solution, *see* Organ preservation

Vascular access, 237-245

WEB 2086 BS, 459

Xenograft, 459, 469, *see also* Islet transplantation

DEVELOPMENTS IN SURGERY

1. J.M. Greep, H.A.J. Lemmens, D.B. Roos and H.C. Urschel (eds.): *Pain in Shoulder and Arm.* An Integrated View. 1979 ISBN 90-247-2146-6
2. B. Niederle: *Surgery of the Biliary Tract.* 1981 ISBN 90-247-2402-3
3. J.A. Nakhosteen and W. Maassen (eds.): *Bronchology: Research, Diagnostic and Therapeutic Aspects.* 1981 ISBN 90-247-2449-X
4. R. van Schilfgaarde, J.C. Stanley, P. van Brummelen and E.H. Overbosch (eds.): *Clinical Aspects of Renovascular Hypertension.* 1983 ISBN 0-89838-574-1
5. G.M. Abouna and A.G. White (eds.): *Current Status of Clinical Organ Transplantation.* With some Recent Developments in Renal Surgery. 1984 ISBN 0-89838-635-7
6. A. Cuschieri and G. Berci (eds.): *Common Bile Duct Exploration*, 1984 ISBN 0-89838-639-X
7. F.M.J. Debruyne and Ph.E.V.A. van Kerrebroek (eds.): *Practical Aspects of Urinary Incontinence.* 1986 ISBN 0-89838-752-3
8. H.G. Gooszen, H.O. ten Cate Hoedemaker, I.I. Weterman and M.R.B. Keighley (eds.): *Disordered Defaecation.* 1987 ISBN 0-89838-891-0
9. S. Bengmark (ed.): *Progress in Surgery of the Liver.* Pancreas and Biliary System. 1987 ISBN 0-89838-956-9
10. J.M. Dubernard and D.E.R. Sutherland (eds.): *International Handbook of Pancreas Transplantation.* 1989 ISBN 0-89838-399-4
11. G.M. Abouna, M.S.A. Kumar and A.G. White (eds.): *Organ Transplantation 1990.* 1991 ISBN 0-7923-1191-4

KLUWER ACADEMIC PUBLISHERS – DORDRECHT / BOSTON / LONDON